# ERRATUM

J. R. Hudson, The Prevention of Retinal Detachment, p. 390.

Replace Figs. 1, 4, 5 and 6 as indicated.

Fig. 6 should be Fig. 5.

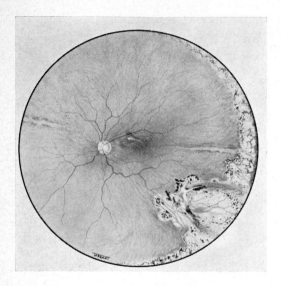

Fig. 1.

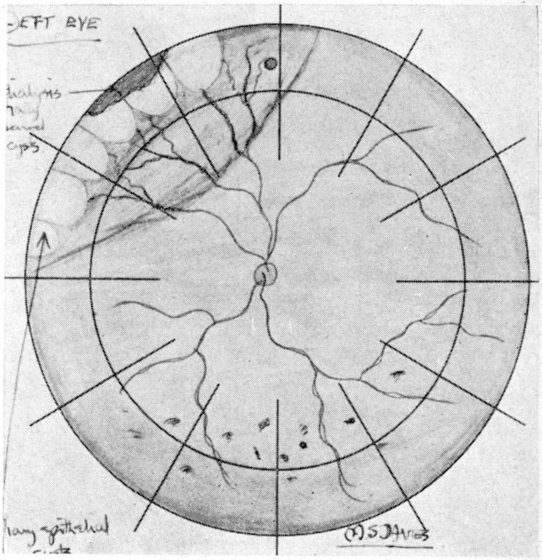

Fig. 6.

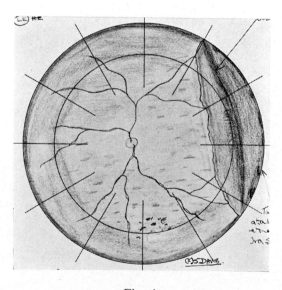

Fig. 4.

# ERRATA

p. 82,  col. 2, 9 lines from bottom change: 1961 to 1952.

p. 83,  col. 1, middle of page change: (1952–61) to (1952; 1955–61).

p. 86,  col. 2, middle of the page change: 1962 to 1961.

p. 130,  col. 2, line 16 from bottom should read: "...zone takes time to..."
line 12 from bottom should read: "...choroidal sclerosis (15) should also be suspect;..."
line 10 from bottom should read: "...punctate keratitis—bearing in mind that Jones (16) describes 35 clinical types of punctate keratitis—can be added."

p. 144,  col. 2, paragraph 2, line 4, should read: "Where life is bearable, vector control should not be recommended, even though the relative proportion of blindness due to onchocerciasis may be as high as 20%, and the skin infectivity from this condition as high as 78%... This too is selective prevention." Last sentence of the paragraph should be deleted.

p. 309,  col. 2, line 10, should read: "On the average, 2.4 coagulation operations were given over a..."

p. 358,  col. 1, line 20 change: "very red" to "irregular."
line 15 from bottom change: "nevritis" to "neuritis."

p. 525,  col. 1, middle of page should read: "...convalently linked to polypeptide residues..." Delete sentence beginning, "The disaccharide..."
col. 2, line 11 from bottom should read: "...complex (CSC) and an insoluble residue, the polymeric stroma (PS) (13). Previous studies have shown that the soluble fractions..."

p. 526,  col. 1, line 4 from bottom change: "soluble" to "structural."

p. 527,  legend to Fig. 3: add "...spots detected by autoradiography."

p. 534,  line 18 from bottom change: "(18)" to "(19)."
line 14 from bottom change: "(21)" to "(22)."

p. 536,  ref. 19 should read: HARDING JJ. Nature and origin of the urea-insoluble protein of human lens. *Exp Eye Res* **13**: 33, 1972.

p. 547,  col. 2, paragraph 2, line 4 delete: "and fluorescence in Fig. 2." Last entry in Table 1 should read: "Guanidine-dithiothreitol insoluble protein Group IV cataracts, age > 60 years."

p. 549,  col. 1, line 1 add: "Fig. 2."
Fig. 5, insert double bonds at appropriate places in benzene ring.

p. 550,  Fig. 7 legend, add: "The solid line without any symbols represents the absorption spectrum of N'-formylkynurenine."

p. 551,  col. 2, end of paragraph 2, delete: "Table 5."
Table 4, footnote a should read: "Performed for 2.5 hr at 10 v/cm, 50 ma, Whatman 3 MM paper, pH 2.
last column, add [b] to second, fourth and fifth lines.

p. 552,  legend to Fig. 10 should read: "Shaded area 100%; ...94%; – – – – 87%.
col. 2, paragraph 2, line 7, change: "black" to "shaded."

CAUSES AND PREVENTION OF BLINDNESS

# CAUSES AND PREVENTION OF BLINDNESS

Proceedings of the Jerusalem Seminar on the Prevention
of Blindness
25 to 27 August 1971, Jerusalem

*Edited by*

I. C. MICHAELSON, D.O.M.S., F.R.C.P. Glas., Ph. D. Glas.

Chairman, Department of Ophthalmology, Hadassah University Hospital and
Professor of Ophthalmology, Hebrew University – Hadassah Medical School,
Jerusalem, Israel

and

ELAINE R. BERMAN, Ph. D.

Head, Biochemistry Section, Sir Isaac and Lady Wolfson Ophthalmic
Research Laboratories, Hadassah University Hospital and
Associate Professor of Human Biochemistry, Hebrew University–Hadassah Medical School,
Jerusalem, Israel

Academic Press                     New York / London

Academic Press, Inc.
111 Fifth Avenue
New York, N. Y. 10003


Distributed in the United Kingdom by

Academic Press (London), Ltd.
Berkeley Square House
London WIX 6BA

Library of Congress Catalog Card No. 72-84281
ISBN 0–12–493650–4


The publication of these Proceedings has been supported in part by
the National Library of Medicine, Public Health Service, U. S.
Department of Health, Education and Welfare, Bethesda, Maryland
and the Israel Academy of Sciences and Humanities, Jerusalem.


Printed in Israel at Central Press, Jerusalem

# CONTENTS

Preface   1

Sponsoring institutions and chairmen   3

Symposium photographs   5

Welcome   I. C. MICHAELSON   7

Chairman's opening remarks   A. E. MAUMENEE   8

Greetings   G. VON BAHR   10

Greetings   J. FRANÇOIS   11

Keynote address   J. WILSON   12

## PUBLIC HEALTH OPHTHALMOLOGY

### BETWEEN THE NATIONS

The role of the World Health Organization in the prevention of blindness   M. L. TARIZZO   17

Governmental foreign aid in ophthalmology   J. FRANÇOIS   21

International organizations for the blind: Activities for the prevention and cure of blindness   J. WILSON   25

The role of missionary societies in the prevention of blindness   N. E. CHRISTY   28

A decade of progress   J. J. LAWLOR   30

The ophthalmological services of MEDICO. A service of "CARE"   R. O. SCHOLZ   32

Discussion   34

### WITHIN THE NATIONS

Introduction   G. VON BAHR   37

Australia   I. MANN   40

Canada   E. SHENKEN   43

Hawaii   W. J. HOLMES   44

India   G. VENKATASWAMY   46

Italy   G. B. BIETTI   49

Japan   A. NAKAJIMA   50

Kenya   G. G. BISLEY   53

Netherlands J. Schappert-Kimijser 54

South Africa M. H. Luntz 55

## ORGANIZATION FOR TEACHING RESEARCH AND INFORMATION

A contribution to the teaching of ophthalmologists from a developing country
I. C. Michaelson 57

Contact lens practice G. P. Halberg and A. Schlossman 59

Training and functions of ophthalmic assistants

India G. Venkataswamy 61

Kenya G. G. Bisley 62

Africa I. Ben-Sira and Y. Yassur 63

Ethiopia I. Feitelberg 64

Auxiliary ophthalmic training

The Joint Commission on Allied Health Personnel in Ophthalmology A. Schlossman 66

Auxiliary ophthalmic training in Canada H. A. Stein and B. Slatt 68

Training of orthoptists in Israel I. Nawratzki 68

Education for ophthalmic nursing in developing countries J. Steiner-Freud 69

The National Eye Institute. An international research resource C. Kupfer 72

Planning a film library for information on the prevention of blindness A. B. Rizzuti 77

Discussion 78

## CLINICAL PROBLEMS IN DEVELOPING COUNTRIES

### TRACHOMA

Natural history and diagnosis of trachoma G. B. Bietti 81

Chemotherapy of trachoma M. L. Tarizzo 87

Rifampicin, an antitrachoma antibiotic Y. Becker 90

Some aspects of trachoma control and provisional estimates of the cost of vaccine production
L. H. Collier 94

Some aspects of immunity in trachoma G. B. Bietti, M. Soldari, A. M. Isetta,
C. Intini and M. Ghione 104

Local antibodies to trachoma agent Z. Zakay-Rones, R. Levy and B. Maythar 110

The molecular biology of trachoma agent. Studies on the nature of trachoma obligate
parasitism Y. Becker 114

Discussion 118

### ONCHOCERCIASIS

Parasitology and diagnosis of onchocerciasis. With special reference to the outer eye
A. E. Gunders and E. Neumann 119

Epidemiology and natural history of onchocerciasis D. P. Choyce 123

Ocular lesions of onchocerciasis F. C. Rodger 130

Epidemiology of ocular onchocerciasis in French-speaking countries of West Africa
J. Lagraulet 133

A comparative study of 500 cases of onchocerciasis and 500 controls with regard to posterior segment lesions in the eye I. BEN-SIRA and Y. YASSUR 136

The posterior segment lesion of ocular onchocerciasis. Histological aspects E. NEUMANN and A. E. GUNDERS 138

Selective preventive treatment of onchocerciasis F. C. RODGER 143

Topical diethylcarbamazine in ocular onchocerciasis E. AVIEL and R. DAVID 146

Discussion 149

**KERATOMALACIA**

The biological role of vitamin A in maintaining epithelial tissues J. A. OLSON 150

Cornea in hypovitaminosis A and protein deficiency C. H. DOHLMAN and V. KALEVAR 159

Clinical aspects of keratomalacia J. TEN DOESSCHATE 164

 G. VENKATASWAMY 170

 Y. YASSUR, S. YASSUR, S. ZAIFRANI, U. ZACHS and I. BEN-SIRA 172

Prevention of blindness due to hypovitaminosis A H. A. P. C. OOMEN 175

The prevention of childhood blindness by the administration of massive doses of vitamin A J. A. OLSON 179

Keratomalacia in Haiti M. L. SEARS 187

Surgical treatment of active keratomalacia by "covering graft" I. BEN-SIRA, U. TICHO and Y. YASSUR 189

Discussion 191

**HERPES CORNEA**

The natural history and diagnosis of herpes cornea H. E. KAUFMAN 192

Studies on the molecular biology of herpes simplex virus Y. BECKER 196

The effect of the antibiotics distamycin A and congocidine on the replication of herpes simplex virus Y. BECKER, S. NEUMAN and J. LEVITT-HADAR 205

Medical treatment of herpes H. E. KAUFMAN 211

Surgical treatment of herpes cornea R. STEIN and A. ROMANO 215

Discussion 218

**CATARACT SURGERY — DEVELOPING COUNTRIES**

Mobile eye clinics
The challenge V. C. RAMBO 219

Mobile eye hospitals and cataract surgery in India A. CHATTERJEE 219

The function of a mobile eye clinic S. FRANKEN 223

Mobile eye units in Kenya G. G. BISLEY 225

Eye camps
Cataract extractions in a Pakistani village hospital. Organization, techniques and results N. E. CHRISTY 230

Screening for amblyopia                    S. Delthil and J. Sourdille    453

Treatment of amblyopia
Amblyopia therapy in an underdeveloped area                A. M. Potts    454

Treatment of amblyopia                              I. Nawratzki    455

Classification and treatment of amblyopia in Nigeria            I. Réthy    460

Stimulus deprivation amblyopia                          K. Wybar    462

Prevention of amblyopia caused by incomplete congenital cataract      S. Merin
and J. S. Crawford    468

Significance of nystagmus in suspected blindness in infancy        K. Wybar    472

Experimental amblyopia                        G. K. von Noorden    476

Discussion                                              480

## BASIC LABORATORY STUDIES

### CORNEAL OPACIFICATION: PHYSIOLOGY OF CORNEAL TRANSPARENCY

The function of the corneal endothelium in relation to corneal dehydration and nutrition
S. Mishima and M. Hayakawa    487

Synthetic activity of corneal endothelium    M. V. Riley, S. A. Hodson and H. T. Orr    499

The active control of corneal hydration    S. Dikstein and D. M. Maurice    503

Discussion                                              509

### CORNEAL OPACIFICATION: EXPERIMENTAL AND CHEMICAL PATHOLOGY

Growth stimulating effects of proteolytic enzymes on corneal tissues    V. L. Weimar
and K. H. Haraguchi    511

Collagenolytic enzymes in corneal pathology                S. I. Brown    517

Polysaccharide chemistry in corneal opacification              A. Anseth    523

Structural macromolecules of the corneal stroma: Embryonic development and biosynthesis
M. Moczar and E. Moczar    525

Discussion                                              529

### CATARACT: CHEMICAL AND EXPERIMENTAL PATHOLOGY

Cataract. An introduction                              A. Pirie    530

Mechanism of development and possible prevention of sugar cataracts    K. H. Gabbay
and J. H. Kinoshita    537

New aspects of cataractogenesis        H.-R. Koch, O. Hockwin and E. Weigelin    542

Photo-oxidation of proteins and comparison of photo-oxidized proteins with those of the
cataractous human lens                              A. Pirie    547

Discussion                                              554

Aggregation of α-crystallin and its possible relationship to cataract formation    A. Spector    557

Lens proteins and fluorescence                          S. Lerman    563

Effects of near-UV irradiation on lens and aqueous humor proteins     S. ZIGMAN,
J. B. SCHULTZ, T. YULO and D. GROVER    570

Induction of cataracts in mice by exposure to oxygen     S. S. SCHOCKET, J. ESTERSON,
B. BRADFORD, M. MICHAELIS and R. D. RICHARDS    576

Discussion    582

## EXPERIMENTAL ASPECTS OF RETINAL DISEASES

Measurement of retinal adhesion     H. ZAUBERMAN    584

The possible role of pigment epithelial cell enzymes in retinal detachment     E. R. BERMAN
and G. BACH    595

Synthesis of fatty acids by normal and diabetic retinal tissue     S. FUTTERMAN
and M. H. ROLLINS    601

Purification and immunological identification of bovine retinal aldose reductase
K. H. GABBAY    606

Experimental diabetic retinopathy     A. PATZ    610

The retinopathy of sucrose-fed rats     L. YANKO, I. C. MICHAELSON and A. M. COHEN    612

Discussion    617

## AN ANALYSIS OF PREVENTION POSSIBILITIES

**SUMMARIES OF SCIENTIFIC SESSIONS**    621

**PLANNING FOR THE FUTURE**    642

Joint resolution by Edward Maumenee and John Wilson    642

**POST-SEMINAR DEVELOPMENTS**

Central Agency for Onchocerciasis    645

Xerophthalmia Club    647

Author Index    651

Subject Index    653

# PREFACE

The Jerusalem Seminar on the Prevention of Blindness was held from 25 to 27 August 1971. It was immediately preceded by the 2nd Conference of the International Society for Geographical Ophthalmology. The two meetings were held in the adjoining and pleasant premises of the Israel Academy of Sciences and Humanities and the Van Leer Foundation. The Seminar was sponsored by the Academy and by the Hadassah Medical Organization.

There were at least two circumstances leading to the convening of this meeting, the first large-scale seminar on the prevention of blindness. One was the recent progress in the basic knowledge required for prevention, (i.e. etiology and recognition of early clinical signs); while the other was the growing awareness of the need for ophthalmic services in developing countries and the present efforts being made to meet it. It seemed natural to hold this seminar in Jerusalem because half of Israel's population has come from developing countries while the other half originates from developed countries. Israel's experience in helping developing countries with their eye problems was another reason for convening the seminar in this country.

There were about 450 participants from 45 countries who delivered about 150 papers and also spoke in the many panel discussions. The participants represented perhaps all the rungs in the ladder of events leading to the prevention of blindness including scientists, clinicians, epidemiologists, public health officials, senior medical administrators of the World Health Organization and spokesmen for international nongovernmental organizations such as the International Association for the Prevention of Blindness, the Royal Commonwealth Society for the Blind, the American Foundation for Overseas Blind, missionary societies, the International Eye Foundation and MEDICO.

Clinical sessions were divided into those dealing with a) the major preventable eye diseases in developing countries such as keratomalacia, onchocerciasis, corneal opacification and trachoma and b) the problems of developed countries such as diabetic retinopathy, glaucoma, amblyopia and retinal detachment. Laboratory sessions dealt with the physiological, biochemical and pathological problems of the cornea, lens and retina. The teaching session dealt with the training of medical, paramedical and auxiliary personnel for developing countries; there were also talks on research and public information.

The seminar concluded with the enthusiastic adoption of a resolution presented by Dr. A.E. Maumenee, Professor and Chairman of the Department of Ophthalmology, Johns Hopkins University School of Medicine and Mr. John Wilson, CBE, Director of the Royal Commonwealth Society for the Blind. The resolution called for the formation of an International Committee for the Prevention of Blindness and special subcommittees for onchocerciasis, xerophthalmia and the training of personnel for developing countries. It is an indication of the timeliness of this seminar that the participants decided that

1

this should be the first of a series of similar international meetings to be held at regular intervals.

The editors wish to express their gratitude to the Israel Academy of Sciences and Humanities and the Hadassah Medical Organization who sponsored the seminar, to the Academy and the Van Leer Foundation who placed their premises at its disposal, to the Department for International Cooperation of the Israel Ministry for Foreign Affairs and to Yad Hanadiv for their encouragement and financial help. The editors also wish to thank the National Library of Medicine, Bethesda, Md. and the Academy for their support of the publication of the proceedings, Professor Moshe Prywes, Editor-in-Chief of the ISRAEL JOURNAL OF MEDICAL SCIENCES and his wonderful staff, especially Mrs. Shulamith Toledano and Mrs. Rebekah Ben-Yitzhak, for their invaluable help.

I. C. MICHAELSON
ELAINE R. BERMAN

# JERUSALEM SEMINAR ON THE PREVENTION OF BLINDNESS

25 to 27 August 1971

Under the auspices of the
ISRAEL ACADEMY OF SCIENCES AND HUMANITIES

Cosponsors:

THE HADASSAH MEDICAL ORGANIZATION
THE ISRAEL OPHTHALMOLOGICAL SOCIETY

**Chairman**

A. E. MAUMENEE, M.D., USA

**Scientific Advisory Committee**

G. VON BAHR, M.D., Sweden
E. R. BERMAN, Ph.D., Israel
G. B. BIETTI, M.D., Italy
J. CHARAMIS, M.D., Greece
J. FRANÇOIS, M.D., Belgium
W. J. HOLMES, M. D., Hawaii
A. E. MAUMENEE, M.D., USA

G. MEYER-SCHWICKERATH, M.D., Germany
A. NAKAJIMA, M.D., Japan
A. SORSBY, M.D., England
P. THYGESON, M.D., USA
A. H. TOWNSEND, USA
J. F. WILSON, C.B.E., U.K.

**Organizing Committee**

I. C. MICHAELSON, M.D., Convener
I. BEN-SIRA, M.D., Secretary
W. FELSENTHAL, M.D.

O. KURZ, M.D.
E. NEUMANN, M.D.
R. STEIN, M.D.

# CHAIRMEN

G. B. Bietti, Italy
S. I. Brown, USA
J. Charamis, Greece
A. Chatterjee, India
D. P. Choyce, U.K.
L. H. Collier, U.K.
J. Dobree, U.K.
C. H. Dohlman, USA
L. Fison, U.K.
J. François, Belgium
E. Friedman, USA
M. Goldberg, USA
W. J. Holmes, Hawaii
J. R. Hudson, U.K.
H. E. Kaufman, USA
J. H. King Jr., USA
T. Kuwabara, USA
M. E. Langham, USA
S. Lerman, Canada
H. Lincoff, USA
E. Linnér, Sweden

M. H. Luntz, South Africa
I. Mann, Australia
D. M. Maurice, USA
D. Mishima, Japan
A. Nakajima, Japan
O. Olurin, Nigeria
A. Patz, USA
A. Pirie, U.K.
A. Potts, USA
I. Rethy, Nigeria
M. V. Riley, USA
F. C. Rodger, U.K.
M. L. Sears, USA
A. Sloane, USA
A. Spector, USA
P. D. Trevor-Roper, U.K.
G. Venkataswamy, India
G. von Bahr, Sweden
G. von Noorden, USA
K. Wybar, U.K.

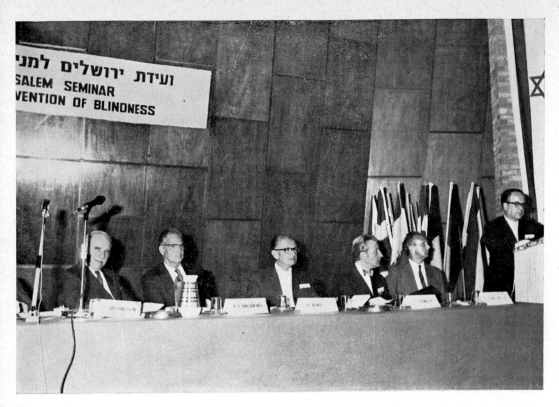

Opening Session of the Jerusalem Seminar on the Prevention of Blindness at the Hebrew University of Jerusalem. On the dais from left to right: I. C. Michaelson (Israel), A. E. Maumenee (USA, Chairman of the Seminar), O. Kurz (Israel), J. François (Belgium), J. F. Wilson (U.K.) and G. von Bahr (Sweden).

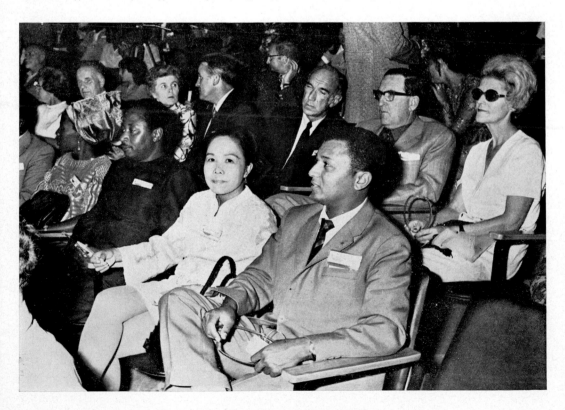

Participants in a working session.

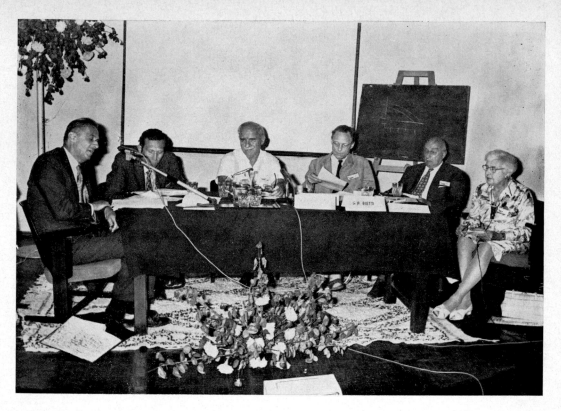

"Within the Nations"—a working session at the Seminar. From left to right: W. J. Holmes (Hawaii), M. Luntz (South Africa), I. C. Michaelson (Israel), V. Clemmesen (Denmark), G. Bietti (Italy) and I. Mann (Australia).

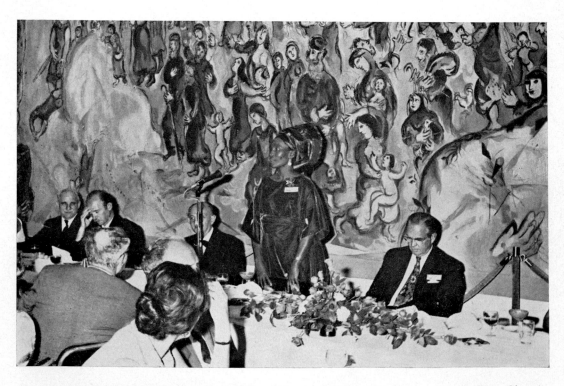

The closing banquet held in the main hall of the Israel Knesset (Parliament) under a tapestry by Marc Chagall. From left to right: I. C. Michaelson (Israel), V. Shem-Tov (Israel Minister of Health), R. Stein (Israel), O. Olurin (Nigeria) and A. E. Maumenee (USA).

# WELCOME

## I. C. MICHAELSON

### Convener

It is my great pleasure to welcome you all to this Seminar on the Prevention of Blindness. You have come here from over 40 countries in all the continents. I especially wish to welcome those coming from the developing countries, and among them Mr. Chessala from Malawi and Dr. Thomas from Liberia who represent the important group of senior medical planners in whose hands lies the future of medicine in the developing continents.

I do not know how many of you have organized conferences in the past, but those who have will well understand me when I say how happy and relieved I am to have you all at last collected into one room; happy and fit and looking well and ready for the strenuous sessions ahead.

In ophthalmology as in other specialities of medicine there are three types of doctors, or rather three main types of doctoring, because most of us combine them all in different degrees: the scientist who studies the physical, chemical or molecular process; the clinician whose world is the individual person with his complaints and his need for relief as quickly as possible; and finally the doctor who wants to prevent disease. I think for the sake of efficiency that comes with simplicity and directness we should call him the "preventist." The idea of prevention is associated with social medicine and public health. But

it is not a specialty. It is an attitude that runs through all the specialties. I am emboldened to make the suggestion when I remember that the word "scientist" was first used as recently as 1840.

To the scientist medicine is a branch of biology; to the clinician it is a kindness—a treatment of himself as well as his patient; to the preventist it is a nuisance and should not exist.

All these doctors have their satisfaction, but the preventist's goal is "no medicine." When he sees illness that could have been prevented, he is an angry man, and because there is so much illness and blindness that could have been prevented, preventists as a class are angry people.

So were the prophets angry people, and when you think of it prophecy and prevention have a common basis. A knowledge of evil things to come, and a passionate feeling for the injustices involved, and surely blindness is the greatest of all injustices.

I now have great pleasure and confidence in handing over the meeting with its high hopes to Prof. A. E. Maumenee of the International Society for the Prevention of Blindness, chairman of the Department of Ophthalmology, Johns Hopkins Medical School who, together with Prof. François and Mr. Wilson, who are on this platform, is the inspirer, encourager and adviser of this meeting.

# CHAIRMAN'S OPENING REMARKS

## A. E. MAUMENEE

### Chairman

The importance of this meeting is indicated by its being sponsored by the Israel Academy of Sciences and Humanities, the Hadassah Medical Organization, and the Israel Ophthalmological Society. I would like to thank all of you, particularly those who are contributing to the program, for taking time from your busy schedules to attend this seminar. I am certain that the thoughts and energies which the participants have put into the development of their presentations will assure the success of this meeting.

Obviously, such a gathering has to have a leader and in this instance, Dr. Isaac Michaelson has conceived the idea, organized the subject matter, arranged for the local accommodations, obtained funds, and has invited his friends from throughout the world to participate. Only someone with Dr. Michaelson's charm, ability, knowledge of ophthalmology, interest in international prevention of blindness and energy could have accomplished this.

The title of the meeting, Jerusalem Seminar on Prevention of Blindness, might be questioned. A review of the participants and content of the material clearly indicates the international nature of the seminar.

The phrase, prevention of blindness, is somewhat misleading, for prevention implies the preclusion of something which will cause a loss of vision. In this seminar we will also discuss the cure of blindness. Finally, blindness implies a severe loss of vision, down to no light perception. During this meeting we will be concerned with more subtle changes, for as the industrialization of the world has proceeded, man's need for vision has increased to the point where reduction to the level of 20/40 will impair his abilities in many jobs or social activities.

In arranging this program, Dr. Michaelson has understood these facts and has selected the subject matter to encompass these problems. He has realized that a scientific discovery, no matter where observed, which would lead to an elucidation of the pathogenesis or etiology of a disease is applicable in other parts of the world. This is true primarily for highly developed or industrialized countries, for in these areas loss of vision is due more to a lack of knowledge of the cause and process of disease than to the delivery of medical services.

In the lesser industrialized or developed countries, however, the prevention and cure of blindness is frequently more a question of delivery of health care services than it is of the understanding of the disease processes. This was brought out by Dr. Gehrig, Deputy Chief Delegate of the United States to the 22nd World Health Assembly of WHO in July of 1969. He stated that an estimate of the number of blind persons in the world was difficult to obtain because data and statistics were incomplete. However, it was estimated that in 1964 there were 14 million totally blind people and that unless decisive action was taken, the number would reach 16 million by 1975 and 20 million by the end of the century. The cost of these blind persons to the world, apart from their personal suffering, was even more difficult to estimate, for neither the number of blind nor their cost to society was based on adequate data.

Dr. Alfred A. Buck, Professor of Epidemiology at the Johns Hopkins University School of Public Health, has made a study during the past ten years of the natural history of disease in such countries as Afghanistan, Chad, Ethiopia, Indonesia, Korea and Peru. From his experience in these studies, he stated that eye disease should be placed high on the list of health problems which he had encountered.

The Director General of the World Health Organization, Dr. Candau, said on World Health Day in April of 1962 that "More than half of the world's blindness is preventable. With proper treatment by drugs and surgery, sight could be restored to millions who are now losing it; preventive measures can ensure that in the future the numbers of the blind will be a third or less of what they are today....

"On this World Health Day, I would urge governments, health administrations, and people everywhere to review what is being done and what could be done to prevent needless loss of sight. The knowledge is there—it remains to apply it on a wide enough scale to protect the sight of millions who, without this help, are doomed to darkness."

On the basis of this testimony and that of others, Dr. Smartt from Malawi proposed a resolution at the 1969 meeting which requested the Director General 1) to undertake a study of the information which is at present available on the extent and causes of preventable and curable blindness and to propose activities in this field which the organization would carry out within its program of work; and 2) to collaborate, as may be required, with other organizations having an interest in this domain, including a number of governmental organizations in relation with WHO. This resolution was approved and transmitted to the Health Assembly in the committee's second report and adopted as Resolution WHA 22.29.

The purpose of our meeting today is not merely to present scientific facts, but to suggest and initiate ways in which to translate this knowledge into action on an international basis. Dr. Michaelson has emphasized this by having a single session, with no conflicting meetings, on Wednesday afternoon during which material on "Organization and Prevention" will be presented. This concept will be further stressed in the sessions on Thursday afternoon on the "Teaching of Ophthalmic Personnel in Developing Countries" and on the "Planning of Research." Additionally, this approach should be incorporated in the clinical discussion of the various topics. Finally, on Friday morning, the chairmen of the divisions should be prepared to summarize not only the scientific significance of their sessions, but also to indicate how this information can be put to practical use. Included in this should be the cost, the priority and the organization for accomplishing this task.

If these goals are reached, this seminar will be considered an important accomplishment not because of its success as a scientific exchange, but rather because it will be a catalyst to organize ophthalmic and administrative knowledge into action and to foster other such sessions, in the near future, where progress will be reported.

# GREETINGS

## GUNNAR VON BAHR

President, International Association for Prevention of Blindness

We all know that many millions of people are suffering from blindness or severe visual impairment, but nobody can tell really how many they are. There has also been information indicating that the number is increasing.

From geographical ophthalmology we know that the frequency of blindness and its causes vary much between various parts of the world. Historical ophthalmology, however, teaches us that it need not be so. Many causes of blindness can be eliminated by preventive measures and many diseases impairing vision can be cured.

Even if effective methods to prevent blindness are known and have been successfully practised in some parts of the world, they are not sufficiently used in others. The reason for this may be lack of knowledge, lack of economic means, lack of personnel, or psychologic or even religious obstacles.

In spite of all advances in medicine we are well aware that much remains to be investigated on new methods to prevent and to cure blindness. It is a tragedy of medicine that even medical advances can be responsible for an increased frequency of blindness. Deplorably it is not only the increased average time of living that has the consequence of an increased number of persons blind from the eye diseases common in old age, it is also the introduction of therapeutics that are only partly effective, as insulin for diabetes, or therapeutic measures intended to cure severe illness or to save life, as oxygen to premature babies, that can severely impair vision.

So, alas, the problems we have to regard and to solve are manifold. As a spokesman for the International Association for the Prevention of Blindness I am happy to see that so many experts in this field have come here to discuss these problems. It may be regretted, however, that the deplorable political conditions prevent some of our co-workers in this human task from joining us, but it is admirable that our Israeli friends, in spite of these conditions, have been able to arrange this seminar so well. It is significant that we shall meet in the building of the Academy of Sciences and Humanities, for our task really is one of Science and Humanity combined.

We have some days of earnest and urgent work before us. I trust that they will give us much new knowledge and stimulate us all to more effective work in order to diminish that suffering to mankind that is blindness.

# GREETINGS

## JULES FRANÇOIS

President, Concilium Ophthalmologicum Universale

It is my agreeable duty to wish, on behalf of the International Council of Ophthalmology and in my own name, great success to this symposium on the prevention of blindness.

Prevention of blindness is an ideal which must be the first goal of ophthalmology. The old adage has it that "Prevention is better than cure." Ophthalmology, as well as medicine, will have only achieved its most important object when physicians no longer need to treat and to cure diseases, but to prevent them. Earth will become a paradise the day that diseases, and of course war, will have disappeared.

Evidently, this ideal in relation to blindness is already partly realized. Adequate treatment of glaucoma, uveitis or many other ocular diseases prevents an evolution towards blindness, even if it cannot prevent the disease itself. For some infectious diseases, such as trachoma or conjunctivitis of the newborn, hygienic and antiseptic measures can even prevent the affection itself.

However, these treatments may not be the prerogative of certain populations, but should be applied to all without distinction of race, religion or politics. That is why a very special effort must be made in favor of the developing countries. This for three principal reasons:

1) Lack of hygiene: Although good hygiene follows in the wake of civilization and prosperity, it also has to be taught.

2) Lack of medical and social personnel: This personnel has not only to teach, but also to help apply the necessary measures.

3) Lack of finances: Medical help is very expensive and the countries which need it most cannot support such a financial burden.

We must, therefore, hope that this symposium will incite the governments and the private and official organizations of the rich and developed countries to start, to continue and to increase their humanitarian welfare action by helping the developing countries. This action must not only consist of financial help, but it must also consist in sending social and medical personnel with the aim of bringing to these countries the necessary education and the possibility of improving their health conditions. In this connection, the prevention of the ocular diseases, which may end in blindness, is of primary importance.

My sincere hope is that this symposium may contribute to the realization of at least part of these goals. If so, it may be proud to have performed not only useful, but also humanitarian work.

# KEYNOTE ADDRESS

## JOHN WILSON, C.B.E.

Director, Royal Commonwealth Society for the Blind

As a blind person, and as the representative of the World Council for the Welfare of the Blind, I suppose I may claim at this Seminar to be a spokesman for that multitude of blind people—a vast and growing multitude—for whom the prevention of blindness is not just an academic question or an administrative task, but a matter of immediate personal concern. On their behalf, may I congratulate the Academy and the sponsors of this Conference and express the hope that this week's work will have its impact on the future. May I go further and, on behalf of the world's blind welfare organizations, urge that action must be taken to halt the advance in the number of blind people, to mobilize the knowledge and skill of science, the mechanism of international cooperation, and the techniques of communication which can give this cause the priority it deserves.

The facts are not in dispute. There are at least 15,000,000 blind people in the world and this number is increasing with population growth so that, unless decisive action is taken soon, there could be over 20,000,000 blind people by the end of this century; that is more than the population of many member states of the United Nations.

Most of this blindness is in the developing countries. More than half of it is preventable and there are millions of blind people whose sight could even now be restored. The causes of blindness and the means of controlling them are known with sufficient certainty. What we lack are the resources in money, personnel and organization and the public determination to apply, on an unprecedented international scale, remedies which have already transformed the situation in some advanced countries.

In human terms, the cost of blindness is incalculable. In economic terms it is astonishing.

Ten years ago, we calculated the cost in North America, Western Europe and the Soviet Union of providing education, rehabilitation, pensions and welfare services for the blind. The total that year came to $220,000,000. The comparative figure today would be in excess of $300,000,000, and that is simply the direct cost in a small part of the world; it takes no account of loss in potential production or of the astronomical cost entailed by eye disease and eye injuries.

What then is the cost of blindness among the massive populations of the developing countries? In the most impoverished village, it must cost at least $1 a week to provide food, clothing and shelter for a blind dependent. Assume a minimum of 8,000,000 such dependents and we have an annual expenditure just on basic maintenance of $400,000,000. The cost in lost production would certainly be a figure at least equal to that amount.

If you add together figures such as these—and obviously they represent only a fraction of the real cost—you very soon reach a figure in excess of a billion dollars a year. You might say that the world's blindness is more expensive than a substantial war, but that the amounts spent on concerted international action to prevent blindness would hardly buy a modern warship.

It is of course only in the past few years that it has been possible to accumulate the information necessary to see this problem on a world scale, and to begin to bring the whole thing to life as a major interest of parliaments and international assemblies. You ophthalmic surgeons were the first to recognize the possibilities and you continue, most notably through gatherings such as this, to make your invaluable contribution to a world effort for the prevention of blindness which grows in strength as it recruits other forces and personnel: scientists of various disciplines, administrators and legislators, opinion formers, publicists and fund raisers, and the complex apparatus of international action.

The United Nations, and particularly the World Health Organization, now has the major role, but it can act only in response to a national request and within a sympathetic climate of opinion. This, I am sure, is why nongovernmental action has proved so successful in this field: particularly the partnership between world organizations of ophthalmologists and organizations concerned with blindness internationally. The cooperation should now be made even more effective by the creation, in countries where they do not already exist, of powerful national organizations for the prevention of blindness.

In this formidably professional audience, I am acutely conscious of my inexpertness, but perhaps it enables me to say some things more emphatically just because I have no professional axe to grind.

The first of these must be the most urgent need for increase in the number of ophthalmic surgeons and allied workers and in the status of ophthalmology, particularly in the developing countries. The figures are well-known. In the United States there is one ophthalmic specialist to every 22,000 people. In Nigeria, the figure is 1:4,000,000 and there are countries of Africa and Asia without a single eye specialist.

It is a question not just of number but also of distribution. Over the past ten years, the number of ophthalmologists in the United States has increased by about 400 each year. This is more than the total annual increase in all the developing countries of the world. Last year's 400 new recruits doubtless added to the excellence of an already superb service in North America, but in rural Asia or Africa could have transformed the whole ophthalmic service of a continent.

Staff training must be the first priority but, for decades to come, it is unlikely that there will be enough ophthalmic specialists to meet the growing needs of the developing countries. Effective use of trained auxiliaries, of mobile teams, of techniques of mass treatment are not just a temporary and regrettable expedient but an essential feature in the extension of a profession whose destiny surely is not just to treat a privileged few but, if necessary, to go out into the wilderness and save the eyes of the world. Already we see the modern ophthalmic specialist accepting his new role with enthusiasm: as head of a fleet of mobile units dealing with trachoma over a vast area; as partner in an interdisciplinary team conducting research into glaucoma; as the essential expert in a program to eradicate onchocerciasis; as collaborator in a world effort to protect the eyes of undernourished children; and I hope that, in the honored hierarchy of your profession, international acclaim will in the future be given not only to the man who writes the great textbook or demonstrates an exquisite new technique but also to the bush doctor who, in a lifetime of patient pedestrian effort, restores sight to 100,000 blind people.

We have long known that most of the world's blindness is preventable, but it is only in recent years that we have recognized that so much of it is curable. In India and Pakistan, it is estimated that 1,200,000 people are needlessly blind for lack of a cataract operation. Recently, in just one state of Nigeria, it was estimated that there were 6,000 blind people whose sight could be restored by skilled surgery. I have visited most of the schools for the blind in Africa and Asia and I am sure that a great many of these children, who are now being lovingly educated in braille, could see again if there was a local surgeon with time and skill to treat them.

It was such a consideration as this which led organizations for the blind to resolve that the prevention and cure of blindness was their concern and to undertake the work which I shall describe tomorrow. One of these organizations, the Royal Commonwealth Society for the Blind, now maintains the largest international sight saving program of any nongovernmental agency in the world; and last year, in 14 countries, sponsored medical teams which performed over 25,000 sight restoring operations.

Interest on a world scale is stirring as never before. A conference such as this could do so much to generate action and to add a new dimension to our task. Where we have thought in hundreds, we must think in scores of thousands; where we have been concerned with a single institution, we must project whole national systems. Where we have worked within the framework of a single, illustrious profession, we must look out over the boundaries and welcome every partner who brings knowledge or resources to the task.

Throughout the ages, this city has had its vision of human value and of the rights of man. May we not claim, that, among those rights, is the right to see: the right of any man anywhere not to lose his sight needlessly or, being blind, not to remain so if, by any human skill, he can recover his sight. Between the affirmation of that right and its realization is a long and arduous journey but where better to start than here in Jerusalem—in this city whose restless dreams have changed the world.

# PUBLIC HEALTH OPHTHALMOLOGY

# THE ROLE OF THE WORLD HEALTH ORGANIZATION IN THE PREVENTION OF BLINDNESS

## M. L. TARIZZO

Virus Diseases, World Health Organization, Geneva, Switzerland

I greatly appreciate having the opportunity of starting this session and would like first of all to convey to you the Director-General of the World Health Organization's wishes for the success of the seminar and to summarize briefly the activities of the World Health Organization with regard to prevention of blindness.

I am also well aware of the fact that much of what has been done by WHO in this field has been possible because of the active collaboration of distinguished workers from many countries, some of whom are present today. Furthermore, I would like to acknowledge the contributions to the subject, made by several of my present and past colleagues within the Organization, which it is my privilege to represent today.

The preamble to the Constitution of the World Health Organization, states: "Health is a state of complete physical, mental and social well-being and not merely the absence of disease or infirmity. The enjoyment of the highest attainable standard of health is one of the fundamental rights of every human being without distinction of race, religion, political belief, economic or social condition."

Good vision is obviously part of this state of well-being, and its protection has been one of the concerns of WHO since its establishment in 1948. Because of its basic orientation towards public health, as opposed to individual-oriented clinical medicine, the approach of WHO to the problem of blindness and loss of vision, as well as to other problems, has been etiologically oriented, with emphasis on acting on the causes of diseases rather than on their manifestations or consequences.

In 1969, the Twenty-second World Health Assembly adopted a resolution requesting the Director-General to undertake a study on the extent and causes of preventable and curable blindness, to propose activities to be carried out in this field by the Organization and to develop its collaboration with other organizations interested in this domain. This resolution reflects the growing awareness of the importance of the problem and has focused attention on an integrated approach for its solution. Some of the activities now in progress or planned in implementation of this resolution are pertinent to the subject of this session, but before describing them I shall briefly review the main WHO programs related to prevention of blindness carried out so far which deal with trachoma, onchocerciasis and xerophthalmia.

Although no accurate figures are available, it has been estimated that there are more than 400 million cases of trachoma in the world and trachoma and its complications are considered to be the single, most important cause of preventable loss of vision on a world-wide basis. Measures for the control of trachoma were already advocated by a joint OIHP/WHO Study Group on Trachoma in 1948, and the need for them was endorsed by the Fourth World Health Assembly in 1951. Extensive campaigns of treatment were started shortly afterwards, after preliminary pilot trials, and benefited from substantial help from other international agencies and organizations, especially UNICEF. The basic principles of mass treatment of trachoma are outlined in the Reports of the three Meetings of the Expert Committee on Trachoma held in 1952, 1955 and 1961. These represent the basis of the assistance provided to date in this field, to 21 countries, by WHO. In addition, technical advice has been given and preliminary surveys have been carried out in other countries by WHO consultants and staff members; fellowships and training grants have been provided; support has been given to various research programs; and conferences on trachoma control were organized in 1958 (Dubrovnik), 1959 (Tunis), 1961 (Istanbul) and 1962 (New Delhi).

Control activities are based essentially on the treatment of active cases of trachoma and associated infections with locally applied broad spectrum antibiotics, but also include health education, environmental sanitation and training at different levels. Methods and criteria have recently been revised on the basis of the experience acquired so far and a field guide has been prepared. Emphasis is now put on reduction of severity, increased coverage of cases, training of paramedical personnel and the use of uniform diagnostic criteria to allow for proper evaluation of the results. The final objective of treatment campaigns is always to reduce trachoma endemicity to a level at which it does not represent a public health problem, but the success of treatment is now measured not only in terms of cure rates, but also of reduction in the severity of the cases and of prevention of complications likely to cause visual impairment.

In addition to control activities, the WHO trachoma program includes support for research aimed at improving diagnostic and therapeutic methods. This research program is carried out through the WHO International Reference Centre for Trachoma, in collaboration with laboratories in all continents, and in close contact with most of the workers active in this field.

Onchocerciasis is the main cause of blindness in parts of Africa, and it occurs also in Central and South America. It is estimated that 20 million people are infected, most of them in Africa. In areas where the disease is endemic, more than a third of the population may have impaired vision, and many of them are totally blind. Onchocerciasis as a cause of blindness will be discussed by other speakers, and it will be enough to mention here that WHO has been and is involved in a number of activities dealing with control and research on this subject. A series of scientific meetings and conferences have been sponsored by WHO and in 1965 the Expert Committee reviewed the epidemiology, public health and economic significance of the disease, as well as methods and techniques for its control. After the Conference held in Tunis in 1968, in collaboration with OCCGE and USAID, it was concluded that control of onchocerciasis is today technically feasible, and it was decided to establish a large scale control program in West Africa. Emphasis of this program and of other programs in other regions is on vector control, and stress is also being put on the epidemiological and socioeconomic aspects of the problem. Technical advice has been provided to African and Latin-American countries, and significant developments have resulted from WHO-assisted field and laboratory activities.

Xerophthalmia has already been the subject of a separate session. Pertinent information and recommendations for action were included in several reports of the Joint FAO/ WHO Expert Committee on Nutrition, from 1955 to 1967. A global survey organized by WHO in 1962/63 confirmed that vitamin A deficiency significantly contributes to the prevalence of blindness in parts of South and East Asia, North Africa, the Near East and Latin America. On the basis of the results obtained by the periodic administration of massive doses of vitamin A in preliminary trials supported by WHO, the government of India is now carrying out an extensive program for the prevention of xerophthalmia.

A number of other WHO activities, not specifically aimed at prevention of blindness or loss of vision or both, have, however, an indirect effect on this problem. Among them are the programs on smallpox, leprosy, venereal diseases, diabetes, vascular diseases, occupational health and human genetics.

A sight-saving program was started by the WHO Regional Office for Europe in 1968 and led in 1970 to a study of methods for the early detection of blinding eye conditions. Its concern with noncommunicable causes and its highly specialized approach to the problem reflect the differences in priorities which exist in different parts of the world. This study, which will be discussed in greater detail by others, may well be an indication of future priorities also for countries where communicable diseases and malnutrition are still the main cause of morbidity.

In order to attempt a definition of the extent of the problem and of its geographical implications, a first compilation of the number of cases of blindness in the world was prepared by WHO in 1953. In 1966, data available in the literature were summarized and tabulated, and provides what is still the most comprehensive set of data on the subject, even if available data are fragmentary and uneven. These data indicate that blindness rates per 100,000 population are general-ly below 200 in Europe, America and Oceania, and around this value in some of the more developed countries in Africa and Asia. In less developed countries in Africa and Asia, and sometimes in Europe, this rate is considerably higher, and reaches values above 1,000.

In approximately one-third of the cases, the cause of blindness is unknown or undetermined. When it is known, noninfectious causes are predominant in the more developed countries, while the ratio between noninfectious and infectious causes is completely reversed in the less developed countries. As an example, in Africa, 26% of the total is attributed to infectious causes and less than 5% to noninfectious causes; in Europe, 5% to infectious and 32% to noninfectious causes. Noninfectious causes include degenerative and hereditary conditions and accidents. Sixty-five definitions of blindness are listed in this report.

Other compilations of available data, on onchocerciasis and trachoma, have been prepared by WHO.

WHO has maintained official relations for a number of years with two nongovernmental organizations active in this field, the International Association for Prevention of Blindness and the International Organization against Trachoma. Frequent contacts have also been maintained with other international and nongovernmental organizations.

As a first step in implementation of the resolution adopted by the World Health Assembly in 1969, an attempt has been made to bring the available information up to date. A questionnaire was sent to all member states in March 1970, requesting them to provide WHO with detailed information on the definition of blindness, number of blind persons, causes and age at onset of blindness and on agencies dealing with the problem. Seventy-five answers were received.

Highly qualified consultants, some of them

present here, were then asked to evaluate this information and to prepare a report on the subject. This has now been drafted and will be presented at the Twenty-fifth World Health Assembly to be held in May 1972. It will include an assessment of the problem of preventable and curable blindness, a proposal for a generally acceptable definition of blindness and impairment of vision, and specific recommendations concerning the activities which WHO should carry out in this field. Plans have also been made to convene a Study Group on Prevention of Blindness later in 1972, to provide further guidance in the formulation and implementation of the WHO program.

It would not be possible or appropriate at this time to enter into the details of the report and of the recommendations which will be submitted. In fact, it is quite possible that the conclusions reached at this Seminar may influence some of the recommendations. However, it is evident that efforts should be made to obtain more complete and more accurate data on the number of persons with impairment of vision and on the cause of partial or total loss of vision before priorities can be defined. Existing data, even if fragmentary, indicate that rates of blindness are very high in the less developed countries, notwithstanding the fact that the average age of the population of these countries is relatively low, and that degenerative and cardiovascular diseases, the more frequent known causes of blindness in the more developed countries, are less frequent than in developed countries.

Another point which is likely to be emphasized in the future is the need for a multidisciplinary approach to the problem. The ophthalmologist will always be required for the early detection of cases and their treatment, and for unravelling the mechanism of the processes leading to loss of vision. However, in order to arrive at an adequate solution, the collaboration of other specialists such as microbiologists, parasitologists, nutritionists, epidemiologists, internists, sociologists, geneticists, administrators, etc. will be necessary.

The role which WHO has played so far and which it is likely to play in the near future in connection with prevention of blindness has thus been outlined in its essential features. This role is in keeping with the basic functions of WHO, which are to act as a coordinating agency, to maintain effective collaboration with other groups and organizations, to provide information and to promote and conduct research. The resources of WHO are limited, especially when compared to existing needs, and the active collaboration of others is therefore essential—the role of WHO being thus often limited to that of a catalyst. WHO cannot and does not intend to supplant or duplicate existing and successful programs, but because of its relative ease of access to information and its world-wide perspective, WHO may play a useful role in helping to establish and maintain priorities and in preventing as much as possible the further widening of the technological gap. This function of WHO conforms with one of the basic principles which appear in its Constitution, and which may appropriately conclude this presentation: "The extension to all people of the benefits of medical, psychological and related knowledge is essential to the fullest attainment of health."

# GOVERNMENTAL FOREIGN AID IN OPHTHALMOLOGY

JULES FRANÇOIS

International Council of Ophthalmology, Ghent, Belgium

We present here a general outline of the technical assistance that some countries provide to the developing countries in the field of ophthalmology, where this information is available.

This ophthalmological assistance can be divided into two groups: 1) integrated foreign aid and 2) varied foreign aid.

### INTEGRATED FOREIGN AID

Israel's foreign aid in ophthalmology is chiefly integrated and may serve as an example.

*Organization.* The Department for International Cooperation, Mashav (Foreign Office).

*Varied aid.* Trachoma in Ethiopia for several years (set teaching courses in Gondar for medical assistants, treatment control in 51 stations throughout Ethiopia).

Child blindness in Cyprus. Periodic visits to the island. Ninety percent of child blindness in Cyprus is genetically determined. Research on the possibilities of prevention has been carried out.

*Integrated aid.* The purpose of this program is to integrate eye services in a developing country with training of ophthalmologists and nurses, and with research. This is done for the given country during a period of seven to eight years, divided into three stages.

Stage 1: An ophthalmic survey of the receiving country is carried out following which suggestions are made for eye service including plans for a department and the listing of necessary equipment. Two qualified nurses come to Jerusalem for six months of training in eye nursing, especially in surgery.

Stage 2: Together with the returning visiting nurses a team of two Israel specialists together with, if possible, an optician-optometrist goes to the receiving country. This team after two years is succeeded by a similar team—this stage lasting a total of four years. During this stage the third stage is being prepared. A doctor from the receiving country comes to Jerusalem for two years of study in ophthalmology. This doctor will be the future head of the department which is being developed.

Stage 3: The personnel for this stage consists of one Israel eye specialist and the eye specialist-in-training from the receiving country, who returns to his country from Jerusalem at the beginning of this stage. This stage lasts about two years, at the end of which the Israel doctor returns to Jerusalem and the local doctor is left in charge—perhaps assisted for a year or two by an Israel doctor who is junior to him.

The plan is shown in Table 1.

The policy of the integrated program is for the Israelis to serve, teach and leave.

TABLE 1. *Schematic presentation of Israel's integrated aid program*

| Stage 1 (1 year) | Stage 2 (4 years) | Stage 3 (2 to 3 years) |
|---|---|---|
| Preparation of eye clinic (inpatients and outpatients) | First Israel team serves for two years | Mixed team consisting of a receiving country doctor and one from Israel |
| Ordering of equipment | Second Israel team for two years in receiving country | |
| Two qualified nurses from the receiving country train in Jerusalem for six months | (Each team consists of eye doctors and if possible optometrist) | |
| | Doctor from receiving country in Jerusalem | |

The salaries of the Israel doctors are paid basically by the host country but supplemented by Israel. The nurses and doctors from the receiving country studying in Jerusalem receive scholarships from the Israel Government.

Research studies are encouraged, in order to benefit from the results and to encourage initiative. These research grants now constitute a good percentage of the income of the specialists serving abroad. The Israel Government and Hadassah Medical Organization have set up special funds for these grants. This integrated form of service has been carried out in Liberia (1960), in Tanzania (1962), in Malawi (1969) and in Rwanda (1966). In the last country the service has been taken over by Belgium.

The Israel doctor going to serve in the receiving country has his research program approved before he goes. In fact he describes himself as a research scholar sent to tackle a problem for a fixed period, as well as a clinician sent to tackle a clinical problem.

### VARIED FOREIGN AID

We have selected only a few programs. There are obviously many more countries helping the developing countries.

*Belgium.* Organization: Administration of the developing cooperation (Foreign Office) and universities.

In Belgium: Scholarships are awared to students in medicine, but not for postgraduate training in ophthalmology.

Abroad: The Government sends technical personnel to the developing countries: Latin America; Africa with the exception of South Africa; Asia with the exception of Japan, USSR and China; Oceania with the exception of Australia. There are cooperative agreements with Zaire, Rwanda, Burundi, Morocco, Tunisia, Peru, Chile, Malaysia, Ivory Coast and Senegal. The candidates are recruited by the Belgian foreign office and submitted for the approval of the developing country. The technical personnel are paid by Belgium according to the official Belgian scale supplemented by an adjustment coefficient. At the present time there are approximately 100 doctors, of whom 60 are in Zaire. There is only one ophthalmologist in Bonaké (Ivory Coast).

The Belgian universities cooperate with the universities in Zaire and Rwanda. The University of Ghent cooperates with Butare (Rwanda), and sent an ophthalmologist; Louvain cooperates with Kinshasa and also sent an ophthalmologist; Liège with Lumumbashi, where an ophthalmologist is working.

*Britain.* Organization: Overseas Development Administrations (Foreign and Commonwealth Office).

In Britain: Postgraduate training, currently

16 scholarships in ophthalmology; awards through various organizations.

Post-registration training scholarships for nurses are available (including ophthalmic nursing).

Abroad: University staff at all levels. The overseas universities provide basic salaries and Britain supplements these with allowances.

Advisors on specific problems for relatively short visits advise on specific problems or on the establishment of particular university departments. The receiving government is expected to provide accommodation and transport. An ophthalmologist was sent to Makerere University (Uganda) to advise on the development of ophthalmic services.

Equipment is occasionally supplied.

Research projects approved by the Tropical Medical Research Board of the Medical Research Council in Britain, e.g. Trachoma Research Unit in Fajara (The Gambia) and in Iran.

Financial assistance to voluntary bodies, e.g. the Royal Commonwealth Society for the Blind and the Order of St. John in Jerusalem (ophthalmic hospital).

*France.* Organization: Foreign office. Organisme de Coopération et de Coordination pour les Grandes Endémies (OCCGE).

Organisme de Coopération des Etats de l'Afrique Centrale (OCEAC).

Fond Européen de Développement.

In France: There are scholarships not only for students, but also for doctors who specialize in ophthalmology.

Abroad: Eye service: 21 ophthalmologists are sent to 14 French-speaking countries in Africa (Burundi, Cameroon, Central African Republic, Congo-Brazzaville, Ivory Coast, Dahomey, Gabon, Upper Volta, Malagasy Republic, Mauritania, Niger, Senegal, Chad and Togo).

Mobile unit in Upper Volta with one ophthalmologist, for the treatment of onchocerciasis and trachoma. In 1965 this unit treated 48,475 cases of onchocerciasis and 24,301 cases of trachoma.

Institut d'Ophtalmologie Tropicale (Institute for Tropical Ophthalmology) in Bamako, Mali. This institute for research and treatment has two ophthalmologists. Sixty percent of the expenses ( $180,000) are paid by France and 40% by OCCGE.

This is only part of what France is doing. The total amount of money devoted to the developing countries is $400,000.

*Germany.* Two ophthalmologists were sent to Lomé (Togo) and one to Addis Ababa (Ethiopia). There is a project of DM 1,554,000 for the development of ophthalmology in Sabata (Ethiopia).

*Holland.* Organization: Universities; private organizations.

In Holland: Neither training nor instruction.

Abroad: Help given by aid to voluntary bodies and private agencies.

Universities: Rotterdam Medical Faculty: Aid in running Dr. Jap Eye Hospital and training staff (Djakarta, Indonesia).

University of Leiden: Training program for residents and senior staff in Undaan Eye Hospital (Surabaja, Indonesia) and Suriname University Eye Department.

University of Amsterdam: Training of optometrists for Indonesia.

Private agencies: Medical aid in tropical countries: Regular supply of ophthalmic equipment to Undaan Eye Hospital (Surabaja, Indonesia).

Prof. Weve Foundation: New Eye Center in Mukuma (Kenya). Training of doctors, medical assistants and nurses.

Flying doctors service and mobile eye units in Kenya (affiliated with the Kenya Society for the Blind).

Equipment for the Eye Department of Bawku Hospital (Ghana).

Mobile eye units in Malawi.

Eye Department of Laela (Tanzania): supply of salaries and equipment.

23

Financial support for the Institute for the Blind (Agua de Dios, Colombia).

Private agency: Running of the school for the blind in Suriname.

Dutch Reformed Church: Eye department of Agogo (Ghana).

Lutheran and Reformed Churches: Support to the Eye Department of the Christian Medical College in Ludhiana (India).

The ICCO (Utrecht) supports the Blind Rehabilitation Center in Kabul (Afghanistan) and the Private Overseas Office in Isfahan (Iran).

Research project: Rotterdam Medical Faculty: Research on retinotoxic effects of chloroquine—medicated salt. Pilot study on onchocerciasis in Tanzania.

### CONCLUSIONS

When we compare the two types of program, the varied and the integrated, we come to the conclusion that the integrated aid is the most efficient.

As many developed countries as possible must assist the developing countries to create effective ophthalmological services, to give good ophthalmological teaching and at the same time to promote interesting research—in brief to give integrated eye service.

*Ophthalmological service.* One must not forget that in many developing countries there are no departments. We must help them in this field by sending personnel and equipment till they become independent of out-side eye help. Besides the setting up of a permanent eye department, mobile ophthalmic units must also be organized.

The ophthalmic service means that we not only have to send ophthalmologists to these countries, but also that local doctors have to come to developed countries to receive specialized training.

*Teaching program.* A teaching program not only for doctors but also for nurses and medical assistants is essential. Medical assistants play an important role in African medicine and necessarily so because of the grave shortage of African doctors. Moreover they are very efficient especially in prevention work.

*Research.* Besides specific ophthalmological help, more specialized help can be given, for example with respect to trachoma or to onchocerciasis. The combination of extensive clinical fields in Africa and of a parent department with laboratory facilities in a developed country, together with a staff which has experience in both places, is clearly likely to stimulate original and useful investigation.

As Professor I. C. Michaelson wrote in 1968 in "World Hospitals," the plan for foreign aid in medicine and especially in ophthalmology must be "to serve, teach and leave."

This survey would have been impossible without the help of Professor I. C. Michaelson, who obtained most of the information I needed. Therefore I thank him very warmly.

# INTERNATIONAL ORGANIZATIONS FOR THE BLIND

## ACTIVITIES FOR
## THE PREVENTION AND CURE OF BLINDNESS

JOHN WILSON

Royal Commonwealth Society for the Blind, Commonwealth House, Haywards Heath, Sussex, England

Organizations for the blind resolved some years ago that, in addition to their traditional role in the education, rehabilitation and welfare of the blind, they must concern themselves with the prevention and cure of blindness. Since then they have become a major factor in an expanding international movement. The work of three organizations functioning in this field—the World Council for the Welfare of the Blind, the American Foundation for Overseas Blind and the Royal Commonwealth Society for the Blind—is summarized in this report.

### THE WORLD COUNCIL FOR THE WELFARE OF THE BLIND

The World Council for the Welfare of the Blind (WCWB) is our world assembly, made up of delegations from 56 countries which together can speak effectively on behalf of organized work for the blind in practically every country in the world. The Council maintains contact with the whole family of United Nations agencies and with international nongovernmental organizations.

Its coverage is remarkable—North and South America, Europe, Asia, Africa, Australasia, with strong and valuable delegations from the Soviet Union and countries of East-ern Europe. We have a secretariat in Paris and an Executive which maintains regular supervision of all aspects of the Council's work, and the World Assembly, which meets every five years.

Almost from the foundation of WCWB, the prevention of blindness was included as one of our major international objectives. At our second World Assembly a standing committee for the prevention of blindness was established of which I have since been Chairman. At a subsequent World Assembly all national affiliates were urged to undertake active interest in the prevention and cure of blindness and, if necessary, to amend their constitutions to enable them to do so.

This expansion of our role, both national and international, resulted from recognition that the blind population of the world was increasing; and that, particularly in the developing countries, the concept of rehabilitation would be frustrated unless a vigorous effort was made for the prevention and cure of blindness. It also seemed to us that there was something fundamentally absurd in the spectacle of the world spending a billion dollars on welfare for the blind, but only a minute sum on international action to reduce blindness.

Having reached this point, we made immediate contact with the World Health Organization and the International Association for the Prevention of Blindness (IAPB). The first result of that partnership was the launching in 1962 of the international effort of publicity which was associated with World Health Day. The object was to draw the attention of international agencies, national governments and of the general public to the facts of needless blindness.

*World Prevention of Blindness Committee.* That cooperation convinced us that the active nucleus in this international work for the future should be an amalgam of three elements: the ophthalmic organizations, the organizations concerned with blindness and the United Nations Agencies. Accordingly an informal group was formed which was called the World Prevention of Blindness Committee consisting of representatives of WCWB, the IAPB, and the secretariat of WHO. This group took the initiative in promoting a resolution on the prevention of blindness which was adopted at the Boston World Health Assembly in 1969. More recently, in April of this year, we collaborated with the secretariat of UNICEF in urging the UNICEF Executive Board to promote coordinated action to protect children from the consequences of vitamin A deficiency.

This mechanism of cooperation, though the best we have, is still inarticulate and insufficiently purposeful. It is evident at this conference that there is a potential world interest waiting to be channelled into action; and I hope that one result of this week's gathering may be to review the organization and give it a more dynamic impulse.

### THE AMERICAN FOUNDATION FOR OVERSEAS BLIND

I come now to the second international organization in our field, the American Foundation for Overseas Blind (AFOB). It is characteristic of the confident cooperation which exists between our organizations that though AFOB is represented here today by Dr. John Ferree, he has asked me to include his material in my presentation.

AFOB, allied to the central organization for the blind in the United States, has a great tradition. Over many years it has pioneered education and rehabilitation for the blind in many countries, particularly of Asia, Central and South America. Three years ago it decided to expand its work to include an international program for the prevention of blindness. Potentially it is one of the most important recent developments in our field, that this organization with its great tradition, its substantial resources and excellent management team has added this new dimension to its work.

So far, understandably, its activities have been exploratory. It has supported rural treatment in East Africa and last year its consultant, Dr. John Holmes, traveled throughout Asia and the Middle East and advised on the Foundation's future program. He recommended that priority should initially be given to the prevention of xerophthalmia among children. More recently, a representative and expert group at the organization's headquarters in New York has been considering policy, priorities and resources. It has endorsed in general terms Dr. Holmes' recommendation and is now formulating a project, the details of which will be announced later, for the control of xerophthalmia, probably in a selected country of Central America.

### ROYAL COMMONWEALTH SOCIETY FOR THE BLIND

The third organization is the Royal Commonwealth Society for the Blind (RCSB) of which I am Director and which I helped to found 21 years ago. This organization works throughout the Commonwealth, but this is an extensive parish covering roughly one quarter of the world's population. Last year the Society sponsored 161 projects in 32 countries. From the outset in 1950, we recognized that the prevention and cure of blindness must be our major priority. We have had the great benefit of constantly being advised on our program by an expert committee under the Chairmanship of Sir Stewart Duke-Elder. Our first research project was a four-year study of the causes of blindness and the control of onchocerciasis in West Africa. We had the good fortune of selecting as leader of that project Dr. F. C. Rodger, whose subsequent work on onchocerciasis has been so conspicuous.

That was the beginning of an interterritorial program of enumeration in which we endeavored to ascertain the extent and causes of blindness over a large part of Africa and the Near East. We later modified this program when we realized that it cost almost as much to count heads as to cure eyes. However, this early program led us into the whole field of the control of trachoma and subsequently into our Asian program, with the emphasis on rural treatment and the cure, on a massive scale, of needless blindness resulting from cataract.

One considerable asset of our organization is that we work with and through Commonwealth governments and with national affiliated organizations in 28 countries. A typical example of this is the organization in Kenya, represented at this Seminar by Dr. G.G. Bisley. That organization early began a program of prevention which now involves the use of five mobile units treating scores of thousands of village people each year.

I cannot here go into the details of our Society's program. To anyone who wishes to study it I will gladly send a copy of our Annual Report. Last year, in 14 countries, medical teams sponsored by RCSB examined 629,000 patients, treated 272,000 of them for various eye conditions, performed 25,599 operations for the restoration of sight and 14,223 operations for the prevention of imminent blindness.

This year, our program is being further expanded. We are sponsoring over 300 eye camps in eight States of India, doubling the number of mobile units in Pakistan, setting up new projects in Nigeria, Sierra Leone, India and Malaysia, undertaking research into vitamin deficiency and into the use of techniques of applied nutrition.

This, somewhat to our surprise, has become the largest international sight-saving program of any nongovernmental agency in the world. I say that not with any sense of satisfaction, but in the conviction that far greater efforts are essential if we are to make a significant impact on this problem. Much greater resources in money, personnel and organizations must be mobilized if we are to touch more than the margin of this world problem.

This, then, is a brief account of the work being done by organizations for the blind. We are anxious to collaborate on a broader scale with the United Nations, with the world organizations of ophthalmology, and with national agencies, to bring to this enterprise any capacity we may have for enthusiasm, for organization and promotion. I believe that there are here all the elements of a great international movement for the prevention of blindness. We have to combine those elements in an enterprise in which we can all collaborate intelligently and purposefully. If this can be the result of this conference it will indeed be a landmark in the prevention of blindness.

# THE ROLE OF MISSIONARY SOCIETIES
# IN THE PREVENTION OF BLINDNESS

NORVAL E. CHRISTY

Christian Hospital, Taxila, Pakistan

Historically, missionary societies have played a significant role in the development of health care in many countries, particularly in those which have achieved independence within the past 30 years. Some of these hospitals, founded and operated by mission societies, were among the first, and, in certain areas, among the only hospitals. Although the medical technical assistance programs of the United Nations and of foreign governments have increased in the past 20 years while the support of medical mission societies has probably decreased in terms of numbers of medical personnel and of sums expended, the treatment and relief of disease by medical missions remains, at least as far as American effort is concerned, the largest single component in medical technical assistance. Those devoted physicians and their colleagues have been important for the maintenance of personal medical services in tropical African countries and will continue to be for many years until local African physicians can be taught in much greater numbers than is the case today.

Exact personnel and expenditure figures for 1971 are not available, but by combining data from several sources and by making certain approximations, I have compiled the following estimates of the work being done at present by mission societies in about 90 countries. Mission societies operate over 3,000 hospitals with about 200,000 beds, and have the services of approximately 5,000 missionary doctors at their disposal. The number of local doctors in these institutions is not known to me, but it is certainly much larger than the number of foreign doctors. For example, in the mission society with which I am affiliated, the number of local doctors is 27 times as great as the number of foreign doctors in the 56 hospitals we operate. An estimated 4,000,000 patients are admitted annually into these mission hospitals and an estimated 30,000,000 patients are treated in their outpatient clinics. These institutions vary in size from medical colleges with several hundred doctors on their staffs, to small village hospitals having only one doctor, or smaller clinics without the full-time services of a doctor. Some of these institutions have eye departments which are staffed by ophthalmologists certified by the Royal College of Surgeons, the American Board of Ophthalmology or other foreign certifying bodies. Others have doctors who practice ophthalmology with little or no specialized training. At least one of these hospitals specializes in the treatment of eye diseases only, while others may stress eye work. For example, in the general hospital with which I am associated, of 10,500 operations performed annually, 9,000 are eye operations. In the mission-affiliated medical colleges there are departments of ophthalmology in which ophthalmologists are trained. Almost all of the mission hospitals have to treat patients who have sore eyes or other eye complaints, or instruct mothers about the care of their children's eyes.

Some mission hospitals have programs which are specifically geared to preventive medicine. An outstanding example of this is the Ludhiana Department of Preventive Medicine of the Christian Medical College, Ludhiana, India. This department was established in 1953 by Dr. Carl E. Taylor who is currently the Chairman of the Department of International Health of Johns Hopkins University.

The chief emphasis of the present report is to point out the potential of this large group of well-established hospitals, which treat millions of patients annually. These are staffed by a group of devoted, highly motivated, able people, including several thousand foreigners, and thousands of local nationals. The latter have not had to face the problem of cultural shock, and understand the psychology, customs and background of their people as no foreigner can hope to do.

These institutions and people represent resources which can and should be utilized to prevent blindness. This is an educational process, requiring among other things, some shift of emphasis. Traditionally, mission hospitals have been concerned mainly with curative medicine and treatment of the individual. However, mission societies have in recent years become more aware of the importance of preventive medicine and of the fact that in many situations the time, energy and resources available to a medical team are exploited more efficiently in the prevention of disease than in its cure.

If the mission societies could be given the vision and advice for preventive ophthalmology, they would be an effective force in the prevention of blindness. In this, assistance along certain lines is needed, such as a training program to teach doctors and other workers preventive ophthalmology. Most of the staff of mission hospitals are already overworked, so that additional personnel will be needed in many cases. These might be short-term helpers from outside, although long-term help is usually more effective. This may be in the form of additional staff hired and trained by the institution. For such help, and for the new materials needed for such programs, financial aid will be needed. Some mission hospitals are financially self-sufficient, but few, if any, have any appreciable surplus for instituting new programs which, by their nature, are not productive of income.

Were the motivation and vision, the personnel and training, and the materials and financing to be provided, this large potential force could be mobilized more actively in the prevention of blindness.

# A DECADE OF PROGRESS

JAMES J. LAWLOR

International Eye Foundation, Washington, D.C., USA

In October 1961, a team of three American ophthalmologists departed from San Francisco for Hong Kong on what was to be the first surgical teaching mission of the newly established International Eye Foundation (IEF). Drs. John Harry King Jr. of Washington, D.C., John M. McLean of New York and Charles E. Iliff of Baltimore were the first surgeons sent abroad by the IEF to teach and operate in areas where their skills were desperately needed, because of the heavy volume of surgical cases and the few ophthalmologists available to perform the surgery. During the course of this program, over 40 ophthalmologists from the Hong Kong area and throughout Asia were on hand to observe surgery. IEF doctors operate only where there are other ophthalmologists in the area who can be taught to perform these operations and to carry on the program after they leave.

The IEF was founded as a charitable, non-profit organization in February 1961, for the broad purpose of preventing and curing worldwide blindness. The headquarters are at Sibley Memorial Hospital, Washington, D.C., and John Harry King Jr. was the founder and is medical director of the IEF. Since its inception, the IEF, through its International Eye Bank program, has provided 2,012 fresh eyes and 4,304 preserved corneas for corneal transplants in areas where there are no eye banks and where eye tissue is extremely scarce. This tissue has been made available to 55 countries through the cooperation of 60 American eye banks, all members of the Eye Bank Association of America. The International Eye Bank serves as a clearing house for all eye bank operations outside the continental United States. There are currently many more demands for eyes than can be met.

The IEF has a many-sided approach to worldwide blindness. The first phase consists of a fellowship program through which qualified foreign ophthalmologists are brought to the United States to learn the latest eye surgical techniques and eye patient care as practiced there. After three months of study at the IEF headquarters in Washington and other eye centers such as Johns Hopkins University, Wills Eye Hospital, Duke University and the University of Florida, they return to their own countries.

The second phase consists of sending young American doctors into developing countries on three- to six-month fellowships to help these nations set up their own eye banks and hospital procedures.

To date the IEF has provided a total of 323 fellowships, 170 young ophthalmologists have been sent to other countries from the United States and 153 ophthalmologists have been brought for training to the United States from other countries. The young Americans who are sent abroad have usually just completed their residency training and are able to assist with the patient load, to help instruct eye residents, nurses and technicians and to help establish new eye banks where they are needed.

Twenty-nine eye banks are now operating in 26 countries as a result of IEF programs. In order to aid these banks initially, fresh eye tissue is flown from the United States in special containers developed by the IEF so that local publicity may be received, which assists in obtaining eye pledges and support for the new eye bank.

Another important phase of the IEF program is support of the surgical teaching teams mentioned earlier. Highly qualified eye surgeons, nurses and technicians are sent to areas where there is a need for ocular surgery to be performed. The local ophthalmologists are trained in the latest operating techniques; where necessary, using eye tissue furnished by cooperating eye banks in the United States. It is often possible to start an eye bank movement which continues with support from the local population. Since 1961, these teams have been sent from the United States to more than 20 countries throughout the world. The ophthalmologists who serve on these teams are usually men with professorial rank, connected with a university teaching program.

A new training program for paramedical personnel (ophthalmic aides) has been established. The first two courses are scheduled to be held this year in Indonesia and Pakistan. The graduates of the three-month course will be able to assume many of the responsibilities

for minor treatment and diagnosis. We are committed to expand our work in the Western Hemisphere through increased funding for fellowships for young Latin American ophthalmologists to attend the Basic Science Course in Ophthalmology given in Spanish at the University of Puerto Rico. We anticipate that as many as 40 young eye surgeons from most Latin American countries will be attending this course each year beginning in 1972. In addition, Latin American programs will be expanded through new Eye Bank units and exchange fellowships scheduled for Haiti and Honduras.

In order to gain additional support for these programs, the IEF recently established the Society of Eye Surgeons, which now has over 800 members throughout the world, and whose purpose is to promote the science of ophthalmic surgery among all peoples and nations by the following means: 1) sponsoring fellowships in eye surgery to young ophthalmologists now in training or who have recently completed training; 2) sponsoring teaching teams and visiting professors to and from certain countries to present lectures, courses and operating demonstrations to improve eye surgical care and for the interchange of scientific knowledge; 3) sponsoring social intercourse among interested physicians and scientists, skilled in ophthalmic surgery and research; 4) sponsoring periodic eye congresses, symposia, panels or other meetings in order to report new eye surgical techniques, modifications of standard techniques, statistical verifications of techniques and research involving eye surgery.

# THE OPHTHALMOLOGICAL SERVICES OF MEDICO

## A Service of "CARE"

ROY O. SCHOLZ*

Department of Ophthalmology, Johns Hopkins School of Medicine, Baltimore, Maryland, USA

MEDICO (the initials of Medical International Cooperation Organization) is a service of "CARE," one of the largest charitable organizations in the United States. Founded by Peter A. Comanduras and Dr. Thomas A. Dooley in 1958 as an organization of medical and paramedical personnel practicing in the United States and Canada, it became the medical arm of CARE in 1962. Its aim is to share its abilities where needed, without regard to race, religion or political persuasion.

Half of the world's population lives and dies without ever seeing a doctor (Table 1) let alone an ophthalmologist. Since sight is necessary for the adequate functioning of any individual in society, the provision of ophthalmic services is of considerable importance to a nation's economy. The world-wide shortage of ophthalmologists and the nature of the problem are well known.

Medical ophthalmology is a part of the overall services of medical care provided by MEDICO. The ophthalmological service of MEDICO is an extension of the basic assistance and rehabilitation provided at very low cost. MEDICO works only in countries where CARE also has a program. This permits balanced and comprehensive assistance, such as feeding in conjunction with medical programs. Following a preliminary survey, a medical team is sent to determine specific needs and to develop a program tailored to these needs. The host government contracts with MEDICO to attempt to provide continuation of medical supplies, counterpart physicians, nurses and technicians for training, and assistance in maintenance of the MEDICO team. MEDICO then recruits personnel to serve for two years, as well as short-term volunteer specialists, and establishes a team in an existing hospital. Additional supplies and equipment are dispatched to ensure an effective effort.

The team is relieved when host facilities become adequate and sufficient trained medical personnel are available adequately to con-

TABLE 1. *Number of inhabitants
per practicing physician in various countries*

| Country | Ratio inhabitants/physician |
| --- | --- |
| United States | 658 |
| Afghanistan | 21,360 |
| Algeria | 8,550 |
| Dominican Republic | 2,514 |
| Honduras | 5,556 |
| Indonesia | 29,480 |
| Tunisia | 8,780 |
| Western Malaysia | 5,320 |

* Author's address: 11 East Chase St., Baltimore, Maryland.

tinue local medical care. In Prof. Michaelson's phrasing, we too "serve, teach and leave."

The primary advantages of such programs lie in the cooperative utilization of the host government's facilities, together with those provided by MEDICO, to train local personnel on the spot, in their own environment and in the treatment of their local diseases. We train not only physicians, but also the paramedical personnel who constitute part of the complete medical team. As more local trainees become qualified to instruct their compatriots, the availability of medical personnel increases, with a minimum permanent loss of brainpower to the host country. With experience, we have been able to structure our programs to offer advanced training in medicine, surgery and other specialties over several years. In some places, with the local government's approval, we have been able to award certificates to our trainees. This has been done in surgery and medicine, as well as in paramedical fields such as nursing.

Costs are important, as Prof. Michaelson has suggested, and we feel that we are quite efficient. We have supplied well over 100 doctor-years since 1958 in all specialties, with ophthalmology listed second in priority. Support is derived partly from individual donations from the United States, the money being used to support volunteer and full-time paid physicians who receive approximately $300 to $400 a month. In addition, we are indirectly supported by large donations of equipment and medicine by the United States drug industry. These resources become reasonably adequate when combined with donations by the host government of cash or, more generally, of housing, gasoline and facilities. Such cooperation benefits everyone concerned.

We make the following suggestions as to problems in the implementation of health services, although we are aware of certain pitfalls involved.

Firstly, we feel that the most important project is the construction of an accurate central registry for all medical assistance programs, a step which is absolutely necessary in order to avoid the unnecessary but increasing duplication of programs and services. We urge this conference to consider seriously the setting up of such a registry, with a view to coordinating effort, particularly in countries most in need of help.

Secondly, most of us are traditional thinkers when it comes to providing ophthalmic care, and host countries are rightfully proud of their small, tradition-oriented systems. We need rethinking, experiment and persuasion in order to introduce new methods of health care to these populations. "Those who cannot be reached cannot be served." Some ideas which have been considered and which should be explored further are:

1) The use of ophthalmic assistants with less education than physicians, who would dispense medication and screen patients. We are beginning this training program in the United States, and the ophthalmic assistants completing the course may be utilized in controlled situations. 2) The feasibility of training technicians capable of doing specialized, specific tasks such as cataract surgery. Such technicians would have to perform under close supervision and control. 3) Expansion of the mobility of international and local medical services in order to provide seasonal but regular health care. 4) Improvement of methods for bringing more patients to existing facilities, as well as improvement of these facilities, themselves. The most important of all requirements and probably our most difficult problem is the expansion and improvement of public health measures.

# DISCUSSION

DR. H. M. THOMAS (*Liberia*): Among the main causes of blindness in developing countries is ignorance. The average African does not know what to do when he has an eye infection and he goes about trying all the means he can find. Only as a last resort, does he go to the hospital. To complicate this further, there are the tribal customs. I wish to emphasize that we could eliminate much of the blindness from our population if we could develop a rigid program of health education. We are fortunate that Dr. Michaelson has established a very sophisticated eye clinic in Monrovia, but I am afraid that it is not enough. The WHO has given priorities to certain diseases, but unfortunately the blind have been forgotten. I have a problem and I hope the experts can help me. With our limited means, we must decide whether to give priorities to the training of paramedical staff or to a census of the blind. I believe that we can prevent 70% of our problems of blindness.

DR. I. C. MICHAELSON (*Israel*): These interesting reports from today's session show that there are three types of prevention of blindness: 1) prevention before the disease occurs, for example, proper nutrition as a means of preventing xerophthalmia; 2) prevention when the disease is present but is in its early stages with little functional loss, for example glaucoma prior to field loss; and 3) prevention after the disease has caused notable organic and functional change, such as blindness from cataract. In other words, there are cases of prevention where the patient cannot know, does not know, or does know but can do nothing about his condition. As for the third type of prevention, a cataract operation performed in New York is not a preventive act, but the sending of staff for this purpose to many areas of the world is. There are two basic problems of personnel in developing countries: that of paramedical personnel, and that of doctors. There is a growing number of ophthalmologists in developing countries, but this number will need to be supplemented for years to come. Are the doctors who come to help ready to carry out curative measures or are they prepared to practice only public health ophthalmology? It will be difficult to persuade many doctors to go out and work in public health ophthalmology, a field which is unassociated with the hospital or with the private curative ophthalmology to which they will return. It will however be possible, from my experience, to send doctors who are prepared on the one hand to run a curative clinic and on the other hand to work in public health ophthalmology, perhaps as part of a multidisciplined WHO team.

DR. J. FRANÇOIS (*Belgium*): I wish to emphasize the very different natures of the many aspects of the prevention of blindness. In onchocerciasis, although a doctor may help his patient, there is a greater need for biologists and research. In other diseases, the village teacher or an evangelical paramedical man is needed. In yet others, an agriculturist is the most important person. Prevention of blindness to me includes all these things, much more than, for example, the clinical achievement of removing a cataract. I think it is important to emphasize this to an audience such as this one.

DR. V. RAMBO (*India*): The medical colleges in India lack transport among other things. We need mobile eye hospitals staffed not only by assistants, but by professors of ophthalmology. Dr. van Ketter is an example. For these units to do good work, they need to be properly equipped with slit lamps, etc. We have three such units in the field. Many medical schools should have an overseas department such as the one at Hadassah Hospital in Jerusalem with Dr. Michaelson and his wonderful team. But most of the blind people of the world live not in the towns but in the villages, where they sit with their blindness which is usually unnecessary and curable. How many children with congenital cataract sit in these places, at the edge of a playground picking up the sand from the ground and letting it run through their fingers. Let's cure them. If they do not need instruction, they need Braille. If there is a sacrifice to be made, let us give the personal example.

DR. A. PIRIE (*England*): I have listened with great admiration to the account of what ophthalmologists and volunteer organizations have done and are doing to cure and help those already afflicted with eye disease, but I was sad that there was so little mention of research. I am a scientist and I want to help and be associated, and I want scientists to help and be associated with this work toward prevention of blindness. As you know, there is always a debate among scientists on the comparative virtues of pure versus applied research. Which is the more worthy? In my view, the genius is a law unto himself and must always remain so. But most ordinary scientists want to feel that their work is useful. In my country, however, the young scientist is not told nor is it explained to him that research into the prevention of blindness is both useful and enormously exciting. In fact, there is little money available for permanent posts for any one who wishes to devote himself to this work. It is my belief that the most fruitful hope for the study of eye diseases and their prevention comes from collaboration between ophthalmologists, pediatricians, and, also, scientists of all varieties. I would like to see an enormous growth of this kind of collaboration. The discovery of the trachoma virus needed biologists. The prevention of retrolental fibroplasia needed experimental pathologists. The elucidation of the role of vitamin A in the visual cycle needed biochemists. Knowledge of the cause of diabetic retinopathy will, I am sure, need ophthalmologists, biochemists, physiologists, endocrinologists, name the lot. I do not believe that this sort of work can be done by ophthalmologists alone. It will come through collaborative research. Research for prevention, I think, is a worthwhile aim and I would like very much to see it developed in this coming decade.

DR. I. FEITELBERG (*Israel*): Thank you very much, Dr. Thomas, for making us aware of the ignorance of the African population with regard to eye diseases. This and the apathy of the village population is a major cause of blindness. I found in Ethiopia that 70% of the patients with eye conditions come to the clinics for other reasons. You spoke, Dr. Rambo, of quality. In India you do have personnel but in Africa personnel is almost nonexistent. Much of the work on the prevention of blindness and of the research associated with it should be done by paramedical and nursing staff. The large central hospitals will require most of the services of the ophthalmic surgeons.

DR. G. G. BISLEY (*Kenya*): I have worked in Kenya for about 25 years and one impression which has always remained very strong in my mind is that about 15 years ago, when I was doing a survey of trachoma in the Northern Frontier districts of Kenya and finding there an incidence of trachoma between 90 and 100%, I was at a little primary school right in the center of this area and examined about 60 little boys and girls. To my amazement, the incidence of trachoma there was about 30% and the disease was very mild. I asked the headmaster of the school "How is it your little boys and girls look so clean and healthy and there is so little eye disease?" He took me down to the bottom of the plot and there was a lovely little stream in this very dry country and this was a permanent stream. He told me that every morning and evening he took the children down to the stream and had them wash their faces and eyes in the water. Much research is necessary but much of our prevention is just a matter of soap and water. When we think of the field of prevention we should also widen our area of exploration and we need water engineers and educators to help us.

DR. N. CHATTERJEE (*India*): People here have been speaking of the lack of medical personnel in the developing countries. Now, the state of Punjab from which I come is the size of New Jersey and we have four medical colleges and one postgraduate institute. We train at least 20 or 25 residents in ophthalmology every year and they find it very difficult to find jobs. Most people won't believe me, but it is very true. In my department, if I have one vacant post for a lectureship, there are 12 applicants for it. I know at least 10 ophthalmologists in the Punjab who are working in family planning because there is no job available in the government service. We don't require personnel but money.

DR. M. E. LANGHAM (*USA*): I would like to put in a word about the multidisciplinary attack.

read and discussed. An important medium for distributing information on these problems has been the *Journal of Social Ophthalmology* (*Journal d'Ophthalmologie Sociale*) published in both English and French. In 1962 it adopted a coding system for the causes of blindness, recommended for international use, and employed in several recent investigations on the causes of blindness.

Although a considerable amount of work has been done to prevent blindness, and in many countries it has met with remarkable success, blindness is still far too common. There is still an immense amount of work to do, most of which must fall on national authorities and organizations. Nevertheless, our Association feels that it ought to do much more. For this and other reasons the Association has been reorganized, and new statutes were adopted at an Assembly Meeting held during the International Congress of Ophthalmology in Mexico City in 1970. The aims of the Association are thus redefined as follows:

a) To study through international organizations the causes, direct and indirect, that may result in blindness or impaired vision. b) To encourage and promote measures aimed at eliminating such causes. c) To promote action for the rehabilitation of blind persons. d) To distribute information on all matters pertaining to the care and use of the eyes.

However, the resources of the Association required to fulfil its goals are at present rather scarce. Our intention is to collect and distribute information on the frequency of blindness, its causes and methods of prevention by arranging symposia and meetings on these problems and by publishing the data. A joint conference between the International Diabetic Federation and the IAPB is now being planned. The Association should act as advisor to international and national organizations and authorities and should, if possible, send out consultants or even teams of practical workers in the field. At present,

however, the Association lacks the means for such enterprises, yet it hopes to be of some help to national organizations.

Prevention of blindness has two aspects: one is to prevent conditions leading to deterioration of vision, the other is to cure states that have caused visual impairment. The latter is the task of ophthalmologists or other doctors with some knowledge of ophthalmology. They can be helped to some extent by paramedical staff. Medical problems of this kind are discussed at the ophthalmological congresses, but should not be dealt with at this seminar because we intend to discuss problems of a more administrative kind: how can the treatment necessary for restoring sight be given to all those who need it? As you know, the causes of blindness are manifold: hereditary malformations or diseases, diseases of mothers during pregnancy, nutritional deficiencies, infectious diseases, idiopathic and general eye diseases, accidents and intoxications. The relative importance of these causes differ widely in different countries. Nowadays some are practically unknown in certain countries, even if they had previously been prevalent. In preventing conditions that will lead to deterioration of vision the ophthalmologists often have to act mainly as initiators. We make the diagnosis, point out the cause of the disease and give advice about what should be done in order to eliminate it. In other cases, such as glaucoma, we also have to treat in order to prevent visual impairment. However in many cases, and often in the majority of cases, the preventive measures must be undertaken by other specialists such as those in general hygiene and contagious diseases, nutritionists, pediatricians and specialists in various branches of medicine. The possibilities for doing this are greatly dependent upon economic and administrative conditions. The responsibility falls heavily on governments and their institutions.

The ideal prevention of blindness should

include genetic advice and even eugenic measures such as sterilization, as long as we cannot change the genes; preventive care of mothers before and during pregnancy, adequate nutrition to all, especially children; excellent general hygiene; effective eradication of the vectors of infectious diseases; preventive vaccinations and systematic health examinations, especially of children. In short, good medical care should be available to everyone. Every doctor ought to have some knowledge of ophthalmology and should understand the influence of some general diseases on vision. The law should enforce eye protection in industrial work and prohibit minors from acquiring shooting weapons and other explosives. General education programs should include lectures on the risks and accidents to eyes during childhood, in sports and at work.

To carry out such programs requires good economy, a wise government with an effective administration, and well-educated and energetic persons to do the field work. In the most developed countries many of the prerequisites for the prevention of blindness are quite well fulfilled even if much still has to be done, but in other countries even basic measures have not yet been undertaken. This may be due to the magnitude of the tasks to be performed, to lack of economic means and qualified personnel, to lack of interest or even to ignorance by the leaders of the state or its administrative institutions of what should be done. Therefore, the methods to improve the program of prevention of blindness will differ in different countries. The appropriate measures will depend mainly on local authorities and institutions. They will have to find out which causes of blindness are the most prevalent in their regions, and which measures should be undertaken. In developed countries this will depend mainly on the government and its institutions. In others, private charity organizations have to take on the main burden; and in some, international support is needed. In some countries the ophthalmological societies are interested in the problems of prevention of blindness and they have taken the initiative in promoting action. In others, public organizations regard this as their task. In most countries this cause might best be served through a National Association for Prevention of Blindness, which would include ophthalmologists as well as other people involved in these complex problems. These national associations should be in close contact with other institutions and organizations for public health. An exchange of knowledge and experience between the various national organizations is essential, and the International Association for Prevention of Blindness wishes to serve as a center for this.

I am convinced that many of you possess broad knowledge and vast experience in these matters, acquired in various parts of the world. It will be of great value if you would let us share your knowledge, your experience and your plans for future work. That will give us an opportunity to exchange ideas, which is the main purpose of this seminar. This in turn would stimulate effective work in this field in the years to come.

# AUSTRALIA

IDA MANN

56 Hobbs Avenue, Nedland, Western Australia

Australia is more complex than it appears. It is as large as the United States (excluding Alaska) and is divided politically and administratively into five states and two territories. The climate varies from the snow and ice of Tasmania to the extreme dry heat of the deserts of the center and north. Its population is between 11 and 12 million. The inhabitants are of two distinct stocks, Aborigines and European settlers. However, the anthropologists tell us that both are Caucasian in origin. This probably accounts for the rapidity with which the deep skin pigmentation of the full blooded Aborigine disappears on miscegenation with Europeans, the quarter-cast often being fair haired and blue eyed. The cultural levels of the two groups are, however, very separate and distinct, as are their ophthalmic problems. Little or no notice had been taken of these until the 1950s when a series of surveys was undertaken, principally by the Flying Doctor Service and the Public Health Department of Western Australia. These surveys disclosed the great disparity between the eye diseases of the two groups.

*Diabetic retinopathy.* This, in Australia as elsewhere in the "civilized" world, is increasing among the white population with the increased expectation of life for young diabetics. Among the Aborigines it is not yet a problem. Their native diet is high in protein, with practically no carbohydrates; and diabetes is rare. However, under the policy of integration at present recommended, the diet is changing to the European pattern and the tall, lean, muscular tribal Aborgine is giving place to an overweight, sedentary type addicted to white bread, refined sugar and, in or near towns. alcohol. This will be a problem in the future,

*Glaucoma.* The incidence of both narrow and wide angle glaucoma in the white population is similar to that elsewhere among Caucasians. There is strong evidence that both types are genetic and in view of the relatively small population, one would expect a gradual increase. A strong campaign for early diagnosis and treatment, initiated and supported by private enterprise, is in progress. The public spirited Lions Clubs conduct diagnostic surveys free of charge and supply information and referrals for treatment. The general public is now aware of the disease and seeks advice freely. There should be no need for government intervention here.

Neither is the disease a problem among the Aborigines. In a survey of 2,185 persons with Aborigine blood, carried out in 1954, only five cases of glaucoma simplex were found (0.2%), one in a woman of mixed blood. This survey did not go into the finer points of glaucoma diagnosis, but if the disease were as common as it is in the white population, one would expect to find many more persons blind from it in the aboriginal population, since they have received no treatment whatsoevers In European and North American popula. tions glaucoma accounts for roughly 10% of blindness and is as high as 16% in white person-in Australia (1). Glaucoma therefore poses no problem in Aborigines and is being efficiently dealt with in white persons.

*Amblyopia ex anopsia.* In Australia there is also a great disparity between the white and the aboriginal populations in this condition. In analyses of series of patients seeking advice, the incidence of convergent strabismus varies between 3.5% (New South Wales) and 8% (Western Australia). There is everywhere a strong genetic factor. Among Aborigines convergent strabismus is rare. It was not once found in 1,680 full blooded Aborigines examined (2) but occurred five times in 507 Aborigines of mixed blood. The treatment of convergent strabismus and amblyopia was very inadequate in 1954 when I began my surveys, but has steadily improved. Infant Health Clinics and the School Medical Services now weed out the cases and refer them for treatment by ophthalmologists and orthoptists. The standard is constantly rising as both general practitioners and parents are alerted to the situation.

There is no problem among the Aborigines and most children of mixed blood have access to medical attention.

*Retinal detachment.* The standard of treatment for this condition is now very high in Australia. The incidence is not great. Redmond reports it as 0.45% in New South Wales. In my practice among white West Australians 0.7% of the population was affected. There are no figures for its incidence in Aborigines but it is certainly rare.

*Senile cataract.* The incidence in white persons is as in Europe and there are full facilities for operation and the prescribing of spectacles. Among Aborigines, the incidence in our first survey before treatment was available was 51 (3%) in 1,678 full bloods examined. All these required operation. The type of cataract was almost invariably a nuclear sclerosis. Since the increasing myopia counteracts the presbyopia in the early stages, no complaint is made until the disability is great. Today, through the Flying Doctor Service and the Royal Perth Hospital, these cases can all be dealt with.

*Corneal opacities.* We now come to the great problem of the Australian Aborigine,

trachoma and the visual disability it entails. Until the 1950s the presence of trachoma among the aboriginal population was not suspected. It was even stated in WHO publications that Australia was free of the disease, though the older ophthalmologists knew this to be untrue.

In 1952 and 1953 the Royal Flying Doctor Service reported the existence of an ophthalmic problem in the Kimberley district of Western Australia. The area was served by District Medical Officers, none of whom had received any postgraduate ophthalmic training nor had they ever seen a case of trachoma, since they had been trained in medical schools in large cities in Australia or England. In 1953 the Service (Victorian Section) offered to defray the expenses of the air travel which would be involved in carrying out a survey of the area. The Public Health Department offered additional road transport and personnel (a health inspector, a physician and an ophthalmologist). The area surveyed was almost the size of the British Isles, and the work took approximately three months. This involved 5,500 miles of road travel, 4,000 miles of flying and 200 miles by sea.

The situation discovered shocked the authorities and was received at first with incredulity. In all, 2,866 persons were examined; 1,678 full blooded Aborigines, 507 mixed bloods and 681 whites. An overall incidence of 42% of trachoma was found. Seventeen were blinded in one eye by trachoma and 96 in both. The figures for infection were somewhat deceptive as the incidence of trachoma in white persons in the district was only 6.14% while in the mixed blood it was 44.38% and in the full blooded Aborigines 56.49%. All the patients who had sought treatment at the district hospitals had been treated simply as conjunctivitis cases without being understood. Surveys were continued through the rest of the State, and similar figures were obtained. Indeed, in the temperate southern parts of Western

Australia, in the agricultural areas around and south of Perth, the incidence in colored and in full blooded Aborigines was sometimes between 60 and 70%, so that the condition was not confined to the tropical north.

The problems of trachoma treatment and control in this State (area, 975,920 square miles) have proved almost insuperable. We aimed at implementing the WHO recommendations of a preliminary survey. This was done and it merely emphasized the problem. Pilot treatment projects were then instituted but here difficulties arose. The Aborigines are nomadic and very philosophical, enduring much hardship as being part of life, and not very easily convinced of the value of western medicine. We aimed at starting a mass campaign but this has proved very difficult. The patients cannot be trusted to use the treatment properly. The children may pretend to swallow the tablets and later may spit them out. The parents will forget to apply the ointment. The supervision required simply cannot be done by the limited nursing staff available for covering large areas. We began by instructing doctors, nurses, health inspectors, missionaries, school teachers and some native affairs officers in the elements of diagnosis. We prepared a series of Kodachrome slides for teaching. Scarcity of personnel and lack of trachomatologists made supervision of large areas impossible, and only in certain cooperating institutions, such as schools, missions, or cattle stations with an enthusiastic manager did we achieve results. We soon learned from an experience with a convent boarding school for Aborigine children that the disease responded well to standard treatment while the children were living in the school. However, when they returned from the long summer holidays spent in native camps and on cattle ranches, they were nearly all reinfected.

At first we were unable to convince the other States of the urgency of the problem.

It was considered to be a matter for Western Australia alone, and no help was offered by the Federal Government. We suggested an application to WHO for advice and assistance but were firmly told by Canberra that Australia was not one of the depressed areas in need of help. Australia was a donor nation pledged to help less fortunate emergent nations and therefore quite unable to accept the role of recipient nation.

Gradually the other States became interested, and due to the private enterprise of ophthalmologists and university departments, further surveys were done. Virologists were interested and Perret of Western Australia cultivated the chlamydozoon in eggs (3). In order to convince the Public Health Departments that the disease was in fact trachoma, it then became necessary to fulfill Koch's postulates by transferring the agent from eggs to a human volunteer. This proved very difficult as there was strong opposition in Western Australia against the use of human volunteers. However, the State of Victoria was more forward looking, and through the influence of ophthalmologists and of the Ophthalmic Research Institute of Australia in Melbourne, Dr. Perret and I were able to perform the crucial experiment of culture, human infection and recovery of virus (4). This necessitated flying material from Perth to Melbourne (2,000 miles) and back. The various States of Australia are practically autonomous units and there is little agreement or collaboration among them. However, South Australia also became interested, and the Institute of Medical and Veterinary Science in Adelaide undertook surveys and laboratory investigations similar to ours.

The situation in Western Australia was politically very difficult. To admit that the problem existed among the Aborigine population was necessary but distasteful, since the disease has been stigmatized by various organizations as one of poverty, ignorance and dirt. Australia is a land of opportunity, of great growing potential; and to be included with Egypt, Africa and India as in need of reform was naturally displeasing. So many departments and interests were involved that no overall plan for a mass campaign seemed possible. The Public Health Department continued to fight with insufficient staff. The Native Affairs Department, at first unwilling to be involved, was unable to cope effectively with matters of housing and welfare. The Education Department, realizing that instruction and treatment could with some success be mediated through schools, came up against the Teachers' Union who proved uncooperative. The Aborigines themselves were unable to grasp that the relatively minor symptoms in children were the precursors of blindness in later life.

The Public Health Department has battled against odds for 15 years with but little success, since it has become increasingly clear that only by raising the standard of living of the Aborigines can the disease be controlled. This appears impossible at the moment for the following reasons: lack of trained personnel, lack of funds, lack of understanding of the Aborigines' point of view and the fact that most white Australians are town dwellers and are hardly aware of the problem of the Aborigines. The Aborigines themselves find it hard to cooperate, largely because their conception of life is more or less the opposite of ours. They are nonagressive, nonacquisitive, unconvinced of the value of work and, through missions and attempted education, deprived of their own culture and unable to accept the validity of ours. These problems are at least well recognized today by the white authorities and by the more progressive and politically conscious of the (usually half-caste) Aborigines.

I see the problem of trachoma control in Australia as only one facet of the complex native problem which is just beginning to worry everyone.

### REFERENCES

1. YATES PC. Blindness in Australia, 1953 to 1958. *Med J Aust* **50**: 828, 1963.
2. MANN I. Western Australia Public Health Department reports, 1954–1956.
3. PERRET D and MANN I. Isolation of virus from embryonate eggs inoculated with material from a case of trachoma in Western Australia. *Br J Ophthalmol* **44**: 503, 1960.
4. MANN I, GREER CH, PERRET D and McLEAN C. Experimental trachoma produced by a West Australian virus. *Br J Ophthalmol* **44**: 641, 1960.

# CANADA

## ELLIS SHEKEN

2, St. Clair Avenue West, Toronto, Canada

Newfoundland is an outlying area of Canada which has long lacked access to health services. This is due in part to its remote location and in part to its sparse population. In Newfoundland there are more than 1,200 small scattered communities, such as small fishing villages. There are only six certified ophthalmologists on the island caring for half a million inhabitants. It is necessary to exercise ingenuity in developing facilities and bringing medical and clinical services to the people living in such areas. An example of this concept of bringing the latest technological developments and medical care to those who need them is the Canadian National Institute for the Blind's mobile eye care unit. The members of the Lions Club of Weston, Ontario, bought the unit and presented it to the Canadian National Institute for the Blind. The unit had to be planned to carry the highly specialized ophthalmological equipment safely over rough terrain. It had to be self-powered, heated, air-conditioned, with hot and cold running water, lighting and sterilization facilities. Indeed, all the services easily available in an eye doctor's office were planned for and installed after careful thought and consultation. Portable, but safe, access steps to entrance and exit doors were essential, and these were so designed as to be set up or taken down in 10 to 15 min by the driver. On uneven ground the unit could be stabilized by four jacks and adjustment of the stair ramps.

The team consists of an ophthalmologist who serves for a month, a registered nurse who is a supervisor of the Canadian National Institute for the Blind eye services and a driver-clerk specially trained to handle the vehicle, set up and close down the clinic and sign in patients. The Lions Club in each outport is an integral part of the operation and helps its members in the organization of each tour.

Large numbers of children may be screened by the public health nurse in the schools prior to the unit's arrival. This saves time and energy on the part of the unit oculist who then examines all suspected cases picked up by the nurse. In the same manner, general practitioners or public health nurses can screen adults for glaucoma by tonometry. The suspected cases may be properly examined when the unit sets up. Certain conditions were extremely prevalent in this particular area, e.g. pterygium and albinism. Infants with strabismus were also very commonly found.

Screening for glaucoma and amblyopia complement the general advantages of having ophthalmic care made proximate. This is an example of a prevention of blindness service dependent on bringing existing ophthalmic services closer to a widely spread population by means of a mobile ophthalmic unit and a small team of enthusiasts.

If the unit succeeds in the objective of bringing eye care services to inaccessible areas, the original mobile eye care unit will, it is hoped, expand into a wide ranging mobile eye care and blindness prevention program carried on from a fleet of mobile clinics specially designed to carry these services to remote areas across Canada or any other country.

# HAWAII

## WILLIAM JOHN HOLMES

International Association for the Prevention of Blindness, Honolulu, Hawaii

The Hawaiian Archipelago is a group of islands, reefs and shoals strung out from the southeast to the northwest for 1,600 miles, with a population of about 700,000. Prevention of blindness in the State of Hawaii is a joint effort of the federal, state and county governments, industry, nongovernmental organizations, service clubs, foundations, public and private schools and concerned individuals.

*Genetic counseling.* Preventive advice on genetic grounds against diseases and anomalies is available at the Birth Defects Center of the Children's Hospital. The service is available to people intending to marry or who are already married, and is concerned with genetic prognosis for possible children in the given parental combination. Advice is also available to pregnant mothers of blind children on eugenic indications of induced abortion and sterilization.

*Retrolental fibroplasia.* The Hospitals and Facilities Branch of the State Health Department has established standards regarding the optimum concentration of oxygen that may be administered to premature infants. The recommended dosages are 32 to 34% concentration of oxygen for large and 28 to 32% concentration for small babies. Ophthalmoscopic examination of infants under 2,000 g birth weight who have received oxygen treatment is carried out through dilated pupils. The first examination is done at the hospital prior to discharge and the second, at three months of age.

*Preschool and school vision screening.* Through the Bureau of Crippled Children of the State Health Department, vision screening is carried out among preschool children enrolled in kindergarten. This office also funds corrective eye surgery, provides glasses and maintains a learning disability clinic. The federally funded Office of Economic Opportunity, better known as Project Headstart, looks after preschool children from low income families. It provides each child with a comprehensive pediatric examination, which includes vision testing, and the identification of all physical and mental health problems, as well as learning problems. Through the office of the Maternal and Child Health Division the State Health Department further arranges for vision tests for preschool children and refers those in need of correction to qualified specialists. Preschool, gradeschool and high-school vision screening is the responsibility of the School Health Department of the Hawaii State Board of Health. The tests administered include distance visual acuity using the Snellen chart plus lenses, the cover-uncover test and Ishihara color vision tests.

*Education of children with learning disability.* Special classes are operated by the Department of Education. Such education is also available through the Variety Club, a private, nonprofit organization to meet the educational needs of children with a learning disability due to neurological dysfunction.

*Visual motor defects.* The assessment of visual motor development in the preschool and early primary grades and the evaluation of deviations in visual motor functioning during the developmental process is offered through the facilities of the California Hawaii Elks Major Project, Inc.

*Amblyopia screening.* This is a project of certain Jaycee Clubs and their women's auxiliaries. The tests follow those recommended by the Neurological and Sensory Disease Control Program of the United States Department of Health, Education, and Welfare.

*Orthoptic clinic.* A trained orthoptic technician is attached to Queen's Medical Center in Honolulu. Her office is equipped with major amblyoscopes. She provides both diagnostic and therapeutic assistance to children and adults with oculomotor problems.

*Eye protection in industry.* According to the revised statutes of the State of Hawaii dealing with industrial safety, every employer is required to furnish and use safety devices and safeguards, and to adopt and use practices, means, methods, operations and processes which are reasonably adequate to render such employment and place of employment safe.

*Glaucoma detection.* A state-wide Glaucoma Detection Clinic is cosponsored by the Department of Social Services and Housing, Vocational Rehabilitation and Services for the Blind Division, Services for the Blind Branch; the Hawaii Lions' Eye Foundation and Lions Club of Hawaii; ophthalmologists of the Hawaii Eye, Ear, Nose and Throat Society; and the Department of Health, Medical Health Services Division, Chronic Diseases Branch.

*Premarital Wassermann test.* This test is necessary to obtain a marriage licence. If an unwed mother seeks prenatal care she must, by law, submit to a Wassermann test. If she is indigent, the Maternal and Child Health office of the State Health Department will provide prenatal, obstetrical and postpartum care.

*Credés treatment.* Following birth, law requires the instillation of 1 % silver nitrate into newborn babies' eyes. Moral standards of the population are changing. During recent years, a few hippies have delivered without the attendance of a physician, nurse or midwife. Babies born to infected women may be blinded. One case of gonococcal conjunctivitis developed in Hawaii last year. Treatment of infected infants consists of isolation, systemic penicillin, mydriatics and saline irrigations.

To reduce the incidence of gonococcal conjunctivitis in newborns, routine vaginal smears and cultures should be taken from the mother late in pregnancy.

# INDIA

## G. VENKATASWAMY

Madurai Medical College, Madurai, S. India

A recent survey by the Indian Council of Medical Research at Madurai, South India, has shown that 1.3% of the population in Madurai are blind in both eyes, and 1.12% are blind in one eye from cataract. In addition, 0.21% are totally blind because of incurable conditions. In rural areas, where 80% of the Indian population lives, and where ophthalmic services are not easily available, the incidence of blindness is considerably higher. India, with a population of 510 million, will have more than 10 million blind people if preventive measures are not taken.

The major steps so far taken are a) application of penicillin or silver nitrate drops to newborn infants to prevent ophthalmia neonatorum; b) introduction of a National Smallpox Eradication Program; c) use of antibiotics to reduce blindness caused by syphilis and gonorrhea; and d) formation of a National Trachoma Control Program to treat school and preschool children in all districts where it is endemic.

*Present position of eye care in Tamil Nadu State.* As early as 1819, an Eye Infirmary was started in Madras. This institution has trained eye surgeons for both India and the Far East. At present there are 10 medical schools in the State of Tamil Nadu. Each has an eye department, some well-equipped and others not.

The State of Tamil Nadu has a population of 41 million divided among 14 districts. In addition to the medical schools, each district hospital has a small eye department, usually of 10 to 15 beds. The Government Ophthalmic Hospital at Madras and the Ophthalmic Department attached to the Madurai Medical College organize mobile eye camps, as does the Christian Medical College, Vellore. A total of nearly 700 beds is available for eye patients in all the State Hospitals in Tamil Nadu. In addition, there are two eye hospitals run by Christian missionaries and an eye department attached to the Swedish Mission Hospital. The State of Tamil Nadu now has nearly 200 ophthalmologists.

*Malnutritional blindness.* Malnutrition is still one of the major causes of blindness in many Indian States, accounting for 5 to 10% of all incurable blindness. In recent years the government has been distributing vitamin A to pregnant mothers and infants in all of its health centers. Unfortunately, some authorities question the effectiveness of prophylactic vitamin A in preventing keratomalacia, and so it is not used everywhere.

In 1970, the Royal Commonwealth Society for the Blind set up a Nutritional Rehabilitation Center at Madurai for preventing malnutritional eye diseases. This is the first center in the world to concentrate on the prevention of malnutritional eye diseases. The main problem faced at this center is that mothers do not realize that conditions such as keratomalacia and marasmus are due to malnutrition. Many of them try quack remedies before bringing the children to the hospital. Because of poverty, they cannot afford to buy protein-rich foods. The center is educating the mothers by recommending cheaper foods with high protein content. Hitherto, the center has been nonresidential, the mother or guardian bringing the child for a light meal and advice. Recently, it has been converted into a residential center where the mother can stay with the child, and both are given meals. This experience has encouraged us to plan to bring this program into rural areas in the near future.

*Glaucoma.* No attempts have been made to educate people on glaucoma, which accounts for about 28% of all incurable blindness. Although screening of the public for glaucoma is rarely done in India, we have had this program in our Eye Department and in the Eye Camps for about five years. Nevertheless, many general practitioners are not aware of this problem, and acute attacks of closed angle glaucoma are often missed.

In November 1970 a comprehensive glaucoma demonstration center was opened at the Erskine Government Hospital, Madurai. This is the first attempt in India to make people "glaucoma conscious" and to train general practitioners and medical students to look for early signs, so that cases can be referred to glaucoma clinics. Many cases are mistakenly diagnosed as cataract, and patients delay medical help until the glaucoma is almost absolute. Screening and education of the public is essential, but unfortunately very few eye clinics in India are equipped for gonioscopy, applanation tonometry, etc.

*Cataract.* Nearly $2\frac{1}{2}$ to 3% of the population are blind in one or both eyes due to cataract. With the help of the Royal Commonwealth Society for the Blind, the Eye Department of the Government Erskine Hospital, Madurai has been organizing large eye camps for cataract surgery. In 1970 12 such camps treated nearly 6,000 patients for cataract. Because of their success, there is a great demand for more camps in many areas.

Efforts are being made to start mobile ophthalmic units at all medical schools. Since the public has felt the need for them, the time has come for the State, with the help of associations such as the National Society for Prevention of Blindness, to extend eye relief work.

At present there are both qualified nurses and opticians, as well as eye surgeons, available to staff these camps. The administration can be carried out by voluntary organizations, and the surgeons' time can be utilized entirely for technical work. In this way, it is hoped, more eye camps can be organized and more people can be helped. Operating on a patient for cataract, feeding him for eight days and giving him aphakia glasses costs about $4.00. This includes other costs such as advertising, sanitation, water supply and medicines.

*Blindness due to infection.* Trachoma and bacterial infections of the conjunctiva and cornea are responsible for nearly 14% of blindness in India. Environmental hygiene has to be improved and facilities for early treatment of infections made available in all areas. Even now we find cases in which quack remedies have worsened the condition and even brought on blindness.

*Increase in the output of eye doctors.* At present the output of eye doctors is insufficient to meet the demands of the community. In Tamil Nadu two medical colleges for postgraduate training accept eight candidates each year and at four medical schools there are 30 places for training in ophthalmology each year. However, not all are filled, possibly because ophthalmology does not seem to attract young doctors. Another problem is that during the training period, doctors do not get any remuneration and must be subsidized from home. Were they to receive a training grant, we might attract larger numbers.

*Expansion of hospital facilities.* There are plans to open new eye hospitals in the main towns of Tamil Nadu and at Taluk headquarters because at present such eye clinics are available only at district headquarters hospitals. In some towns, organizations such as the Lions Club or industrialists are ready to support such new eye hospitals. Given the necessary encouragement, it should be possible to build 50 or 60 of them from public donations alone. They could then be taken over and run by the government.

*Ophthalmic equipment for the eye hospital.* At present, ophthalmic institutions find it extremely difficult to obtain equipment such as slit lamps and ophthalmoscopes. Some efforts have been made to manufacture them locally, but the quality has not come up to international standards. Some operating instruments are also made in India, but they too are of poor quality. Until these industries develop, much of our equipment must be purchased from abroad, and our supplies of hard currency are limited. Therefore, equipment which is not in use in some of the developed countries should be donated to institutes in Tamil Nadu. War surpluses also provide a potentially good source not only of instruments, but also of generators, sterilizers, tents and other items required for mobile eye hospitals.

The Madurai Eye Bank Association was set up in 1966 and has subsequently expanded its activities through both public donations and Government grants. It has used this money to build a new wing for eye patients at the Government Erskine Hospital and to help organize eye camps. This is an example of what we can do locally. International organizations such as the Royal Commonwealth Society for the Blind, the American Foundation for the Overseas Blind, the International Eye Foundation and CARE-MEDICO. could help us to achieve our objectives as soon as possible.

# ITALY

## G. B. BIETTI

Clinica Oculistica, University of Rome, Italy

For many years, trachoma was a very serious problem in Italy. However, due to improved sanitation, living standards, economic conditions and more effective treatment, the disease is at present regressing markedly both in incidence and severity in Italy as well as in other European Mediterranean countries. The incidence of trachoma in southern Italy was first established by examining elementary school pupils. This could not be done in central and northern Italy since there were only sporadic cases in 1939, and no statistical data were available. In 1939, Italy was found to have 645,000 cases of trachoma. Nine percent of the inhabitants of southern Italy were active cases. In Sicily and Sardinia, the incidences were 7 and 8%, respectively.

Further information about the distribution of trachoma in Italy was obtained at a much later period from the Ministry of Health's reports on the sanitary conditions of the Italian Republic. They showed that in 1959–60 the percentage of trachoma cases in the lowest grades of the elementary schools had dropped from 9 to 3.48% in southern Italy and from 7 to 2.62% in Sicily. In contrast, the rate in Sardinia remained high, nearly 7.4% as compared to 8% in 1939. Five years later the figures were even lower: 2.1% in southern Italy, 2.62% in Sicily and 4.85% in Sardinia. In 1967 a further decrease in the incidence of trachoma in the elementary schools was recorded: 1.05% in southern Italy, 0.66% in Sicily and 1.72% in Sardinia.

The clinical aspects of the disease have also changed considerably, with a shift toward milder forms that are more amenable to chemotherapy. In this connection, I some-times sense a tendency to minimize the contribution of chemotherapy in eradicating the trachomatous infection, and to emphasize instead the social and economic factors. Though I fully agree with the importance of these factors, it would be erroneous to ignore the impact of chemotherapy. I personally have witnessed how the 40 beds for trachoma, as well as the antitrachomatous outpatient dispensary of the University Eye Clinic of Rome, had to be closed after the introduction of sulfonamides during the period 1937–39. Great improvements in social and hygienic standards could surely not have taken place in such a short period of time. In addition to the lowered trachomatous index in the schools, a corresponding decrease in the number of outpatients in the trachoma dispensaries was observed, with attendance dropping from 40,000 in 1964 to 15,000 in 1968 (Fig. 1). These data for the civilian population find their counterpart in the figures supplied

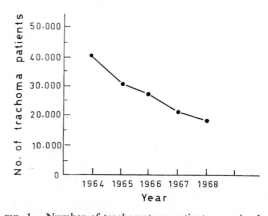

FIG. 1.   Number of trachomatous patients examined in the provincial antitrachoma organizations during the period 1964–68.

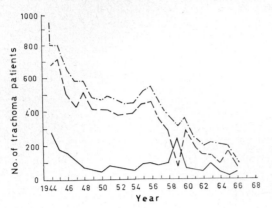

FIG. 2. Incidence of trachoma among army recruits showing: —·—·, number of exemptions due to trachoma out of 300,000 new recruits; ———, new recruits (previous years); – – –, new recruits (20 years).

by the military authorities on young draftees from all over the country. Out of 300,000 inductees examined in 1944, about 1,000 were trachomatous; whereas in 1966–67, there were fewer than 100 (Fig. 2).

Better use of the funds originally intended for the fight against trachoma has recently been proposed by the Ministry of Health. Following a suggestion of the Supreme Council of Health, to which I belong as an ophthalmologist, certain other eye conditions are also being considered as specially important today. These include strabismus, amblyopia, glaucoma, retinal detachment and heredo-degenerative changes of the retina and optic nerve.

The first task of these new services will be to screen children of school and preschool age for visual defects (e.g. amblyopia and strabismus). The examination will include not only checking of the general ocular state, but also testing of visual acuity (with Albini's E in preschool age, and Landolt's ring for elementary school children). This type of ophthalmological screening has already been accepted in several important centers such as Naples, Caserta, Sassari, Benevento, Salerno and Bari and is now being organized in the remaining trachomatous provinces. These activities are particularly important because medical facilities are generally less developed in the provinces of southern and insular Italy. It is here that the need for a better ophthalmic service is particularly great. Whenever possible (especially in the larger centers), special classes or schools are arranged for the treatment of amblyopia and disorders of ocular motility, as well as for the teaching of partially sighted children. The latter comprise about 1 to 2 ‰ of the children. A bus service helps in transporting pupils living in peripheral areas.

We also expect in the near future to expand the tasks of these ophthalmic units in order to cover the whole field of social ophthalmology and of the prevention of blindness. In northern and central Italy, where anti-trachomatous units are not in operation, services for "social ophthalmology" should be started from the beginning.

# JAPAN

## AKIRA NAKAJIMA

Department of Ophthalmology, School of Medicine, Juntendo University, Bunkyo-ku, Tokyo, Japan

First, I would like to express my sincere gratitude and admiration to the effort of our Israel colleagues and officers of the International Association for Prevention of Blindness, for organizing such a useful and timely seminar. As far as I know, this is the

TABLE 1. *Blinding diseases of the eye*

| Type of disease | Examples |
|---|---|
| Preventable and curable | Infection, trauma, malnutrition |
| Not preventable but curable | Cataract, retinal detachment, glaucoma, uveitis, corneal degeneration |
| Preventable but not curable | Trauma, infection, malnutrition, some congenital anomalies, diabetic retinopathy (?) |
| Not preventable and not curable | Retinal degenerations, high myopia, congenital malformations, optic atrophy |

first major seminar devoted to the prevention of blindness, though there have been sessions on this topic at previous congresses.

*Classification of eye diseases causing blindness.* The prevention of blindness is not quite the same as the prevention of blinding diseases. Even though we do not know how to prevent a disease, the patient can still have his vision restored if the disease can be treated successfully. Senile cataract is the best example of this. The prevention of a disease requires knowledge of the etiology and causal inducing factors; whereas for its treatment, an understanding of the mechanism is very important.

A curable disease may become incurable if it is discovered too late. Knowing these variations, blinding diseases may be classified into four groups (Table 1). This classification is meant to serve mainly as a guide. The diseases in the first three categories are controllable to a certain degree even in our present state of knowledge, but for those in the last category, only rehabilitation is possible. By means of research we can hope to transfer a disease from the last to another category. The prevention of blindness caused by the conditions in the first three categories is not only a problem of science and research, but also of other social and administrative factors.

*Organization.* A famous ancient Chinese philosopher said, "If we get necessary information about the enemy as well as ourselves, we shall never lose the war." The prevention

of blindness is a large project whose purpose is clearly defined. Some suggestions for the organization of this project are shown in Table 2. Among them, I would like to stress the importance of the fifth item, public education. Disease or blindness is above all a problem for the individual. In most cases, a final decision for either treatment or prevention resides with the individual. An enlightened public is therefore essential. Japan has one of the highest rates of compulsory education as well as a highly advanced and widespread mass communications system. October 10 is Eye Hygiene Day, and mass eye examinations as well as campaigns to distribute information are organized for that day.

For those patients who notice changes in sight, early detection of eye disease is relatively easy. However, there are diseases that require mass examination for early detection. Although public awareness and cooperation are important, there are additional factors, such as availability of medical care and ex-

TABLE 2. *Suggestions for organization*

A center or organizer or both to carry out the project
A proper flow of necessary information
Planning, organization and evaluation of projects
Coordination of prevention and treatment
Public education (school, mass media, Eye Hygiene Day, etc.)
Education of necessary manpower
Facilities (efficiency, expense)
Research activities (both prevention and treatment-oriented)

pense. Setting up of a medical service easily accessible to the people is therefore very important.

Over 90% of the population in Japan is covered by medical insurance. We have one ophthalmologist per 22,000 population, and no optometrist system. However, a certified orthoptist system has recently been started. Okinawa, which will soon be returned to us, is made up of some 60 islands. Income per capita in Okinawa is less than half of that in Japan, and there is practically no medical insurance. The number of ophthalmologists per person is only one-seventh that in Japan. And yet, the blindness rate is nearly the same as in Japan. There are many factors responsible for this; and I hope this does not suggest that ophthalmologists in Japan are lazier than those in Okinawa! It may in fact indicate that there may be an optimal threshold for the number of ophthalmologists per person. If that number is very small, even a slight improvement in eye care, if properly organized, will have a significant impact on the prevention of blindness. But if the number of ophthalmologists per person approaches a maximum threshold level, much greater effort is needed to achieve a further reduction in the rate of blindness.

*Information.* There are several sources of information on the prevalence of eye diseases in the population on the one hand, and of information on ophthalmic services on the other. Nearly all Japanese are examined at birth by gynecologists or midwives, at three years of age by pediatricians, and at six or more years of age nearly every year until they retire from work. These mass examinations are useful in the early detection of eye diseases. In addition, a Government survey of 1% of the population is done every five years in order to obtain basic figures for the planning of welfare aid for handicapped people. At present, however, the survey is not geared to pick up problems related to the prevention of blindness.

*Congenital rubella.* After the rubella epidemic of 1965, a survey on congenital rubella was carried out in the main island of Okinawa and in Mayako and Yaeyama which have about the same population. It was found that the incidence of congenital rubella in Yaeyama was about half that in Miyako, in spite of the fact that the rubella epidemics were of equal intensity on both islands. Although this difference may be only chance variation, the staff that took part in the survey discovered that in Yaeyama a gynecologist who knew the work of Sir Norman Gregg warned the inhabitants about the danger of congenital rubella as soon as there were signs of a rubella epidemic. He performed induced abortion at request in suspected cases. This preventive measure was not taken in Miyako. This is a good example of how knowledge about the congenital rubella syndrome, early detection of rubella epidemics, warning the public about the danger and the existence of laws allowing artificial abortion can reduce the incidence of the congenital rubella syndrome.

*Purulent ulcer.* Another survey was carried out on the incidence of purulent corneal ulcer. It was concluded that immediate and proper first aid after injury to the cornea, public knowledge about the possible danger of even minor corneal injury, especially in relation to chronic dacryocystitis or conjunctivitis, are all important for the prevention of this condition.

# KENYA

## G. G. BISLEY

Department of Ophthalmology, Kenyatta National Hospital, Nairobi, Kenya

All developing countries need external help in terms of skilled manpower, materials and especially finance. However, much of this aid is not used in the best possible way, or may even be misused or indeed lost, because of failure to plan the organization to bring it to maximum effect. Assistance may falter for a variety of reasons: 1) Lack of knowledge on the part of the donor country about the local situation and the best ways of providing the necessary help. 2) Lack of adequate liaison between the donor and the recipient countries. Initial consultation between the donor organization and the government of the recipient country must, of course, be carried out. But difficulties of communication, and perhaps a failure to grasp the true issues involved can give rise to delays, misunderstandings and frustrations. 3) There may be unexpressed emotional feelings on the part of the recipient country as to the true motivation of the donor country. The donor's motives may be of the highest, and the aims and objectives impeccable, but to the developing countries, independence is a very precious thing, and who can blame them if they ask the question—"is this project entirely an altruistic one, or are there any hidden motives?" In other words, is this aid entirely "without strings," or does it contain an element of neo-colonialism? I feel sure that this emotional content may impede some of the most excellent of development schemes.

How can we best resolve these problems?

How can we make the wheels of aid go round? The answer, I am sure, lies in the creation of two bodies: 1) A strong national nongovernmental organization to promote the prevention and treatment of blindness which is properly and legally constituted, and in which there is adequate representation of both government and nongovernment membership. If this organization has good leadership and fosters good public relations, it will rapidly gain the respect and confidence of the government, and the latter will turn to it increasingly for advice and help in its development projects. 2) In all areas of blindness prevention there must be close cooperation between this local organization and the government, such as a Prevention of Blindness Committee. In this way plans would be coordinated and the best possible use would be made of available resources.

How does this work out in practice? In Kenya, we have aid in our Kenya Ophthalmic Programme from Great Britain, the USA and, more recently, from the Netherlands, and we hope in the very near future from Canada as well. All this aid is channeled through our local Kenya Society for the Blind, and because of this we have been able to establish a coordinated program of development in full accord with the Government of Kenya, and in line with the call of our most respected President Mzee Jomo Kenyatta of "Harambee"—or "pulling together" for the benefit of the people.

# NETHERLANDS

JOHANNA SCHAPPERT-KIMIJSER

Netherlands General Association for Prevention of Blindness, The Hague, Netherlands

Holland is the only country in Europe which has a national society for the prevention of blindness. This organization was founded about 35 years ago. In developed countries many external causes of blindness have nearly disappeared during the last decades, and been replaced in importance by other causes. Therefore, a new survey on the causes of severe visual impairment was undertaken between 1954 and 1958. "The causes of Blindness in the Netherlands" was published in 1959 and reports on 4,382 cases. One of the consequences of this survey was the establishment of the following committees:

*Committee for Partially Sighted and Blind Children.* This group includes ophthalmologists from all institutions for partially sighted and blind children. The causes of severe visual impairment in about 1,400 children were analyzed. The children could be divided into three groups: a) mentally normal and blind; b) mentally normal and partially sighted; and c) visually and mentally handicapped children. Differences have already been found in the causes of blindness and in the percent distribution in the three groups. In the future special attention will be given to the etiology of these eye conditions.

The European Committee on Causes of Blindness and Partial Sightedness was established three years ago by the International Association for Prevention of Blindness. It can, in a sense, be considered as an extension of the Dutch society.

*Committee for Retinoblastoma.* This group is engaged on two problems. First, it classifies all patients suffering from this disease, either in the past or currently, and keeps in contact with patients and members of their families threatened with the disease. Secondly, research is being conducted with the aim of distinguishing the hereditary form of the disease from the spontaneous form.

*Committee for Glaucoma.* Two investigations have been carried out to date by this group: a) Frequency distribution of intraocular pressure in the Netherlands; and b) a five-year follow-up of subjects with intraocular pressures of 22 to 30 mm Hg but not showing anomalies of the optic nerve or the visual field. The follow-up will be continued for a second period of five years.

*Committee for Genetics.* In close cooperation with the eye departments in the Netherlands, investigations of several hereditary eye diseases causing blindness were undertaken, and the results published.

Since tapetoretinal degeneration is still the principal cause of blindness in both children and adults in the Netherlands, special attention was paid to this disease. Hereditary diseases related to other parts of the eye, e.g., the optic nerve, choroid, lens and uvea were also investigated.

Three new committees have recently been added to the original ones. They are:

Committee for the Prevalence of Blindness and Partial Sightedness in Persons Aged 65 Years and Older. A preliminary conclusion is that about 11,000 of the 1.3 million inhabitants aged 65 years and over (about 0.85%) have severe visual handicaps. Committee for Prevention of Amblyopia and Committee for Prevention of Severe Eye Lesions Caused by Traffic Accidents.

In addition to this the Netherlands General

Association for Prevention of Blindness occupies itself with social activities, such as the issuing of warnings against the possible consequences of fireworks and of dangerous toys for children.

Finally the close cooperation between our society and the organizations working for the blind must be emphasized. The Netherlands General Association is the link between the medical and the blind communities. For about 20 years the secretary of our association has also been a member of the board of the Netherlands Society for the Blind. Every two years a new edition of the bulletin "Addresses and Suggestions for the Benefit of the Partially Sighted and the Blind" is published by our association. One of the great advantages of this close cooperation is that the ophthalmologists become better informed of the needs of the visually handicapped, and more aware of the extension of their task in this direction.

# SOUTH AFRICA

MAURICE H. LUNTZ

Department of Ophthalmology, University of Witwatersrand, Johannesburg, South Africa

Hospitals in Africa must serve unusually wide sections of the population and must be multipurpose, serving their own community in addition to taking preventive medical services to the rural population. This paper describes the organization of such a hospital, the St. John Eye Hospital in Johannesburg. One of its important functions is to collect accurate information of disease patterns in the African population. In the past, inaccurate statistics have often distorted our concepts of disease, especially in the South African Negro. Thus we have wrongly accepted that some diseases, for example angle closure glaucoma, are rare in Negroes; and others, such as open angle glaucoma, are more prevalent. The use of better research methods is exposing and correcting these misconceptions.

The hospital is integrated with other organizations involved in the prevention of blindness. In South Africa these are highly developed, and activities are undertaken by central, provincial and local governments as well as by voluntary organizations, in particular the South African National Council for the Blind. The latter has made a major contribution to the detection, treatment and prevention of blindness from trachoma. The statistical information collected in their records is a valuable indication of the prevalence of eye disease in rural areas.

The St. John Eye Hospital is a 100-bed teaching hospital within the complex of teaching hospitals attached to the University of Witwatersrand, Johannesburg, and has been organized to play a major role in the prevention of blindness in the Negro community of the Transvaal Province. It is situated at Baragwanath, adjacent to a predominantly Negro city, Soweto, with a population of 750,000, on the outskirts of Johannesburg.

*Medical services to rural areas.* Extension of the hospital services to the rural community is achieved by integrating the hospital staff with the mobile unit service organized by the South African National Council for the Blind and its Bureau for the Prevention of Blindness. The National Council mobile unit has an operating theater capable of major surgery and carries with it all the necessary equipment for a general outpatient service. Field workers, including trained ophthalmic nurses and social workers, are sent ahead by the Bureau to the area selected for a tour by the mobile unit. Whenever possible a site near a mission hospital is selected so that the hospital's operating theater and facilities for postoperative care can be used. The field workers set up the operating theater and an outpatient clinic, advertise the arrival of the unit and the offer of an ocular health service. This is done through close liaison with the local authority and by means of the regional radio station, which has proved a very effective medium. By the time the ophthalmologist arrives, all is ready. Any complex surgical procedures are referred to the central teaching hospital. The nurses assist the doctor with minor surgery and special tests, e.g., visual field examination, and remain behind after the doctor has left so as to provide postoperative care. These tours are undertaken throughout the year in different areas, in this way covering virtually the entire Transvaal Province, and a considerable portion of the other three provinces. Eleven tours were undertaken in 1970. An average tour, in which 2,360 patients are seen and 108 operations performed, costs $3,150. This cost is met by the South African National Council

for the Blind, under a subsidy from the Central Government.

*Services to neighboring countries, e.g., Swaziland.* We believe that the facilities of the teaching hospital should be extended to surrounding countries if requested. An ophthalmic service is provided to the Swaziland Government once a month. There are well equipped hospitals in each of the larger centers in Swaziland; and an ophthalmologist is flown to Swaziland together with a team of other specialists and gives a clinical service using a Government hospital as his base.

The Royal Commonwealth Society for the Blind also provides a medical service to the Swazi people through its mobile unit, and during 1970 treated 33,213 patients.

However, invaluable as these services are to the Swaziland Government, the ideal way of preventing and treating blindness in this and other countries with predominantly rural populations would be to train doctors, nurses and auxiliary personnel to take over the eye care of their own countrymen. Subject to the approval of the Swaziland Government, we will therefore provide a teaching service to the general practitioners in the country from 1972. The problem of training selected Swazi doctors as specialist ophthalmologists at the St. John Eye Hospital is being actively investigated at the present time.

# A CONTRIBUTION TO THE TEACHING OF OPHTHALMOLOGISTS FROM A DEVELOPING COUNTRY

I. C. MICHAELSON

Department of Ophthalmology, Hadassah University Hospital, Jerusalem, Israel

Certain problems are involved in the specialist training of doctors from developing countries, some of which are general and some largely confined to ophthalmology. The trainee specialist has in many instances already been an expatriate of his country for about six years and an extension of this period of time by another few years may have undesirable psychological and social consequences and may often lead to yet a further extension of the period of his stay abroad. Moreover, each trainee, after the first few months of training and during the next few years, could contribute progressively and quite considerably to the ophthalmic services in his home country, which often needs such help more than does his host country. Such problems are general to all cases of prolonged residence abroad for purposes of specialization.

The problems peculiar to ophthalmology include the fact that there is often no tradition of popular ophthalmic services in the trainee's country, while traditional methods of an unsatisfactory nature are sometimes widespread. Moreover, there may be no senior ophthalmologist to turn to for guidance, the fledgling ophthalmologist being the first of his kind and the responsible founder of a new tradition. Ophthalmology is dependent on equipment and on its maintenance perhaps more than any other clinical specialty.

Every ophthalmologist in a developed country knows well the importance of these circumstances, which are of course aggravated in most developing countries by the shortage of electricians and mechanics and small repair factories. I once asked my colleagues who had served in developing countries what proportion of inefficiency could be attributable to a shortage or to the breakdown of equipment. The answers varied from 10 to 50%.

I am therefore of the opinion that the training of ophthalmologists for developing countries is an especially delicate and responsible matter. For the reasons stated I believe that the trainee ophthalmologist should spend as little time abroad as possible, and that the instructor should preferably come to the developing country to teach and train.

The method used by the Department of Ophthalmology of the Hadassah University Hospital, Jerusalem has already been referred to by Prof. François. The trainee in ophthalmology serves his first two years in Jerusalem, where he is introduced to the basic aspects and practice of ophthalmology. During this time he attends 240 hr of lectures and 800 hr of seminar training. The following two years of training are spent in his own country, where he studies under the Jerusalem ophthalmologists who have set up a central department and clinics. The training now continues in the trainee's own country, with his own people as his patients and with the available standard of equipment. In due time he will formulate his demands for the acquisition of equipment of a higher standard. There will be more surgery to perform, and he will begin to operate under guidance earlier and advance more gradually. Not having been away for very long from his country, he will be more involved in and sensitive to its social problems than a colleague who has been absent longer.

Finally, a more junior trainee may come from Jerusalem for a one-year period to help the head of the department in the receiving country. The latter is thereafter launched alone on his tasks until another candidate from his country is found to participate in the training program.

There are other advantages to our program. The Jerusalem-based period of the training is facilitated by the fact that the teachers have practically all visited his home country, so that they are familiar with the circumstances of ophthalmic practice there and can accordingly better direct his training. In addition, this help can be continued by correspondence after the trainee returns home.

# CONTACT LENS PRACTICE

G. PETER HALBERG* and ABRAHAM SCHLOSSMAN

International Contact Lens Council of Ophthalmology, New York, N.Y., USA

Contact lenses are worn daily by millions of patients and their use is increasing. The fitting of contact lenses to the human cornea is a medical task with all the attendant risks and responsibilities. The medical aspects of contact lens fitting have been emphasized by the introduction of new types of contact lenses, and also by the various therapeutic applications of hard and soft contact lenses in certain pathologic conditions of the anterior segment of the eye.

Although discomfort is natural during the initial phase of contact lens fitting, persisting discomfort or pain is always a sign that something is wrong and grave danger exists if the patient perseveres. Severe, sometimes permanent, corneal damage may ensue. The pathology induced by ill-fitting contact lenses is often characterized by chronic epithelial or stromal edema or both, and staining with fluorescein of the defective epithelium including the 3 and 9 o'clock staining syndrome. The traumatized cornea may become the portal of entry for bacterial, viral or fungal infections. It is obvious that many of the factors which have to be dealt with before, during and after fitting of contact lenses are strictly in the medical ophthalmologic area.

Fortunately, more and more ophthalmologists accomplish the entire fitting procedure in their own offices, thus avoiding a dangerous gap in supervision of technical help. This trend has been accelerated by the fact that many large ophthalmic centers and teaching hospitals have made contact lens management an integral part of their teaching schedules, so that graduates from these residency programs have adequate knowledge of this important discipline of ophthalmology.

A distinct improvement in the management of the contact lens problem came about in 1963 with the formation of the Contact Lens Association of Ophthalmologists in New York. Today, this Association has 1,400 members throughout the United States and includes many leading ophthalmologists abroad who fit contact lenses.

Together with its sister organization, the Japan Contact Lens Society under the leadership of Professor Nakajima, the Contact Lens Association of Ophthalmologists enjoyed early support from American and world leadership in ophthalmology. A constructive cooperation exists between the American Academy of Ophthalmology and Otolaryngology and the Contact Lens Association of Ophthalmologists, thanks to the wisdom of leaders like Professor Maumenee, President of the Academy, who takes great personal interest in this problem. The Contact Lens Association of Ophthalmologists has surveyed the training programs in the United States

* Address for reprints: 40 West 77 Street, New York, N.Y., 10024, USA.

and offers regular courses for ophthalmologists and for assistants and technicians working under ophthalmologic supervision.

In 1964, the International Contact Lens Council of Ophthalmology was formed. This Council has Professor François as its Honorary President and is officially sponsored by the International Contact Lens Council of Ophthalmology which serves as liaison between the different national medical contact lens organizations. In the seven years since its inception, many countries of the world have joined the Council, thus greatly speeding the global exchange of information and knowledge among ophthalmologists. This Council has no individual members. Only medical ophthalmologic organizations may belong and are represented by delegates. Different regions of the world are served by Regional Secretaries, who usually represent the specific language areas. Because of its unique status, the International Contact Lens Council is eager to offer advice and guidance to any nation or teaching center in the world desirous of aid in setting up or improving contact lens programs.

In its short history, the Council has been instrumental in organizing the International Contact Lens Symposia which were associated scientific events of the XXth International Congress in Munich, and the XXIst International Congress in Mexico City. The Organizing Committee of the XXIInd International Congress of Ophthalmology has already invited our Council to plan the International Contact Lens Symposium to be associated with the International Congress which will meet in Paris in 1974. The Contact Lens Symposium will take place in Lyon with the cooperation of Professor Bonamour, and under the honorary Presidency of Professor François.

In 1970, the International Council of Ophthalmology and the International Federation of Ophthalmologic Societies, under the leadership of Professor François, took a firm position on the problem of contact lens fitting: "The indication, the prescription, the clinical and optical adaptation, and the control of contact lenses must remain medical acts, of which only the ophthalmologist has to assume the responsibility. Nonmedical technicians, even those specialized in optics, may only participate in the optical adaptation as medical assistants in the doctor's office. These assistants have to be submitted to all the restrictions fixed by the regulations concerning medical auxiliaries." This decision does not mean that most technicians who have been active for many years should be forbidden to function within the field, but only that they should be brought under medical supervision.

# TRAINING AND FUNCTIONS OF OPHTHALMIC ASSISTANTS

## INDIA

G. VENKATASWAMY

Madurai Medical College, Madurai, S. India

*Optometrists.* Schools for optometrists in several states in India have been in existence since 1958 and are all attached to ophthalmic institutions where students receive training for two years in refraction, grinding of lenses and fitting of spectacles. At present they are not allowed to practice independently, and work only with ophthalmologists. Unfortunately some of the schools for optometrists have been temporarily closed because of unemployment among the qualified graduates.

The optometrists assist the ophthalmologists in several ways. In the Eye Department of Madurai Medical College, there are 12 optometrists. With some extra training, they can assist in determining tensions, doing tonography and measuring visual fields. Optometrists also work in the Neuroophthalmology Department where they measure visual fields and exophthalmos and assist the neuroophthalmologists in keeping case records. In the hospital and eye camps, they do most of the refractions. Two optometrists have been trained for low vision aid work and in the fitting of contact lenses.

At present there are seven schools for optometry in India. The total yearly admission is 100 students, some of whom receive stipends. For lack of funds, the state medical depart-

ments are not able to employ all the qualified optometrists. However, we hope this will improve in the future. Opportunities for employment with private practicing ophthalmologists are good but this field has not yet been fully exploited.

*Orthoptists.* There are seven schools for orthoptists in India in which the period of training is two years. These schools which are attached to ophthalmic institutions admit 60 candidates every year. The training is good and the graduate students are employed in the orthoptic departments. Nevertheless, many of our qualified orthoptists are unemployed because only a few eye departments in India have orthoptic departments. Many of the ophthalmologists have not had training in orthoptics, and hence it is difficult to open new orthoptic departments. If a short term course (not exceeding three months) could be given to ophthalmologists in all the medical colleges then more orthoptic sections could be opened and the services of the orthoptists could be fully utilized.

*Ophthalmic nursing.* There is no special course in this field, and the nurses are trained in ophthalmic hospitals. It has been proposed that special nine-month training courses be started in ophthalmology. These nurses assist in eye operations, examine the patency of the lacrimal passage, remove foreign bodies, etc. Given additional training the nurses could be used for determining tension, measuring visual fields and also for giving facial and ciliary block for eye surgery. In some states in India there is currently acute unemployment of these nurses. However, it is hoped that in the future, their training can be utilized to the fullest extent for all types of eye relief.

# KENYA

## G. G. BISLEY

Department of Ophthalmology, Kenyatta Hospital, Nairobi, Kenya

There are two primary essentials which must be observed: 1) The selection and assessment of each candidate must be undertaken by the ophthalmologist himself, and must never be delegated to a junior colleague. 2) Unless the ophthalmologist is prepared to devote considerable time to training and subsequent regular supervision, the project will most certainly fail and should not be undertaken.

With regard to selection, all candidates should have completed a full general medical and surgical course at a recognized training center. In Kenya, this would be the Government Medical Training Center. They should have had at least a further year's experience in general clinical work, preferably in a district hospital or health center, proving to be energetic, resourceful and honest, with a real interest in eye work, and able to get on with all types of people.

It is better not to advertise vacancies for eye training, but to select candidates known personally by the ophthalmologist, or recommended by other doctors with sound judgment.

The ophthalmic training course in our country lasts for one year. The trainees are taught as often as possible by the ophthalmologist himself, as apprentices working in the clinic with the ophthalmologist. Formal didactic teaching is useful, but less emphasis is placed on this, 1 hr a week being allocated for such instruction.

During the year's training, each candidate spends short periods in the theater learning the essentials of sterilization, theater technique and care of instruments. During the last six months, the candidates spend two periods of one month each, attached to different mobile units, working with regular teams and learning how to work in the field.

*Functions.* This will depend on the local situation and the specific requirements of the particular scheme for the prevention of blindness. Good medical assistants are very adaptable people and will be able to perform the majority of routine tasks normally performed by a doctor.

However, sustained performance will depend on: a) the ophthalmologist maintaining an active personal interest in each candidate; b) prompt and sympathetic handling of personal problems; c) regular visits during which the ophthalmologist works in the field with the candidate; d) promotion to a somewhat higher salary scale than that of a general medical assistant, and if possible a specialist title such as Medical Assistant (Ophthalmic).

In other words, the ophthalmologist must not only be a good doctor but a good commanding officer!

# AFRICA

I. BEN-SIRA and Y. YASSUR

Department of Ophthalmology, Hadassah University Hospital, Jerusalem, Israel

The physician to population ratio in Africa is approximately 1 in 20,000 except in the Arab countries and South Africa. It has been estimated that in order to bring the average ratio up to 1 in 10,000, 13,000 doctors would have to qualify every year for the next 10 years. However, since the optimal ratio is 1 in 1,000, much is left to be desired. The problem of lack of doctors and other medical staff is, therefore, very serious and it has to be solved efficiently and quite rapidly.

One way of tackling the problem of the gap between needs and available personnel is the creation of a cadre of medical assistants and paramedical personnel. These should form an extension arm of one body or team in which the doctor plays a central role in treatment, supervision and training.

The aim of medical assistants' education is the production of persons with factual information, practical knowledge and technical skill. The curriculum for ophthalmic medical assistants should include preventive medicine, hygiene and nutrition as well as theoretical and practical teaching in the ward and clinic, and basic extraocular surgery.

The scope of work of these ophthalmic medical assistants should encompass several fields:

1) Health education. This is an extremely important aspect of the work. A medical assistant whether visiting a clinic, a school or a village begins his visit with a lecture on the preventive cure of eye diseases. The talk should be based on the following points: a) The causes of eye diseases, e.g., infection, malnutrition, changes in old age; b) the importance of cleanliness; c) the spread of eye diseases; d) how eye diseases can be treated; how trachoma can be cured; how a child with measles who has sore eyes should receive urgent medical attention; how blind people with cataract can see again; how people with entropion should have a simple operation before their eyes are blinded by ingrowing lashes; and when to refer patients to the eye clinic.

2) School visits.

3) Case finding: Old people and young children especially will not voluntarily come to a dispensary for treatment. Therefore, the medical assistant has to seek them out in their villages and to explain to them how they can be helped.

4) Follow-up of cases.

5) Registration of the blind.

6) Treatment at the clinic: This is mainly for external diseases and includes selection of cases to be transferred to the ophthalmic hospital department.

7) Operating on cases (especially trichiasis, injuries and enucleations).

The university should be responsible for the curriculum since it is a question of fitting it into the medical curriculum in an overall plan. The medical assistants must be taught certain skills, and the local doctor must be instructed how to supervise them. This can only be done if the medical schools take the responsibility for this medical assistant training. Those responsible for formulating the curricula in the medical schools must be convinced of the importance of organizational structures in medicine. In this way they could help in achieving the goal of creating efficient ophthalmic medical assistants.

ETHIOPIA

I. FEITELBERG

Eye Clinic, General Sick Fund, Jerusalem, Israel

During my service in Ethiopia as Head of the Communicable Eye Diseases (CED) and Trachoma Control Project my main tasks were: 1) to teach ophthalmology in general and, in particular, to instruct the senior student health officers and nurses of the Public Health College in Gondar in the fight against trachoma; 2) to give refresher courses to the health officers and nurses, who had graduated from the school since 1958, and were already established in health centers throughout the country; 3) to train groups of advanced dressers to recognize trachoma in order to enable them to help health officers examine school children.

The importance of these tasks cannot be overstressed, considering the scarcity of doctors, and especially eye doctors, in this large country with a population of 20 million. In 1964 there were in the whole Empire, except Eritrea, four ophthalmologists, three of them in Addis Ababa, working in hospitals or private practice. Accordingly, my task was to train these health officers to organize and execute eye work on their own. They had to be given authority to work, within the limits of their training, as heads of teams in health centers, schools or in the field. However, they were under the supervision of the center in Addis Ababa and the provincial medical authorities. In contrast, the dressers were auxiliary workers, specially trained to examine eyes for trachoma and to assist the paramedical health officers.

The Gondar Public Health School and Training Center was established in 1954 to train health officers and community nurses. Health officers received a secondary school education plus four years of theoretical and practical training in preventive medicine, basic clinical medicine, health administration, various aspects of community development and methods of education and public information. The community nurses had had 8 to 10 years of secondary schooling plus three years of advanced training including maternity, child health and midwifery, as well as general nursing skills.

In 1962, the training program of the health officers became a degree course leading to the award of a Bachelor in Public Health. The curriculum was increased to five years with greater stress on academic subjects, there being 24 hr per week of theoretical anatomy and pathology compared with 15 hr for the nurses. In addition, small groups of health officers and nurses together received 12 hr of practical training in schools, pediatric clinics and the outpatient department of the Gondar Hospital. Dressers received the same practical training, but only 8 hr of theory per week.

The refresher courses to the personnel of the health centers spread throughout this extensive country had necessarily to be given on the spot. Over a period of three years I visited most of the 52 existing health centers, remaining at each for two to four days. The personnel had already received training in CED and ophthalmology during their school years in Gondar. The course was given to the team as a unit and consisted on the first day of 4 hr of theory, especially CED and the effects of trachoma on the individual, and on the national and economic plan. My theme was always: "Many sick people form a sick nation."

The other half of the day was devoted to random examination of the eyes of all the outpatients who came to the clinic for any reason. It was amazing how many patients were found to be suffering from eyes diseases without having previously been aware of this. First aid and traumatology of the eyes were also discussed.

During the next day and the following, if necessary, schoolchildren were examined. The routine of the examinations, diagnosis and treatment and the writing of correct reports to the center was explained. Each member of the team was taught to correctly overt the upper lid. This scheme worked quite well, and until the end of my service I received reports on about 35,000 children. The dressers were particularly helpful to the health officers in the provincial towns, where the number of schoolchildren reached many thousands.

In conclusion, the concept of preparing health officers is sound and there should be many more schools like the one in Gondar. Most of the health officers can do their work very well especially if the following three conditions are met: 1) There must be constant and rigorous supervision by an ophthalmologist. 2) Health officers must have a sense of responsibility, initiative and a high degree of willingness to do their work properly. 3) There must also be encouragement by the proper authorities for the young health officer who has to go straight from school and face grave responsibilities alone in his new health center often very far from home and friends.

# AUXILIARY OPHTHALMIC TRAINING

## THE JOINT COMMISSION ON ALLIED HEALTH PERSONNEL IN OPHTHALMOLOGY

A. SCHLOSSMAN

Department of Ophthalmology, State University of New York, Downstate Medical Center, Brooklyn, New York, USA

The necessity of providing medical eye care for the 200 million people in the United States who are demanding ever more sophisticated and comprehensive ophthalmologic treatment has long been of concern to the large medical societies and organizations of ophthalmologists in America. Because of the cost and difficulty of training medical specialists in the United States, only about 400 ophthalmologists a year are graduated from residency training programs. The productivity of these ophthalmologists can be augmented by the employment of medical auxiliary personnel, who work under supervision as part of a team.

The Joint Commission on Allied Health Personnel in Ophthalmology (JCAHPO) was created to encourage the establishment of training programs, to develop standards of education, to provide examinations for certification, and to stimulate continuing education of allied personnel in ophthalmology. It is hoped that many of the developing countries which have relatively few ophthalmologists and must depend even more on allied health personnel than we do in the United States will find some application to their own problem in this communication on the Joint Commission.

JCAHPO was organized in 1969 as the joint effort of five associations, each represented by three commissioners, the American Academy of Ophthalmology and Otolaryngology, the American Medical Association, the Association of University Professors in Ophthalmology, the Contact Lens Association of Ophthalmologists, and the Society of Military Ophthalmologists. The personnel trained and certified under the sponsorship of JCAHPO must perform their allied health occupations under the supervision of ophthalmologists. There should be no misconception; these physicians' assistants are not authorized to exercise any independent judgment over whether to treat, refer or dismiss patients. This may contrast with the situation in some developing countries where there are too few ophthalmologists to care for the complete needs of the population, and where allied personnel may take on greater responsibility.

There is an immediate need for an estimated 6,000 allied ophthalmic aides to work in ophthalmologists' offices, hospitals, medical groups and eye research and training centers. With the increased demand of the American public for eye care, this number may even treble in the not too distant future.

For the purposes of training and certification there are three categories: 1) ophthalmic assistant, 2) ophthalmic technician and 3) ophthalmic technologist. Those with sufficient training may take examinations for certification in any of these categories. Ophthalmic assistants may qualify on the basis of written examinations alone. The technicians and technologists must take oral examinations too. The candidate receives a certificate after passing the appropriate test.

JCAHPO has attempted to design and modify its proposals for curricula in such a way as to encourage "career-ladder" training. Thus, upward movement of the trainee is stimulated, because curricula proposed for training at one level will have academic credits which can be applied to an educational program at a higher level. In this way there is incentive for the assistant to become a technician, assuring him of higher salary, and at the same time upgrading the reservoir of trained ophthalmic health personnel in the country.

The ophthalmic assistant category is the lowest rung on the career ladder and has the largest number of certified trainees. The assistant has had at least one year of practical accredited training. The program includes introduction to diseases of the eye, elements of ophthalmic assistance, ocular screening techniques, introduction to optics, knowledge of the responsibilities of the physician and technician in the delivery of eye care and their relationship to the community. Last and perhaps most important is the clinical experience of the candidate.

The ophthalmic technician has at least two years of classroom and apprentice training. He has more advanced education in such areas as ocular anatomy, physiology, pharmacology and embryology. Physiologic and geometric optics are studied in some detail and the candidate is given some knowledge of motor and sensory anomalies of the visual

system and is taught simple laboratory tests in microbiology. Tonometry and tonography are important in the curriculum.

The ophthalmic technologist should have four years of approved formal training and experience in an accredited eye training center leading to a baccalaureate degree. Up to the present time the Joint Commission has not certified any individual in this group. However, there are many technicians in ophthalmology who work in areas of electrophysiology, ocular photography, biochemistry and physics who will eventually be certified.

Each training center is inspected periodically to ensure the maintenance of minimum standards. A basic factor in determining the need for repeated visits is the performance of the applicants in the examinations. At present about 10 centers are training candidates for certification. In addition, the American Association of Ophthalmology has a home study course which has proven valuable and effective.

During the past year the American Orthoptic Council, which serves a function similar to that of the Joint Commission in standardizing training and holding examinations for certification of orthoptic technicians, has formed a liaison with the Joint Commission. It is debatable whether it is not better to train a technician to perform all necessary tasks as part of the ophthalmologic team than to train an expert in orthoptics alone; and the same may be true, to an even greater extent, of contact lens assistants. It is my opinion that medical auxiliary personnel should be trained in all aspects of ophthalmic procedures in which they can be of help to the ophthalmologist.

The program of JCAHPO is designed for developed rather than for developing countries. However, it is hoped that some of our experiences can be adapted to developing countries.

# AUXILIARY OPHTHALMIC TRAINING IN CANADA

H. A. STEIN and B. SLATT

University of Toronto, Medical School, Toronto Canada

*Functions of the ophthalmic assistant.* These include: 1) preschool and school screening programs in which the ophthalmic assistant is more likely to be successful with the visual acuity tests than the school nurse because of his greater experience; 2) glaucoma detection tests, particularly in surveys during which the ophthalmic assistant can do tonometry and measure visual fields; 3) mass screening of ophthalmic conditions in which a group of ophthalmic assistants may be helpful—each carrying out a step in a series of investigations which are later to be assessed by the ophthalmologist; 4) work in the ophthalmologist's office in which his duties include surgical assistance, visual fields, low-vision examinations, tonometry, tonography, photography, etc.

*Training of the ophthalmic assistant.* This should include specially conducted intensive whole day courses lasting several weeks, evening classes in the larger centers spread over two years and finally preceptorships in hospital clinics.

Our experience in training ophthalmic assistants may be of help to others. We began the training program with correspondence courses. This failed, however, because of the lack of opportunities for practice. Then we began a six-week summer course. In addition to doctors we had to employ non-medical personnel as teachers. Finally, we have opened a two-year night course in town in which most of the teachers are other ophthalmic assistants.

# TRANING OF ORTHOPTISTS IN ISRAEL

I. NAWRATZKI

Department of Ophthalmology, Hadassah University Hospital, Jerusalem, Israel

The importance of the orthoptist's contribution to progress in the treatment of strabismus and amblyopia is generally recognized. Most ophthalmologists simply do not have the time for the routine work required in this field. Apart from this, an orthoptist is specially trained to examine children and to measure their visual acuity, both of which are very time-consuming tasks. They also play an important role in the various screening programs involving preschool and school children.

Orthoptists are usually trained in perimetry, tonometry and tonography, so that in smaller departments they can participate in the work of glaucoma clinics.

In countries like the United States, England and France, schools of orthoptics with a full curriculum lasting two or three years have long been established. Moreover, most ophthalmological centers have an orthoptics department. In contrast, work in strabismus is considerably handicapped in small or developing countries owing to the scarcity of trained personnel. Such countries rely mainly on help from outside, either by inviting an orthoptist from abroad or by sending students to foreign countries. However, this is not always possible because of language difficulties and financial problems.

In Israel there was, until several years ago, a severe shortage of orthoptists; but in 1966 a two-year training program for orthoptists was introduced in the existing orthoptic department at the Hadassah University Hospital.

The present training program consists of one year of theoretical study in the Orthoptics Department of Hadassah Hospital and a second year of practical training. Two hundred and fifty lectures are given by various members of the staff on basic ophthalmology, orthoptics, optics, eye pathology and symptomatology and neurology. In addition, there are daily sessions in practical orthoptics.

Second-year students either continue to work at Hadassah or are referred to former graduates of the course now working in orthoptics departments of other hospitals. They work with patients in the department. In addition, the students are introduced to the problems of amblyopia. For this purpose they regularly attend mother-and-child clinics. In the past, three pupils were accepted each year, but this has proved to be too small a class. We now plan to accept six students every two years.

Three rooms of 50 square meters are required for a course with three students. This is the size of an average orthoptics department. In addition a lecture room is necessary.

For teaching and to cope with routine work, two full-time orthoptists are necessary in our clinic, but one full-time and one half-time orthoptist may suffice for a smaller teaching department.

# EDUCATION FOR OPHTHALMIC NURSING IN DEVELOPING COUNTRIES

JUDITH STEINER-FREUD

Henrietta Szold–Hadassah School of Nursing, Hadassah University Hospital, Jerusalem, Israel

A survey of health problems in developing countries reveals a high prevalence of eye diseases and health problems associated with the eye. Here in Israel, we find proof of this in the fact that the first nurses to come from abroad for training were ophthalmic nurses. It seems important, therefore, to stress the preparation of nursing personnel in ophthalmology and, in particular, in preventive work through public health activities.

While many countries are developing a corps of paramedical personnel and auxiliaries other than nurses to work in ophthalmology, we believe that highly specialized nurses with a basic broad general training are needed. Comprehensive care is needed in this field, and today's nurse must have a sound background in many branches of the behavioral and medical sciences, in addition to nursing skills and knowledge. In addition to carrying out orders for the patient, such a nurse also does professional work in her own right, including health education and rehabilitation as well as physical care and some of

# THE NATIONAL EYE INSTITUTE

## AN INTERNATIONAL RESEARCH RESOURCE

CARL KUPFER

Na ional Eye Institute, National Institutes of Health, Bethesda, Maryland, USA

Diseases of the eye and visual system know no geographical boundaries and research progress in one country ultimately confers universal benefits. Therefore, it is appropriate that the research programs of the National Eye Institute be discussed at an international Seminar such as this.

The National Eye Institute is part of the National Institutes of Health, itself the major resource for the support of biomedical research in the United States.

### HEW-NIH ORGANIZATION

The basic organization of the U.S. Department of Health, Education and Welfare may be described as follows: The Secretary of the Department, Elliot L. Richardson, is one of 12 secretaries or department heads who comprise the President's cabinet. Under him are a number of Assistant Secretaries including the Assistant Secretary for Health and Scientific Affairs, Dr. Merlin K. Duval. Under Dr. Duval's supervision come the Public Health Service, which consists of the Food and Drug Administration, the Environmental Health Service, the Health Services and Mental Health Administration and the National Institutes of Health.

The National Institutes of Health today consist of a Bureau of Health Manpower Education which supports undergraduate medical, nursing, dental and allied health education, and the National Library of Medicine, in addition to traditional research Institutes and Divisions. The oldest and probably best known of the latter is the National Cancer Institute. There are ten research institutes. Each is concerned with a particular disease or group of diseases, such as heart disease, arthritis and allergy.

### MISSION OF NIH

The mission of NIH is to advance health and well-being through support of research on the diseases of man, of education of manpower for research and service, of institutions engaged in medical research and education and of biomedical communications.

The National Institutes of Health have their headquarters on a 300-acre campus located in Bethesda, Maryland in suburban Washington, D.C. Over 11,000 people work in the laboratories, clinics, offices, and service areas of nearly fifty buildings on the NIH grounds. The National Eye Institute conducts its laboratory and clinical studies in a large red-brick Clinical Center. New laboratory space for the Institute is now under construction.

The support of vision research by the National Eye Institute transcends national boundaries in seeking those investigators who can potentially contribute to the prevention, diagnosis and treatment of eye diseases and disorders of the visual system.

The establishment in 1968 of the National Eye Institute as the newest part of the National Institutes of Health represented an unprecedented acknowledgement of the importance of the support of vision research to public health in the United States. In the hearings before the U.S. Congress to create the Institute, testimony was presented which clearly indicated the significance of blindness and visual disability as a major public health problem. These discussions convinced the legislature of the need for an independent organization to be created within the National Institutes of Health, which would mount a national vision research program.

Inherent in the creation of the Institute was also the recognition that additional basic knowledge of vision and visual disorders would have to be gained before major advances could be made in the prevention of many of the leading visual disorders. There was need for improved methods of early diagnosis and the development of preventive measures even for many of those conditions which the ophthalmologist could adequately treat.

## MISSION OF NEI

The general mission of the National Eye Institute is to conduct, foster and support research and research training related to disorders of the visual system in order to increase the knowledge available to prevent, diagnose and treat these diseases, and to foster research on rehabilitation of the blind and partially seeing.

The specific objectives of the Institute are to
- improve prevention, diagnosis, and treatment of visual disorders;
- understand the functioning of the visual system;

- foster research on the rehabilitation of the visually handicapped;
- apply research knowledge to clinical practice.

It is necessary to emphasize that the National Eye Institute's sole concern is with the conduct and support of vision research and research training. It provides no medical services to the public at large, nor does it support the provision of services for the rehabilitation of the visually handicapped. It is not involved in the payment of welfare assistance to the needy blind. These are functions of other organizations.

## NEI ORGANIZATION

The administration of the National Eye Institute is embodied in the Office of the Director, which is concerned with general administration of the Institute and in the planning of research programs and provisions for public information. An Office of Biometry and Epidemiology has also been established. The remainder of the Institute is divided between extramural and intramural programs. Extramural programs include research support for individuals at universities, medical schools and hospitals. Intramural programs include work at the research laboratories in Bethesda where NIH is located. An Associate Director for Extramural Research has the responsibility for all research programs wherever they may be. At present, 10 Eye Institute research grants are active outside the United States.

Apart from its support of research in universities, medical schools and hospitals, which accounts for the largest share of our budget, the Institute is developing a national resource at Bethesda for the conduct of vision research. At present there are 38 research and ancillary staff working in laboratories in Bethesda, with nine ophthalmologists conducting research in the Clinical Branch. Within the Clinical Branch are 26 hospital beds, outpatient facilities and research laboratories for the study of patients having certain eye diseases. These patients are referred from the United States or from abroad by ophthalmologists. In general, such patients represent diagnostic problems or have failed to respond to conventional treatment of their eye disease. The clinical research studies are intended to develop better diagnostic techniques and methods of treatment.

Clinical studies take place within the Clinical Center, a 14-story, 516-bed research hospital designed to bring scientists working in 1,100 laboratories into close proximity with clinicians caring for patients, so that laboratory investigators and research physicians may collaborate on problems of mutual concern.

Concerning the referral of patients to the Clinical Center, the expense of transportation is the only charge to the patient. Otherwise, there is no cost whatsoever to the patient for hospital care or room and board while at the Clinical Center. A publication listing the current clinical studies of all the Institutes is published twice a year and can be mailed free of charge to physicians on request.

At the present time the NEI is accepting three groups of patients:

1) Patients with glaucoma who are resistant to medical therapy or in whom the diagnosis is in doubt.

2) Patients with retinal degenerations and dystrophies in whom additional diagnostic studies such as Ganzfeld electroretinography and retinal function testing are indicated.

3) Patients with inflammatory disease, with particular emphasis on Behçet's syndrome and sympathetic ophthalmia.

A major contribution of the clinical program over the past five years has been the introduction of the use of immunosuppressive and antimetabolite drugs in the treatment of uveitis. During the next year, the clinical research program will be expanded to include corneal diseases and the diagnosis of intraocular tumors using a radioactive chloroquine analog.

## VISION RESEARCH

The other major component of our intramural program is the Laboratory of Vision Research. Here laboratory studies are conducted which include the biochemistry of rhodopsin, embryology of the lens and cornea, physiology of color vision, the coding of visual information from the eye to the brain, as well as the pharmacology of aqueous humor dynamics.

The Office of Biometry and Epidemiology is interested primarily in reviewing, coordinating, and conducting statistical and epidemiological studies of human populations. Comparing sick persons with healthy controls, studying disease variability in twins and observing treated and untreated cases for disease progression are among studies of this type conducted at the Institute. Mr. Harold A. Kahn, Chief of the Office of Biometry and Epidemiology, is present at this meeting and would welcome discussions concerning research opportunities in other countries, such as might result from particularly high or low incidence or prevalence of certain eye diseases within specified population groups.

Scientists from abroad may participate in our intramural research activities as either guest workers or participants in the visiting program.

## GUEST WORKERS AND VISITORS

A Guest Worker is not an employee of NIH but is sponsored by another organization, and has requested and been granted permission to carry on a specific research project of his own, or to participate in a program already established at NIH. Guest workers are employed for at least one year and are provided with laboratory space, equipment and materials. However, salaries are paid by another source, either an institution or foundation in the United States or a similar body in the scientist's home country.

The fundamental purpose of the Visiting Program of NIH is to broaden the utility of the physical facilities and intellectual environment of NIH as an international resource. Each NIH Institute takes the initiative in inviting scientists to visit Bethesda. These scientists may be young men and women who come as Visiting Fellows to receive further advanced training in research. This is essentially a training appointment and one to three years of appropriate postdoctoral education is a prerequisite for appointment.

In addition, scientists may come as Visiting Associates or Visiting Scientists to conduct research on their own and take part in the research program of NIH. Visiting Associates must have more than three years' postgraduate experience. Visiting Scientists must have more than six years' postgraduate experience as a prerequisite for the appointment.

During 1970 there were 53 Guest Workers at NIH from 20 countries. There were 178 scientists in the Visiting Program, representing 31 nations.

The most frequently used mechanisms for international research support are grants and contracts. Since not all may be familiar with these terms as used by NIH, these are briefly discussed.

Research grants account for the largest share of the total NIH budget devoted to research support. In applying for grants, scientists design their own research proposals and submit them to NIH for review and approval. Review is done first by a study section, on the basis of scientific merit. Study section members are experts in various aspects of the biomedical sciences.

Most of the research supported by the National Eye Institute is reviewed by a panel of experts in vision research. This panel or study section is usually chaired by an ophthal-

mologist. Chairmen have included Drs. Irving H. Leopold, Mansour F. Armaly, Edward W. Norton, and most recently Arthur J. Jampolsky. Study section review is based primarily on the scientific merit of the proposal, keeping in mind the relative importance of the problem to be studied.

The second major review is done by the National Advisory Eye Council. Again, these are experts in the visual sciences, practitioners and also representatives of the public.

The Advisory Council relies in great part upon the judgment of the study section, but its primary concern is that the research proposal fit the policies and objectives of the Institute.

## INTERNATIONAL
### RESEARCH GRANTS AND CONTRACTS

Research grants awarded to applicants outside the United States must meet five criteria in addition to meeting the general requirements for domestic projects: 1) the results must be likely to make a significant contribution to the health sciences in both the United States and the country of the applicant; 2) the proposal should be outstanding or original in concept; 3) the research must be carried out outside the United States because of unusual personnel or material resources available; 4) the proposal must constitute a timely research opportunity which would be lost if not supported at this time; and 5) research of the specific nature proposed should not be underway in the United States.

A second method of support at NIH is the contract, sometimes referred to as collaborative research. At the National Eye Institute we are only just beginning to use this mechanism, which is viewed as an extension of our own direct research operations. Contracts, unlike grants, are used to attain a specified objective or to reach a stated goal. The research is useful primarily in those areas where laboratory knowledge is available, and where all indications are that real and significant progress will be made through the targeted application of laboratory results to a clinical problem.

The same criteria that apply to international research grants also apply to the awarding of contracts.

Another means of international support is through the Special Foreign Currency Program authorized under the Agricultural Trade Development and Assistance Act of 1954, designated as Public Law 480. This Act authorizes the use of U.S.-owned foreign currencies derived from the sale of surplus agricultural commodities to foreign markets. P.L.-480 funds can support a variety of scientific activities outside the United States which are of common interest to NIH and to the host country, its institutions and investigators.

Through utilization of these various programs, it should be possible to extend the opportunities available through the National Eye Institute across international boundaries.

It would be appropriate to contact the present author concerning the Guest Workers and Visiting Program. For the grants and contracts, either Dr. Brooks or Dr. Schwartz should be contacted. For projects in biometry and epidemiology, Mr. Kahn would be the appropriate source of information.

In conclusion, these mechanisms available from the National Eye Institute should certainly be considered. They offer a virtually untapped source for the support of outstanding research projects outside the United States, and have potential for greatly strengthening international cooperation and endeavor in vision research.

# PLANNING A FILM LIBRARY FOR INFORMATION ON THE PREVENTION OF BLINDNESS

A. B. RIZZUTI

Corneal Service, New York Medical College, New York, New York, USA

An important element in the cause of blindness is the ignorance of the public, especially in developing countries, but to a certain extent too in developed countries. One of the most effective means of overcoming this is the distribution of films supplying information on common ocular conditions leading to blindness. The subjects which are most suitable for this method of exposition are keratomalacia, onchocerciasis, amblyopia, glaucoma and cataract.

A limited number of films on these subjects is available from the Society for Prevention of Blindness, New York, The Eye Bank Association of America (Manhattan Eye and Ear Hospital, New York) and the International Film Library, New York. There is no doubt that one of the activities potentially most useful for a group engaged in the prevention of blindness is to increase the number of available films and to broaden the aspects of the prevention of blindness with which they deal.

The anticipated audiences would be both students and the general public. For the latter, the degree of sophistication would depend on whether the films are destined for developed or developing countries. If we succeed in completing a wide series of films, their availability, together with a fairly detailed synopsis of contents, should be made known to all concerned, particularly to all national societies for the prevention of blindness.

# DISCUSSION

Dr. Y. Stohlman (*Israel*): I object to the omission of optometrists from the framework of para-ophthalmic training. In the U.S., optometrists go through a six-year curriculum and represent a large body of adequately trained nonmedical eye practitioners. It is not necessary for the ophthalmologists to train the optometrists as ophthalmic assistants since they have already received training of their own and are licensed by the state in which they work.

Dr. I. C. Michaelson (*Israel*): I wish to define the functions of the ophthalmic auxiliary as being a person who helps the eye doctor and consults him on every case, as opposed to the para-ophthalmologist in the developing countries who does not need the ophthalmologist's constant supervision and proximity. The discussion should be limited to the subject of training of para-ophthalmologists in developing countries.

Dr. H. Wyatt (*Canada*): I have worked among the Canadian Indians in Alberta and in the Northwest Territories. The Canadian government requires some system of evaluation of the trainees after the training program. How can the usefulness of the paramedical worker best be assessed?

Dr. A. Schlossman (*USA*): In the U.S., assessment is by a written examination at the lower level and by a written and oral examination at the higher level. Prof. Peter Evans of Georgetown University, Washington, D.C. is in charge of these examinations.

Dr. Wyatt: It is necessary to know the effect of using paramedical personnel in existing care programs.

Dr. B. Slatt (*Canada*): Ophthalmic assistants can improve the efficiency of ophthalmologists by a factor of 10 since they can screen all patients, treat the simple cases, refract and refer the 10% of patients needing more complex care to the ophthalmologist.

Dr. Schlossman: The public health offices in Indian reservations in the U.S. constitute a possible reservoir of information.

Dr. J. Ten Doesschate (*Holland*): The ophthalmologist may find it too burdensome to give sufficient attention to the supervision of his ophthalmic assistants.

Dr. Michaelson: The degree of supervision can be laid down and be well understood by the doctor and his assistant, alike. In Malawi, where throughout the country, there are various ophthalmic substations manned by an ophthalmic assistant, an exact definition of the activities of the ophthalmic assistant makes smooth operation of the system possible.

Dr. P. Quana'a (*Ethiopia*): The four-year training for ophthalmologists in Israel is too long for African demands. It should be shortened to three years. We have found that ophthalmic assistants do not enjoy the financial status and legal standing to which their functions entitle them in the community. An example of this is given by the trachoma workers in Ethiopia who were trained by an Israel doctor during his stay there. These assistants often consult the ophthalmologist when they have problems. An exact classification of medical and paramedical status in the developing countries is called for.

Dr. Michaelson: I, on the other hand, favor the four-year training program in ophthalmology. This period is more suited to the great challenges that will confront the young ophthalmologist in his developing African country.

# CLINICAL PROBLEMS
# IN DEVELOPING COUNTRIES

# NATURAL HISTORY AND DIAGNOSIS OF TRACHOMA

G. B. BIETTI

Clinica Oculistica, University of Rome, Italy

Trachoma is one of the classical ophthalmological diseases. This audience consists not only of ophthalmologists, well acquainted with trachoma, but also of oculists from countries where the disease is infrequent. In addition, we have many participants who do not belong to the ophthalmological world, but who are interested in trachoma problems because of their affiliation with public health services. Therefore, I believe that it would be useful to open this meeting with a brief description of the clinical and pathological characteristics of trachoma, its evolution in special epidemiological and environmental conditions, its classification and its diagnosis.

## GENERAL CHARACTERISTICS

Trachoma is an inflammatory contagious disease of the conjunctiva provoked by a specific agent. Although basically characterized as a chronic disorder, it may nevertheless be accompanied by acute phenomena, both at the onset and during its development. Conjunctival granulations ultimately lead to cicatrization if there is no early treatment. These conjunctival alterations are associated with changes in other ocular tissues, especially the cornea, which influence both the course and the sequelae of the disease. This generic definition of trachoma describes essential features, common to all areas where the disease is present.

However, the separate clinical features listed above are not necessarily pathognomonic of trachoma. Some also characterize other diseases which can be differentiated from trachoma only by virtue of other associated elements. Moreover, environmental conditions vary from country to country and affect the course of the disease.

The origins of trachoma go back to earliest times. There is ample evidence of its existence in many archaeological and historical documents. The disease is practically universal, although there may be regions of high endemicity adjacent to relatively trachoma-free areas. The number of trachomatous patients throughout the world may be about 400 or 500 million.

Interest in trachoma lies not only in its many peculiar biological and clinical problems, but also in the fact that it is increasing in incidence in some developing countries, where social problems are particularly urgent.

The pathology of trachoma consists essentially of a diffuse cellular infiltration of the adenoid layer of the conjunctiva accompanied as a rule by the presence of lymphoid follicles undergoing necrotic changes, by invasion of macrophages and by papillary hypertrophy. These elements are gradually replaced by newly formed connective tissue leading to cicatrization. The most striking characteristics of trachoma are the follicles, the papillary hypertrophy and the diffuse involvement of the mucous and submucous tissue which are capable of leading to the formation of cicatricial tissue. These, when considered individually, are, however, not specific for trachoma since they are also observed in other conjunctival diseases that can also lead to cicatrization. For example, scarring is observed in diphtheric conjunctivitis where it is due to a loss of tissue substance. In contrast to this, such losses are very moderate, or even insignificant, in trachoma. The reason for this marked tendency toward conjunctival cirrhosis is unclear, especially if—as accepted today—the dehiscence of the trachomatous nodule occurs less frequently than we formerly believed. In fact, one of the characteristics differentiating the granulomatous tissue of trachoma from that of the gumma and of the tubercle is a lesser tendency to necrosis in the center of the focus.

## CLASSIFICATION

The appearance, development and cicatrization of the follicles, and the presence of infiltration of the conjunctival mucosa correspond to certain clinical stages of the disease. Although intermediate phases undoubtedly exist, the evolution still consists mainly of four stages: 1) initial stage; 2) florid trachoma; 3) scarring and 4) complete cicatrization. This last stage represents the healing phase which is a clinical, but not an anatomical, recovery owing to the absence of a *restituto ad integrum* of the conjunctival mucosa.

Although the most striking phenomena of trachoma develop in the subepithelial adenoid layer, the opinion that the point of attack occurs in this layer has in recent years undergone some modifications. In fact, typical trachomatous inclusions are found only in the epithelium and this has permitted us to locate the site of the infection exclusively in the epithelial cells, whereas the subepithelial changes (infiltration, necrosis and scarring) are secondary

phenomena, possibly caused by toxic products originating in the diseased epithelium. Alternatively, they may be the consequences of an allergic reaction or, more possibly, a delayed hypersensitivity reaction to the antigen.

Trachoma follicles develop mainly in the area underlying the epithelial zones where Prowazek and Halberstaedter inclusion bodies are localized. The epithelial inclusions represent microcolonies of the trachoma agent undergoing a developmental cycle from elementary to initial bodies and cytoplasmic inclusions, stainable with Giemsa, iodine and acridine orange. New elementary corpuscles originate in these bodies. The trachoma agent may be cultivated not only on the yolk sac of the fertilized chicken egg, but also in various types of synthetic cell culture media.

The subdivision of trachoma into four stages is based on the well-known classification of MacCallan. With a few specific additions, it is still widely used today both for clinical and epidemiological purposes. It has also been accepted by WHO. MacCallan's original classification included specific aspects of conjunctival trachoma, such as the predominance of follicles or papillary hypertrophy. However, it completely disregarded the usefulness of recording both the conjunctival and corneal lesions, either in the active or in the evolved stage.

The first attempt to record the principal manifestations of trachoma at the level of both cornea and conjunctiva was at the first meeting of the WHO Trachoma Expert Committee in 1961. The following definitions were emphasized: 1) The term trachoma dubium (Tr D) for cases where a definite diagnosis of the disease cannot be made in spite of the presence of clinical signs suggesting trachoma.

2) Prototrachoma or prefollicular trachoma (Pr Tr) in cases of confirmed trachoma. In these cases, there are clinical signs of the first phase of conjunctival reaction to the infec-

tious agent, the latter being confirmed by appropriate microbiological tests.

3) Tr I usually designates cases where immature follicles (F) are present on the upper tarsal conjunctiva, including the central zone. In addition there are early corneal alterations, properly called initial trachoma.

4) Tr II designates cases where the follicles are soft, mature and fully developed, and where a papillary hyperplasia (P) coexists with pannus and corneal infiltrations starting from the upper limbus. The extent of follicular involvement (F) is evaluated by three degrees of gravity: 1, 2 and 3.

5) In stage III (Tr III), in addition to the follicular (F) and papillary (P) involvement, the letter C is used to indicate the presence of scars, also evaluated in three degrees of gravity.

6) In stage IV of cicatrized trachoma, obviously only the symbols indicating different degrees of cicatrization are recorded.

The classifications of Geneva (1952–61) not only codified the conjunctival state, but also pointed out the various types of corneal involvement such as infiltrates (i), opacities (kop) and vascularization (v). A form of trachoma associated with other conjunctival manifestations is indicated by the letter *m*. The existence of a trichiasis, whether operated or not, is also recorded. Indications that cultures of the agent were successful are also considered.

The suggestions of the WHO Expert Committees, of which I have always been a member, are particularly important for evaluating the role played by trachoma as a cause of visual impairment or of blindness. This is in fact one of the most important aspects of trachoma for in highly endemic areas, the incidence of blindness is higher than in nonendemic regions and in some places, trachoma may even be the principal cause of blindness. Hence, it is extremely important to evaluate not only the endemicity but also the severity.

This aspect was dealt with in great detail by the third WHO Experts' Committee which emphasized the necessity of distinguishing between the relative intensity of trachoma and its relative severity. The former is an expression of the degree of activity in the patient while the latter describes the complications and sequelae which, if they are present but are not treated, will result in functional impairment.

The evaluation of the severity, which is closely linked to the prognosis, is obviously based on both the presence and the extent of conjunctival and tarsal scars, trichiasis, pannus and corneal opacities. A formula has been elaborated which takes into account these elements and, within certain limits, permits an evaluation of the severity of trachoma in a given area. A scoring system to evaluate the intensity has also been proposed by the fourth WHO Trachoma Study Group. Consideration was also given to evaluation of the severity of the disease in terms of the degree of both conjunctival and corneal involvement.

A more comprehensive evaluation of trachoma should also take into account the factor of time in the evolution of the disease since this greatly influences the prognosis. From the clinical point of view, the development of trachoma through all of its stages usually takes many years. Various types of exacerbations may cause the active phase (generally at stage III) to persist during the patient's whole life. Similarly in those cases carefully followed up for a long time (e.g. in experimental trachoma), the evolution from the early to the final phase always requires many months. There is no doubt that chemotherapy markedly enables us to modify the course of the disease, both in the time of its resolution and in the gravity of the sequelae. It is in fact possible today to observe a trachomatous patient, who had undergone early treatment, reach the final stage (IV) of the disease practically cured, i.e. without visible scars and without passing through stages II and III.

### GEOGRAPHICAL AND EPIDEMIOLOGICAL ASPECTS

Elements accelerating or decelerating the healing process, and thus influencing the gravity of the picture, may be broadly identified with the factors responsible for the gravity of the disease. Among these are the geographical aspects of trachoma. When we speak of "geographical differences," we do not mean that it is possible, from the observation of any individual case, to attribute its provenance to a given country. However, we can collect data on some of its manifestations, such as age of onset, frequency of the cicatricial phenomena, incidence and severity of pannus, importance of the conjunctival hypertrophy, presence and type of corneal (e.g. Herbert's pits) and palprebal (trichiasis) complications and sequelae, and incidence and type of associated (mainly microbial, but also vernal, phlyctenular and viral) conjunctivitis. In considering a rather large community, we note geographical differences not only between one country and the next, but also within the same region.

A survey of the literature shows that differences in the incidence of these manifestations are sometimes very marked in different areas. In general, however, findings have not been discussed both in relation to the geographical problem and as an expression of the gravity of the disease in the area under consideration.

For example, pannus, is reported to vary from 2 to 70%. It may even reach 90% if the investigation is carried out carefully. Such wide variations have also been reported for the entropion-trichiasis which I have reported previously. In one such study the factors producing geographical differences in the severity and clinical morphology of trachoma fell into broad groupings such as ecological, individual variation and specific properties of the infecting agent. These play an important role in influencing the epidemiological picture. The factors are as follows: 1) age of onset of the disease; 2) association with other conjunctival, mainly bacterial, infections; 3) degree of endemicity in the area; 4) hygienic habits and degree of infectivity in the specific environment; 5) climatic factors; 6) economic and social conditions; 7) racial factors; 8) properties of the trachoma agent; 9) treatment carried out previously or in progress in the affected area and 10) modes of transmission.

1) The age of onset varies from a few months to several years of life. Roughly speaking, the higher the extent of endemicity, the earlier the infection occurs. Thus, in some Arab, African and Oriental populations, the onset of trachoma occurs in most cases by the age of one year, whereas in Italy and in several regions of Japan, the time of onset is at about three years of age.

Different modalities exist regarding the onset of trachoma. The classical form is characterized by an insidious onset, with the symptoms of follicular or initial trachoma (Tr I). It is also possible to observe a pure acute onset (that is, with massive infection or highly virulent trachomatous material) with the sudden development of a Tr II. We may also observe a pseudoacute onset, for example, the development of trachoma after a bacterial episode such as often occurs in regions having seasonal epidemics of bacterial conjunctivitis. Together with my co-worker, Ferraris-De Gaspare, I checked the occurrence of these three types in 250 newborn Arab children in Jerusalem and found an absolute prevalence of the first modality.

2) The association of trachoma with conjunctivitis, mainly bacterial, is well known. Such an infection not only facilitates the penetration and spread of the trachoma agent, but it also provokes corneal complications. The most common bacterial conjunctivitis is that due to the Koch-Weeks' bacillus which may be very severe. Such a superimposition accounts for the high number of blind people

found in certain regions. Other complications from various forms of hyperplastic conjunctivitis (especially vernal conjunctivitis) are well known.

3) The degree of endemicity of trachoma in a given area has a decisive influence on some geographic differences. The importance of the endemicity is really the essential basis of the geographical differences and is responsible for the precocity of the disease, for cicatrization and for granulations.

In fact, the more widespread the disease, the earlier is its onset. These cases have more significant granulations and more severe and earlier cicatrization. My own observations in Sardinia, Java, East Africa, the Philippines, Australia, USA, Japan and among Arab refugees confirm this. Thus, the trachomatous school index in Sardinia was 4.6%, with scars present in 4.5 and 13.5% of the children in the lower and upper elementary schools, respectively. In contrast to this, the Arab refugees of Palestine in 1950/51 had a trachomatous index of 78%. Scars were present in 34 and 88% of the pupils in the lower and upper elementary schools, respectively. Many other investigators have confirmed these data in other geographical areas.

The incidence of spontaneous recovery with moderate sequelae also seems to be conditioned by the endemicity and the severity of the disease. The effects of chemotherapy are less satisfactory when the endemicity index in the area is very high.

These findings may be explained in terms of a mechanism which I will try to illustrate.

It is my opinion, based on 40 years' experience in various countries, that trachoma persists and worsens when the patient is continuously exposed to unsatisfactory environmental conditions. In fact, the spontaneous recovery of a trachoma patient is not unusual if he is removed from his environment. In contrast to this, the disease persists and worsens in his relatives who remain in the same highly infected environment.

This may well be explained by the low degree of local immunization left by the trachomatous infection. This is so even if repeated reinfections give way to a diminishingly severe clinical picture after each reinoculation. On the other hand allergic factors, which may play an important role in the development of pannus by the precipitation of antigen-antibody complex, cannot be ruled out.

4) On the basis of what I have said above, it is obvious that the hygienic habits of a community lower the possibility of infection, and thus favorably influence the severity of the disease and diminish the incidence as well as complications from secondary infections, reinfections and allergic stimulation. This accounts for the moderate severity of trachoma, in spite of the high endemicity, in some Japanese populations having excellent hygienic habits.

5) Owing to insufficient data, we cannot draw definitive conclusions on the role played by climatic conditions in the spread and severity of trachoma. However, in the light of other factors (economic and social development, environment, secondary bacterial infections, etc.), such an influence cannot be denied. The forms of trachoma are in general less severe in temperate climates than in tropical and subtropical ones, though there may be some exceptions to this.

In any case, bacterial conjunctivitis, which permits the entry of secondary infections and aggravates the already existing trachoma, has a definite seasonal occurrence. This is usually in spring and autumn, and affects only certain countries with subtropical climates. Mechanical irritations may also aid the entry of the trachoma agent and aggravate it.

6) Similar considerations may be applied to socioeconomic conditions. In regions where trachoma exists, the disease is less widespread

The effect of sulfonamides and antibiotics on chlamydiae is related to the relative complexity of the metabolism of these microorganisms. Sulfonamides act by interfering with the synthesis of folic acid and not all chlamydiae are susceptible. Some of them, especially those of avian origin, are capable of utilizing the folic acid synthesized by the host cell, and this difference together with other metabolic and immunological properties is utilized for differentiating chlamydiae into two subgroups. Among the most commonly used antibiotics, the tetracyclines and some of the macrolides are the most effective (1). They act as inhibitors of protein synthesis at the ribosomal level. On the other hand, the presence of cell wall mucopeptides in chlamydiae makes them susceptible to some of the penicillins less, however, than to broad spectrum antibiotics. Other antibiotics effective on chlamydiae are the rifamycins, which have been discussed in detail by others.

Both sulfonamides and antibiotics can be used systemically or by local applications. Systemic administration would be the method of choice whenever extraocular localizations are present or suspected. When the infection is limited to the eye and its annexes, topical applications are more logical and economical, and are less likely to cause untoward reactions. Experience over a number of years and in many countries has shown that antibiotic preparations are better tolerated and are more effective than sulfonamides when locally applied.

In order to be effective, treatment must be given over a period of several weeks or months and must often be repeated. The reason for this is probably the one that has so far prevented the development of an effective vaccine: the low antigenicity of the trachoma agent. Infection does not result in adequate immunological response by the host, and all chlamydiae therefore tend to cause latent infections. Chemotherapy is thus not supplemented by inhibition of the agent by immune response, and exposure of the agent to sufficiently high concentrations of the medicaments must be prolonged. This need is further enhanced by the fact that not all phases of the development cycle of the agent are equally susceptible to the medicaments.

The need to prolong treatment increases the risk of improper administration, and relapses may occur. In endemic areas, reinfection must also be taken into consideration when evaluating the success of treatment.

A distinction must be drawn between the treatment of individual cases and the treatment of the disease, where it is endemic, on a large scale.

Treatment of individual cases usually implies that adequate supervision can be exercised. Both sulfonamides and antibiotics can be used, the former systemically and the latter systemically or locally or both. Long-acting sulfonamides may be preferred because of their ease of administration, but short-acting compounds present less risk, should toxic or allergic reactions occur. Dosages according to body weight must in any case be accurately established, and special attention must be given to renal function. Antibiotics can also be given by mouth, but in this case as well, the need to continue treatment over relatively long periods increases the possibility of cumulative effects and adverse reactions.

The only method which can be recommended for large scale campaigns, (when close supervision is usually impossible because of a lack of adequate facilities and personnel), is the local application of antibiotic preparations. Systemic sulfonamides or antibiotics should not be used under these conditions because, in addition to the risk of toxic or allergic reactions and to the need for accurate dosages for maintaining effective concentrations without cumulative effects, there is the possibility that they might be misused and that drug-resistance might be induced in other microorganisms which may be present, and for which no alternate treatment would be available.

As for the type of preparations, ointments have been used for many years with satisfactory results. Preference is now being given to oil suspensions of antibiotics, which are easier to administer and better accepted. They are still somewhat more expensive, although waste is to a certain extent reduced.

Any large scale therapeutic campaign requires a certain amount of investment and organization as well as a sustained effort. The seriousness of the problem must therefore justify the undertaking and it must be compatible with other priorities and warranted by the expected results. All these points are interrelated and although they might seem obvious, the level at which they become critical may vary significantly according to local conditions. With regard to the results, it has been stated on previous occasions that treatment may be considered successful even if a complete cure has not been achieved, provided that complications are prevented and the disease becomes self-limited and mild. From a pragmatic point of view, the reason why a treatment is successful may be disregarded. It has been shown, however, in a number of countries that the effect of treatment, if carried out well, goes beyond the immediate and essential objective of reducing the severity of the cases. The cumulative effect of large-scale treatment is also to reduce the amount of infectious agent released and thus to diminish the risk of transmission, the incidence and eventually the prevalence of the disease in the region being treated.

The indirect effect of large-scale therapeutic campaigns on health consciousness of the population is an added benefit which is difficult to measure. In some instances, the setting up of trachoma control measures has been the first step in the development of efficient public health services, and it has often been possible to combine trachoma control with other programs.

The present trend to integrate trachoma control activities into general health services and to use available personnel and facilities makes it possible to expand coverage and to increase efficacy without undue increase in operational costs.

As for the future, available methods may be further improved by comparative trials on the relative efficacy of known antibiotics or of different schedules of treatment. Work is now being carried out in various laboratories on the use of new antibiotics and of long-acting preparations which may diminish the need for frequent applications. Finally, new approaches to treatment may result from research now in progress on the basic properties of chlamydiae.

In conclusion, there is as yet no simple, rapid and totally effective treatment of trachoma. But the disease may and should be brought under control with available methods. Definition of objectives and a clear understanding of what is achievable may avoid disappointments, while a hypercritical approach may hinder positive action.

REFERENCE
1. TARIZZO ML and NATAF R. The treatment of trachoma. *Rev Int Trachome* **46/47**: 7, 1970.

# RIFAMPICIN, AN ANTITRACHOMA ANTIBIOTIC

YECHIEL BECKER

Department of Virology, Hebrew University–Hadassah Medical School, Jerusalem, Israel

*The prokaryotic nature of trachoma agent.* Studies on the molecular biology of trachoma agent (1) reveal that the agent is a prokaryotic parasite of eukaryotic cells. Trachoma agent develops in the cytoplasm of the host cell but utilizes its own ribosomes for the synthesis of its proteins during its complicated life cycle. Due to its need to develop in the eukaryotic cell, trachoma agent has developed a growth cycle which consists of the formation of small, rigid structures with a diameter of 0.3 nm called elementary bodies, and a large inclusion body in which the elementary bodies are formed (2). The elementary bodies, infectious progeny of the trachoma agent, can exist outside the cells but can develop only inside a host cell. Analysis of the elementary bodies demonstrated that each particle contains a DNA genome of $660 \times 10^6$ daltons molecular weight (3), ribosomal subunits (50S and 30S subunits of the bacterial type) (4) and a large number of proteins (1). The trachoma elementary bodies contain an enzyme, DNA-dependent RNA polymerase, which is responsible for RNA synthesis. The elementary bodies contain not only the DNA genome but also the machinery for RNA synthesis (the RNA polymerase) and protein synthesis (ribosomes). Nevertheless, the elementary bodies cannot develop *in vitro* but must penetrate into a host cell in order to initiate their growth cycle. This property of the trachoma agent indicates a requirement for host cellular functions. Trachoma agent depends on mitochondrial functions which make possible the development of the trachoma elementary bodies into inclusion bodies. Thus, in the absence of macromolecular processes in the mitochondria after treatment with ethidium bromide, trachoma elementary bodies fail to develop (5).

The developmental cycle of trachoma agent in the infected cells is characterized by active RNA synthesis. Analysis of the RNA species synthesized in the developing agent demonstrates that ribosomal RNA (23S and 16S species) as well as 5S and 4S RNA molecules are synthesized. The synthesis of the trachoma ribosomal RNA resembles that of bacterial cells. A precursor to 16S RNA (designated 17.2S) is synthesized prior to the formation of the mature ribosomal RNA species (6).

Trachoma agent is thus a prokaryotic organism and hence should be sensitive to antibiotics which inhibit bacteria.

*Properties required of an antitrachoma antibiotic.* Various antibiotics tested for their inhibitory effect on trachoma agent were recently summarized by Tarizzo and Nataf (7). Although a large number of antibiotics inhibit the development of trachoma agent in infected cells, only a small number, mainly tetracyclines, are used for the treatment of trachoma patients. Growing knowledge of the molecular biology of trachoma agent makes it possible to suggest which properties of the antibiotics might be of advantage in the treatment of trachoma. Some of these requirements are given below: a) The antibiotic should inhibit a trachoma-specific enzyme which is essential for the development of the agent, preferably one which functions at an early stage in the trachoma developmental cycle. b) The antibiotic should bind irreversibly to the enzyme so that when the antibiotic is removed trachoma development is not reversed. c) The antibiotic should be trachoma-specific and should not be toxic to the eukaryotic host cell. d) The antibiotic should be effective at low doses *in vivo*. e) The antibiotic should have two modes of anti-trachoma activities due to different sites on the antibiotic molecule. The semisynthetic antibiotic rifampicin (8) seems to have properties making it a good candidate as an anti-trachoma antibiotic.

*Inhibition of trachoma agent by rifampicin.* The finding that trachoma agent synthesizes RNA throughout the developmental cycle (6) suggests that rifampicin, which binds to bacterial DNA-dependent RNA polymerase molecules in the bacterial cell might be effective against trachoma agent as well. Addition of different quantities of rifampicin to trachoma-infected FL cells, immediately after infection shows that the formation of inclusion bodies is inhibited by 0.01 µg/ml. The antibiotic penetrates through the host cell and the trachoma membranes, and inhibits the development of the agent (9–11). Further studies on the mode of antitrachoma activity of rifampicin (12, 13) show, that the trachoma DNA-dependent RNA polymerase is inhibited by the antibiotic. Under these conditions the synthesis of trachoma RNA is prevented.

The effect of rifampicin on the developmental cycle of the trachoma agent in cultured cells was investigated (9). Rifam-picin inhibits trachoma development when added at any time during the initial 24 hr after infection. During this stage RNA synthesis takes place in the developing inclusions. When the rate of RNA synthesis later declines and the progeny of the elementary bodies appear, the sensitivity to rifampicin gradually declines.

The effect of rifampicin and other derivatives of rifamycin SV on the development of trachoma agent in the yolk sacs of embryonated eggs was studied as a model for an *in vivo* system where it was shown that rifampicin was highly effective in inhibiting trachoma agent. All strains of trachoma agent studied were sensitive to rifampicin regardless of their geographical origin. Thus different strains of trachoma agent resemble each other in their sensitivity to rifampicin. Other TRIC agents and psittacosis agent (6BC strain) were somewhat less sensitive than trachoma agent and a larger amount of the antibiotic was needed for complete inhibition of their development.

The efficacy of rifampicin the treatment of trachoma infections *in vivo* was studied both in infected embryonated eggs and infected monkey eyes. Injection of rifampicin into infected embryonated eggs prevented further embryonic death after some of the embryos had already died of trachoma infection (10). This study suggested that the antibiotic might be effective in eyes previously infected by trachoma. Indeed, application of a solution of rifampicin to monkey eyes experimentally infected with a trachoma agent (10) cured the disease. The trachoma infection was stopped by daily treatment with a solution of rifampicin and was completely cured within one week. Addition of rifampicin to uninfected monkey eyes had no deleterious effect on the conjunctiva.

In order to evaluate the value of rifampicin in comparison to that of tetracyclines, trachoma-infected cells were treated with either

**91**

rifampicin, achromycin or erythromycin. The antibiotics were removed at different time intervals from the infected cultures, which were then reincubated, and the infectious progeny was determined. Whenever the tetracyclines were removed from the infected cells, the development of trachoma progeny occurred (1). This did not happen with rifampicin or its derivative (compound 33). When these antibiotics were removed, trachoma development did not occur. Thus, rifampicin irreversibly inhibits the development of the trachoma agent and therefore is more effective than the tetracyclines, achromycin or erythromycin.

The use of several derivatives of rifampicin (14, 15) indicated that two sites on the rifampicin molecule are effective in the inhibition of trachoma agent. The major activity is due to the site which binds to the DNA-dependent RNA polymerase. The second site is the hydrazone sidechain. The 8-0-acetylrifamycin S, which does not bind to *Escherichia coli* RNA polymerase, is also inhibitory to trachoma agent. These findings suggest that the appearance of trachoma mutants which are resistant to rifampicin might be extremely rare, since a very low mutation frequency to antibiotics with more than one inhibitory site has been observed (16).

## CONCLUSIONS

The studies on rifampicin and trachoma agent tend to suggest that rifampicin might be a suitable antibiotic for the treatment of trachoma infections in human eyes. It is possible that rifampicin can eliminate the trachoma agent in treated trachoma patients and thus not only reduce the severity of the disease but also limit its spread. Controlled studies in human beings are still needed in order to evaluate the efficacy of rifampicin in the treatment of trachoma (14).

I wish to thank my colleagues Drs. Z. Zakay-Rones, I. Sarov, B. Maythar, Mrs. N. Himmel, K. Press, Y. Asher, H. Loker and Mr. B. Gutter for their enthusiastic collaboration and contributions to the development of this study.

Rifampicin and rifamycin SV derivatives were a gift from Dr. L. Zeller, Prof. L. Silvesti and Prof. P. Sensi, Gruppo Lepetit, Milan, Italy. The derivatives 8-0-acetylrifamycin S, rifamycin B and compound VIII were a gift from Drs. Staehelin and Bickel, CIBA Ltd., Basel, Switzerland.

The study was supported by grants from the World Health Organization, Geneva, Switzerland, the National Institutes of Health, Bethesda, Md., USA, and by a grant from Gruppo Lepetit, Milan, Italy.

## REFERENCES

1. BECKER Y, LOKER H, SAROV I, ASHER Y, GUTTER B and ZAKAY-RONES Z. Studies on the molecular biology of trachoma agent, in: Nichols RL (Ed), "Trachoma and related disorders caused by chlamydial agents." *Excerpta Med Int Cong Series no 223*, Amsterdam, 1971, p 13.
2. BERNKOPF H, MASHIAH P and BECKER Y. Correlation between morphological and biochemical changes and the appearance of infectivity in FL cells infected with trachoma agent. *Ann NY Acad Sci* **98**: 62, 1962.
3. SAROV I and BECKER Y. Trachoma agent DNA. *J Mol Biol* **42**: 581, 1969.
4. SAROV I and BECKER Y. RNA in the elementary bodies of trachoma agent. *Nature (Lond)* **217**: 849, 1968.
5. BECKER Y and ASHER Y. Synthesis of trachoma agent proteins in emetine treated cells. *J Bacteriol* **109**: 966, 1972.
6. GUTTER B and BECKER Y. Synthesis and maturation of ribosomal RNA during the developmental cycle of trachoma agent, a prokaryotic obligate parasite of eukaryocytes. *J Mol Biol* **66**: 239, 1972.
7. TARIZZO ML and NATAF R. The treatment of trachoma. *Rev Int Trach* **47**: 7, 1970.
8. SENSI P, MARGALITH P and TIMBAL MT. Rifamycin, a new antibiotic. Preliminary report. *Farmaco [Sci]* **14**: 146, 1969.
9. BECKER Y and ZAKAY-RONES Z. Rifampicin—a new antitrachoma drug. *Nature (Lond)* **222**: 851, 1969.
10. BECKER Y, ASHER Y, HIMMEL N, ZAKAY-RONES Z and MAYTHAR B. Rifampicin inhibition of trachoma agent *in vivo*. *Nature (Lond)* **224**: 33, 1969.
11. BECKER Y, ASHER Y, HIMMEL N and ZAKAY-RONES Z. Antitrachoma activity of rifampicin and rifamycin SV derivatives. *Nature (Lond)* **225**: 454, 1970.
12. SAROV I and BECKER Y. DNA dependent RNA polymerase in the trachoma elementary bodies. in: Nichols RL (Ed), "Trachoma and related disorders caused by chlamydial agents." *Excerpta Med Int Cong Series no 223*, Amsterdam, 1971, p 27.
13. SAROV I and BECKER Y. DNA dependent RNA polymerase in purified trachoma elementary

bodies: effect of NaCl on RNA transcription. *J Bacteriol* **107**: 593, 1971.

14. BECKER Y. Cure and eradication of trachoma agent by the antibiotic rifampicin. XXI Concilium Ophthalmologicium, Mexico City, 1970. *Excerpta Med. Int Cong Series, no 222,* Amsterdam, 1971, p 1921.

15. BECKER Y. Antitrachoma activity of rifamycin B and 8-0-acetylrifamycin S. *Nature (Lond)* **231**: 115, 1971.

16. KNÜSEL F, BICKEL H and KUMP W. A new group of rifamycin derivatives displaying activity against rifampicin resistant mutants of *S. aureus. Experientia* **25**: 1207, 1969.

very general terms, the passage of the organism from one person to another is best prevented by environmental measures aimed at improving general hygiene. Attack on the source of infection involves treatment of the active disease with antibiotics or sulfonamides, while the protection of those at risk is the point at which vaccination might prove most useful. However, no clear-cut lines can be drawn between these three facets of trachoma control.

### ENVIRONMENTAL MEASURES

It is chastening to reflect that today, more than 60 years after Halberstaedter and von Prowazek (5) first identified the trachoma agent in the conjunctival epithelium, we still have no conclusive evidence of the way in which it travels from eye to eye. There are circumstantial grounds for supposing that close physical contact may be an important factor. Moreover, the agent can survive for up to 90 min on cloth, so that recently infected fomites such as clothing and bed coverings may be a source of infection (2). In some countries, especially those in which epidemics of conjunctivitis due to hemophilus bacteria occur, reduction of the fly population diminishes the incidence of trachoma. This may be because flies primarily help to spread bacterial conjunctivitis and the resulting copious secretions from a suitable medium for spreading the trachoma agent (3). On the other hand, trachoma is highly endemic in The Gambia, where epidemic bacterial conjunctivitis does not occur and there is comparatively little fly infestation, so that these factors are by no means essential to its dissemination.

Although "improvements in hygiene" and "raising of living standards" are somewhat vague terms, there seems little doubt that they play a major and often decisive role in the disappearance of trachoma. In The Gambia for example, we have observed during the last 15 years a dramatic diminution of prevalence in the more rapidly developing areas near the coast, despite the absence of any mass treatment campaign likely to affect this disease. It is difficult, if not impossible, to identify precisely the variables responsible; improved education, water supplies and access to treatment centers and drug supplies, facilitated by better communications and increased income, may all contribute. Unfortunately, however, the results of attempts by various workers to define the role of social factors have sometimes been inconclusive or have contradicted the findings of others, so that control of infection by specific modifications of the environment is still at the empirical stage.

### THE MASS TREATMENT CAMPAIGN

*Organizational factors.* The approach to treatment of active cases of trachoma representing the source of infection is governed by the degree of endemicity. In general, the more developed countries with reasonable medical facilities are likely to have a comparatively low prevalence rate and a comparatively high average age of onset. Treatment programs based on systematic case-finding and follow-up are suitable under these circumstances, and may be further helped by the existence of a good school system with its "captive" population of children already infected or at risk. By contrast, in the less-favored regions where endemicity is high, blanket treatment of whole communities may be the more economical and efficient method. In such areas, however, the age of onset is likely to be very low, so that the main reservoir of infection is the young preschool child. In countries where such children are secluded with their mothers it may be difficult to gain access to them, especially if there is a shortage of female medical and paramedical workers. Again, the less developed the country, the worse communications are likely to be, so that regular access to isolated communities may be difficult or impossible, and may also be periodically hindered by unfavorable climatic conditions.

*Application of antibiotics and chemotherapy.* The principles of treating active infectious trachoma are well understood, but understandably the efficiency of therapy diminishes somewhat in proportion to the number of patients that have to be dealt with. At one extreme, the treatment of an individual to whom tetracycline or sulfonamides can be given by mouth or by injection is usually straightforward and rapid. Difficulties arise in mass treatment campaigns in which skilled personnel may not be able to supervise such treatment. Under such circumstances the wholesale distribution of orally-administered drugs carries a serious risk that tablets may not be taken at all, may be taken in excessive doses or may be given or sold to others, often for treating diseases for which they are not intended. Thus topical therapy with tetracycline ointment is still the only safe method for large-scale treatment in developing countries. The World Health Organization has pioneered a number of schemes in which communities are treated at regular intervals by mobile teams. Later, as a result of intensive education and health propaganda, people are encouraged to buy the ointment at a subsidized price and to treat themselves and their families. The onus for continuing such schemes must eventually be transferred to the government concerned, and the degree of success in eradicating trachoma will depend on the efficiency with which this responsibility is discharged. In some countries campaigns may be prosecuted so effectively that within the space of a decade or so the impact on the prevalence of trachoma is dramatic. In others, the initial momentum may diminish to such an extent that the tide of trachoma starts to rise again. This is not really surprising, because the mass treatment of trachoma with tetracycline ointment alone is a relatively inefficient, time-consuming and ex-

pensive operation that makes heavy demands both on medical personnel and on patients.

## VACCINATION AGAINST TRACHOMA

### The case for immunization

Although general improvement in living standards and mass treatment campaigns both contribute materially to the control of trachoma, a method of dealing with the third element in the chain of transmission, the person at risk, would be an extremely valuable weapon. One way of protecting such people is the regular use of antibiotic eye ointment during the course of a blanket-type treatment campaign; but such a method holds obvious disadvantages and it is at this point that a trachoma vaccine might prove useful. The truism, "prevention is better than cure," applies to trachoma as to any other disease but, in addition, a vaccine that conferred long-lasting immunity might have a considerable advantage over antibiotic therapy in terms of ease of administration in areas with scattered communities and poor communications (6). Immunoprophylaxis could also be used as an adjunct to antibiotics or sulfonamide therapy, a technique which has already been tried, notably by Italian workers in Ethiopia (see, e.g., ref. 7).

### Results of field trials

After reviewing the progress made by various groups of investigators in developing trachoma vaccines and testing them in man (8), I concluded that "…a fully effective vaccine has not yet been reported. Although a measure of protection can be obtained against both experimental and naturally occurring trachoma, and there is some evidence of therapeutic effect, there is no assurance of solid immunity; and several reports suggest that any beneficial effect is of comparatively short duration." This opinion received additional support from the results of field trials subsequently published. Dhir and co-workers (9) tested two formalin-inactivated vaccines in India. Although the degree of protection afforded one year after vaccination was still statistically significant, it was observed to diminish progressively over this period. A long-term follow-up of a trial in Taiwan (10) showed that the formalin-inactivated vaccines employed had effected a substantial reduction in the incidence of trachoma two years after vaccination, but protection subsequently started to wane and was no longer demonstrable by the sixth year. In The Gambia it was found that a live vaccine incoporated in mineral oil adjuvant induced a barely significant measure of protection six months after the first dose, but despite a second dose given at the time of this follow-up examination, no protection was demonstrable one year after the start of the trial (11). An aqueous live vaccine failed to induce any immunity. Guerra et al. (12), working in Ethiopia, considered that a beneficial therapeutic effect of vaccination on active trachoma was still evident $2\frac{1}{2}$ years later. By contrast, it was found in Taiwan that vaccination used as an adjunct to chemotherapy did not improve the cure rate (13).

On reading these reports, one is struck by the fact that even when protective or therapeutic effects of vaccination are demonstrable, they are never dramatic in clinical terms, and are rarely so obvious that they are apparent without resort to statistical tests of significance. However, one encouraging feature is that even though immunization may be much less than fully effective in preventing the acquisition of trachoma, the average number of inclusions in vaccinated children who do become infected may be significantly less than in control subjects (14), or the proportion of inclusion-positive patients may be lower than in the control group (12, 15). Vaccination, like antibiotics, might therefore be able to play a part—perhaps an important one—in

reducing the infectivity of active trachoma, and hence its transmission rate.

On the deficit side, there are disquieting reports that vaccination against trachoma may actually be deleterious. Under certain circumstances vaccinated monkeys (16, 17) and baboons (18) may respond more severely than control animals to a challenge dose of live trachoma/inclusion conjunctivitis (TRIC) agent inoculated into the eye. According to an analogous finding in The Gambian field trial (11), two years after vaccination with a live vaccine in aqueous suspension the incidence of trachoma was similar in the vaccinated and the control groups, but the severity of the disease was on average worse in the immunized children. These untoward effects are almost certainly the result of delayed hypersensitivity induced by the vaccine. A result that is rather more difficult to explain in these terms is the higher attack rate reported in vaccinated than in control Taiwanese children (10).

### THE PRODUCTION COSTS OF TRACHOMA VACCINE

From what has been said, it is apparent that much more research must be undertaken before a vaccine is produced that is both effective and safe; and any realistic view of the future role of immunization in the control of trachoma must take into account not only the resources in terms of scientific manpower and funds that can be applied to research and development, but also what production costs are likely to be, and how the cost-effectiveness of immunization compares with that of other methods of control.

#### Factors affecting cost

There are so many ways in which a trachoma vaccine could be manufactured that at first sight the problems of making any sort of financial estimate seem insuperable. Nevertheless, with the aid of some informed guesswork about the scientific aspects, combined with the expertise of some of my colleagues who deal with vaccine production at the Lister Institute, it has been possible to make order-of-magnitude estimates for various eventualities.

*Scientific considerations.* Many subsidiary factors such as method of purification, use of adjuvants, safety test requirements and storage problems may affect production costs; but the single most important element is the dose of antigen needed. The mode of administration, whether vaccine is live or inactivated, and choice of host cell are also significant factors, and all are related to the central question of dose. I shall deal with them first.

Mode of administration: Papers presented at the International Congress on Trachoma and Allied Diseases, held in Boston in 1970, suggested a revival of interest in the old idea of stimulating immunity by applying inactivated, or perhaps live attenuated trachoma agent directly to the conjunctiva. Should such vaccines prove successful, the manufacturing costs are likely to be less than the costs of injected vaccines, since the dose would probably be much smaller and the safety tests less stringent. However, so little is known about the potentialities and practical details of such a method that any attempt at costing would be quite impracticable at this stage. I shall therefore confine what follows to a consideration of conventional types of vaccine.

Live vs. inactivated vaccine: In our hands, vaccines made from live TRIC agent (19) proved much better immunogens than those inactivated by heat, formalin or ultraviolet light (20). This may be because the inactivating procedures impair immunogenicity or because multiplication of live TRIC agent results in a more effective antigenic stimulus. We have administered live vaccine without ill effects to some hundreds of children (11 and unpublished observations) and to large numbers of baboons; but the subsequent find-ing that live TRIC agent can multiply in the skin and lymph nodes and sometimes in the spleens of baboons injected parenterally (21, 22) dictates caution in the large-scale use of live vaccine in man, at least until more is known about the effects of TRIC agent multiplication in the primate host.

Choice of host cell: So far, all vaccines used in man have been prepared from chick embryo yolk sacs. For production purposes, this substrate has the advantage of yielding comparatively large amounts of antigen. The main disadvantages are that specific pathogen-free eggs are very expensive, and that yolk sac suspensions are not as easily purified as cell culture material. In baboons, vaccines prepared from infected cell cultures are as immunogenic as comparable yolk sac vaccines (19). For use in man, cell culture vaccine would have to be prepared from an approved diploid cell line, such as WI-38.

Coupled with the general trend towards cell culture vaccines seen in the field of virology, the two main advantages are ease of purification and a short inoculation-to-harvest time of 48 hr, compared with at least a week for chick embryos; but the second of these advantages is illusory in that it reflects the much more limited multiplication that takes place in cell cultures, and hence a comparatively low yield. Furthermore, the use of diploid cell lines demands constant surveillance of karyological characteristics to guard against the appearance of transformed, potentially neoplastic cells.

Dose of antigen: If a live vaccine is used, the minimal effective antigenic mass might be attained by multiplication of the organism so that the dose actually injected need not be large, but as we have seen, there may be objections to the use of such vaccines. Furthermore, the safety tests would be more elaborate and expensive than if an inactivated vaccine were employed. Assuming the use of an inactivated preparation, what dose of antigen

**99**

would be needed? There is not a great deal of information on this point. In an experiment with vaccines prepared in HeLa cells (19), three doses of $5 \times 10^7$ inclusion-forming units protected two of five baboons, whereas doses 10 or 100-fold less failed to protect any animals. Particle counts were not done on these vaccines, but $5 \times 10^7$ inclusion-forming units are equivalent to between $10^8$ and $10^9$ elementary bodies of the strain of TRIC agent employed. In a later experiment (18) three doses of HeLa cell vaccine with a particle count of $2 \times 10^{10}/$ ml protected all of six baboons, so that the minimal effective dose is probably somewhere between $10^9$ and $10^{10}$ elementary bodies. These tests were done with live vaccines. The immunity induced did not last more than a matter of months, and it may be that larger doses are needed. The minimum dose of an inactivated vaccine would presumably not be less, and might be much more.

It seems reasonable to approach the problem by taking as a guideline the amount of antigen in a dose of one of the established bacterial vaccines. Typhoid vaccine contains at least $10^9$ bacteria per ml. On this basis, my colleague Dr. J. Garrett made the following calculations of the equivalent dose of trachoma vaccine, and of the quantities of chick embryos or cell cultures that would be needed to yield it.

a) Assume that the dry weight of a typhoid bacillus is similar to that of *S. typhimurium*, i.e. about $3.5 \times 10^{-13}$ g (based on data in ref. 23).

b) On the basis of their respective dimensions, and assuming similar densities, it can be calculated that one TRIC elementary body (EB) weighs about 100 times less than a typhoid bacillus. Hence one dose of typhoid vaccine (say $10^9$ organisms) is equivalent to $10^{11}$ EB.

c) The yield from a heavily infected chick embryo yolk sac is about $10^{10}$ EB so that 10 embryos would be needed to provide a dose

of $10^{11}$ organisms. (Roughly speaking, one dose of most experimental trachoma vaccines used hitherto has been equivalent to the yield from only one embryo).

d) In our laboratory, about $10^{10}$ EB can be obtained from two 250-ml Falcon bottles bearing cell monolayers with a total area of about 200 cm$^2$; hence 2,000 cm$^2$ of monolayer is needed to produce $10^{11}$ EB.

*Nonscientific factors.* Many variables that are only secondarily related to the scientific requirements of the production system will also influence production expenses. They include the costs of a wide range of overheads, such as labor and materials, which may vary widely from country to country. Accounting procedures, for example the apportionment of overhead charges and calculation of depreciation factors, can themselves greatly affect the figure that finally emerges as the "real" cost per dose.

### COST ANALYSIS OF
### TRACHOMA VACCINE PRODUCTION

Taking into account the considerations discussed in the preceding paragraphs, I thought that it might be useful to make cost analyses for vaccines prepared either from chick embryos or from WI-38 cell monolayers. These are based on 1971 costs in the United Kingdom, and on the use of a typical production unit of moderate size, appropriately equipped and operating at near maximum capacity.

*Production in chick embryo yolk sac*
This estimate assumes the use of specific pathogen-free (SPF) chick embryos, and manufacture by the method employed for the vaccine tested in our third Gambian field trial (11). This was a live vaccine. Inactivation by formalin would not increase the cost significantly.

Table 1 shows that the total annual production costs would be about £57,000

TABLE 1. *Estimate of annual production costs for trachoma vaccine prepared in chick embryos*

| | Annual cost | |
|---|---|---|
| | £ | U.S. $ (£ × 2.50) |
| **Area** | | |
| Assume total area excluding washup and media service = | | |
| Production 3,000 sq ft | | |
| Testing 1,500 sq ft | | |
| Total 4,500 sq ft | | |
| suitable for maximum holding of 10,000 eggs with a turnover of 5,000 eggs per week. | | |
| Expenditure inclusive of rates, heat, light, power, telephone, depreciation of buildings and equipment, insurance, direct maintenance, etc. | 4,000 | 10,000 |
| **Staff** | | |
| Assume departmental head (half-time), graduate assistant, 2 senior technicians (1 production, 1 testing), 12 technician-assistants (10 production, 2 testing). | | |
| Expenditure inclusive of employer's contributions to pensions and social security schemes, etc. | 24,000 | 60,000 |
| **Overheads** | | |
| Inclusive of general administration of staff, site maintenance and provision of general amenities, e.g. canteen service, library facility, incineration, sewage disposal, etc. | 7,000 | 17,500 |
| **Materials** | | |
| SPF eggs (fertile) | 15,000 | 37,500 |
| Other materials | 5,000 | 12,500 |
| **Media and washup service** | 2,000 | 5,000 |
| | 57,000 | 142,500 |

TABLE 2. *Estimate of annual production costs for trachoma vaccine prepared in WI-38 cells*

| | Annual cost | |
|---|---|---|
| | £ | U.S. $ (£ × 2.50) |
| **Area** | | |
| Assume total area same as for production in eggs, suitable for maximum holding of 480 Belco roller bottles (six roller machines each holding 40 bottles carrying inoculated cells for harvesting each week, and six similar machines holding bottles for preparation of new monolayers; one bottle = 900 cm²). | 4,000 | 10,000 |
| **Staff** | | |
| As for production in eggs | 24,000 | 60,000 |
| **Overheads** | | |
| As for production in eggs | 7,000 | 17,500 |
| **Materials** | 10,000 | 25,000 |
| **Media and washup service** | 4,000 | 10,000 |
| | 49,000 | 122,500 |

($142,500). Assuming that 10% of inoculated eggs would be lost because of bacterial contamination or "nonspecific" deaths, and that there would be 45 production weeks in the year, the maximum annual turnover of eggs actually used would be 200,000. If 10 eggs are used for each dose (see Scientific considerations section, above), the annual output would be 20,000 doses. Dividing this into the annual cost of £57,000 we obtain a figure of £2.85 ($7.13) per dose. If only one egg is needed per dose, the annual output is increased to 200,000 doses, but the overheads remain materially the same, so that the cost per dose is reduced by a factor of 10 to about £0.29 ($0.71). The costs of filling and packing and of freeze-drying, if required, do not add substantially to these figures.

### Production in WI-38 cell monolayers

The estimated annual production costs are £49,000 ($122,500) (Table 2). If there are 45 production weeks in the year, the maximum output of monolayer will be about $240 \times 900 \times 45$ cm². On the assumption that 2,000 cm² is needed for one dose (see Scientific considerations section, above), the annual output will be 4,860 doses—say 4,500 allowing for contaminated cultures, etc. This figure divided into the total production expenses gives a cost of £10.89 ($27.23) per dose. As with production in eggs, a reduction in the amount of substrate required to produce one dose would mean a proportionate decrease in cost.

### Additional costs

The estimates in the two previous sections do not include research and development costs, or, assuming production by a commercial organization, sales and advertising expenses and profit margin. When considering the cost per patient, it must not be forgotten that more than one dose would almost certainly be needed.

### COST OF TOPICAL ANTIBIOTIC THERAPY

It is interesting to compare the estimated costs of trachoma vaccines with that of the antibiotic preparations employed for mass treatment. The oily suspension of tetracycline now preferred for mass treatment costs about £0.08 ($0.20) for one 4- to 6-ml container,

which is very roughly the amount needed for one cycle of treatment per person. Antibiotic ointment costs only £0.02 to 0.03 ($0.04 to 0.08) per 4- to 5-ml tube.

### CONCLUSIONS

In this paper I have tried to summarize the ways in which the spread of trachoma might be controlled. It goes without saying that the most satisfactory solution would be the raising of living standards to the point at which trachoma dies out. In certain areas, this might even be the best answer in terms of cost effectiveness, provided always that any improvements introduced could be maintained as part of a general betterment of socioeconomic status. However, it would be unrealistic to suppose that such a solution, which is primarily a matter for the politicians, will find general application in the foreseeable future. We are thus left with topical antibiotic treatment as the present mainstay, the possibility of the large-scale use of long-acting sulfonamides if problems of safe administration can be overcome, and the more remote prospects of a trachoma vaccine. Presumably, an effective vaccine would not need to be administered nearly so frequently as antibiotic therapy, with a consequent saving in distribution costs. But unless small doses can be employed, perhaps by local application or by injection with an adjuvant, trachoma vaccine is likely to be expensive, particularly if prepared from cell cultures. It must give adequate value for money in the sense of conferring immunity of reasonably long duration on a substantial proportion of those receiving it. There seems to be little place for vaccines that do not adequately fulfill these criteria.

During the last decade, widespread research has indicated that the mechanism of immunity to trachoma and other diseases caused by the *Chlamydia* organisms is complex and that delayed hypersensitivity and other cell-mediated factors may play important roles both in immunity and pathogenicity. Indeed, the problem of vaccine-induced sensitization may prove more difficult of solution than the enhancement of resistance to infection, and there is no doubt that much fundamental research will be necessary before a trachoma vaccine becomes a viable proposition.

Cost analyses of trachoma vaccine production were kindly undertaken by my colleague, Mr. J. Rodican, Head of the Coordination of Production Department at the Lister Institute, in collaboration with Dr. H. G. S. Murray, Head of the Virus Vaccines Department.

I am indebted to Dr. M. Tarizzo (WHO) for the information on the cost of the oily suspension of tetracycline used in mass treatment.

## REFERENCES

1. BIETTI GB, FREYCHE MJ and VOZZA R. La diffusion actuelle du trachome dans le monde. *Rev Int Trach* **39**: 113, 1962.
2. SOWA S, SOWA J, COLLIER LH and BLYTH WA. Trachoma and allied infections in a Gambian village. *Med Res Counc Spec Rep Ser (Lond)* 1965, no 308.
3. REINHARDS J, WEBER A, NIŽETIČ B, KUPKA K and MAXWELL-LYONS F. Studies in the epidemiology and control of seasonal conjunctivitis and trachoma in southern Morocco. *Bull WHO* **39**: 497, 1968.
4. REINHARDS J. Aspects actuels et problèmes de l'épidemiologie du trachome. *Rev Int Trach* **47**: 211, 1970.
5. HALBERSTAEDTER L and VON PROWAZEK S. Über Zelleinschlusse parasitärer Natur beim Trachom. *Arb Gesundh Amt (Berl)* **26**: 44, 1907.
6. COLLIER LH. Trachoma and allied infections. *Trans Ophthalmol Soc UK* **81**: 351, 1961.
7. FELICI A and PENSO G. The prevention of the experimental human trachoma infection. *Boll Ist Sierot Milan* **44**: 365, 1965.
8. COLLIER LH. The present status of trachoma vaccination studies. *Bull WHO* **34**: 233, 1966.
9. DHIR SP, AGARWAL SP, DETELS R, WANG SP and GRAYSTON JT. Field trial of two bivalent trachoma vaccines in children of Punjab Indian villages. *Am J Ophthalmol* **63**: 1639, 1967.
10. WOOLRIDGE RL, GRAYSTON JT, CHANG IH, YANG CY and CHENG KH. Long-term follow-up of the initial (1959–1960) trachoma vaccine field trial on Taiwan. *Am J Ophthalmol* **63**: 1650, 1967.
11. SOWA S, SOWA J, COLLIER LH and BLYTH WA. Trachoma vaccine field trials in The Gambia. *J Hyg (Camb)* **67**: 699, 1969.
12. GUERRA P, BUOGO A, MARUBINI E and GHIONE M. Analysis of clinical and laboratory data of an experiment with trachoma vaccine in Ethiopia. *Am J Ophthalmol* **63**: 1631, 1967.
13. WOOLRIDGE RL, CHENG KH, CHANG IH, YANG CY, HSU TC and GRAYSTON JT. Failure of trachoma treatment with ophthalmic antibiotics and systemic sulfonamides used alone or in combination with trachoma vaccine. *Am J Ophthalmol* **63**: 1577, 1967.
14. SNYDER JC, NICHOLS RL, BELL SD, HADDAD NA, MURRAY ES and McCOMB DE. Vaccination against trachoma in Saudi Arabia: design of field trials and initial results. *Indust Trop Health* **5**: 65, 1964.
15. COLLIER LH, SOWA S, SOWA J and BLYTH W. Experiments with trachoma vaccines: therapeutic effect on established trachoma. *Orient Arch Ophthalmol* **1**: 67, 1963.
16. WANG SP, GRAYSTON JT and ALEXANDER ER. Trachoma vaccine studies in monkeys. *Am J Ophthalmol* **63**: 1615, 1967.
17. MORDHORST CH. Experimental infections and immunogenicity of TRIC agents in monkeys. *Am J Ophthalmol* **63**: 1603, 1967.
18. COLLIER LH and BLYTH WA. Immunogenicity of experimental trachoma vaccines in baboons. II. Experiments with adjuvants, and tests of cross-protection. *J Hyg (Camb)* **64**: 529, 1966.
19. COLLIER LH and BLYTH WA. Immunogenicity of experimental trachoma vaccines in baboons. I. Experimental methods and preliminary tests with vaccines prepared in chick embryos and in HeLa cells. *J Hyg (Camb)* **64**: 513, 1966.
20. COLLIER LH, BLYTH WA, LARIN NM and TREHARNE J. Immunogenicity of experimental trachoma vaccines in baboons. III. Experiments with inactivated vaccines. *J Hyg (Camb)* **65**: 79, 1967.
21. COLLIER LH and SMITH A. Dissemination and immunogenicity of live TRIC agent in baboons after parenteral injection. *Am J Ophthalmol* **63**: 1589, 1967.
22. COLLIER LH and MOGG AE. Dissemination and immunogenicity of live TRIC agent in baboons after parenteral injection. II. Experiments with a 'slow-killing' strain. *J Hyg (Camb)* **67**: 449, 1969.
23. SCHAECHTER M, MAALOE O and KJELDGAARD NO. Dependency on medium and temperature of cell size and chemical composition during balanced growth of *Salmonella typhimurium*. *J Gen Microbiol* **19**: 592, 1958.

# SOME ASPECTS OF IMMUNITY IN TRACHOMA

G. B. BIETTI, M. SOLDARI, A. M. ISETTA, C. INTINI and M. GHIONE

Clinica Oculistica, University of Rome, Rome and Farmitalia Research Institute, Milan, Italy

Shortly after the isolation and cultivation of the trachoma agent, many investigators became interested in producing an antitrachomatous vaccine and in testing its effectiveness. The first results were reported simultaneously and independently in 1960 by Grayston et al. (1) and by Felici and Vozza (2). These clinical trials were subsequently extended and other researchers in many parts of the world joined in the production and testing of antitrachoma vaccines. The results have been critically reviewed in excellent papers by Collier (3), Jawetz and associates (4), Babudieri (5) and Bietti and Werner (6). According to Collier, although some of the vaccines tested proved partially effective, "much remains to be learned about immunity to trachoma and methods of inducing it artificially."

In the three years that followed, the situation has not changed much and there is still considerable controversy regarding the practical value of an antitrachoma vaccine. This situation has so far not encouraged the WHO to recommend the use of vaccine in antitrachoma campaigns.

The best results have been obtained with inactivated vaccine either in aqueous solution (7) or combined with $Al(OH)_3$ adjuvant (2, 8). As we have already pointed out, however, the protective effects of antitrachoma vaccines observed by various authors were variable and sometimes unsatisfactory in clinical trials.

This probably arises from many factors such as varying degrees of antigen purification, the amount of antigen employed, the adjuvant used, and also the treatment schedule. For example, it seems very important to administer a booster injection. The increased activity of a vaccine observed after a second shot is well known in practice and this agrees well with our immunological knowledge. Differences between the primary and the secondary antibody responses are well documented.

Environmental conditions such as the incidence, severity and gravity of the disease, hygienic habits of the population, differing epidemiological patterns and introduction of chemotherapy into a particular area may all play a role in the variability of response. These points have not yet been carefully examined nor have any comparative investigations of the immunogenicity of the different vaccines been performed.

We carried out double-blind field trials with liotrachomin (9, 10) in Ethiopia on nearly 10,000 people, the largest group so far examined, from 1960 to 1965. Liotrachomin is a vaccine prepared by Farmitalia laboratories which used a trachoma strain, Trachoma 3/ Asmara/1960, isolated in Ethiopia by Felici and Vozza. The vaccine was inactivated with formalin and contained 500 million highly purified elementary bodies. The vaccine had statistically significant preventive and therapeutic effects lasting for two to three years. Neither side effects nor reactions of delayed hypersensitivity were noted. $Al(OH)_3$ was used as the adjuvant. After 40 days, or in some cases even six months, a booster injection of 50% aqueous vaccine was administered.

In spite of these encouraging results, we intend to extend our clinical trials in order to clarify discrepancies between our results and those of other authors, and to analyze the causes for failures. Further planned clinical trials in the Middle East have, unfortunately, so far not been performed. Trained local personnel is lacking in many of these countries.

The chronicity of trachoma, the individual variability, the occurrence of secondary infections and the uncertainties of the clinical scoring systems make it difficult to evaluate the immunological responses to an antitrachoma vaccine on a purely clinical basis.

Our most recent studies, carried out jointly with the Farmitalia laboratories, have therefore been directed towards laboratory investigations of immunity in trachoma. Some of the factors related to the immunological response elicited either by the trachoma agent or by its antigen(s) are here reported.

*Histological features of cellular immunity.* In man, penetration of the infectious agent into the epithelial conjunctival cells causes a conjunctival hyperemia, a cellular exudation initially characterized by polymorphonuclear cells and later by lymphocytes, macrophages and plasma cells (3). This histopathology is essentially similar to that observed in laboratory animals, particularly in the mouse, following i.p. injection of viable suspensions of trachoma agent. In the mouse a peritoneal exudation is readily observed and consists initially of neutrophilic granulocytes, followed by a large number of macrophages, lymphocytes and undifferentiated elements of the reticular endothelial system. The macrophages

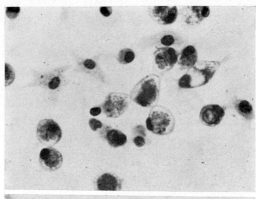
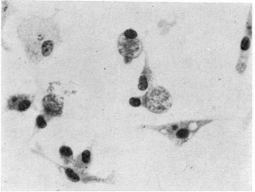

FIG. 1.   Macrophages infected with trachoma agent.

engulf various characteristic stages of the trachoma agent (Fig. 1). This exudate persists for many days (11–13). In the peritoneal exudate of the mouse the infectious agent is found in the macrophages, whereas in the human eye, it is present in the epithelial cells. Such a difference is not surprising because the trachoma agent is able to penetrate into and reproduce in cell lines of mesenchymal origin, both *in vitro* and *in vivo* (11–18).

In the human ocular infection, the persistence of mononuclear cells, even when severe inflammatory phenomena are no longer present and intracellular inclusions are scant or absent, indicates an effective participation of the mesenchymal cells in the necrotic process (3), and represents a hypersensitivity reaction of a delayed or cellular type. In man, the polysaccharide-lipoprotein trachoma antigen is produced in the conjunctival epithelium (3). It stimulates the local mesenchymal cells, macrophages and lymphocytes to multiply *in situ* and to produce immunologically committed cells. Similarly, in the experimental animal, the introduction of the infectious agent or of its antigen(s) elicits a cell-mediated immunological reaction (8, 12, 13, 20–23).

Our findings suggest that the immunization of normal human volunteers with trachoma vaccine (liotrachomin) activates a clone of small circulating T-lymphocytes, or thymus-dependent cells. This activation is revealed by culturing the lymphocytes of the vaccinated subjects *in vitro* in the presence of the specific antigen(s). The percentage of blast cells is then calculated (13). Fig. 2 shows lymphocytes that have transformed into blast cells after contact with the immunizing antigen *in vitro*. These results have been confirmed (24).

This test of lymphocyte activation, positive in all our vaccinated subjects, is widely used today as an index of the onset of cell-mediated immunity. In the mouse, either immunization with trachoma antigen(s) or repeated infection by the i.p. injection of suspensions of viable agent causes activation of the peritoneal macrophages. These cells not only increase their phagocytic efficiency, but also acquire the ability to inhibit the intracellular growth of the infectious agent. The experimental evidence of this immune capacity of macrophages in either vaccinated or superinfected animals was gathered from two sources: a) morphological observation of smears of peritoneal cells stained with May-Grünwald-Giemsa or with fluorescent antibodies and b) measurement of the titer of infectious agent by inoculating samples of peritoneal exudate into embryonated chick eggs (12). These findings are in good agreement with the observations on the ornithosis agent (25) and can be reconciled with the observations of many previous workers (26, 27). Turk (28) gives a detailed discussion

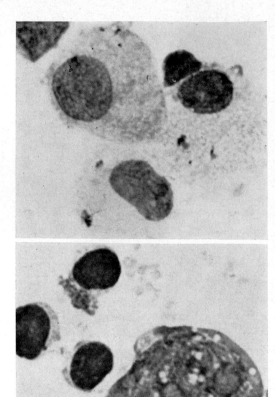

FIG. 2. Lymphocytes transformed into blast cells after contact with the immunizing antigen *in vitro*.

of recent work on the "immune capacity" of "immune macrophages."

Thus, the introduction into the organism of either elementary trachoma bodies or antigen(s) apparently triggers a sequence of immunologic events, basically similar to those elicited by many other antigens (29–31) and consisting essentially of the following stages, some of which have been observed in humans and some in experimental animals: a) engulfing of the elementary body or of the antigen(s) by macrophages; b) activation of lymphocytes or their transformation or derepression; c) proliferation of the activated lymphocyte clone, with formation of new "committed" elements and production of memory cells; d) release by the activated lymphocytes of pharmacologically active substances such as macrophage inhibiting factor, lymphocytotoxins and mitogenic factor(s); e) activation of the macrophages, probably determined by factor(s) released by the activated lymphocytes; and f) onset of a lytic activity, sustained by lymphocytotoxins and directed against the target cells.

Thygeson (32) has pointed out that the development of human trachoma follicles is often characterized by marked necrobiotic modifications with scarring. Although these degenerations have traditionally been ascribed to toxic factor(s) elaborated by the trachoma agent, it is probable that the activated lymphocytes are, in fact, responsible. This series of immunologic events plays an important role in the experimental defense mechanisms against infectious agents, and promotes rapid clearance of the agent from the peritoneal cavity. However, it is not yet clear what role they play in human trachoma, since cell-mediated immunologic phenomena take place only in the anterior segment of the eye and seem to affect the whole organism to a very limited extent.

The topical administration of cortisone, which depresses the immunological response, exacerbates latent or quiescent infections (33–35). Conversely, repeated antigen stimulations can probably promote local exacerbation of the delayed hypersensitivity reactions and may eventually lead to the formation of granulomatous inflammatory foci, i.e., follicles, as well as corneal pannus. Similar reactions play a role in the pathogenesis of other infectious diseases such as tuberculosis and brucellosis, characterized by marked cellular immunity (36, 37).

*Humoral immunity.* Recent investigations suggest that the trachoma infection in man elicits serum or specific antibodies belonging to different classes of immunoglobulins (IgA, IgG, IgE and possibly IgM) either in serum or tears or both (4, 38–47). Complement-fixing and neutralizing antibodies also occur in trachomatous patients and in immunized experimental animals. All attempts to correlate the presence of humoral antibodies with the course of the human disease have so far been fruitless. Thus, complement-fixing antibodies seldom reach high titers. Moreover, a wide range of antibody levels exists within the same community, and even in the same individual, on successive sampling.

In a study on human volunteers treated with the vaccine, we observed neutralizing antibodies in some, but no correlation existed with the experimental data on cell immunity. Complement-fixing antibodies were scarce or absent (13). High antibody titers after infection with trachoma agent or after immunization with trachoma vaccine have been observed in animals (48). We recently observed the immunization of mice with a trachoma antigen administered i.p. in Freund's complete adjuvant. Remarkable quantities of ascitic fluid containing complement-fixing antibodies accumulated. The experimental schedule is simple and ascites appeared after the injection of either suspensions of live elementary bodies or of trachoma vaccine. The precise role played by humoral antibodies in the pathogenesis and course of the human disease is not yet fully understood (4, 41, 44).

Collier (3) suggested that the formation of corneal pannus may result from the precipitation of antigen-antibody complexes at the corneal level (49), as in animals sensitized with an antigen by intracorneal injection. Although this seems improbable, it might be confirmed or denied by the use of the fluorescent antibody stain technique.

### DISCUSSION AND CONCLUSIONS

These investigations strongly suggest that it is possible to obtain a long-lasting state of cell-mediated immunity with a properly prepared antitrachoma vaccine, with the highest pos-

**107**

sible antigenic power and the almost complete elimination of the lipid fraction. In addition, the vaccine apparently induces the production of humoral antibodies. Since the prophylaxis and therapy of trachoma by chemotherapy are still open questions, an immunological approach might be rewarding. At the present stage of our knowledge, the use of a well-tested vaccine appears justified.

The decision to adopt a vaccine should be left to the local health authorities and local ophthalmologists, who are best able to judge what is most suitable to a particular country. Variations in the incidence, severity and gravity of the infection, as well as the priority of this disease among other public health problems, are important factors. We therefore consider that mass vaccination for the prevention of trachoma in early childhood cannot be universally recommended at the present time. However selective vaccination of individuals exposed to the infection, such as public health workers, missionaries, nurses, doctors, families with affected relatives and travelers should be considered, and has in fact already proved to be justified.

A combination of vaccination with chemotherapy not only accelerates the healing process and minimizes undesirable sequelae, but also has a consistent effect of some duration against the reinfections or recurrences so common in highly endemic areas. This combination of treatments is recommended in individual cases. For example, if I had trachoma, I would surely want to receive an antitrachoma vaccination parenterally in addition to local or oral treatment, or both, with tetracycline, erythromycin, rifampicin or long-acting sulfonamides.

## REFERENCES

1. GRAYSON IT, WANG SP, WOOLRIDGE RL, YANG YF and JOHNSTON BP. Trachoma studies of etiology, laboratory diagnosis and prevention. *JAMA* **172**: 1577, 1960.
2. FELICI A and VOZZA CR. Ricerche virologiche sul tracoma. *RC Ist Sup Sanita* **23**: 1242, 1960.
3. COLLIER LH. The immunopathology of trachoma: some facts and fancies. *Arch Gesamte Virusforsch* **22**: 280, 1967.
4. JAWETZ E, JUCHAU V, NABLI B, SCHACHTER J, and HANNA L. Immunoglobulin nature of antibody responses to chlamydial infections in man and monkey. *Int Conf Trachoma, Boston*, 17–20 August, 1970.
5. BABUDIERI B. La vaccinazione contro il tracoma. *Rev Int Trach* **43**: 27, 1966.
6. BIETTI GB and WERNER GH. "Trachoma. Prevention and treatment." Springfield, Illinois, CC Thomas, 1967.
7. SYNDER JG, BELL SD and MURRAY ES. Attempt to immunize a volunteer with formalin-inactivated virus against experimental trachoma induced by Saudi Arabia strain 2. *Ann NY Acad Sci* **98**: 368, 1962.
8. GRAYSTON JT, KIM KSW, ALEXANDER ER and WANG SP. Protective studies in monkeys with trivalent and monovalent trachoma vaccines. *Int Conf Trachoma, Boston*, 1970.
9. BIETTI GB, GUERRA P, VOZZA R, FELICI A, GHIONE M, LOLLI B, BUOGO A, SALOMONS R and KEBRETH Y. Results of a large scale vaccination against trachoma in East Africa (Ethiopia) 1960–1965. *Am J Ophthalmol* **61**: 1010, 1966.
10. GUERRA P and BUOGO A. Données récentes sur les résultats de la vaccination antitrachomateuse en Ethiopie. *Rev Int Trach* **1**: 64, 1968.
11. CASAZZA AM, INTINI C, SOLDATI M and GHIONE M. Étude de l'infection expérimentale par voie intrapéritoneale dans la souris par l'agent du trachome. *Rev Int Trach* (in press).
12. SOLDATI M, INTINI C, ISETTA AM and GHIONE M. Further studies of the experimental infection of the mouse with trachoma agents. *Rev Int Trach* (in press).
13. SOLDATI M, VERINI MA, ISETTA AM and GHIONE M. Immunization researches in the field of trachoma. Some laboratory and clinical contributions. *Int Conf Trachoma, Boston*, 1970.
14. CASAZZA AM, INTINI C, VERINI MA and GHIONE M. Preliminary studies on mouse macrophage cultures infected with trachoma agents. *Experientia* **25**: 327, 1969.
15. GORDON FB and QUAN AL. Occurrence of glycogen in inclusions of the psittacosis-*lymphogranuloma venereum*-trachoma agents. *J Infect Dis* **115**: 186, 1965.
16. LASSALLE J. Effet cytolytique de l'agent du trachome et de l'agent de la conjonctivite à inclusions sur cultures de fibroblastes embrionnaires humains. *CR Acad Sci [D] (Paris)* **257**: 2562, 1963.
17. OH JO, TARIZZO ML and YONEDA C. Growth of trachoma agent in primary cultures of rabbit corneal endothelial cells. *J Bacteriol* **97**: 1502, 1969.
18. POLLARD M and TANAMI Y. Cytochemistry of trachoma virus in tissue cultures. *Ann NY Acad Sci* **98**: 60, 1962.
19. COLLIER LH and BLYTH WA. Immunogenicity of experimental trachoma vaccines in baboons. I. Experimental methods and preliminary tests with vaccines prepared in chick embryos and

in HeLa cells. *J Hyg (Camb)* **64**: 513, 1966.

20. COLLIER LH and BLYTH WA. Immunogenicity of experimental trachoma vaccines in baboons. II. Experiments with adjuvants and tests of cross-protection. *J Hyg (Camb)* **64**: 529, 1966.

21. JONES BR. Immunological specificity of conjunctival follicles in conjunctivitis due to *Molluscum contagiosum*, adenovines, and catscratch disease. *Int Conf Trachoma, Boston,* 1970.

22. KUO CC, WANG SP and GRAYSTON JT. Delayed hypersensitivity with trachoma and related organism. *Int Conf Trachoma, Boston,* 1970.

23. OH JO, OSTLER HB and SCHACHTER J. Effects of typhoid endotoxin and synthetic polynucleotides on ocular lesions produced by trachoma agent in rabbits. *Int Conf Trachoma, Boston,* 1970.

24. COONROD JD and SHEPARD C. Lymphocyte transformation in rickettsiases. *J Immunol* **106**: 209, 1971.

25. ORFILA J and LEPINAY A. Étude de l'ornithose expérimentale de la souris blanche infectée par voie intrapéritonéale. *Ann Inst Pasteur (Paris)* **116**: 111, 1969.

26. LURIE MB. A correlation between the histological changes and the fate of living bacilli in the organs of reinfected rabbits. *J Exp Med* **57**: 181, 1933.

27. METCHNIKOFF E. "Immunity in infective diseases." London, Cambridge University Press, 1905.

28. TURK JL. "Delayed hypersensitivity." Amsterdam, North Holland Publishing Co, 1967.

29. HERSH EM and HARRIS JE. Macrophage-lymphocyte interaction in the antigen-induced blastogenic response of human peripheral blood leukocytes. *J Immunol* **100**: 1184, 1968.

30. MOLLER G. Situations leading to lymphocyte activation, in: Lawrence HS and Landy M (Eds), "Mediators of cellular immunity." New York, Academic Press, 1969, p 1.

31. SILVERSTEIN AM. Varied effects of lymphocyte products ranging from destruction of target cells to activation of lymphocytes and macrophages, in: Lawrence HS and Landy M (Eds), "Mediators of cellular immunity." New York, Academic Press, 1969, p 321.

32. THYGESON P. Trachoma and inclusion conjunctivitis, in: "Viral and rickettsial infections of man." Philadelphia, JB Lippincott Company, 1948, p 365.

33. FREYCHE MJ and NATAF R. Sur l'emploi de la cortisone comme test de guérison du trachome. *Rev Int Trach* **29**: 3, 1952.

34. ORMSBY HL, THOMPSON GA, COUSINEAU GC, LLOYD LA and HASSARD J. Topical therapy in inclusion conjunctivitis. *Am J Ophthalmol* **35**: 1811, 1952.

35. THYGESON P. Criteria of cure in trachoma with special reference to provocative tests. *Rev Int Trach* **30**: 450, 1953.

36. DANNENBERG AM. Cellular hypersensitivity and cellular immunity in the pathogenesis of tuberculosis. *Bacteriol Rev* **32**: 85, 1968.

37. LURIE MB. "Resistance to tuberculosis: Experimental studies in native and acquired defensive mechanisms," Cambridge, Massachusetts, Harvard University Press, 1964, p 77.

38. GRAHAM DM. The immune response of rabbits and mice to trachoma agents. *Int Conf Trachoma, Boston,* 1970.

39. HATHAWAY A and PETERS JH. Characterization of trachoma antibodies in human eye secretions. *Int Conf Trachoma, Boston,* 1970.

40. ISA AM. Characterization of serum antibodies in the monkey following experimental ocular infection with Chlamydia (LGV) agent. *Int Conf Trachoma, Boston,* 1970.

41. McCOMB DE, PETERS JH, FRASER CEO, MURRAY ES, MacDONALD AB and NICHOLS RL. Response in owl monkeys to topical application of killed trachoma antigens. *Int Conf Trachoma, Boston,* 1970.

42. MOGG AE, COLLIER LH and HARRIS R. The antibody response to primary and repeated intravenous injections of TRIC agent. *Int Conf Trachoma, Boston,* 1970.

43. MURRAY ES and CHARBONNET LT. Experimental conjunctival infection of guinea pigs with the guinea pig inclusion conjunctivitis organism. Appearance of IgA antibodies in eye secretions correlating with resistance to rechallenge. *Int Conf Trachoma, Boston,* 1970.

44. MURRAY ES, FRASER CEO, PETERS JH, McCOMB DE and NICHOLS RL. The owl monkey as an experimental primate model for conjunctival trachoma infection. Studies on the clinical course, antibody rise in eye secretions and serum, and resistance to rechallenge with homologous and heterologous trachoma strains. *Int Conf Trachoma, Boston,* 1970.

45. WANG SP and GRAYSTON JT. Local and systemic antibody response to trachoma eye infection in monkeys. *Int Conf Trachoma, Boston,* 1970.

46. WANG SP. A new microtiter immunofluorescence technique. *Int Conf Trachoma, Boston,* 1970.

47. ZAKAY-RONES Z and BECKER Y. Antibodies to trachoma elementary bodies. *Int Conf Trachoma, Boston,* 1970.

48. VERINI MA, ISETTA AM and GHIONE M. Quantitative approach to trachoma serology. *Rev Int Trach* **44**: 218, 1967.

49. WESSELY K. Über anaphylaktische Erscheinungen auf der Hornhaut. *Munch Med Wochenschr* **58**: 1713, 1911.

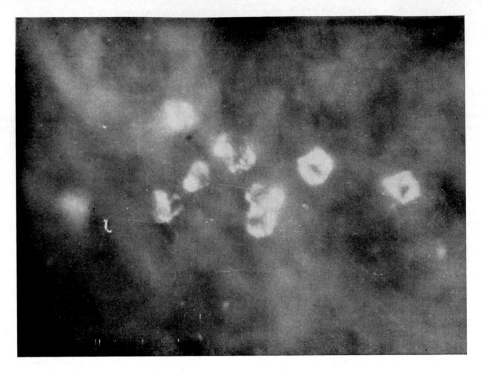

FIG. 1. A section of conjunctiva obtained from topically immunized guinea pigs, stained with fluorescent antibodies. × 1,200.

body, either topically or i.m. (Table 3). Topical administration induced the appearance of local antibodies in the conjunctiva of the guinea pigs as well as in their serum. Cells containing antibody were found in frozen sections of conjunctivas of topically immunized guinea pigs (Fig. 1). No antibodies were detected in the eyes of i.m. immunized animals, even after six injections of antigen, but humoral antibodies were found in them (4).

These results justify the consideration of local immunization as an effective method of vaccination against trachoma. However, one cannot deal with local immunization separately from other aspects of the problem.

The role and function of the local anti-

TABLE 4. *Trachoma antibodies in lacrimal fluids*

| Age group | No. of patients | Reciprocal of fluorescent antibody titer | | | | | | | | Average reciprocal titer |
|---|---|---|---|---|---|---|---|---|---|---|
| | | 0 | | 2 to 10 | | 10 to 20 | | 40 to 80 | | |
| | | No.ᵃ | % | No. | % | No. | % | No. | % | |
| I 0 to 6 | 8 | 1 | 12.5 | 0 | 10 | 5 | 62.5 | 2 | 25 | 25 |
| II 7 to 14 | 42 | 0 | 0 | 6 | 14.3 | 21 | 50.0 | 15 | 35.7 | 25.8 |
| III 15 to 40 | 39 | 4 | 10.2 | 2 | 5.1 | 18 | 46.2 | 15 | 38.5 | 25.8 |
| IV 41 to 60 | 47 | 7 | 14.9 | 10 | 21.3 | 20 | 42.5 | 10 | 21.3 | 16.8 |
| V 61 to 80 | 58 | 22 | 38.0 | 11 | 18.9 | 21 | 36.2 | 4 | 6.9 | 8.5 |
| VI 0 to 14 | 34 | 5 | 14.7 | 5 | 14.7 | 18 | 52.9 | 6 | 17.6 | 13.2 |

ᵃ No. of patients.
Group I to V include trachoma patients; Group VI includes children without any clinical signs.

TABLE 5. *Trachoma antibodies in lacrimal fluids of two families living in an endemic community*

| Family | Age of patient (years) | Stage of trachoma | Fluorescent antibody titer |
|---|---|---|---|
| I | 6 | IV | 4 |
| | 5 | — | 10 |
| | 3 | — | 40 |
| | 1½ | — | 10 |
| | 34 | IV | 10 |
| II | 6 | — | 10 |
| | 1½ | — | 30 |
| | mother | IV | 20 |

bodies and their ability to confer immunity in susceptible animals without causing damage is one question of importance. But, even if this type of vaccination were found to be successful, it may still not be effective in elderly people. There is a sequential diminution in the level of local antibodies due to aging, and the percentage of negative samples increases (Table 4). The decrease starts at the age of 40 (Group IV) and becomes more prominent in the group of people aged 61 to 80 (Group V). A different situation seems to exist in the younger age groups. Antibodies could be demonstrated in about 85% of the lacrimal fluid samples collected (Table 4, Group VI)

from a group of children living in an endemic community and having no sign of clinical trachoma. In Table 5 an example of two families is shown; the older members of the family have trachoma, sometimes even in its active stage, while the infants who lack any clinical symptoms, have antibodies even at a titer of 1:30, 1:40. The role of these antibodies is not yet clear, but it may be that in the young age group local antibodies play some role in the defense mechanism, especially against the primary infection.

Supported by grants from the National Institutes of Health, Bethesda, Md. and from the Robert Szold Center for Applied Science and the Michael and Rose Tenzer Memorial Fund of Fight for Sight Inc. New York.

## REFERENCES

1. BERNKOPF H, ORFILA J and MAYTHAR B. Fluorescent antibodies in the fluid of the conjunctival sac of trachoma patients. *Nature (Lond)* **209**: 725, 1966.
2. MOULDER JW. "The psittacosis group as bacteria." New York, John Wiley and Sons Inc., 1964, p 86.
3. TOMASI TB Jr and BIENENSTOCK J. Secretory immunoglobulins. *Adv Immunol* **9**: 1968.
4. ZAKAY-RONES Z, LEVI R, MAYTHAR B and BECKER Y. The antibody response of guinea pigs to topical and intramuscular administration of trachoma antigens. *J Immunol* **102**: 1290, 1969.

# THE MOLECULAR BIOLOGY OF TRACHOMA AGENT

## STUDIES ON THE NATURE OF TRACHOMA OBLIGATE PARASITISM

YECHIEL BECKER

Department of Virology, Hebrew University–Hadassah Medical School, Jerusalem, Israel

Trachoma agent is a prokaryotic obligate parasite of human conjunctival cells. The infectious entity of trachoma agent, designated as the "elementary bodies" (e.b.), develods only in the cytoplasm of a sensitive eukaryotic cell. Outside of the host cell the e.b. are inert particles. The particles are small (0.3 μm in diameter) prokaryotic cells enclosed within a rigid cell wall. The trachoma e.b. contains a) the complete circular genome of the agent, $660 \times 10^6$ daltons mol wt (1); b) the 23 S, 16 S and 5 S ribosomal RNA (2) present in the form of 50 S and 30 S ribosomal subunits (3); c) transfer (4 S) RNA molecules; d) DNA-dependent RNA polymerase molecules which transcribe RNA from the DNA template (4, 5). Thus, the trachoma e.b. contain an enzymatic system for the transcription of the genome into RNA chains, as well as the machinery for translation of the genetic information into peptides. However, the inability of the trachoma e.b. to develop outside a host cell indicates that the trachoma e.b. lack the enzymatic systems necessary for free development, which are probably supplied by the host cell. In the present paper the early development of trachoma e.b. is analyzed and the cellular systems participating in the process are indicated. The development of trachoma agent was found to depend on the presence of active mitochondria in the infected host cells.

*Initiation of the developmental cycle of the trachoma agent.* a) Adsorption and penetration of trachoma e.b. to host cells: The elementary bodies of trachoma agent were regarded as "large viruses" for many years (6) before their molecular composition and prokaryotic nature were determined. One of the reasons for this misidentification was the ability of trachoma agent to infect eukaryotic cells very much like viruses. Indeed, the kinetics of the adsorption and penetration of trachoma e.b. to cultured host cells resembled that of herpes simplex virus (7, 8). Trachoma e.b. become attached to the cell membrane by the same electrostatic forces responsible for the attachment of herpes simplex virions. Both herpesvirions and trachoma e.b. are detached from the cell membrane by heparin. Thus, the trachoma e.b., though covered with a cell wall, can effectively adsorb to and penetrate into a eukaryotic cell. This property, however, is mainly confined to elementary bodies of trachoma strains adapted to growth in cultured cells. New isolates are not very efficient in this respect, and must be centrifuged onto the cultured eukaryotic cells in order to facilitate the entrance of the e.b. into host cells.

114

Under optimal conditions, the adsorption process takes about 3 hr. Later, after an additional 3-hr period, most of the e.b. start to develop, and lose their ability to infect cells. Part of the e.b., however, retain their infectivity for at least 24 hr (9). The reason for the inability of part of the e.b. to initiate their development is not known. These particles initiate development at a later stage.

b) Initiation of morphological changes in the e.b.: The development of trachoma agent can be detected both chemically and morphologically. Electron microscopy of the early recognizable changes in the e.b. (10) revealed that the electron-dense region in the e.b. disappeared and the particle lost its rigid shape. The next recognizable developmental stage in the host cytoplasm was a larger structure within a membrane, which contained the trachoma agent cytoplasm, in which ribosomes were detectable. This suggested that metabolic changes occur in the e.b. starting at about 6 hr after infection, which involve a probable conformational change of the macromolecules inside the e.b., removal of the cell wall and, most probably, the synthesis of macromolecules.

c) Initiation of molecular changes in the e.b.: The change in macromolecular synthesis was detected by staining the trachoma-infected cells with acridine orange and viewing them in an ultraviolet microscope (11). Acridine orange yields a red fluorescence when it binds to RNA molecules, and a green fluorescence after binding to DNA molecules. The trachoma e.b. showed a green fluorecence prior to and after entry into the host cells. However, after 6 hr the green fluorescence gave place to a bright red fluorescence, which was retained by the developing inclusion until green-fluorescing e.b. of the progeny were formed. Thus, the initiation of development of trachoma e.b. is associated with the synthesis of RNA. Since the molecular processes which occur in the developing trachoma

e.b. constitute only a small portion (less than 10%) of those of the host cell, it is impossible to measure these processes without completely inhibiting the host cell processes. Until such inhibition is achieved, the conclusion that initiation of the developmental cycle of the trachoma e.b. is associated with the activation of RNA synthesis must be retained. The ability of rifampicin, an inhibitor of DNA-dependent RNA polymerase, to inhibit the development of trachoma e.b. (12) also provides evidence that a) the synthesis of RNA is one of the initial processes which occur in the developing trachoma e.b.; and b) the e.b. carry DNA-dependent RNA polymerase molecules (4, 5). An *in vitro* study of the trachoma RNA polymerase might provide information regarding the initiation of this process *in vivo* (4, 5).

In vitro *RNA synthesis by the trachoma e.b.* a) Site of RNA polymerase in the e.b.: Incubation of purified trachoma e.b. *in vitro* in the presence of $H^3$-uridine triphosphate ($H^3$-UTP) resulted in the incorporation of the isotope into RNA chains. This study (4) demonstrated that the e.b. contain enzyme molecules capable of synthesizing RNA chains on the DNA template. Actinomycin D, which binds to the DNA, prevented RNA transcription (12). It was also demonstrated (4, 5) that most of the RNA polymerase molecules were attached to the DNA template. Only part of the molecules were released from the e.b. after treatment with 2-mercaptoethanol. Furthermore, the antibiotic rifampicin, which binds only to free DNA-dependent RNA polymerase molecules, did not inhibit the initiation of RNA synthesis *in vitro*. It was therefore concluded that the enzyme molecules are attached to the DNA genome, most probably to the initiation site. They can be activated and can synthesize RNA under *in vitro* conditions.

b) The need for the four nucleoside triphosphates: In order to initiate the synthesis

**115**

of RNA *in vitro* it was essential to supply salt solutions containing $Mn^{++}$ or NaCl and the four nucleoside triphosphates to the e.b. treated with 2-mercaptoethanol (5). Omission of one of the four nucleoside triphosphates resulted in the inhibition of $H^3$-UTP incorporation into RNA chains. Even under conditions which permit protein synthesis, the requirement for the four nucleoside triphosphates is obligatory. The trachoma elementary bodies must therefore either lack the ability to synthesize the four nucleoside triphosphates, or the precursors for the synthesis of the nucleoside triphosphates are not available *in vitro*. Further studies are required to determine whether the trachoma e.b. depend on the supply of nucleoside triphosphates from the host.

c) Effect of salt on RNA transcription: The synthesis of high molecular weight RNA was achieved by the e.b. *in vitro* only in the presence of 0.2 or 0.3 M sodium chloride. While it is assumed that the initiation of RNA synthesis was not affected by the salt, the transcription of DNA by RNA polymerase was improved, to yield RNA chains of about $1 \times 10^6$ daltons mol wt (23 S RNA molecules).

*Initiation of protein synthesis.* a) Ribosomal subunits and protein synthesis in the trachoma e.b.: Analytical and morphological evidence demonstrated that the e.b. contain ribosomal subunits. As ribosomal subunits, and not complete ribosomes, associate with mRNA molecules to form polyribosomes, it is assumed that the initiation of protein synthesis by the e.b. ribosomal subunits follows the initiation of RNA synthesis. The ribosomal subunits of the e.b. are 50 S and 30 S, and resemble the ribosomal subunits of prokaryotic cells. In the latter, the initiation of peptide chain synthesis is carried out by N-formyl-methionyl-tRNA$_F$.

A similar process probably takes place in the developing e.b. The elementary bodies contain 4 S RNA molecules (2), but the various 4 S RNA species have not yet been characterized.

b) Effect of trimethoprim on protein synthesis by the trachoma agent: An indication that the initiation of protein synthesis in trachoma agent requires the formylation of methionyl-tRNA$_F$ was obtained by studying the effect of trimethoprim on trachoma agent. The addition of trimethoprim (which inhibits the formylation of methionyl-tRNA) to trachoma-infected cells inhibits protein synthesis in the trachoma inclusion bodies (Y. Becker, unpublished results). The initiation of peptide chain synthesis in the e.b. may be carried out in a similar way to that in bacterial cells.

c) Amino acid requirement: The trachoma e.b. synthesize proteins in the cytoplasm of the host cells during their entire developmental cycle (12, 13). This could involve either the *de novo* synthesis of amino acids, or the acquisition of essential amino acids from the cytoplasm of the host cell. The finding (14) that trachoma agent requires the amino acids arginine, histidine and lysine for its development indicates the need for a supply of those amino acids which cannot be synthesized by the developing agent.

*The role of host cell mitochondria in the development of trachoma e.b.* a) The development of trachoma agent in the absence of host cell protein synthesis: Although trachoma agent depends on the host cells for the supply of amino acids, the synthesis of host cell proteins was not required. Treatment of host cells with the ipecac alkaloid, emetine (15), inhibited 98.5% of the cellular protein synthesis. Nevertheless, the development of trachoma agent was stimulated (13). The development of trachoma agent is therefore not dependent on the proteins of the host cell. The stimulation of the yield of the infectious trachoma progeny suggests that the trachoma agent had to compete with the host's cytoplasmic protein-synthesizing system.

**116**

Emetinc inhibited cytoplasmic protein synthesis, but did not affect protein synthesis in the mitochondria (16). The mitochondria were therefore suspected of being associated with the initiation of trachoma e.b. development.

b) Mitochondria and trachoma development: To study the role of mitochondria in the development of trachoma agent, the eukaryotic cells were treated with ethidium bromide, which binds to mitochondrial DNA. The synthesis of macromolecules in the mitochondria is thereby inhibited (16). Treatment of cells with ethidium bromide prior to, or at the time of, trachoma infection results in the prevention of the development of the trachoma elementary bodies (17). If the ethidium bromide-treated cells are reincubated for 24 hr in fresh medium without the drug, they regain the ability to support trachoma development. The sensitivity of the developing inclusion bodies to ethidium bromide gradually decreases with the progression of the developmental cycle.

These results supported the conclusion that active mitochondria are essential for the initiation of trachoma development.

Supported by grants from the National Institutes of Health, Bethesda, Md., USA, and World Health Organization, Geneva, Switzerland.

## REFERENCES

1. SAROV I and BECKER Y. Trachoma agent DNA. *J Mol Biol* **42**: 581, 1963.
2. GUTTER B and BECKER Y. Trachoma agent RNA synthesis. *J Mol Biol* **66**: 239, 1972.
3. SAROV I and BECKER Y. RNA in the elementary bodies of trachoma agent. *Nature (Lond)* **217**: 849, 1968.
4. SAROV I and BECKER Y. DNA-dependent RNA polymerase in trachoma elementary bodies, in Nichols RL (Ed), "Trachoma and related disorders caused by chlamydial agents." Amsterdam, Excerpta Medica, 1971, p 27.
5. SAROV I and BECKER Y. DNA-dependent RNA polymerase in purified trachoma elementary bodies: effect of NaCl on RNA transcription. *J Bacteriol* **107**: 593, 1971.
6. MOULDER JW. The relation of the psittacosis group (Chlamydiae) to bacteria and viruses. *Annu Rev Microbiol* **20**: 107, 1966.
7. BECKER Y, HOCHBERG E and ZAKAY-RONES Z. Interaction of trachoma elementary bodies with host cells. *Isr J Med Sci* **5**: 121, 1969.
8. HOCHBERG E and BECKER Y. Adsorption, penetration and uncoating of herpes simplex virus. *J Gen Virol* **2**: 231, 1968.
9. BECKER Y and ZAKAY-RONES Z. Rifampicin—a new antitrachoma drug. *Nature (Lond)* **222**: 851, 1969.
10. BECKER Y, MASHIAH P and BERNKOPF H. Electron microscope observations on the growth cycle of a trachoma agent in FL cell cultures. *Bull Res Counc Isr E* **10**: 160, 1963.
11. POLLARD M and TAMAMI Y. Cytochemistry of trachoma virus replication in tissue cultures. *Ann NY Acad Sci* **98**: 50, 1962.
12. BECKER Y, LOKER H, SAROV I, ASHER Y, GUTTER B and ZAKAY-RONES Z. Studies on the molecular biology of trachoma agent, in: Nichols RL (Ed), "Trachoma and related disorders caused by chlamydial agents." Amsterdam, Excerpta Medica, 1971, p 13.
13. BECKER Y and ASHER Y. Synthesis of trachoma agent proteins in emetine treated cells. *J Bacteriol* **109**: 966, 1972.
14. OSSOWSKI L, BECKER Y and BERNKOPF H. Amino acid requirements of trachoma strains and other agents of the PLT group in cell culture. *Isr J Med Sci* **1**: 186, 1965.
15. GROLLMAN AP. Inhibitors of protein biosynthesis. V. Effects of emetine on protein and nucleic acid biosynthesis in HeLa cells. *J Biol Chem* **243**: 4089, 1968.
16. ZYLBER E, VESCO C and PENMAN S. Selective inhibition of the synthesis of mitochondria—associated RNA by ethidium bromide. *J Mol Biol* **44**: 195, 1969.
17. BECKER Y and ASHER Y. Studies on the obligate parasitism of trachoma agent; lack of trachoma development in ethidium bromide treated cells. *Antimicrob Agents Chemother* **1**: 171, 1972.

# DISCUSSION

DR. G. B. BIETTI (*Italy*): Dr. Collier, in your description of the production of vaccine, it was not clear how many elementary bodies per ml of dose you consider optimal.

DR. L. H. COLLIER (*U.K.*): From our experience we believe that the minimum effective dose is of the order of $10^9$ elementary bodies per ml. What I was trying to point out was that our trachoma vaccine contains only about 1% of the amount generally used in bacterial vaccines. What was the strength of the vaccine used in your studies, Dr. Bietti?

DR. BIETTI: We used only $10^6$ bodies per ml, at least for the initial dose. This makes our vaccine much cheaper and, we believe, just as effective as those using larger concentrations of elementary bodies.

DR. P. QUANA'A (*Ethiopia*): Ten thousand people were vaccinated against trachoma in Ethiopia during a two-year period. My question concerns the criteria used to evaluate the efficacy of the vaccine. I ask this because if complement fixation was used for evaluation, the results must be carefully reviewed, due to the high incidence of lymphogranuloma in Ethiopia. Such individuals have high titers of complement-fixing antibodies which give misleading results in evaluating the efficacy of trachoma vaccine.

DR. BIETTI: Some laboratory investigations were carried out during that study as well. It is curious, however, that the antibody titer in the serum did not always correspond to the clinical observations. Moreover, a high percentage of trachoma patients given placebos did remarkably well. We have been very puzzled by this observation. I bring up these points to show that infection with lymphogranuloma is not the only complicating factor in evaluating the effectiveness of trachoma vaccine.

# PARASITOLOGY AND DIAGNOSIS OF ONCHOCERCIASIS

## WITH SPECIAL REFERENCE TO THE OUTER EYE

A. E. GUNDERS and E. NEUMANN

Department of Medical Ecology, Hebrew University–Hadassah Medical School, Jerusalem, and Eye Department, Rothschild Municipal–Government Hospital and Aba Khoushy School of Medicine, Haifa, Israel

*Onchocerca* is a disease-causing filarial roundworm that infects man. Other filariae include *Wuchereria bancrofti*, *Brugia malavi* and *Loa loa*. The first two live in the lymphatic vessels and glands, and their progeny, the microfilariae (mf.) are found in the bloodstream. These two species do not affect the eye. The adult worms of *Loa loa* wander in the subcutaneous tissue where they cause transient fungal swellings. They may occasionally pass in front of the eyeball and across the bridge of the nose. However, neither the adult worms nor their mf. penetrate the eye.

Onchocerciasis was first recognized as a human disease by a German medical missionary in 1893. The worms, which were found in tumors of two inhabitants of what was then the Gold Coast, were named *Filaria volvulus*. Further cases were later described in Sierra Leone, Central Africa, the Cameroons, Nigeria and Liberia. We know today that the disease occurs in Africa south of the Sahara in a wide belt stretching across the continent, extending from about 15° N, from Senegal across to Ethiopia, down to Angola in the west and Tanzania in the east. Small foci have also been reported in the northern part of the Republic of Sudan and in Yemen. According to recent WHO publications, this is only an approximate estimation of the distribution. Further information is required in order to yield a more precise determination.

The disease is believed to have reached the American continent with African slaves; and, in consequence, important foci now exist in Mexico, Guatemala and Venezuela. The world prevalence of onchocerciasis is estimated to be at least 19.8 million, of whom 19 million are in Africa (1).

Only one species of *Onchocerca* is known to infect man, namely *O. volvulus*, though at one time the Guatemalan worm, *O. caecutiens*, was considered to be a distinct and possibly infectious species (2). Other species of *Onchocerca* occurring in cattle (e.g. *O. gutturosa* and *O. armillata*) are, like *O. volvulus*, transmitted by *Simulium*. In contrast, *O. cervicalis* and *O. gibsoni*, which infect horses and cattle, respectively, are transmitted by *Culiocoides*. The fact that species of *Onchocerca* infecting nonhuman hosts exist and are transmitted by *Simulium* is of great importance in the interpretation of epidemiological data.

Finally, while *O. volvulus* is the only species of *Onchocerca* infecting man, it may perhaps have other hosts in nature. For example, a gorilla infected with *O. volvulus* has been found in the Congo (3); and in our laboratory, the chimpanzee has been used experimentally for the intraocular inoculation of both living and dead mf. (4).

The worm is transmitted to man by the bite of small blackflies of the genus *Simulium*. The species found in Africa are *S. damnosum* and *S. naevi*; and in America, *S. ochraceum*, *S. metallicum* and *S. callidum*. The life cycle (5) may be divided into three stages: 1) the uptake by *Simulium* of mf. from the skin of an infected person; 2) the development of mf. in the thoracic muscles of the insect through two ecdyses; and 3) after a minimum of six days, the appearance of infective larvae which may be transmitted with the next bite.

The incubation period (i.e., the time from the infective bite until the appearance of mf. or nodules) is unknown. However, nodules have been found in infants less than a year old, and even under three months of age.

The adult worms which develop in subcutaneous tissue are whitish-opalescent in color and have characteristic conspicuous transverse striations. The male worms measure 19 to 32 mm in length and 0.13 to 0.21 mm in width. The females are much larger, measuring 335 to 500 mm in length and 0.27 to 0.41 mm in breadth. In the subcutaneous tissue they may either remain free or concentrate in typical "nodules" called onchocercomata. The latter are hard fibrous nodes varying in size from that of a pea to a walnut, and each containing several entwined and tangled worms. *Onchocerca* is an ovoviviparous worm. Fully embryonated mf. may be found inside the uterus within the eggshell. After emerging from the shell, they migrate freely in the skin as nonsheathed mf. Some adult worms may live for as long as 16 years (6). The life span of mf. (of the forest strain) of *O. volvulus* is 6 to 30 months (7).

The nonencapsulated worm causes no clinical symptoms, but nodules may sometimes be tender and painful, particularly if they are situated over pressure points. In Africa and Venezuela, nodules are nearly always situated about the pelvic girdle, on the legs and over the ribs. A few may occasionally be found on the head. In contrast to this, in Mexico and Guatemala, the nodules are usually found on the head and on the upper extremities.

The clinical manifestations of onchocerciasis are caused by both living and disintegrating mf., and include pruritus, pigmentary changes and atrophy and loss of elasticity of the skin. In the American variety, they cause "erisipelas de la costa" and "mal morado." Lymphoedema and hydrocele are infrequently encountered in areas of high endemicity in Africa.

It is mainly the ocular consequence of onchocerciasis that has won for it the popular name of "river blindness." Onchocerciasis has caused the depopulation of many areas where blindness rates of 30% or more have been recorded. However, *O. volvulus* infection may not be the sole cause of blindness in such a region. All parts of the eye are affected by mf. which have been found even in the optic nerve.

Diagnosis may be exceedingly simple or very difficult. The best parasitological diagnosis of onchocerciasis is the direct demonstration of mf. Freely moving adult worms cannot be diagnosed nor can the presence of nodules be accepted as proof until they have been surgically removed and examined for worms or mf. A diagnosis of onchocerciasis should not be made on the basis of skin changes alone, even if these seem convincing (e.g. pruritus, loss of elasticity, depigmentation and occasionally lymphadenopathy with hydrocele). Blood changes such as eosinophilia and serological or intradermal skin tests are nonspecific and unreliable.

The presence of mf. in the skin or in the anterior chamber of the eye is diagnostic. The former requires removal of a small piece of skin, a so-called "skin snip," obtained by inserting a fine needle into the skin, lifting the needle and cutting the skin below the needle. The biopsied skin is placed in saline and examined periodically under a low-power objective for the presence of active mf. When a quantitative assessment is required, the biopsied snip can be accurately weighed; and, if many mf. are present, it may be transferred into successive drops of saline in order to obtain a more accurate count. The skin snip is finally teased in order to liberate any trapped mf. The distribution of mf. at various body sites and at different times has been studied by several investigators (8–12). In Africa, where *S. damnosum* is the vector, the highest concentration is found on the lower extremities, i.e., calf, upper thigh and buttock. Only in very severe infections, and in cases where a head nodule (or worm) is present, are high counts obtained on the upper extremities, including the outer canthus of the eye. The mf. counts in the outer canthus are best correlated with those found in the forearm and least correlated with counts in the hip and calf, the usual sites used for establishing the presence of infection (10).

Mf. can also be found in conjunctival biopsies, which are a more reliable indication of microfilarial invasion of the eye than skin snips of the outer canthus (13). The conjunctival biopsies can be performed with tetracaine (PANTOCAINE®) or cocaine administered locally. Neither anesthetic affects the mf. count; and in fact, both have a positive chemotaxic effect on the mf.

In the eye itself, mf. can be identified with the slit lamp in the cornea, where they are relatively immobile. More often, however, they are seen moving about actively in the anterior chamber and, when present in large numbers, appear in the form of a large octopus-like mass of entangled mf. We have reported three cases where mf. were partially embedded in the anterior capsule of the lens,

while parts of their bodies were lashing about in the anterior chamber. In aphakic eyes, mf. were also seen in the vitreous, sometimes in very large numbers (14).

In most surveys of ocular onchocerciasis, the most commonly reported lesion is that of punctate keratitis. However, from our early observations in Liberia, we had the impression that this lesion was of viral origin in the majority of cases, but its predilection for the limbal area was highly suggestive of a coexisting onchocercal infection (15). This suspicion was subsequently confirmed in Kenya where the vector, *S. naevi*, had been eliminated 11 to 18 years prior to the survey. The prevalence of punctate keratitis was similar in all age groups examined, including young were children who had never been exposed to infection with *O. volvulus*.

## REFERENCES

1. STOLL NR. This wormy world. *J Parasitol* **33**: 1, 1947.
2. BRUMPT E. Une nouvelle filaire pathogène parasite de l'homme (*Onchocerca caecutiens* n. sp). *Bull Soc Pathol Exot* **12**: 464, 1919.
3. VAN DEN BERGHE L, CHARDONE M and PEEL E. The filarial parasites of the eastern gorilla in the Congo. *J Helminthol* **36**: 349, 1964.
4. NEUMANN E, LUCAS C and GUNDERS AE. Experimental ocular lesions of *Onchocerca volvulus* in the chimpanzee; effects of microfilariae. *Am J Ophthalmol* **57**: 217, 1964.
5. BLACKLOCK DE. The development of *Onchocerca volvulus* in *Simulium damnosum*. *Ann Trop Med Parasitol* **20**: 1, 1926.
6. ROBERTS JMD, NEUMANN E, GOCHEL CW and HIGHTON RS. Onchocerciasis in Kenya, nine, eleven and eighteen years after elimination of the vector. *Bull WHO* **37**: 195, 1967.
7. DUQUE BO and MOORE PS. The contribution of different age groups to the transmission of onchocerciasis in a Cameroon forest village. *Trans R Soc Trop Med Hyg* **62**: 22, 1968.
8. KERSHAW WE and DUKE BO. Studies on the intake of microfilariae by their insect vectors, their survival and their effect on survival of their vectors. *Ann Trop Med Parasitol* **48**: 340, 1954.
9. RODGER FC and BROWN JA. Assessment of the density of infection with onchocerciasis and the probable level of safety from its ocular complications. *Trans R Soc Trop Med Hyg* **51**: 271, 1957.
10. MILLER J and GUNDERS AE. Studies on onchocerciasis in Liberia. *Proc Sixth Int Cong Trop Med Malaria* **2**: 300, 1958.

11. LAGRAULET J. Les maladies d'importation. *Bull Soc Pathol Exot* **57**: 902, 1964.
12. OVAZZA M, RENARD J and BALAY G. Etudes des populations de *Simulium damnosum* Theobald 1903 en zones de gites non permanents. 3. Correlation possible entre certains phenomènes metèorologiques et la reapparition des femelles en début de saison des pluies. *Bull Soc Pathol Exot* **60**: 79, 1967.
13. GUNDERS AE and NEUMANN E. The effect of PANTOCAINE® and cocaine anaesthesia on the findings of microfilariae of *Onchocerca volvulus in vitro* and in conjunctival biopsies. *Am J Trop Med Hyg* **12**: 767, 1963.
14. NEUMANN E and GUNDERS AE. Ocular lesions of onchocerciasis in Liberia. *Am J Ophthalmol* **56**: 573, 1963.
15. GUNDERS AE and NEUMANN E. A controlled study of the ocular findings in Liberian subjects with microfilariae of *Onchocerca volvulus* at the outer canthus of the eye. *Am J Trop Med Hyg* **12**: 761, 1963.

# EPIDEMIOLOGY AND NATURAL HISTORY OF ONCHOCERCIASIS

D. P. CHOYCE

Hospital for Tropical Diseases, London, England

Onchocerciasis occurs throughout the greater part of tropical Africa, especially in the rain forest regions and the Savannah belt that stretches for more than 4,000 miles from the Atlantic coast of Senegal to the Indian Ocean in Tanzania. This is the primitive home of the disease, the great endemic area where more than 30 million people are infected. Other foci occur in Yemen, Guatemala, Mexico, Venezuela and Colombia. Infected expatriate Europeans seen in London and elsewhere are by no means uncommon.

### GEOGRAPHICAL DISTRIBUTION OF
### *Onchocerca volvulus*

In the past, many extensive endemic areas escaped detection because the local medical staff, with a doctor-patient ratio of less than 1 to 50,000, had to deal with many other pressing problems. The very few trained ophthalmologists in the tropics are almost all confined to urban areas where there is no onchocerciasis. In the rural areas many thousands of people with onchocercal eye disease remain undiagnosed because they never have the opportunity of being examined by anyone competent to make a specific diagnosis. Most of the so-called "new" foci have been discovered fortuitously.

The extensive focus in Kenya, including the famous "Valley of the Blind" at Kodera, was discovered quite by chance when a pathologist found an *O. volvulus* adult worm in a "tumor" sent for examination to the central pathology laboratory in Nairobi (1).

We should never forget that it was Robles (2) and his ophthalmologist colleague Pacheco-Luna (3) who described the blinding onchocercal keratoiridocyclitis in Guatemala several years before the same phenomenon was observed in Africa: the Congo (4), Sudan (5), the former British West African territories (6–8) and in the former French African territories (9–13). These are only a few of the many reports that have helped to map the extent of the disease in Africa.

A superb example of scientific serendipity occurred in 1958 when Dr. Mario Giaquinto, who was on an official visit from the World Health Organization, discovered a focus of transmission almost within the compound of the Vector-Borne Diseases Institute at Amani in Tanzania. At that time the nearest known focus was several hundred miles away, but it is now known that the disease is widespread in Tanzania (14). Amani is situated among thickly wooded hills with swift flowing streams and plenty of shade. Anyone

Address for reprints: 9 Drake Road, Westcliff-on-Sea, Essex, England.

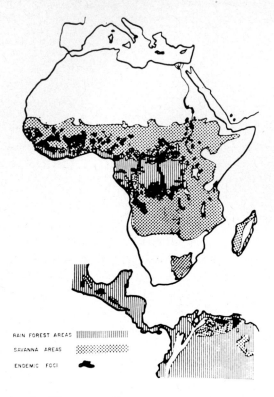

RAIN FOREST AREAS |||||||||||||||||||||||||

SAVANNA AREAS

ENDEMIC FOCI

FIG. 1. The geographical distribution of onchocerciasis in man (kindly supplied by Prof. G. S. Nelson).

Africa differ quite markedly in their vector infectivity, their infectivity to chimpanzees and in their general epidemiology and clinical manifestations (15–19). There are also marked differences in the clinical manifestations of onchocerciasis in West and East Africa.

It is difficult to see how the parasite could have become established in Central America except by a mass movement of population from endemic areas such as occurred with the slave trade, or by the transfer of the infection to man from a primary animal maintenance host, of which there is no evidence whatever. There are three possible explanations of the Central America foci of onchocerciasis: 1) a genuine multicentric origin; 2) a primary focus in Equatorial Africa which spread to Central America with the slave traffic; 3) though Central American onchocerciasis was indigenous, it became considerably modified by contact with the African variety after its arrival with the slave traffic. On the whole, I consider that the balance of evidence supports the second theory.

Attempts have been made to infect the eyes of nonhuman species of primates and of a variety of laboratory animals with *O. volvulus*, but so far without success. Duke and Anderson in Kumba (Nigeria) have, however, claimed some success with rabbits (personal communication).

interested in landscape epidemiology would have suspected that there might have been transmission of onchocerciasis in this area. Further studies will doubtless show that onchocerciasis is far more widespread than is indicated in Fig. 1. It should be looked for in all parts of the world where Simuliids bite man. The disease may not occur in Arctic regions but there is a possibility that it will be found in other areas, especially in Asia and South America where the rivers flowing from the great mountain chains are often ideal breeding places for Simuliids. There are differences between the African and American forms of *O. volvulus*. There is also much clinical and pathological evidence suggesting that there are several variants of *O. volvulus* in different parts of the world and in Africa itself. The savanna and forest forms in West

PATHOGENESIS OF ONCHOCERCIASIS IN MAN

*Adult worms and nodules.* Irrespective of the strain of parasite, the most severe clinical manifestations of onchocerciasis are due to reactions to the presence of the microfilariae (mf). The adult worms are usually of secondary importance. It takes nine months for a larva to change into a fertile female worm.

*Production of mf.* At that point, the female worm produces a large number of mf which infiltrate the skin and the tissues. Female worms are known to have a life span of approximately 15 years and to produce about

2,500 mf daily, that is almost a million a year or 14 million in their life span! In an infant, the daily mf output would be sufficient to populate the skin with one mf to every 4 mm$^2$ of skin within a month (20).

The evident longevity of adult female worms is confirmed by numerous case records at the Hospital for Tropical Diseases in London, which include a significant number of patients who have not been exposed to reinfection for over 10 years, but who regularly produce fresh crops of skin lesions with positive biopsies with or without fresh spots of onchokeratitis and mf in the anterior chambers. The latter indicate the presence of living, fertile, adult female worm(s) within their tissues (though not necessarily in the form of palpable nodules).

Nelson's studies on *Onchocerca gutturosa* in the cow indicate that the mf have a well developed directional mechanism which determines their final position in the skin. They do not merely "sit around" in the skin close to their parent worms but migrate through the tissues to the skin, where there are the best opportunities of being picked up by the vectors. Irrespective of the position of the adult worms, the mf in naturally infected cattle migrate preferentially to the umbilicus where they accumulate in large numbers (Fig. 2). This is a beautiful adaptation to transmission, because more than 90% of the vectors (*Culex nubeculosus*) bite around the umbilicus.

One may ask if mf involvement in man exhibits a similar directional mechanism with the anterior segment of the eye as its preferred site. This would be of no advantage to the parasite because the fly vector does not bite the conjunctiva or the cornea. We may speculate that perhaps the worms are attracted by the temperature gradient or the greater degree of light present in the translucent cornea than the skin.

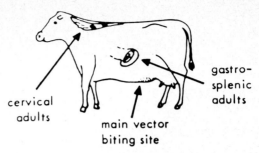

FIG. 2. The distribution of mf *Onchocerca gutturosa* in the skin of naturally infected cattle (kindly supplied by Prof. G. S. Nelson).

ONCHOCERCAL EYE LESIONS
AND THEIR NATURAL HISTORY

The most severe eye lesions are seen in the drier regions of Africa and also in Central America. Blindness is less common in the rain forest regions even though infection rates are often very high and there is intensive transmission. In one of the rain forest areas of the Cameroons, Duke (21) obtained data on the biting and infection rates of *Simulium damnosum*. He calculated that a single person exposed all day and every day for a year would be bitten by 14,000 infective *S. damnosum* capable of transmitting more than 92,000 infective larvae. Yet the blindness rate is less than 1% compared with more than 10% in the savanna regions, where the biting rate of *S. damnosum* is often less intense.

During the past 20 years, I have visited endemic areas in Guatemala and Mexico

TABLE 1. *Ocular findings in 800 onchocercal cases (Hospital for Tropical Diseases, 1952–63)*

| Ocular lesion | Percent |
| --- | --- |
| Onchokeratitis | 43 |
| Mf in anterior chamber | 5 |
| Mild anterior uveitis | 2 |
| Posterior uveitis | 0 |
| Chorioretinal degenerations | 0 |
| Loss of vision | 0 |

**125**

TABLE 2. *Comparison of onchocerciasis in Central America, Africa and the British Isles*

|  | Central America | Africa | British Isles |
|---|---|---|---|
| Erysipela de la costa | + + | Nil? | Nil |
| Intensity of infection: |  |  |  |
| a) General | + + | + + + | + |
| b) Periocular | + + + | + + | + |
| Location of nodules | 2/3 above waist | 2/3 below waist | 2/3 below waist |
| Total number infected | 200,000 | 50,000,000 | 2,000 |
| Total blind | 2,000 (1 %) | 500,000 (1 %) | Nil |
| Age of blind | Usually over 50 | Children and adults | — |
| Main cause of onchocercal blindness | Anterior segment | Anterior and posterior segment (ratio varies from place to place) | — |
| Treatment | Nodulectomy | Control of Simulium | Nodulectomy; filaricidal drugs |
| Other filarial diseases | Nil | Common | Common |
| Nutrition | Generally good. Some lack of vitamin A and animal protein | Variable. May be deficient in vitamin A, vitamin B complex and animal protein, especially in savanna regions | Excellent |

TABLE 3. *Ocular onchocerciasis in Central America, Africa and the British Isles*

|  | Central America | Africa | | British Isles |
|---|---|---|---|---|
|  |  | Savanna | Forest |  |
| Anterior segment lesions |  |  |  |  |
| Trachoma | Rare | + + | Rare | Rare |
| Conjunctival lesions | + | + + | + | Slight injection |
| Keratitis | + + | + + + | + | + |
| Iridocyclitis | + + + | + + | + | + |
| Posterior segment lesions |  |  |  |  |
| Primary optic atrophy | Not seen | + + | + + | Not seen |
| Secondary optic atrophy | Possibly + | + + | + | Not seen |
| Postinflammatory chorioretinitis |  |  |  |  |
| 1) Anterior | Probably +[a] | + + | + | Not seen |
| 2) Posterior | + | + + | + | Not seen |
| Posterior degenerative lesions | Few and ill-defined | + + | + | Not seen |

[a] Obscured by occluded and down-drawn pupils and complicated cataracts.

and various parts of East, West and Central Africa, where I examined many hundreds of onchocercal and nononchocercal patients. Ind have also seen about 1,500 cases of onchocerciasis at the Hospital for Tropical Diseases in London.

Table 1 gives the ocular findings in about half the cases in the Hospital for Tropical Diseases. The figures for the other half, although not complete, are very similar. Substantial differences were noted between the Central American, the African and the British human onchocercal cases (Table 2). The anterior segment lesions exhibited similar differences and the posterior segment lesions were also dissimilar (Table 3).

a) The cornea. The opacities vary according to the type of patient and his age; from the fluffy, nummular or snowflake opacities typical of European cases at the Hospital for Tropical Diseases, particularly in children or young adults, to much smaller opacities

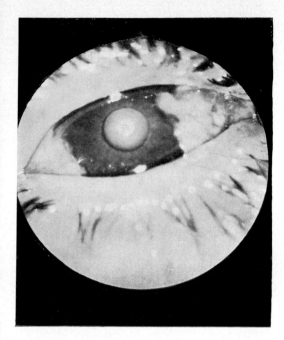

FIG. 3. Pseudopterygium formation, very characteristic of Central American onchocerciasis.

in the African patients, to pseudopterygium which typically appears in the Amerindians of Central America. This limbitis or pseudopterygium formation (Fig. 3) was a very striking finding in Central America, and in those cases the punctate keratitis tended to fade out over the age of 40, being replaced by pseudopterygium formation. Do these morphological differences represent varying degrees of personal, and perhaps racial, immunity to dead mf?

b) The anterior chamber. Interest centers upon the presence, number and behavior of mf. Patients with numerous mf in their anterior chambers nearly always had photophobia and furrowing of the brows, and either complained of ocular irritation or admitted to it on direct questioning. This is in general agreement with observations on European patients at our Hospital for Tropical Diseases, but contrasts with Amani and Bonjongo (Cameroon) patients, in whom it was quite common to see completely asymptomatic eyes with numerous intracameral mf.

The lack of extraneous mesodermal tissue in the anterior chambers made recognition of mf easier in Guatemala. The mf were often observed attached by the blunt (mouth) end not only to the iris stroma, especially to the lower nasal and lower temporal quadrant, but also to Descemet's membrane in these areas. Their behavior is then strongly reminiscent of the behavior of a windsock at an airfield in a light breeze. Fixed by the larger end, the rest of the mf demonstrates its usual constant movement and is at the same time extended, as it were, by the aqueous flow. In the lower nasal quadrant, the flow was down and slightly towards the nose. Temporally, it was down and slightly towards the outer canthus.

This phenomenon was observed several times, and presumably the same mf were observed there, attached to the same part of Descemet's membrane, on consecutive days on several occasions. I am not familar with the amount of suction exerted by the mouth end of these mf, but I am satisfied that this observation is probably the explanation of the limbitis. This trauma, however slight, is repeated over long periods of time, and must locally weaken Descemet's membrane, permitting a transudation of aqueous through the altered membrane into the deeper layers of the corneal stroma. There could thus be a localized corneal dystrophy even resulting in a minor degree of bullous keratopathy, which would in turn promote the formation of a protective pterygium. In my view, this is the explanation of the limbitis and the later pterygium formation so commonly observed in these onchocercal patients both in Guatemala and Africa.

c) The iris. Between 1915 and 1919, Pacheco-Luna and Robles described the painful and blinding ocular consequences of onchocerciasis, centering around the exudative

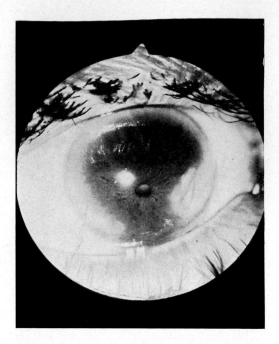

FIG. 4. Advanced onchocercal keratoiridocyclitis with ring synechiae, small down-drawn pupil and complicated cataract in a Guatemalan patient.

fibrinous iridocyclitis. In spite of the nodulectomy campaign which has been going on in Guatemala for nearly 40 years, the blinding iritis is still very evident. It is still the major cause of blindness in a heavily infected community. The first synechiae were observed in patients around the age of 20; with advancing age, they become denser and creep around the circumference of the pupil. The youngest patient blinded in this way was aged 37, but a more usual age is 50 to 60 (Fig. 4). Though some immobile pupils were central, most were displaced downward, with the narrow pear-shaped or slit-like appearance described by Pacheco-Luna (3) and also by Bryant (5) and Ridley (6).

In several cases the iritis was so severe that there was literally no pupil to be seen, and only careful examination with a corneal microscope usually permitted a guess as to where it lay. This finding must surely be unique to onchocerciasis. By the time the iritis is really severe, punctate keratitis is rare, and mf in the anterior chamber are distinctly uncommon. Thus, Central American ocular onchocerciasis starts, as in Africa, as a benign parasitosis, with mf swimming harmlessly about in the anterior chamber and a few equally harmless spots of keratitis. Possibly due to an immune reaction, more and more of the mf die liberating their well-known necrotizing toxins. These particularly affect the iris and also the ciliary bodies; hence the chronic, insidious, blinding iritis.

The down-drawing and eventual obliteration of the pupil is, in my experience, not such a common finding in Africa.

d) The lens. Torroella (22) has observed mf attached to the anterior lens capsule. There is general agreement that this capsule constitutes an impassable barrier for the mf. In some parts of Africa, especially in Ethiopia, Anderson (personal communication) observed a high incidence of exfoliation of the lens capsule, in association with onchocerciasis, which he did not observe in other parts of Africa. This is a chance observation, which has yet to be explained. The incidence of senile cataract does not appear to be related to onchocerciasis as such, though complicated cataracts in association with the onchocercal keratoiridocyclitis described above are very common.

ECONOMICS OF CONTROL

Is control desirable? It is clear that probably the vast majority of patients are in no danger of blindness and in no great discomfort, apart from a troublesome recurrent skin irritation. They therefore have a low priority as regards prophylaxis, treatment or control of blindness. Nodulectomy, which has been widely practiced in endemic areas such as Guatemala and other Central American foci, is reasonable in the case of nodules close to the eye, and should be continued. It is not, however, an attainable or even helpful objective in Africa.

The third and probably the best method of control is elimination of the vector fly. With the knowledge at our disposal it is possible to eliminate selectively one particular vector, for example *Simulium neavei*, as was successfully done by McMahon in an area of 6,000 square miles in Kenya. He accomplished this without interfering with other vectors, and thus without dangerously interfering with the local ecology. This was, however, a very expensive exercise.

## REFERENCES

1. PRESTON PG. Report of a case of human onchocerciasis in Kenya. *J Trop Med Hyg* **38**: 81, 1935.
2. ROBLES R. Onchocercose humaine au Guatemala produisant la cecite et l'"Erysipèle du littoral." *Bull Soc Pathol Exot* **12**: 442, 1919.
3. PACHECO-LUNA R. Filarial tumors. *Am J Ophthalmol* **3**: 805, 1918.
4. HISETTE J. Memoire sur l'*Onchocerca volvulus* Leuckaert et sur manifestations oculaires au Congo belge. *Ann Soc Belg Med Trop* **12**: 433, 1932.
5. BRYANT J. Endemic retino-choroiditis in Anglo-Egyptian Sudan and its possible relationship to *Onchocerca volvulus*. *Trans R Soc Trop Med Hyg* **28**: 523, 1935.
6. RIDLEY H. Ocular onchocerciasis. *Br J Ophthalmol* (Monogr Suppl) **10**: 1945.
7. BUDDEN FH. Natural history of onchocerciasis. *Br J Ophthalmol* **41**: 214, 1957.
8. RODGER FC. "Blindness in West Africa." London, HK Lewis & Co, 1959.
9. PUYUELO R and HOLSTEIN MM. L'onchocercose humaine en Afrique noire francaise; maladie sociale. *Med Trop* (*Mars*) **10**: 397, 1950.
10. D'HAUSSY R, RIT JIM and LAGRAULET J. Contribution à l'étude des lesions du fond d'oeil dans l'onchocercose. *Med Trop* (*Mars*) **18**: 340, 1958.
11. QUERE MA, BASSET A, LARIVIERE M and RAZAFINJATO R. Statistical study on the frequency and specificity of ocular complications of onchocerciasis. *Bull Mem Fac Mixte Med Pharm* (*Dakar*) **11**: 238, 1963.
12. TOUSSAINT D and DANIS P. Retinopathy in generalized Loa-Loa filiariasis. *Arch Ophthalmol* **74**: 470, 1965.
13. LAGRAULET J, BAUMONT R and COULAND L. Aspects epidemiologiques de l'onchocercose dans le moyen-chari (Tchad). *Bull Soc Pathol Exot* **60**: 173, 1967.
14. RAYBOULD JN. Change and the transmission of onchocerciasis. *East Afr Med J* **45**: 292, 1968.
15. DUKE BOL, LEWIS DJ and MOORE JP. *Onchocerca-Simulium* complexes. I. Transmission of forest and Sudan-savanna strains of *Onchocerca volvulus* from Cameroon by *Simulium damnosum* from various West African bioclimatic zones. *Ann Trop Med Parasitol* **60**: 318, 1966.
16. DUKE BOL, MOORE JP and DE LEON RJ. *Onchocerca-Simulium* complexes. V. The intake and subsequent fate of microfilariae of a Guatemalan strain of *Onchocerca volvulus* in forest and Suda-savanna forms of West African *Simulium damnosum*. *Ann Trop Med Parasitol* **61**: 332, 1967.
17. LEWIS DJ and DUKE BOL. *Onchocerca-Simulium* complexes. II. Variation in West African female *Simulium damnosum*. *Ann Trop Med Parasitol* **60**: 337, 1966.
18. DUKE BOL. *Onchocerca-Simulium* complexes. III. The survival of *Simulium damnosum* after high intakes of microfilariae of incompatible strains of *Onchocerca volvulus*, and the survival of the parasites in the fly. *Ann Trop Med Parasitol* **60**: 495, 1966.
19. DUKE BOL. *Onchocerca-Simulium* complexes. IV. Transmission of a variant of the forest strain of *Onchocerca volvulus*. *Ann Trop Med Parasitol* **61**: 326, 1967.
20. MILLS AR. A quantitative approach to the epidemiology of onchocerciasis in West Africa. *Trans R Soc Trop Med Hyg* **63**: 591, 1969.
21. DUKE BOL. Studies on factors influencing the transmission of onchocerciasis. VI. The infective biting potential of *Simulium damnosum* in different bioclimatic zones and its influence on the transmission potential. *Ann Trop Med Parasitol* **62**: 164, 1968.
22. TORROELLA JL. Nota sobre la observacion de microfilarias de *Onchocerca in vivo* en. el ojo humano. *An Soc Mex Oftalmol Otorinolaringol* **9**: 87, 1931.

# OCULAR LESIONS OF ONCHOCERCIASIS

F. C. RODGER

Princess Margaret Hospital, Swindon, Cirencester, England

Newcomers to the field of ocular onchocerciasis are bound to make new observations; they are also bound to make old ones, so the best advice I can give is to read the literature. How many have read the works of Bryant and Kirk of Scotland, Hissette, van den Berghe and Rodhain of Belgium, Pacheco-Luna and Diaz of Guatemala and Strong and Ochoa of the United States?

Misclassification is probably more common in ophthalmology than in any other discipline in medicine. This is true not only of ocular onchocerciasis but also of trachoma, xerophthalmia and other disease complexes of the eye. To avoid misclassification is of paramount importance because if one characteristic is mistakenly taken as representing an ocular complication of onchocerciasis, mathematical errors will creep in and are difficult to rectify later. Damage is done and perpetuated, for it takes courage to alter criteria as the epidemiological data pile up. It is better to err on the side of being overscrupulous rather than in the opposite direction in field work, unsupported as it is by laboratory assays. Where it is possible later to utilize better facilities and greater expertise, the opposite is true. This principle, however, cannot be applied to onchocercal endemic areas. In hospital practice, the number of investigatory procedures into the cause of a uveitis may be as high as 20 or 30, including X-ray as well as serological and other tests although only a few may be worthwhile. Nevertheless, the association with a positive skin biopsy cannot be accepted as diagnostic if the uveitis is nonspecific. Thus, accurate clinical descriptions are as vital now as in the 19th century.

The establishment of criteria for diagnosing ocular lesions as being directly caused by onchocerciasis is, therefore, long overdue. There are only four lesions which have clinical characteristics possessed by no other disease and which can truly be called specific; they represent no more than a tithe of the whole. They include most examples of sclerosing keratitis, some examples of anterior uveitis, one variety of posterior chorioretinitis (or uveitis) and a particular complicated, secondary optic atrophy, rarely found among the welter of nonspecific optic atrophies. While there are many other ocular effects caused by onchocerciasis, they are nonspecific and occur in association only. One cannot, therefore, classify them as examples of ocular onchocerciasis in the field without the risk of grossly misrepresenting the ravages of this disease, until one compares their prevalence with those in comparable nonendemic areas. This has never been done on a large scale by skilled observers.

Three questions arise:

1) *Can fallacies in assessing the density of skin infectivity lead to fallacies in ocular*

*diagnosis*? Epidemiological surveys of skin infectivity, classifying various ocular onchocercal lesions by association, have been the basic means of listing specific onchocercal eye lesions, and indirectly the means of assessing the prevalence rates of blindness or seriously impaired vision caused by this disease (1–10). There has been no agreement in evaluating skin infectivity rates, and so there must be some disagreement about the ocular classification. We should reconsider the techniques and standards best able to give a true prevalence rate of skin infectivity and density of infection in an individual and in a community (4, 11–13). For example, if the pooled estimate of variance in counting skin biopsies is $\pm 27$ (4) then a village in Abuja (13) classed as one in which there is mild skin infectivity $(+)$ could jump two places and become classed as a village in which there is severe infectivity $(+++)$ (14). Shade temperatures and biological variations must also have confused the issue in a number of projects (4, 12, 14).

2) *Which ocular lesions believed to be caused by onchocerciasis might lead to misclassification in field surveys*? The official list (11) is as follows: microfiliariae (mf) in anterior chamber; punctate keratitis; typical sclerosing keratitis alone or combined with anterior uveitis; chronic glaucoma; chorioretinitis; and optic atrophy. No ophthalmologist was a member of the 1965 Expert Committee that determined this list, published in 1966, although I was present in an advisory capacity. The ocular complications were extended arbitrarily by the Kenya Survey team as follows: punctate keratitis (fluffy opacities); sclerosing keratitis; mf in anterior chamber; chronic iritis; chorioretinitis (focal); optic atrophy; secondary glaucoma; cataract (vaguely); luxation or subluxation of the lens and degenerative onchocercal chorioretinitis.

The Abuja follow-up project (14) concluded that accuracy in assessment lay in considering a reduced number of lesions: 1) sclerosing keratitis exhibiting three zones (occasionally combined with large polyhedral punctate corneal opacities); 2) anterior uveitis demonstrating a pyriform pupil or (more important) a blue-milky-white flocculation at the pupil margin, or on the lens surface, in arcs or circles or clots; 3) posterior degenerative chorioretinopathy (Ridley fundus); 4) a complicated optic atrophy, unilateral or bilateral, where the nerve head is spattered with dense black pigment heaped up around a white disk-like heraldic ermine. Often there is an adjacent focus of chorioretinitis. These are the only truly specific lesions.

3) *Which ocular lesion or lesions should be selected as a potential threat to sight*? Even though there may be a risk of misclassification, the following list is presented as a basis for discussion. It can be divided into three; the so-called specific lesions mentioned in the section immediately above, suspicious lesions and lesions worth including in comparison studies, provided that an experienced ophthalmologist is to carry out the job. Thus, the four lesions mentioned above are potential threats and, in addition, early sclerosing keratitis (perhaps not exhibiting the three zones since the basal or peripheral, pigmented zone take time to develop); mf in the anterior chamber or a positive skin biopsy; evidence of any anterior uveitis (keratic precipitate cells, flare, synechiae, floccules) and early choroidal sclerosis (15) should be suspected; optic neuritis with or without a polyneuropathy; punctate keratitis, bearing in mind that Jones (16) describes 35 clinical types of punctate keratitis.

Other speakers suggest that what appear to be primary senile cataract and chronic simple glaucoma (17) may in fact be precipitated by onchocerciasis. If true, this is a most important new concept and widens the field for any extensive program of comparison. We shall also hear further evidence that the posterior degenerative lesion (the Ridley fundus), as distinct from the posterior exudative inflammatory lesion of onchocerciasis, does in fact exist with a rationalized pathogenesis (18, 19) confirming my longstanding views which have never been quoted except by the late Dr. Allan Woods.

Finally we must be absolutely sure about the observations made in Abuja (20) that with a very heavy skin infection and a low intake of one or more members of the vitamin B complex, we are not actually dealing with an optic and peripheral neuropathy.

Despite the lack of uniformity in collecting data, and despite the astounding number–65– of different criteria of blindness, all workers in endemic onchocercal areas have quickly become convinced that this is one of the major blinding disease of the world. Thus, it is important that we quickly reach a global decision as to how we should record blindness. An acceptable definition of blindness will, hopefully, be based on the subjective recording of visual acuities rather than on a socioeconomic or any other standard. The definition should make it possible to record and compare the idea of "seriously impaired vision" also in terms of acuity. Records should be of single eyes for statistical application and for a more accurate analysis of risk. The only method whereby all these aims can be achieved is by using the Landolt-C chart, which excludes guessing and can be understood by a child. If visual acuities are recorded for each eye, standards adopted as locally convenient will produce records directly comparable between one territory and the next. This will be in keeping with WHO's aims to obtain early diagnosis and to screen populations in a practical manner, so as to pursue epidemiological investigations and campaigns to prevent further blindness.

## REFERENCES

1. D'HAUSSY R, BOITHIAL R and BERTHET P. L'onchocercose oculaire. Bull Med AOF spec no 115, 1954.
2. BUDDEN FH. The epidemiology of onchocerciasis in northern Nigeria. Trans Soc Trop Med Hyg 50: 366, 1956.
3. D'HAUSSY R, PFISTER R, RIT J-M and BRETEAU G. Note sur les relations de l'onchocercose et de la syphilis au Soudan. Bull Soc Pathol Exot 50: 314, 1957.
4. RODGER FC. "Blindness in West Africa." London, Lewis, 1959, chap 4.
5. RODGER FC. The pathogenesis and pathology of ocular onchocerciasis. IV. The pathology. Am J Ophthalmol 49: 327, 1960.
6. RODGER FC. The pathogenesis and pathology of ocular onchocerciasis. IV. The pathology. Am J Ophthalmol 49: 560, 1960.
7. LAGRAULET J. L'étude de lésions oculaires dans l'Onchocerca cervicalis du cheval peut-elle apporter des données interessantes sur la pathogénie de l'onchocercose oculaire humaine? Bull Soc Pathol Exot 55: 417, 1962.
8. BUDDEN FH. The incidence of microfilariae in the eye and of ocular lesions in relation to the age and sex of persons living in communities where onchocerciasis is endemic. Trans R Soc Trop Med Hyg 57: 71, 1963.
9. MONJUSIAU AGM, LAGRAULET JD, D'HAUSSY R and GÖCKEL CW. Aspects ophthalmologiques de l'onchocercose au Guatemala et en Afrique occidentale. Bull WHO 32: 339, 1965.
10. WOODRUFF AW, CHOYCE DP, PRINGLE G, LAING ABG, HILLS M and WEGESA P. Onchocerciasis in Tanzania: the disease, its epidemiology and its relationship to ocular complications. Trans R Soc Trop Med Hyg 60: 695, 1966.
11. WHO Expert Committee on Onchocerciasis. Second report. WHO Tech Rep Ser 335: 95, 1966.
12. LARTIGUE J-J. Variations du nombre de microfilaires d'Onchocerca volvulus contenues dans des biopsies cutanées pratiquées à différentes heures de la journée. Bull WHO 36: 491, 1967.
13. DAVIES JB. The Simulium Control Scheme at Abuja, Northern Nigeria, and its effect on the prevalence of onchocerciasis in the area. Bull WHO 39: 187, 1968.
14. RODGER FC. The simulium control scheme at Abuja, North Nigeria and its effect on the prevalence of ocular onchocerciasis in the area. AFR ONCH 17 unpublished WHO document, 1971.
15. CHOYCE DP. Onchocerciasis: ophthalmic aspects. Trans R Soc Trop Med Hyg 60: 720, 1966.
16. JONES BR. Differential diagnosis of punctate keratitis. Int Ophthalmol Clin 2: 591, 1962.
17. BEN SIRA I and YASSUR Y. A comparative study of 500 onchocerciasis cases and 500 controls with regard to the posterior segment lesions in the eye. Isr J Med Sci 8:1156, 1972.
18. NEUMANN E and GUNDERS AE. The posterior segment lesions of ocular onchocerciasis. Histological aspects. Isr J Med Sci 8: 1158, 1972.
19. GUNDERS AE and Neuman 6. Parasitology and diagnosis of onchocerciasis, with special reference to the outer eye. Isr J Med Sci 8: 1139, 1972.
20. SCRIMSHAW NS, TAYLOR CE and GORDON JE. "Interactions of nutrition and infection." WHO Monog Ser 57, 1968.

# EPIDEMIOLOGY OF OCULAR ONCHOCERCIASIS IN FRENCH-SPEAKING COUNTRIES OF WEST AFRICA

## J. LAGRAULET

Institut de Médecine Tropicale, Paris XVe, France

The French-speaking countries of West Africa pay a heavy toll in onchocerciasis, particularly in the endemic areas of Tenkodogo, Diebougou and Ordara in Mali, and in the endemic regions of Kayes, Bougouni, Korosso and Sikasso in Upper Volta. In these areas, both the severity of the eye lesions and the extent of the resulting blindness are well known. Other regions are also affected, but to a lesser degree. These include Senegal, the Tiassale region of Ivory Coast, the Macenta district of Guinea, Dahomey in the Mono valley and Niger. This report describes some of our observations in these regions.

*Savannah onchocerciasis, forest onchocerciasis and ocular lesions.* The *Simulium* vector of onchocerciasis needs running water for the development of its larvae, and their breeding places are therefore on the banks of rivers. This means that the main areas of onchocerciasis are situated in the rich agricultural regions. Unfortunately, irrigation provided by the construction of dams has created new breeding sites and, consequently, new breeding areas.

This is now a very serious problem, especially in the savannah. It is here that the inhabitants themselves have established the cause-and-effect relationship between running water and blindness. This has forced them to abandon these rich farm areas. In the light of this experience, it would seem unwise to develop new areas of artificial irrigation.

We have noted that the ocular lesions in the savannah are much more severe than in the forest areas. Rodger has suggested that there may be a deficiency of vitamin A among the inhabitants of the savannah which could be an aggravating factor. However, a nutritional survey which we conducted revealed no hypovitaminosis A, an observation confirmed by others.

There may possibly be epidemiologically different types of onchocerciasis in these regions, although this has not been established. If the ocular lesions are more severe in the savannah than in the forest areas, it is because the intensity of infestation is higher in the savannah. In the forests, the high humidity allows for a wide dispersion of the female *Simulium*. In the savannah, on the other hand, the *Simulium* are concentrated around their breeding places, and bite the nearby population in great numbers.

*Relationship of the degree of infestation to the proximity of the breeding sites.* In the savannah, the villages are considered to be hyperinfested when 70 to 95% of the population have the disease. These villages are usually situated less than 2 km away from the breeding areas. At 4 km, the degree of infestation is only 10% while at 8 km, it is practically nil.

Although this relationship does not always hold true, nevertheless we can say that in the savannah, the intensity of infestation is generally higher in those villages having the highest rates of infestation.

*Relationship of ocular lesions to intensity of infestation.* There is a direct relationship between the intensity of infestation and the severity of the ocular lesions. Whereas there are no ocular lesions in the early stages, later ones produce severe lesions, such as sclerosing keratitis, iritis and chorioretinal lesions.

It is therefore important to assess the intensity of infestation, especially in the early stages. Two methods are presently available:

1) Total count of nodules or groups of nodules: This is not always easy due to the presence of composite nodules, which makes it difficult to assess the number of individual nodules. On the other hand, both small and large nodules exist, the larger ones being much more productive than the smaller ones, provided that they are still active.

This finding has given rise to the notion of living and dead nodules, both of which may degenerate spontaneously. We have recently shown that about 80% of the nodules in children under 10 years of age showed the degenerative process. Between the ages of 20 and 40, about half of the nodules were still active, whereas in people over 45 years of age, less than 40% contained live worms.

Nevertheless, the nodule is not an obligatory manifestation of onchocerciasis. In Venezuela, for example, only 30% of the affected individuals have nodules, compared with 70 to 80% in Africa. The counting of nodules is therefore unreliable in the evaluation of the degree of infestation.

2) Cutaneous biopsies: These are absolutely essential. Ideally, several should be performed: two on the upper extremities, and two on the lower. In our experience, one can find 60 microfilariae in one biopsy and only one or two in another one taken from the same person. In Africa, biopsies from the lower body (trochanter, iliac crest and calf) are more frequently positive than those from the upper sites.

The best way to perform a comparative count of microfilariae is with a Moria forceps. Circular biopsies measuring 2.2 mm in diameter are thus obtained, nearly all of similar weight. The biopsies remain in a drop of water or physiological saline for 30 min before counting. This method gives a reasonably accurate assessment of the intensity of infestation, provided that several biopsies are performed on the same patient.

*Other factors affecting the severity of the ocular lesions.* 1) Race: Europeans are infested as frequently as Africans, since persons working in the proximity of breeding places are exposed equally to *Simulium* bites. Racial factors do not, therefore, play a role.

2) Sex: Men are more frequently bitten than women because they work outside of their homes. Since they usually present a higher intensity of infestation, they are more frequently affected by severe ocular lesions.

3) Although ocular lesions may appear at any age, they are seldom found in children under the age of four. These lesions are usually benign (punctate keratitis, for example). It is only in the older age groups that we find severe corneal lesions, iridocyclitis or chorioretinitis. The latter condition is very rare in young people under the age of 20.

4) Location of nodules: It has long been held that the ocular lesions are related to the location of the nodules. However, this view has been invalidated by many investigators. Ocular lesions are more frequently seen among Africans in whom the nodules are generally situated on the lower extremities than among Central Americans, in whom the nodules are usually found on the upper extremities. Nevertheless the location of the nodules is a good indicator of the site of the *Simulium* bite. Thus, we have observed that only head nod-

ules are present in African infants. This is because during their first years of life, children can be bitten only on the head, due to the African custom of carrying the wrapped infant on his mother's back.

In Guatemala, *Simulium ochraceum* bites are found only on the upper parts of the body, and the nodules are situated in the same area. But in Venezuela, *Simulium metallicum* bites are present on the lower extremities, and nodules appear only in the lower body regions.

*Types of eye lesions.* Limbal inflammation does not seem to be related to onchocerciasis, nor does onchocercal conjunctivitis exist. In our opinion there may be only a transient hyperemia due to a discharge of toxic substances of microfilarial origin. No conjunctival nodules have been found in over 5,000 affected patients examined by us.

Punctate keratitis, which is the most frequent manifestation, is the characteristic lesion of the disease. It is found in 30 to 50% of the patients. Sclerosing keratitis is sometimes found, but the advanced stage of semilunar and total keratitis has rarely been observed by us.

Microfilariae may be found in the anterior chamber in more than 20% of the patients. It is important to do biomicroscopic examinations since the presence of microfilariae in the aqueous humor may be the only sign of onchocerciasis (5% of patients).

Iritis is usually chronic, although some have frequently observed acute iritis. Iris atrophy is frequently present even in normal subjects, so that only stage III of iris atrophy should be considered as being associated with onchocerciasis. Although the piriform pupil is typical of the disease, it is seldom found.

The fundus may be affected in several stages. The first is the dappled stage, followed by tigroid and "Ridley" stages, the latter being pathognomonic of the disease. The fundus resembles cracked and dried mud. Histologically we find chorioretinitis following the inflammatory lesions. Vasculitis is predominant and is responsible for the degenerative lesions.

*Blindness from onchocerciasis.* Approximately one-third of the blindness is caused by the corneal lesions, another third by iritis and the remainder by chorioretinal degeneration.

*Survey of the savannah and forest areas.* The results of surveys in patients from Upper Volta, a highly endemic savannah district, compared with surveys from forest areas of lower endemicity are summarized in Table 1.

TABLE 1.  *Survey of ocular lesions in patients from a savannah district and a forest area*

| Ocular lesion | % of patients affected | |
|---|---|---|
| | Savannah district (2,170 patients) | Forest area (714 patients) |
| Keratitis | 39.2 | 18.5 |
| Microfilariae in anterior chamber | 21.4 | 6.5 |
| Iris lesions | 6.3 | 2.3 |
| Fundus disturbances | 9.8 | 3.1 |
| Blindness | 8.5 | 1.1 |

# A COMPARATIVE STUDY OF 500 CASES OF ONCHOCERCIASIS AND 500 CONTROLS WITH REGARD TO POSTERIOR SEGMENT LESIONS IN THE EYE

I. BEN SIRA and Y. YASSUR

Department of Ophthalmology, Hadassah University Hospital, Jerusalem, Israel

Epidemiological (1), clinical (2) and histological (3) studies indicate that a cause-and-effect relationship exists between onchocerciasis and certain posterior segment lesions. Regional differences have been noted both in the prevalence and in the clinical appearance of these lesions. The reasons for these discrepancies are poorly understood at the present time. There are as yet no comparative epidemiological studies which take into account the influence of regionally prevalent diseases and the roles played by nutrition and heredity.

We recently described certain aspects of the anterior segment lesions in onchocerciasis (4). The present report, based on the same comparative study, deals with the prevalence and nature of the fundal pathology in Malawi.

## MATERIALS AND METHODS

"Materials and Methods" were the same as those previously described (4). One-third of the cases in the two groups came from a village near the center of the endemic focus, while the other two-thirds were inhabitants of three other villages at the periphery of the focus (5). Onchocerciasis was diagnosed if microfilariae (mf) were present in the skin of the outer canthus of the eye. Those with negative diagnoses of onchocerciasis served as controls. In the controls, there were no clinical signs of infection and six consecutive skin snip examinations given to each person were negative. The fundus was examined using Fison's indirect ophthalmoscope and a Zeiss direct electric ophthalmoscope.

## RESULTS AND DISCUSSION

Abnormal findings resembling onchocercal posterior segment lesions were seen in 25 of 500 patients with onchocerciasis, and in 22 of 500 controls. None of the lesions resembled the so-called Ridley's classical posterior segment lesion. Senile choroidal atrophy and choroidal sclerosis were encountered in eight patients with onchocerciasis and in 10 controls. No significant differences in the nature of the posterior segment lesion were found when comparing the two groups (Table 1).

The prevalence and incidence of onchocercal fundal lesions are controversial points,

TABLE 1. *Principal fundal lesions in 500 patients with onchocerciasis and in 500 controls*

| Ocular lesion | Onchocerciasis group | Control group |
|---|---|---|
| Opaque vitreous | 3 | 0 |
| Pigmentary mascular degeneration | 4 | 2 |
| Choroidal atrophy and sclerosis | 8 | 10 |
| Small pigmented choroidal patches | 2 | 4 |
| Retinitis proliferans | 0 | 1 |
| Glaucomatous excavation of optic nerve | 7 | 4 |
| Optic nerve atrophy | 1 | 1 |

TABLE 2. *Prevalence of posterior segment lesions in cases of onchocerciasis reported in the literature*

| Reference no. | % with lesions | Country |
|---|---|---|
| 10 | 41.5 | Ghana |
| 9 | 6.7 | Chad |
| 2 | 24.0 | Ghana |
| 11 | 0.0 | Malawi |
| 8 | 0.0 | Malawi |
| 7 | 1.0 | England |
| 7 | 1.0 | Tanzania |
| Present study | 5.0 | Malawi |

TABLE 3. *Clinical appearance and description of posterior segment lesions in cases of onchocerciasis reported in the literature*

| Lesions | Ref. no. |
|---|---|
| Inflammatory choroidal sclerosis | 1 |
| Pigmented chorioretinitis | 3 |
| Choroidoretinal degeneration | 2 |
| Posterior exudative uveitis | 6 |
| Choroidal sclerosis and retinal pigmentation | 12 |
| Disseminated choroidoretinitis | 13 |

summarized in Table 2. The variability in the clinical appearance of the posterior segment lesions is reflected in the many different names ascribed to them (Table 3).

The pathogenesis of the posterior segment lesion is by no means clear. Ridley (2) and Hissette (3) think that the lesion is an inflammation, aggravated by the local death of the mf. This view was supported by finding mf in the choroid (3). Rodger (6) described two types of posterior segment lesion, "exudative" and "degenerative", which were etiologically, clinically and histologically distinct. Choyce (7) proposed a genetic origin for some of the lesions, whereas other investigators felt that nutritional factors such as vitamin A deficiency play a role in their development (6). Regardless of the factors involved, the exact nature of the posterior segment lesion is still unknown.

The absence of significant differences in either the prevalence or the nature of the posterior segment lesions in our two groups raises some doubt as to whether there is in fact a direct relationship between onchocerciasis and fundal lesions. This view is supported by a number of reports from East Africa (8 and P. H. Williams, personal communication), Chad (9) and Central America (7) where very few posterior segment lesions were encountered. We think that other comparative epidemiological studies similar to ours may elucidate the mystery of these lesions, especially if the studies are carried out in areas where posterior segment lesions are common. Such investigations should include a comprehensive search for other etiological factors that might be responsible for the lesions.

## REFERENCES

1. BUDDEN FH. Comparative study of onchocerciasis in savannah and rain forest. *Trans R Soc Trop Med Hyg* **57**: 64, 1963.
2. RIDLEY H. Ocular onchocerciasis including an investigation of the Gold Coast. *Br J Ophthalmol* Monograph suppl. 10, London, G. Pulman and Sons Ltd, 1945.
3. HISSETTE J. Ocular onchocerciasis. *Am J Trop Med (Suppl)* **18**: 58, 1938.
4. BEN SIRA I, TICHO U and YASSUR Y. Onchocerciasis in Malawi. Ocular manifestations. *Br J Ophthalmol* (in press).
5. BEN SIRA I, TICHO U and YASSUR Y. Onchocerciasis in Malawi. Distribution and prevalence. *Trans R Soc Trop Med Hyg* **66**: 296, 1972.
6. RODGER FC. Posterior degenerative lesion of onchocerciasis. *Br J Ophthalmol* **42**: 21, 1958.
7. CHOYCE DP. Ocular onchocerciasis in Central America, Africa and the British Isles. *Trans R Soc Trop Med Hyg* **58**: 11, 1964.
8. HARVEY RJ. The early diagnosis and treatment of onchocerciasis. *Cent Afr J Med* **13**: 242, 1967.
9. VON NOORDEN GK and BUCK A. Ocular onchocerciasis, an ophthalmologic. l and epidemiological study in an African village. *Arch Ophthalmol* **80**: 26, 1968.
10. MCLEAN CM. Ocular onchocerciasis in Northern Ghana. *Br J Ophthalmol* **43**: 447, 1959.
11. GOPSIL WL. Onchocerciasis in Nyasaland. *Trans R Soc Trop Med Hyg* **32**: 551, 1939.
12. D'HAUSSY R, RIT JM and LAGRAULET J. Contribution a l'étude des lésions du fond d'oeil dans l'onchocercose. *Méd trop (Mars)* **18**: 340, 1958.
13. SARKIES JWR. Ocular onchocerciasis. *Br J Ophthalmol* **36**: 81, 1952.

# THE POSTERIOR SEGMENT LESION OF OCULAR ONCHOCERCIASIS

## HISTOLOGICAL ASPECTS

E. NEUMANN and A. E. GUNDERS

Eye Department, Rothschild Municipal–Government Hospital and Aba Khoushy Medical School, Haifa, and Department of Medical Ecology, Hebrew University–Hadassah Medical School, Jerusalem, Israel

This study concerns a 25-year-old man who was admitted to the eye clinic of the Monrovia Government Hospital in Liberia due to gradual loss of vision during the past 10 years. The right eye was blind and vision in the left eye was 6/12, but the patient was unable to count fingers in front of his eye because of extreme constriction of the visual field. Intraocular pressure was normal. Live microfilariae of *Onchocerca volvulus* were seen in the anterior chamber of both eyes, and fundoscopy revealed a typical posterior segment lesion of

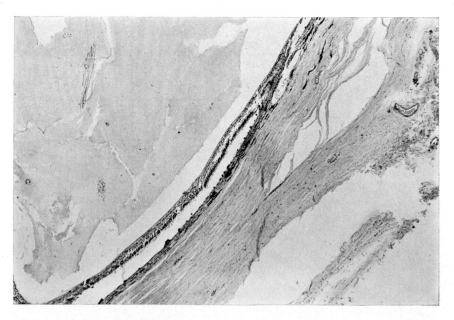

FIG. 1. The edge of the posterior segment lesion of onchocerciasis, showing fusion of the atrophic choroid and retina. The retinal detachment is an artifact. Hematoxylin and eosin. × 30.

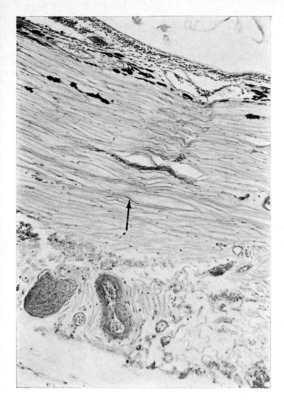

FIG. 2. The fused chorioretinal lesion of onchocerciasis at higher magnification. Clumps of pigment are scattered throughout the atrophic choroid. Almost the entire length of a live microfilaria is seen deep within the sclera (arrow). Hematoxylin and eosin. × 65.

onchocerciasis surrounding a pale, waxy disk.

The skin changes were moderate, and limited to the lower extremities. There were no onchocercomata. Microfilarial skin counts at 12 body sites revealed high counts over the hips and outer canthus of the eye with lower counts on the shoulders and forearms.

The right blind eye was enucleated since there were repeated attacks of pain; microphotographs were taken from serial sagittal sections of the posterior segment. Fig. 1 shows a low-power view of the edge of the chorioretinal lesion surrounding the disk and macula. Within the lesion the choroid

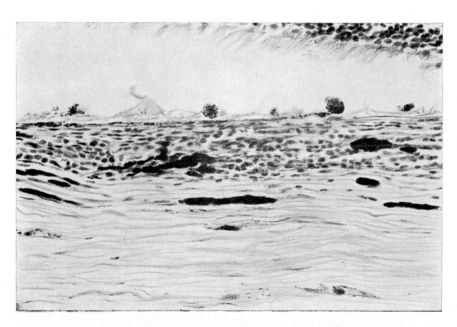

FIG. 3. High power view of the choroid, peripheral to the area of fusion of the choroid and retina. The hexagonal cells are atrophic and the pigment in this layer is aggregated in small round masses. Note the round cell infiltration and the clumps of pigment within the choroid. Hematoxylin and eosin. × 300.

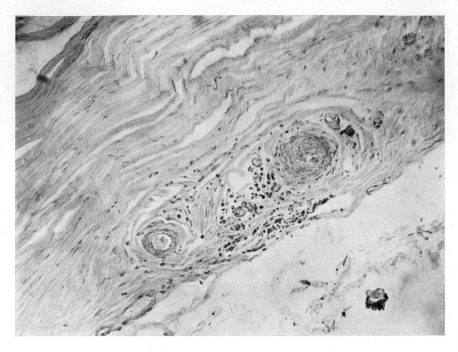

FIG. 4. Marked plasma cell infiltration surrounding posterior ciliary arteries inside the sclera. The larger artery shows a thickened wall with a markedly narrowed lumen. Hematoxylin and eosin. × 75.

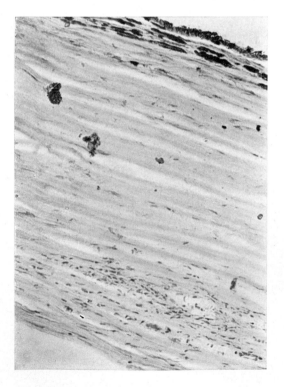

and retina were atrophic and fused to one another. Beyond this area there was an abrupt change to normal choroid and retina. Hence the apparent retinal detachment is an artifact. Higher magnification (Fig. 2) showed that the choriocapillaris and the outer retinal layers were missing, and Bruch's membrane could not be identified. At the center of the lesion (not shown in Fig. 2) only the larger blood vessels of the choroid and retina and the internal limiting membrane remained.

Fig. 3 shows a high power view of the choroid and retina just peripheral to the area of fusion where the cells of the hexagonal pigment layer were atrophic, the pigment was heaped up in masses and the choroidal capillaries were sparse. There was dense, patchy pigmentation of the choroid (see also Fig. 2,

FIG. 5. Plasma cell infiltration surrounding a small blood vessel in the outer third of the sclera underlying the chorioretinal lesion. Hematoxylin and eosin. × 95.

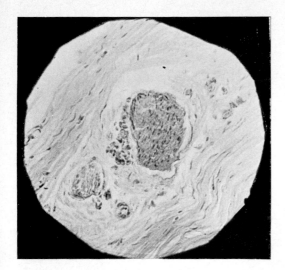

FIG. 6. A crescent of plasma cells adjacent to a posterior ciliary nerve in the sclera. Hematoxylin and eosin. × 80.

5, 8). The retina in this area and throughout the peripheral fundus was normal except for the fact that nuclei were scarce in the ganglion cell layer. The optic nerve was atrophic, with cavernous spaces, columnar gliosis and thickening of the septa.

Foci of round-cell infiltration were present in the choroid surrounding blood vessels and nerves in the sclera especially in its outer third and in the loose connective tissue behind the globe. Basophilic, amorphous debris of microfilariae could be identified in most of the larger infiltrates. Fig. 4 shows marked round-cell infiltration, consisting mainly of plasma cells with a few eosinophils, surrounding two posterior ciliary arteries. The larger artery had a thickened wall and a markedly narrowed lumen. However, serial sections showed all the other posterior ciliary arteries to be fully patent.

One of several infiltrates surrounding the smaller blood vessels in the outer third of the sclera in the area underlying the fused choroid and retina is shown in Fig. 5. A crescent of plasma cells adjacent to a ciliary nerve in the sclera of the posterior pole was also found (Fig. 6).

Live microfilariae of *O. volvulus* were observed outside and within the sclera and occasionally within the chorioretinal lesion. Almost the entire length of a live microfilaria could be seen in the sclera under low power (Fig. 2). Microfilariae were also seen in other

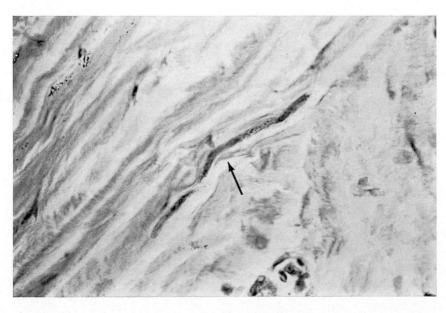

FIG. 7. High power view of a live *O. volvulus* microfilaria deep within the sclera. Hematoxylin and eosin. × 480.

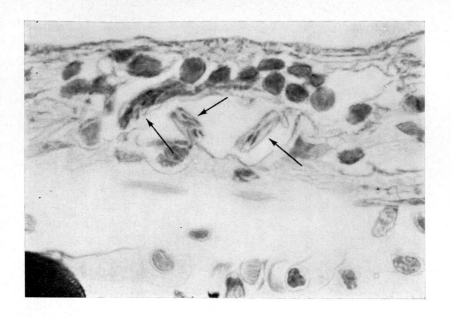

FIG. 8. Three fragments of live *O. volvulus* microfilariae within the atrophic retina (arrows). Clumping of pigment within the atrophic choroid. Hematoxylin and eosin. × 1,200.

parts of the sclera (Fig. 7) and in the chorio-retinal lesion where a section was made passing through three fragments of live microfilariae (Fig. 8).

### DISCUSSION

Histopathological reports on the posterior segment lesion of onchocerciasis are rare, and none of the cases published to date have shown as much inflammatory activity as the present one, nor have they demonstrated the portal of entry of microfilariae into the posterior part of the globe. Our findings indicate that microfilariae penetrate the sclera alongside the posterior ciliary arteries and nerves, and are found in small numbers in the choroid and retina. The chorioretinal lesion is apparently due to an inflammatory reaction caused by the death of microfilariae *in situ*, within the posterior part of the globe; or to the diffusion of toxic products from a disintegrating microfilaria into the choroid and retina. Over a period of years, numerous small inflammatory foci in the fundus would result in the coalescence of areas of chorioretinal atrophy around the optic disk.

# SELECTIVE PREVENTIVE TREATMENT OF ONCHOCERCIASIS

F. C. RODGER

Princess Margaret Hospital, Swindon, Cirencester, England

The public health ophthalmologist knows the answer to the question: "Do we cure the curable or prevent the preventable in onchocerciasis?" The ocular lesions are always irreversible, and we have not yet learned how to interrupt progression from an early lesion to partial sightedness or from the latter to total blindness. There are only a few equivocal case reports of individuals treated under the best of circumstances.

The obvious starting point is to destroy the vector; the next most obvious is to reduce the human reservoir by nodulectomy or chemotherapy. These approaches have been tried for over 20 years, and the results have been disappointing largely because of lack of precontrol data.

There is no drug which kills the adult worm, whose life span was assessed on the basis of two cases in Buenos Aires by Diaz in 1940 to be from 15 to 20 years. This was confirmed in the 1950s by myself in one patient who had settled outside the endemic area. Finally, this was further verified on a large scale by the Kenyan follow-up in which Dr. Neumann of Israel was involved.

Suramin has not proven itself in widespread campaigns. Some people have adhered to their faith in this drug despite the extremely doubtful evidence of its efficacy, the danger to life (it has probably caused more deaths than we know) and its impracticability since it is administered intravenously. Microfilaricides are different—they work and are safe; but the adult filariae continue to produce new larvae in a matter of days or weeks after the course, which has no effect on them. There is no chemotherapeutic cure for half a million people, even if any country could afford one if it were discovered.

Nodulectomy, which is still widely practiced in Guatemala, is harder to evaluate. As in the case of massive campaigns with drugs, lack of ocular data on pretreatment has negated every single trial. Statistics published in Guatemala seem unlikely: in 1935, 17 out of every 1,000 infected by the disease were blind; in 1945, one person per 1,000 infected was blind. This figure was given by Diaz in support of nodulectomy campaigns. In 1965 the number of persons with skin infestation was officially published by the Bureau of Public Health as 25,000, suggesting that there are only 25 people in all Guatemala blinded (on the basis of the 1945 statistics) by onchocerciasis. A follow-up in the same tea plantation in the San Yepocapa district made in the 1960s, 20 years after the first eye survey, revealed no difference in the incidence of blindness from onchocerciasis.

There is only one other obvious option: control of the vector. The fact is that after

20 years and 27 WHO reports on vector control (as compared with 37 WHO reports on the effect of drugs and seven WHO reports on the ocular aspects), it has not accomplished its purpose—reduction of the incidence of blindness or of ocular lesions. There has been a lack of dependable data before control started, and poor evaluation throughout. Nineteen years after the Kenyan eradication program, people are still being blinded because of the long life span of *Onchocerca volvulus*.

A classic example of what vector control means today is the recent project, the Kainji Dam. Evaluation after several years reveals that there were no reliable data on fly densities before control commenced. Ocular data were not given. It was simply felt that treating the dam area would benefit the local inhabitants. A recurrent expenditure of £ 30,000 rising to £ 35,000 annually has had to be maintained by the Nigerian Government for a project originally planned to cover 3,000 square miles but which has grown to over 10,000 square miles, since windborne migration from distant breeding sites (not aestivation) is responsible for the annual reinfestation of the rivers feeding the dam. In this way the scheme has had to be extended a little more every year. Vector control and cost must keep expanding to be effective until the whole endemic area of Africa is treated. I am, therefore, against the indiscriminate use of vector control in endemic areas.

What kind of area requires measures to prevent blindness from onchocerciasis and what should these measures be? There is a great variation in the prevalence of ocular lesions from place to place, which of course bears some relation to the density of the infection but little to the infectivity rate. Onchocerciasis can, in certain areas, account for 100% infectivity and 100% of all the blindness, overlaying other coincident ocular diseases.

In order to decide where one is justified in carrying out control, we must know the incidence, or at least the prevalence and the severity of onchocerciasis ocular lesions and decide if the people otherwise find life unbearable. There may, for example, be an area with only a moderate prevalence of blindness, but associated with excessive biting and intensive itching which, combined, make life unbearable.

Vector control should be recommended when blindness occurs at a certain level and when life is unbearable for the people. This is *selective* prevention. Where life is bearable, vector control should not be recommended, although there might be a relative prevalence as high as 20% onchocerciasis blindness (less than cataract) and a skin infectivity of up to 78%. The objective here should be to improve the quality of life, carry out cataract surgery and improve nutrition. This too is *selective* prevention. Neither approach will necessarily prevent the ocular lesions of onchocerciasis.

Hence, control should not be carried out as a single project since it is not certain that it will do more than reduce biting (maybe itching) for the next 20 years. The hypotheses outlined in general terms in my earlier speech could be tested area against area within "unbearable" and "bearable" areas or compared among different terrains, or races, or diets. It would be interesting to discover if an increase in the quality of life in an "unbearable" area made any difference in the short term, for example, three years, in the prevalence of ocular lesions at least in comparison with a similar area where vector control alone was put into effect.

Some of the severest skin reactions as well as some of the severest ocular reactions to infection are seen in very early cases. Repeated ocular inflammations become either less severe or more severe as time goes on. Thus, we should devise schemes to study the effect of inducing or boosting premunity in children and immunity in young adults.

An example would be to study the effect of a six-monthly or annual short course of diethyl carbamazine (HETRAZAN®) which, by killing a large proportion of the larvae, would boost the antibodies. One group would receive γ-globulin as a supplement and a control group would not receive any. A highly imaginative and sophisticated integrated program of research combined with some of the vector projects is needed in areas selected as "unbearable" and "bearable" or in those in which projects are already planned.

The Volta River Basin Scheme, costing 37 million dollars, incorporates an improvement in the quality of life on a large scale and not vector control alone which would simply turn the Volta Basin into a large DDT powder box with unknown effects on the ecology. Any plan should, however, be preceded by rigorous ocular surveys and evaluated regularly by ophthalmologists, since after the scheme gets under way, these studies will be impossible.

# TOPICAL DIETHYLCARBAMAZINE IN OCULAR ONCHOCERCIASIS

E. AVIEL and R. DAVID

Department of Ophthalmology, Hadassah University Hospital, Jerusalem, Israel

Systemic diethylcarbamazine has been reported to be effective against the microfilariae (mf) of *Onchocerca volvulus* but the exact mode of action of the drug is not clear (1, 2). Topical administration of diethylcarbamazine was first reported in rabbits and no adverse effects were found (3). Clinical trials carried out afterward, using a 5% solution of the drug, suggested that it may be effective in bringing about the disappearance of mf from the anterior chamber (4). This report describes the results of further clinical trials in six patients harboring mf in the anterior chamber.

## MATERIALS AND METHODS

The patients were Africans living in the Cholo district, an endemic area in southern Malawi. The Cholo district in the Shire Highlands is hilly with lush vegetation and includes several fast flowing streams, thus providing a favorable habitat for the black fly vector, *Simulium damnosum*.

All the patients who attended the outpatient department of the Cholo Hospital had skin snips taken from the outer canthus of the eye over a period of three days. The eyes of those patients who were positive for mf were subsequently examined with the Haag Streit slit lamp set at high power. The mf appear in the wide beam of the lamp as snake-like larvae (8 × 300 μm) which actively swim in the aqueous. Skin snips were taken from 750 patients and 65 were positive for mf. Of this latter group, 21 also had mf in the anterior chamber. However, only six of these patients could be persuaded to enter the central hospital in Blantyre (25 miles away) for treatment since none of the patients had eye symptoms and the pressure of agricultural work was great.

Information on the ocular condition of the six patients is shown in Table 1. All the patients had floaters in the aqueous. Nummular and snowflake scars in the cornea as well as pigment invasion of the corneal periphery were present in all but one of the patients. The fundi were normal in four of the patients, but in the female patient suffering from cataract and in one patient with corneal scarring, the fundi could not be properly examined.

A solution of 3% diethylcarbamazine was administered four times daily in the lower conjunctival fornix of the right eye. The left eye was not treated. Treatment continued for 7 to 15 days. In all patients, slit lamp examinations for live mf in the anterior segment of both eyes were made three times daily. This was continued even after cessation of drug treatment. Although more than five mf were occasionally found in one eye, the maximum figure listed in the results does not exceed this number because it is difficult to assess accurately more than five actively motile mf within a single eye.

## RESULTS

Only in Patient 4 did mf disappear from the treated eye 48 hr after the start of the therapy. In this case the anterior chamber remained clear for five consecutive days during treatment, but on interruption of the therapy, mf reappeared the next day. Patients 2 and 5 showed a reduction in the number of mf but

TABLE 1.   Ocular condition of patients before diethylcarbamazine therapy

| Patient no. | Age | Sex | Visual acuity | | Intraocular tension | | Cornea of Both eyes | Presence of mf in anterior chamber of both eyes | Lens of both eyes | Fundi | |
|---|---|---|---|---|---|---|---|---|---|---|---|
| | | | Right eye | Left eye | Right eye | Left eye | | | | Right eye | Left eye |
| 1 | 55 | M | 6/6 | 6/6 | 17.3 | 17.3 | Nummular corneal opacities, pigment invasion | Floaters, mf | Normal | Normal | Normal |
| 2 | 30 | M | 3/60 | 4/60 | 20.6 | 17.3 | Corneal scarring from applications of traditional medicine | Floaters, mf | Normal | Hazy view in both eyes | |
| 3 | 65 | M | 6/12 | 6/18 | 18.9 | 17.3 | Nummular corneal opacities, pigment invasion | Floaters, mf | Normal | Normal | Normal |
| 4 | 23 | M | 6/5 | 6/5 | 14.6 | 14.6 | Normal | Floaters, mf | Normal | Normal | Normal |
| 5 | 35 | M | 6/9 | 6/9 | 15.9 | 15.9 | Nummular corneal opacities, pigment invasion | Floaters, mf | Normal | Normal | Normal |
| 6 | 60 | F | Perception of light | 3/60 | 17.3 | 18.9 | Nummular corneal opacities, pigment invasion | Floaters, mf | Cataract | Not seen | Hazy view |

TABLE 2.   Mf counts in the anterior chamber during trial therapy with diethylcarbamazine

| Patient no. | Eye | No. of days from start of treatment | | | | | | | | | | | | | | | | |
|---|---|---|---|---|---|---|---|---|---|---|---|---|---|---|---|---|---|---|
| | | 1 | 2 | 3 | 4 | 5 | 6 | 7 | 8 | 9 | 10 | 11 | 12 | 13 | 14 | 15 | 16 | 17 |
| 1 | Right | 5,5,5 | 3,2,1 | 1,0,0 | 0,0,1 | 2,1,2 | 3,1,0 | 0,0,0 | 2,1,1 | 2,1,1 | 2,1,0 | 1,1,0 | L 0,0,0 | 0,0,0 | 0,0,0 | 1,1,0 | | |
| | Left | 3,2,1 | 0,0,0 | 0,0,0 | 0,0,0 | 0,0,0 | 0,0,0 | 0,0,0 | 1,1,2 | 1,2,1 | 2,0,1 | 1,0,0 | 0,1,0 | 2,0,1 | 0,2,2 | 0,1,0 | | |
| 2 | Right | 2,1,0 | 1,1,0 | 0,0,0 | 1,1,1 | 2,1,0 | 0,0,0 | 0,0,0 | 0,0,0 | 0,0,0 | 3,1,0 | 0,1,1 | 0,0,0 | 0,0,0 | 3,2,0 | L 2,1,0 | 2,1,1 | 0,0,0 |
| | Left | 3,2,0 | 1,1,4 | 3,1,0 | 2,1,1 | 3,1,0 | 1,0,1 | 1,0,1 | 0,0,0 | 2,1,0 | L 2,1,0 | 2,2,1 | 1,5,4 | 1,2,4 | 3,2,4 | 3,4,4 | 3,3,3 | 0,1,1 |
| 3 | Right | 5,5,5 | 5,5,3 | 5,5,5 | 5,5,5 | 5,5,5 | 5,5,5 | 3,4,5 | 3,3,4 | 3,4,4 | 2,4,3 | 3,2,0 | 5,2,0 | 0,2,3 | 5,3,2 | 5,3,2 | | |
| | Left | 3,5,4 | 4,3,0 | 4,3,0 | 3,5,2 | 2,1,0 | 2,1,1 | L 3,2,1 | 1,0,0 | 0,0,0 | 2,1,1 | 0,1,1 | 1,1,1 | 2,3,4 | 2,1,0 | 2,2,1 | | |
| 4 | Right | 0,0,0 | 3,2,2 | 0,0,0 | 0,0,0 | 0,0,0 | 0,0,0 | 0,0,0 | 0,1,3 | 0,0,0 | 0,1,0 | 0,1,1 | 1,1,2 | | | | | |
| | Left | 1,0,0 | 1,3,2 | 0,0,0 | 0,1,1 | 0,1,0 | 0,0,0 | 0,1,0 | 0,0,0 | 0,0,0 | 0,0,0 | L 0,0,0 | 0,1,1 | | | | | |
| 5 | Right | 2,1,0 | 0,0,0 | 1,1,0 | 0,0,1 | 4,1,0 | 0,0,0 | L 0,0,0 | 0,0,0 | 0,1,0 | 0,0,0 | 0,0,0 | 0,0,0 | 1,3,2 | 1,1,2 | | | |
| | Left | 2,1,0 | 0,0,0 | 1,1,1 | 1,0,2 | 2,0,1 | 1,3,1 | 0,1,2 | 0,0,0 | 2,1,1 | 0,0,0 | 1,1,2 | 1,1,0 | 2,2,1 | 4,1,0 | | | |
| 6 | Right | 5,3,1 | 3,2,2 | 4,2,0 | 1,0,1 | 1,0,1 | 1,0,1 | 0,1,0 | 1,1,0 | 2,1,0 | 4,3,1 | 0,0,0 | 1,3,1 | 1,0,1 | | | | |
| | Left | 2,2,2 | 0,0,1 | 3,1,0 | 1,1,3 | 3,2,1 | 1,0,1 | 0,1,2 | 2,0,1 | 0,0,0 | 0,0,0 | 0,0,0 | 2,1,1 | 1,1,1 | | | | |

Three counts were made each day; the digits in the Table represent the mf counts made. Diethylcarbamazine treatments were started on Day 1; L above the values indicates the last day of drug treatment.

147

TABLE 3.  *Means of mf counts in treated and untreated eyes during therapy*

|  | Patient no. | | | | | |
| --- | --- | --- | --- | --- | --- | --- |
|  | *1* | *2* | *3* | *4* | *5* | *6* |
| Treated right eye | 1.25 | 0.56 | 4.33 | 0.33 | 0.38 | 1.38 |
| Untreated left eye | 0.53 | 1.66 | 1.80 | 0.52 | 0.76 | 1.24 |

TABLE 4. *Means of mf counts during and after therapy*

|  | Patient no. | | | | | |
| --- | --- | --- | --- | --- | --- | --- |
|  | *1* | *2* | *3* | *4* | *5* | *6* |
| During therapy | 1.25 | 0.56 | 4.33 | 0.33 | 0.38 | 1.38 |
| After therapy | 0.22 | 0.67 | 2.47 | 0.73 | 0.44 | 1.11 |

in the latter there was an increase after interruption of therapy. Patients 1, 3 and 6 showed no appreciable reduction in the mf count during the diethylcarbamazine treatment (Table 2).

There were wide variations in the mf count in all of the untreated eyes. In three of the patients, the average count was higher in the untreated eye than in the treated one, whereas the opposite was true in the other three patients (Table 3). A comparison of the means of mf count in the treated eyes during and after therapy showed higher counts in half of the patients and lower counts in the other half (Table 4).

There were no signs of irritation after treatment except in one patient in whom the mf disappeared temporarily from the anterior chamber. Although showing conjunctival infection after the third day of treatment, he experienced no discomfort and the reaction disappeared spontaneously.

## DISCUSSION

In only one of the six patients in the present trial was there apparently a clear effect of diethylcarbamazine therapy on the number of mf in the anterior chamber. If the initial count is high, possibly due to the presence of an onchocercal nodule in the vicinity of the eye, it tends to remain so throughout the duration of the trial irrespective of whether or not treatment is given. Although longer periods of observation were desirable, it was impossible to keep the patients hospitalized further. This may continue to be a major difficulty in any future trials of this type.

The results of the present trial were inconclusive, not only because of the small number of cases but also because of the wide variations in mf counts in the untreated eyes. Also, in the present trial, a 3% solution of diethylcarbamazine was used whereas a 5% solution was used previously (4). The higher concentration caused edema of the lids and conjunctival injection.

More extensive trials are necessary before conclusions can be reached as to the value of topical applications of diethylcarbamazine in the treatment of ocular onchocerciasis.

Supported by a grand from the National Society for the Prevention of Blindness, New York.

## REFERENCES

1. BURCH TA and ASHBURN LL. Experimental therapy of onchocerciasis with suramin and Hetrazan. *Am J Trop Med Hyg* **31**: 617, 1951.
2. HAWKING F. The chemotherapy of filarial infection. *Pharmacol Rev* **7**: 279, 1955.
3. LAZAR M, LIEBERMAN TW, FURMAN M and LEOPOLD IH. Ocular penetration of Hetrazan in rabbits. *Am J Ophthalmol* **66**: 215, 1968.
4. BEN-SIRA I, AVIEL E, LAZAR M, LIEBERMAN TW and LEOPOLD IH. Topical Hetrazan in the treatment of ocular onchocerciasis. *Am J Ophthalmol* **70**: 741, 1970.

# DISCUSSION

MR. J. DOBREE (*UK*): This is the ideal time for a series of long-term studies on the natural evaluation of onchocerciasis modeled after those carried out for glaucoma and diabetic retinopathy. These studies are essential for a proper evaluation of treatment. It is necessary for such studies to be carried out over a considerable length of time by workers who are well equipped and likely to stay in the same area for a sufficient period of time.

MR. F. C. RODGER (*U.K.*): Institutes for such studies do exist in Bamako in Mali and in Kampala where work has been going on for 15 years. It is necessary to incorporate more than one discipline—entomology, helminthology, ophthalmology—in this kind of work.

DR. A. E. GUNDERS (*Israel*): I am afraid that there will be violent reactions to the large-scale use of diethylcarbamazine among the population in endemic areas.

MR. RODGER: From my experience in Ghana, Nigeria and the Cameroons, I can state that no reaction to the drug in the eye ever diminished visual acuity. There was only a surface reaction accompanied by photophobia and lacrimation. Eventually there was an improvement in the symptomatology. The greatest reaction is in the skin and it does not seem to be controlled even by the use of steroids.

MR. D. P. CHOYCE (*U.K.*): An experiment with diethylcarbamazine and suramine in Guatemala done 20 years ago resulted in the death of several people. The large-scale use of these drugs would be risky. More basic information about the epidemiology of onchocerciasis is required, for instance the parallel study of onchocercal and nononchocercal patients in the same area.

DR. I. BEN-SIRA (*Israel*): Such studies are currently being conducted on a large scale in Nigeria.

DR. H. M. THOMAS (*Liberia*): Can prophylactic treatment be instituted on the same lines as for malaria?

MR. RODGER: Prophylactic chemotherapy should be tried.

MR. CHOYCE: I disagree and do not think that this is a practical proposition at all.

MR. RODGER: Yes, mass prophylactic chemotherapy has been shown to be impractical. Mass campaigns of this type have already been carried out in the former French territories. They always fail on such points as good pretreatment data, poor evaluation in the middle, lack of cooperation between units and sometimes falsified reports. It has never been conclusively demonstrated that control by drugs works.

# THE BIOLOGICAL ROLE OF VITAMIN A IN MAINTAINING EPITHELIAL TISSUES

JAMES A. OLSON

Department of Biochemistry, Faculty of Science, Mahidol University, Bangkok, Thailand

Our thinking about the role of any vitamin is usually influenced by historical perspective, that is, by the effects of its deficiency on growth, on the disruption of physiological processes and on changes in biological structure. In vitamin A deficiency a vast array of symptoms appear which ultimately involve almost all tissues of the body (see Table 1). As vitamin A deficiency develops, infection also becomes a problem which exacerbates the severity of xerophthalmia and often causes death. The question therefore arises whether some of the symptoms and tissue changes attributed to vitamin A deficiency might actually be caused by bacterial invasion. The examination of vitamin A-deficient germ-free animals showed that epithelial tissues still keratinize, and bones, glands and endocrine organs are still similarly affected (1–4). However, retardation of growth and loss of weight are less marked and survival is prolonged, sometimes indefinitely (2, 4).

Of various tissues of the body affected by vitamin A deficiency, epithelial tissues show the most extensive and consistent changes (Table 2). Although the precise effects produced by the presence or absence of vitamin A differ for each tissue, certain general similarities can be noted. Thus, in the absence of vitamin A the fraction of squamous and keratinized cells rises, and conversely in its presence, the relative number of mucus-secreting and columnar or cuboidal cells increases (5–8). This shift from keratinizing to mucus-

TABLE 1. *Symptoms of vitamin A deficiency*

| Symptom | Causes and tissues involved |
| --- | --- |
| Loss of appetite | Taste bud degeneration |
| Retardation of growth | Inadequate intake and utilization of food, intestinal obstruction etc. |
| Nervous disorders | Defective myelinization, abnormal growth of bone |
| Follicular hyperkeratosis | Epithelial keratinization |
| Defective reproduction | Testicular degeneration, fetal resorption, hormonal abnormalities |
| Night blindness | Loss of rhodopsin |
| Xerophthalmia | Defects in corneal epithelium, tear duct obstruction, infection |
| Blindness | Rod and cone cell destruction, corneal rupture etc. |
| Generalized infection | Immunological defects, reduced mucus secretion, keratinization of larynx and trachea |
| Death | Infection, volvulus, urinary blockage |

TABLE 2. *Some epithelial tissues affected by vitamin A deficiency*

| Tissue | Effect |
|---|---|
| Cornea | Keratinization |
| Epidermis | Keratinization |
| Trachea | Squamous metaplasia and keratinization |
| Urinary tract | Squamous metaplasia and keratinization |
| Vagina | Cornification |
| Sebaceous glands | Cystic atrophy |
| Hair follicle | Cystic atrophy, hyperkeratosis |
| Salivary gland ducts | Squamous metaplasia |
| Intestinal mucosa | Goblet cell decrease |
| Testes | Degeneration of germinal epithelium |
| Pancreatic ducts | Squamous metaplasia |

secreting tissue in the presence of vitamin A is most dramatically seen in some chemically induced epithelial tumors (9).

Vitamin A may also cause hyperplasia of epithelial tissues and an increase in the mitotic index (10, 11). Since cell division in normal stratified epithelium occurs mainly in the basal cells along the basal lamina (12, 13), vitamin A might primarily stimulate cell division in sensitive tissues leading secondarily to a shift in the population of cells and to a change in tissue structure.

In order to study this process more directly Dr. Adrian Lamb, a colleague in Bangkok, studied the effect of vitamin A on liver regeneration in vitamin A-deficient rats. The liver shows marked histological changes in vitamin A deficiency (1) and it has been postulated that chalone-like inhibitors control cell division in liver (14). However, Dr. Lamb found that the rate of liver regeneration in vitamin A-deficient and normal rats was essentially the same although some biochemical differences were noted (Lamb, unpublished observations). A number of other considerations also argue against a specific role of vitamin A in cell division. First, cell division is a generalized property of all living organisms, many of which have no demonstrable requirement for vitamin A. Second, a large number of factors either stimulate or inhibit cell division, varying from physical contact inhibition, on the one hand, to specific hormones and proteinaceous factors, on

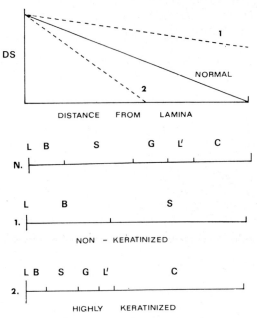

FIG. 1. A continuous gradient model for the control of cell type in stratified epithelium. The top graph expresses the gradient in some differentiation signal (DS) in the normal and in two variant cases. Cells in the field respond to DS to give different cell types in keeping with fixed threshold values. The response of a stratified epithelial tissue such as epidermis to DS in the three cases is given below. Abbreviations are: L, basal lamina; B, basal cells; S, stratum spinosum; G, stratum granulosum; L′, stratum lucidum; C, stratum corneum.

**151**

the other (14). Finally, some tissues, such as the tracheal epithelium, undergo marked hyperplasia in vitamin A deficiency.

It seems more likely that vitamin A somehow directly affects the specific differentiation of cells. Although this idea has great current vogue, only one generalized model for vitamin A action has been suggested (15). This model will be discussed shortly. Similarly, hypotheses that attempt to rationalize the cellular structure of stratified epithelium are almost equally rare. If the effect of vitamin A on epithelial tissue is to be elucidated, we must clearly first know something about the normal control of epithelial tissue patterns.

Based on modern ideas of tissue regulation at least two generalized models for the structure of stratified epithelium might be defined. The first, "the continuous gradient model," is based on Wolpert's concept of positional information (16). In Fig. 1 the simple application of this idea to a stratified epithelial tissue is presented. In essence a signal which determines the nature of cellular differentiation at any point varies in a prescribed way from the dominant region of the tissue which might well be the basal cells along the basal lamina. Cells at different levels "read" the signal and their differentiation depends on its value. Thus, in Fig. 1 three cases are given: the normal case, in which cell types are normally distributed between basal cells on the left and a cornified layer on the right; and two variant cases, in which the differentiation signal has either a more gradual or a more precipitous slope than normal. In the former case a nonkeratinized tissue will form, and in the latter, a highly keratinized epithelial tissue will develop. If we also assume that keratinizing cells produce an inhibitor of mucus

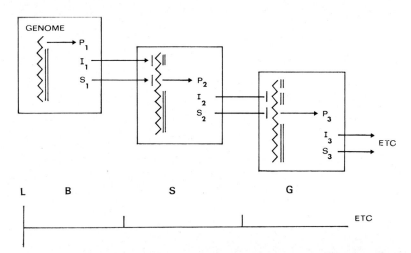

FIG. 2. A cascade model for the control of cell type in stratified epithelium. Basal cells produce both basal cell products ($P_1$) from a derepressed portion of the genome as well as a signaling inhibitor ($I_1$) and stimulator ($S_1$). In the next cellular stratum $I_1$ turns off the formation of $P_1$, $I_1$ and $S_1$. $S_1$ then stimulates the synthesis of type-specific products $P_2$, $I_2$ and $S_2$. Then, $I_2$ and $S_2$ act similarly on the next stratum of cells. In the diagram, the genome is represented by a wavy line, interaction with a specific portion of it by a line to the left and inhibition of its expression by a double line to the right. No attempt has been made to specify any of the details of genome expression nor to indicate the site of control. Abbreviations are: L, basal lamina; B, basal cell layer; S, stratum spinosum; G, stratum granulosum.

secretion which diffuses back towards the basal lamina, the epithelium of the first variant will also become mucus-secreting.

The second hypothesis, which is modified slightly from a suggestion by Mercer (17), is the "cascade model" (Fig. 2). In this case a given cell, let us say a basal cell, produces normal products which include specific inhibitors of its own products and stimulators of other products. These inhibitors and stimulators are transmitted to nearby cells, where they inhibit the formation of products characteristic of basal cells, but give rise to a new set of products which in turn include specific but different inhibitors and stimulators. The latter again similarly affect the next stratum of cells. In this way, cells in a given stratum are alike but differ appreciably from strata above or below their stratum. The net effect is that cells in different strata differentiate differently. A shift from keratinizing to non-keratinizing tissue might also be readily explained by this model through control of the diffusion distance and the rates of synthesis and destruction of various intercellular inhibitors and stimulators. The existence of epidermal growth factor (18), chalones (19) and possibly other mesenchymal factors which affect cellular proliferation and differentiation in epithelial tissues makes both such models attractive for further experimental testing. Vitamin A might possibly affect either the slope of a gradient or the balance in a cascade system, or might possibly alter the response of cells to a given signal.

As mentioned earlier, only one generalized theory for the action of vitamin A on cells has been proposed, namely, the interrupted differentiation model of Hayes (15). This hypothesis is presented in Fig. 3. The idea is that vitamin A-deficient epithelial cells are arrested at the squamous cell stage so that few ciliated and goblet cells are formed, whereas mesenchymal cells differentiate mainly to the blast cell stage. This hypothesis would explain bone overgrowth and the rather puzzling finding that some cells produce excess mucus in vitamin A deficiency whereas others produce a subnormal amount. Arrest of cellular differentiation in the adrenal cortex and primary sex glands might also lead to the reduction in the production of sex hormones observed during vitamin A deficiency. On the other hand, the hypothesis does not attempt to explain the mechanism by which differentiation is arrested nor indeed why the differentiation of epithelial cells involves branching, whereas that of mesenchymal cells is linear.

All other suggestions or hypotheses relating to vitamin A action tend to be partial explanations and some are very narrow indeed, dealing with only a single observation or

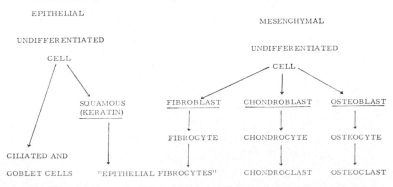

FIG. 3. The interrupted differentiation model of Hayes (15). In vitamin A deficiency the underlined cells tend to increase with respect to more mature forms.

physiological process. For example, a large number of enzymes are markedly depressed in vitamin A deficiency and hence it is supposed that vitamin A might serve as a coenzyme for them. However, since the chemical reactions catalyzed by affected enzymes are quite different, any consistent coenzymic role of vitamin A is difficult to imagine. Furthermore, a coenzymic form of vitamin A has never been identified nor convincingly shown to be essential for any specific reaction. Finally, and most convincingly, the activities of several presumably vitamin A-dependent enzymes are the same in normal and vitamin A-deficient animals when inanition and stress are carefully controlled (20). Future claims for a coenzymic function of vitamin A must therefore rest on more solid and extensive experimental evidence than has been presented in the past.

The second partial hypothesis deals with the role of vitamin A in membranes and particularly in lysosomes (21, 22). At relatively low concentrations vitamin A specifically stimulates the release of lysosomal enzymes into the extracellular space of fetal limb bone rudiments, which results in proteolytic breakdown of the ground substance (22). In this process vitamin A presumably induces a micellar phase change in both the cell and the lysosomal membranes, thereby catalyzing their fusion and stimulating the release of intracellular lytic enzymes. At much higher concentrations of vitamin A, membranes of many kinds are completely disrupted (21). Vitamin A has also been identified in various membrane fractions under physiological conditions (23). Enthusiasm for the membrane-lysosome hypothesis must necessarily be tempered, however, by the knowledge that α-retinol, which contains a double bond in the 4,5- rather than in the 5,6-position of the ionone ring, shows most of the membrane effects of retinol without possessing any biological activity (24). Neither is it immediately

apparent how this action of retinol might explain changes in patterns of tissue differentiation or induced shifts from keratinizing to mucus-secreting epithelia. If vitamin A stimulates secretion through membrane fusion, vitamin A-deficient animals should be less able to secrete mucus and hence should have an increased number of goblet cells. In fact, the goblet cell fraction is markedly reduced in vitamin A deficiency.

The final partial model deals with the synthesis of mucopolysaccharides. The initial suggestion that vitamin A is specifically and generally involved in such synthesis (25) has not been generally confirmed (26, 27). Past contradictory findings are probably due to differences in the nutritional states of experimental animals (20) rather than to differences in the degree of vitamin A deficiency. On the other hand, it has been conclusively shown that the incidence of goblet cells in the intestinal mucosa is reduced in vitamin A deficiency and that a fucose-containing glycopeptide normally produced by goblet cells is concomitantly depressed (28–30). Although rough endoplasmic reticulum was normal in vitamin A-deficient mucosal homogenates, the fraction containing amino acid synthetases and transfer RNA molecules was considerably less active (28). Since vitamin A also stimulates the synthesis of RNA in the colon of vitamin A-deficient rats *in vivo* and *in vitro* (31, 32), and at much higher doses also in the liver (33), some cellular products might be specifically stimulated by the presence of the vitamin. However, since no specific products have as yet been identified, the pertinence of these observations to the process of cellular differentiation is unclear.

We query whether vitamin A acts locally and directly on sensitive cells, or whether its effects are mediated through the endocrine or nervous systems. Certainly vitamin A can act directly on tissues, as shown by its marked effects on cells in tissue culture and the

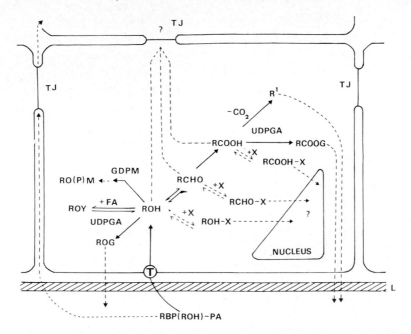

FIG. 4. Possible metabolic relationships in the basal cells of stratified epithelium. Known reactions are indicated by full lines, postulated reactions or transport pathways by dotted lines. Abbreviations are: RBP, retinol binding protein; PA, prealbumin; ROH, retinol; RCHO, retinal; RCOOH, retinoic acid; R′, uncharacterized oxidation products of retinoic acid; ROG, retinyl β-glucuronide; RCOOG, retinoyl β-glucuronide; ROY, retinyl ester; RO(P)M, complex of mannose and a retinol derivative, possibly including phosphate; X, a specific intracellular binding protein; UDPGA, uridine diphosphoglucuronic acid; GDPM, guanosine diphosphomannose; FA, long chain fatty acid; T, membrane transport mechanism; TJ, tight junctions.

localized tissue response to vitamin A *in vivo* (22). When small amounts of vitamin A are injected into a single rat testis, for example, a unilateral local spermatogenic response results (34). On the other hand, a deficiency of vitamin A affects both the structure of endocrine glands and the secretion of hormones from them (1, 35). The ability of pregnenolone and β-estradiol to delay fetal resorption in rats maintained with retinoic acid suggests that endocrine relationships are not balanced in these animals.

Finally, what is the biologically active form of vitamin A? Since retinol and retinal are biologically interconvertible, either form will obviously fulfill all of the necessary physio-logical requirements for the vitamin. On the other hand, retinoic acid is particularly interesting since it fulfills the functions of vitamin A in growth, in the maintenance of normal epithelial tissue and in the normal development of bone and cartilage, but not in vision or in reproduction (37). Since retinoic acid is rapidly metabolized and not stored in tissues, it may indeed be an active form if generated *in situ* from retinol in specific target tissues (38). However, this is certainly not the case in the process of vision, and is probably not true in reproduction either. No other derivative or metabolite of vitamin A with high biological activity has yet been identified.

Some metabolic aspects of vitamin A which might bear on its function in epithelial cells are depicted in Fig. 4. Retinol is transported in the blood as a 1:1 complex with a specific carrier, retinol-binding protein (RBP), which is normally associated with an acidic protein (prealbumin) of plasma (39, 40). Since capillaries do not usually cross the basal lamina of epithelial tissues the RBP must diffuse out of the capillary and across the lamina into the basal cells. Whether this transfer into cells is an active or a passive process is not known. Within the cell, retinol may be oxidized through retinal to retinoic acid which may then be decarboxylated to as yet unidentified products. Retinol may also be conjugated in at least three ways: with uridine diphosphoglucuronic acid to form retinyl β-glucuronide, with guanosine diphosphomannose to form a retinyl mannose complex, which may or may not contain phosphate (41), and with palmitate and possibly other long chain fatty acids to give retinyl ester. Most but possibly not all of these reactions occur in epithelial tissues. Retinol or one of its oxidized products might also interact with a specific intracellular binding protein to form a complex which might then exert biological action. However, specific intracellular binding proteins for vitamin A have not yet been identified.

In moving from the basal lamina into upper layers of the stratified epithelium, the retinol-RBP complex might diffuse through intercellular spaces into cells at various levels of the tissue, or indeed vitamin A might be transported through tight junctions or other contacts between epithelial cells in direct cell-to-cell communication. Quite possibly a gradient in vitamin A concentration might exist in stratified epithelium but we have no knowledge at present about any of these matters. Other aspects of vitamin A metabolism have been considered in detail in recent reviews (42–44).

In summary, the symptoms of vitamin A deficiency are extensive and ultimately involve almost all the tissues of the body, but they particularly affect epithelial tissues. In the absence of vitamin A, epithelial tissues generally form an extensive keratinized layer, whereas in its presence and particularly in an excess of vitamin A, mucus-secreting cells predominate. Two models have been presented for the control of stratified epithelia: 1) a variable gradient model, and 2) a cascade inhibitor-stimulator model. Vitamin A as well as many other factors might influence these overall control systems to give largely keratinized or nonkeratinized tissue.

The only recent generalized hypothesis for vitamin A function is the interrupted differentiation model of Hayes. While intrinsically interesting it is based largely on microscopic observations and does not suggest possible molecular mechanisms for vitamin A action. Other hypotheses dealing with vitamin A function such as the membrane-lysosome concept, the mucopolysaccharide stimulatory concept, and possible specific coenzymic roles of vitamin A explain at best only a portion of the observed effects of vitamin A action.

In a more metabolic sense only retinol and retinal possess the full biological activity of the vitamin, but how they are transported into cells, in what manner they combine with intracellular elements and how they exert their biological effects are still largely unknown.

Vitamin A is only one of a relatively large number of factors, which include several steroid hormones, growth factors and mitotic inhibitors, that influence the size and nature of epithelial tissues. The future unraveling of these interrelationships will hopefully give us insight both into the basic mechanism underlying pattern formation in epithelial tissues and into the function of vitamin A.

The author, a field staff member of the Rockefeller

Foundation, is indebted to Miss Patchari Karnasuta for expert secretarial assistance.

Supported in part by grants-in-aid from the Rockefeller Foundation (GA-BMS-7006) and from the United States Public Health Service, National Institutes of Health (5-ROI-AM-11367-03).

## REFERENCES

1. BEAVER DL. Vitamin A deficiency in the germ free rat. *Am J Pathol* 38: 335, 1961.
2. BIERI JG, MCDANIEL EG and ROGERS WE JR. Survival of germ free rats without vitamin A. *Science* 163: 574, 1969.
3. ROGERS WE JR, BIERI JG and MCDANIEL EG. Vitamin A deficiency in the germ free state, in: DeLuca HF and Suttie JW (Eds), "The fat soluble vitamins." Madison, University of Wisconsin Press, 1970, p 241.
4. RAICA N JR, STEDHAM MA, HERMAN YF and SAUBERLICH HE. Vitamin A deficiency in germ free rats, in: DeLuca HF and Suttie JW (Eds), "The fat-soluble vitamins." Madison, University of Wisconsin Press, 1970, p 283.
5. FELL HB and MELLANBY E. Metaplasia produced in cultures of chick ectoderm by high vitamin A. *J Physiol (Lond)* 119: 470, 1953.
6. LAWRENCE DJ and BERN HA. Mucous metaplasia and mucous gland formation in keratinized adult epithelium *in situ* treated with vitamin A. *Exp Cell Res* 21: 443, 1960.
7. LAWRENCE DJ, BERN HA and STEADMAN MG. Vitamin A and keratinization studies on the hamster cheek pouch. *Ann Otol Rhinol Laryngol* 69: 645, 1960.
8. KAHN RH. Effect of locally applied vitamin A and estrogen on the rat vagina. *Am J Anat* 95: 309, 1954.
9. PRUTKIN L. The effect of vitamin A acid on tumorigenesis and protein production. *Cancer Res* 28: 102, 1968.
10. LAWRENCE DJ and BERN HA. On the specificity of the response of mouse epidermis to vitamin A. *J Invest Dermatol* 31: 313, 1958.
11. SHERMAN BS. The effect of vitamin A on epithelial mitosis *in vivo* and *in vitro*. *J Invest Dermatol* 37: 469, 1961.
12. LEBLOND CP and WALKER BE. Renewal of cell populations. *Physiol Rev* 36: 255, 1956.
13. GREULICH RC. Aspects of cell individuality in the renewal of stratified squamous epithelia, in: Montagna W and Lobitz WC Jr (Eds), "The epidermis." New York, Academic Press, 1964, p 117.
14. BECKER FF. Cell division in normal mammalian tissues. *Annu Rev Med* 20: 243, 1969.
15. HAYES EC. Comments on studies of vitamin A in reproduction and differentiation. *Am J Clin Nutr* 22: 1081, 1969.
16. WOLPERT L. Positional information and the spacial pattern of cellular differentiation. *J Theor Biol* 25: 1, 1969.
17. MERCER EH. Protein synthesis and epidermal differentiation, in: Montagna W and Lobitz WC (Eds), "The epidermis." New York, Academic Press, 1964, p 161.
18. TURKINGTON RW. The role of epithelial growth factor in mammary gland development *in vitro*. *Exp Cell Res* 57: 79, 1969.
19. BULLOUGH WS. The control of mitotic activity in adult mammalian tissues. *Biol Rev* 37: 307, 1962.
20. ROGERS WE JR. Reexamination of enzyme activities thought to show evidence of a coenzyme role for vitamin A. *Am J Clin Nutr* 22: 1003, 1969.
21. LUCY JA. Some possible roles for vitamin A in membranes: micelle formation and electron transfer. *Am J Clin Nutr* 22: 1033, 1969.
22. FELL HB. The direct action of vitamin A on skeletal tissue *in vitro*, in: DeLuca HF and Suttie JW (Eds), "The fat-soluble vitamins." Madison, University of Wisconsin Press, 1970, p 187.
23. ROELS OA, ANDERSON OR, LUI NST, SHAH DO and TROUT ME. Vitamin A and membranes. *Am J Clin Nutr* 22: 1020, 1969.
24. PITT GAJ. Comments on the role of vitamin A in membranes. *Am J Clin Nutr* 22: 1045, 1969.
25. WOLF G and JOHNSON BC. Vitamin A and mucopolysaccharide synthesis. *Vitam Horm* 18: 439, 1960.
26. PASTERNAK CA and THOMAS DB. Metabolism of sulfated mucopolysaccharides in vitamin A deficiency. *Am J Clin Nutr* 22: 986, 1969.
27. KEAN EL. Vitamin A deficiency and glycolipid sulfation. *J Lipid Res* 11: 248, 1970.
28. DELUCA L, LITTLE EP and WOLF G. Vitamin A and protein synthesis by rat intestinal mucosa. *J Biol Chem* 244: 701, 1969.
29. DELUCA L, SCHUMACHER M and WOLF G. Biosynthesis of a fucose-containing glycopeptide from rat small intestine in normal and vitamin A-deficient intestine. *J Biol Chem* 245: 4551, 1970.
30. DELUCA L, SCHUMACHER M and NELSON D. Cellular localization by immunofluorescence of the retinol dependent fucose glycopeptide in the goblet cells of the small intestine. *Fed Proc* 30: 583, 1971.
31. ZACHMAN RD. The stimulation of RNA synthesis *in vivo* and *in vitro* by retinol in the intestine of vitamin A deficient rats. *Life Sci [I]* 6: 2207, 1967.
32. ZILE M. Comments on RNA synthesis in vitamin A deficiency *Am J Clin Nutr* 22: 1089, 1969.
33. JOHNSON BC, KENNEDY M and CHIBA N. Vitamin A and nuclear RNA synthesis. *Am J Clin Nutr* 22: 1048, 1969.
34. AHLUWALIA B and BIERI JG. Local stimulatory effect of vitamin A on spermatogeneses in the rat. *J Nutr* 101: 141, 1971.
35. GANGULY J, POPE GS, THOMPSON SY, TOOTHILL J, EDWARDS-WEBB JD and WAYNFORTH HB. Studies on the metabolism of vitamin A. The effect of vitamin A status on the secretion rates of some steroids into the ovarian venous blood of pregnant rats. *Biochem J* 122: 235, 1971.
36. JUNEJA HS, MOUDGAL NR and GANGULY J. Studies on metabolism of vitamin A. The effect of hormones on gestation in retinoate-fed female rats. *Biochem J* 111: 97, 1969.
37. THOMPSON JN. The role of vitamin A in re-

production, in: DeLuca HF and Suttie JW (Eds), "The fat-soluble vitamins." Madison, University of Wisconsin Press, 1970, p 267.

38. KLEINER-BOSSALER A and DeLuca HF. Formation of retinoic acid from retinol in the kidney. *Arch Biochem Biophys* **142**: 371, 1971.

39. KANAI M, RAZ A and GOODMAN DS. Retinol binding protein: the transport protein for vitamin A in human plasma. *J Clin Invest* **47**: 2025, 1968.

40. PETERSON PA and BERGGARD I. Isolation and properties of a human retinol-transporting protein. *J Biol Chem* **246**: 25, 1971.

41. DeLuca L, ROSSO G and WOLF G. The biosynthesis of a mannolipid that contains a polar metabolite of 15-C$^{14}$-retinol. *Biochem Biophys Res Commun* **41**: 615, 1970.

42. OLSON JA. The metabolism of vitamin A. *Pharmacol Rev* **19**: 559, 1967.

43. OLSON JA. Some aspects of vitamin A metabolism. *Vitam Horm* **26**: 1, 1968.

44. OLSON JA. The metabolism and function of vitamin A. *Fed Proc* **28**: 1670, 1969.

# CORNEA IN HYPOVITAMINOSIS A AND PROTEIN DEFICIENCY

CLAES H. DOHLMAN* and VASUNDHARA KALEVAR

Department of Cornea Research, Retina Foundation and the Cornea Service of
the Massachusetts Eye and Ear Infirmary, Boston, Massachusetts, USA

Hypovitaminosis A and protein deficiency can lead to xerophthalmia and can also result in the rapid ulceration of the stroma, keratomalacia. The pathophysiology of the corneal symptoms in these deficiency states are here discussed in the light of recent findings on the stability of the tear film and on the mechanism of stromal ulceration.

## XEROPHTHALMIA

Xerophthalmia can occur in children and adults who have been on a diet low in vitamin A, or who have for some reason been unable to absorb sufficient amounts of the vitamin from the gastrointestinal tract (1). A degree of protein malnutrition probably coexists when ocular symptoms develop (2).

Histologically keratinization of the corneal and conjunctival epithelium is characteristic. Also, there is an early disappearance of the goblet cells of the conjunctival epithelium (3, 4).

The most striking clinical phenomenon is the lack of luster and the dryness of the ocular surface often in spite of a seemingly adequate amount of tear fluid (Fig. 1). The tears appear unable to wet the eye. During slit lamp examination, one can see how the tear film has lost its stability and has a tendency to break up and to form dry spots immediately after a blink. In more advanced cases, the tears can be seen along the lid margins when they even wet the lashes, whereas the corneal and conjunctival epithelium in the palpebral fissure appears completely dry (Fig. 2). It is likely that the tear film has become altered thus making it unable to wet the underlying epithelial surface properly.

The normal tear film consists of three main layers: the superficial lipid layer derived from the meibomian glands, the aqueous layer orig-

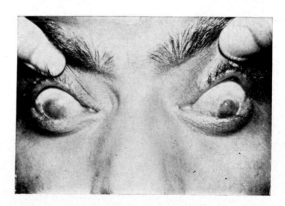

FIG. 1. Xerophthalmia with lusterless cornea and wrinkled, keratinized conjunctiva (courtesy of Dr. P. Siva Reddy, Hyderabad, India).

* Address for reprints: Claes H. Dohlman, M.D., 20 Staniford Street, Boston, Mass. 02114.

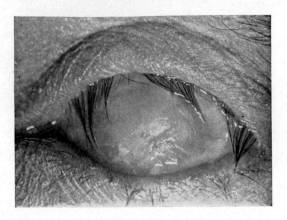

FIG. 2. Xerophthalmia. Note abundant aqueous tears that even wet the lashes; nevertheless the corneal surface appears dry.

inating in the lacrimal glands and the mucus layer (5, 6). The mucus seems to be mostly adsorbed to the epithelium (6, 7). In all likelihood the corneal mucus comes from the conjunctival goblet cells, which secrete mucus into the tears. The mucus is then rubbed into the corneal surface at each blink.

Recent *in vitro* studies in our laboratory on the surface chemistry of the tear film have shown that mucus is essential for the stability of the tear film (8, 9). Mucus can make the normally hydrophobic epithelial surface hydrophilic, and this is necessary for proper wetting with aqueous tears.

A definite correlation exists between lack of stability of the tear film and absence of conjunctival goblet cells in patients (10, 11). Thus, in the Stevens-Johnson syndrome, ocular pemphigus etc. patients may have an adequate volume of aqueous tears, but still the tear film breaks up early, probably due to the deficiency of mucus caused by the lack of goblet cells. The same situation probably prevails in xerophthalmia, due to hypovitaminosis A and other metabolic deficiencies. These patients usually have sufficient aqueous tears (normal Schirmer test) but goblet cells disappear early and insufficient

mucus is therefore secreted into the tear film. Lack of mucus then results in immediate disruption of the tear film between blinks.

When the eye is open, evaporation from the tear film always takes place (12). Where the tear film has broken up and exposed the epithelium, evaporation can instantaneously damage the epithelium. If neglected, this may lead to irregularity and opacity of the epithelium, scarring of the stroma and susceptibility to infection. However, it would probably be wrong to ascribe the well-documented keratinization of the ocular epithelium to evaporative damage. Keratinization also occurs in the respiratory, gastrointestinal, urogenital and other tracts where evaporation is not a factor.

Therapy of xerophthalmia includes the systemic administration of high doses of vitamin A and a protein-rich diet (1). Whether topical delivery of the vitamin has any effect on the eye is uncertain. Ointments containing vitamin A have been extensively used throughout the world for a variety of external conditions of the eye. However, the efficacy of such a topical regimen is poorly documented.

In the chronically mucus-deficient eye, in which no therapy is likely to restore the conjunctival goblet cells, new developments may offer some amelioration. Synthetic and natural polymers with a mucus-like effect have been sought. At present, the two most promising substances are the so-called B-P polymer and gelatin (7), which can both transform corneal epithelium into a hydrophilic and therefore more wettable surface *in vitro*. Undoubtedly, other more effective mucomimetic agents will be found. They can be incorporated in regular tear substitutes, and can be used as eye drops when needed.

Soft hydrophilic lenses are also promising. They create a relatively stable tear film and, in combination with artificial tears, they offer a certain protection to the ocular surface particularly when trichiasis is also present mediated by enzymes, and that this concept should be valid for keratomalacia as well.

Under any circumstances, the initial step in keratomalacia is damage to the epithelium possibly due to localized drying, and resulting in an epithelial defect. Release of proteases may then occur and the enzymes attack the exposed stroma. Still, it is surprising how fast the stroma melts away. The stroma may possibly be abnormally susceptible to enzymatic action as has been shown to occur after alkali burns (22). It is possible that the corneal stroma in keratomalacia (which usually occurs only in severe protein deficiency) has lost normal defenses against enzymatic invasion. Serum is known to contain powerful collagenase inhibitors ($\alpha_2$-macroglobulin and $\alpha_1$-antitrypsin) (23), and such natural inhibitors may possibly diffuse into the stroma and normally protect it from autodigestion. In severe protein deficiency the inhibitor level may go down and expose the stroma to the destructive enzymes. No experimental or clinical investigations along these lines have yet been done on the cornea. The precise pathophysiology of keratomalacia is still unknown. A tentative flow chart for possible events in xerophthalmia and keratomalacia is presented in Fig. 4.

Therapy of keratomalacia usually comes too late. However, intramuscular vitamin A

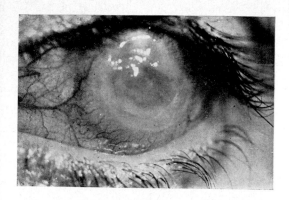

FIG. 3. Ulcerations of the corneal stroma, regardless of the initial etiology, are in all likelihood mediated by destructive enzymes released from the altered cells at the edge of an epithelial defect.

(13). The disadvantages of soft lenses include unpredictable tolerance and a rare infection.

### KERATOMALACIA

Keratomalacia is an acute ulceration of the cornea, usually occurring in children. Vitamin A serum levels are usually very low and protein malnutrition is also present (14). Keratomalacia may or may not have been preceded by xerophthalmia.

Characteristics of keratomalacia are the rapid progression of stromal ulceration (Fig. 3) and the relative lack of ocular reaction to the massive damage. Thus, virtually the entire cornea can melt away in 24 hr and the eye may still appear rather quiescent (14).

In tissue culture corneal epithelium can synthesize enzymes that digest stroma (15), including collagenase and similar proteases, which have been identified by a variety of techniques (16–18). In patients with corneal ulcers and not in normal patients, epithelial biopsy and cultures have demonstrated release of collagenase (19). In addition, collagenase inhibitors, used as eye drops, have a certain inhibitory effect on stromal ulceration in animals and man (20, 21), all suggesting that corneal ulcerations in general are

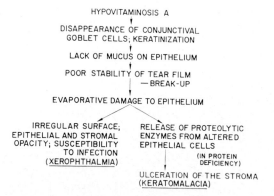

FIG. 4. Flow-sheet of possible pathophysiological events leading to xerophthalmia and keratomalacia.

in large doses should be given immediately and, if the progress of the ulceration has not been too rapid, improvement can set in after 24 hr (1). An ulcerating cornea should be kept clean with antibiotics topically administered. In addition, enzyme inhibitors may be applicable here. EDTA, EDTA-Ca, cysteine and acetylcysteine have all been found to have some effect in preventing or retarding stromal ulceration by inhibiting proteolytic enzymes released from the damaged epithelial cells (24). The action is indisputable but is probably not very strong. One can attempt to treat the eye with either 0.2 M EDTA-Ca every 2 hr or with 0.3 M cysteine every 3 hr, or finally, with 1.2 M acetylcysteine every 3 hr (i.e., waking hours) for three weeks. In the concentrations mentioned, these chelators do not seem to have any toxic effect. It is possible that in the future stronger inhibitors will be found. Under any circumstances, the possibilities of preventing stromal ulceration with enzyme inhibitors is a new and exciting one.

Finally, the cornea in keratomalacia may be covered with a conjunctival flap. If the ulceration has not yet resulted in perforation but is nevertheless severe, a total Gundersen type of conjunctival flap can be immobilized and such a flap will stop further stromal ulceration in virtually all cases (25). However, children with keratomalacia and protein deficiency may be poor risks for general anesthesia.

Prevention is strikingly easy, effective and inexpensive in both xerophthalmia and keratomalacia compared with efforts to rectify the final damage. Public health measures and mass education deserve top priority in the competition for resources in countries where dietary deficiencies cause widespread blindness.

Supported in part by a Public Health Service International Postdoctoral Research Fellowship 1 F05 TW01683–01, Project Center Grant EY-00292, Research Grant EY-00208–11, Training Grant EY-0043– 05, 06, from the National Eye Institute; and by the Massachusetts Lions Eye Research Fund, Inc.

## REFERENCES

1. RODGER FC and SINCLAIR HM. "Metabolic and nutritional eye diseases." Springfield, Ill, CC Thomas, 1969.
2. KUMING BS. The evolution of keratomalacia. *Trans Ophthalmol Soc UK* **87**: 305, 1965.
3. MORI S. Primary changes in eyes of rats which result from deficiency of fat-soluble A in diet. *JAMA* **79**: 197, 1922.
4. KREIKER A. Zur Klinik und Histologie der epithelialen Bindehautxerose. *Albrecht von Graefes Arch Klin Ophthalmol* **124**: 191, 1930.
5. WOLFF E. Mucocutaneous junction of lid margin and distribution of tear fluid. *Trans Ophthalmol Soc UK* **66**: 291, 1946.
6. MISHIMA S. Some physiological aspects of the precorneal tear film. *Arch Ophthalmol* **73**: 233, 1965.
7. HOLLY FJ and LEMP MA. Surface chemistry of the tear film; implications for dry eye syndromes, contact lenses and ophthalmic polymers. *J Contact Lens Soc Am* **5**: 12, 1971.
8. LEMP MA, HOLLY FJ, IWATA S and DOHLMAN CH. The precorneal tear film. I. Factors in spreading and maintaining a continuous tear film over the corneal surface. *Arch Ophthalmol* **83**: 89, 1970.
9. HOLLY FJ and LEMP MA. Wettability and wetting of corneal epithelium. *Exp Eye Res* **11**: 239, 1971.
10. LEMP MA, DOHLMAN CH and HOLLY FJ. Corneal dessication despite normal tear volume. *Ann Ophthalmol* **2**: 258, 1970.
11. LEMP MA, DOHLMAN CH, KUWABARA T, CARROLL JM and HOLLY FJ. Dry eye secondary to mucus deficiency. *Trans Am Acad Ophthalmol Otolaryngol* **75**: 1223, 1971.
12. MISHIMA S and MAURICE DM. Oily layer of tear film and evaporation from corneal surface. *Exp Eye Res* **1**: 39, 1961.
13. GASSET AR and KAUFMAN HE. Hydrophilic lens. *Am J Ophthalmol* **71**: 1185, 1971.
14. OOMEN H. Hypovitaminosis. *Fed Proc* **17**: 103, 1958.
15. ITOI M, GNÄDINGER MC, SLANSKY HH, FREEMAN MI and DOHLMAN CH. Collagenase in the cornea. *Exp Eye Res* **8**: 369, 1969.
16. SLANSKY HH, FREEMAN MI and ITOI M. Collagenolytic activity in bovine corneal epithelium. *Arch Ophthalmol* **80**: 496, 1968.
17. BROWN SI, WELLER CA and WASSERMAN HE. Collagenolytic activity of alkali-burned corneas. *Arch Ophthalmol* **81**: 370, 1969.
18. BERMAN M, DAVISON P, DOHLMAN CH and GNÄDINGER M. Characterization of collagenolytic activity in the ulcerating cornea. *Exp Eye Res* **11**: 255, 1971.
19. SLANSKY HH, GNÄDINGER MC, ITOI M and DOHLMAN CH. Collagenase in corneal ulcerations. *Arch Ophthalmol* **82**: 108, 1969.
20. ITOI M, GNÄDINGER M, SLANSKY HH, FREEMAN M and DOHLMAN CH. Prevention d'ulcère du stroma de la cornée grâce à l'utilisation d'un sel

de calcium d'EDTA. *Arch Ophthalmol (Paris)* **29**: 389, 1969.

21. BROWN SI, AKIYA S and WELLER CA. Prevention of the ulcers of the alkali-burned cornea. *Arch Ophthalmol* **82**: 95, 1969.

22. GNÄDINGER MC, ITOI M, SLANSKY HH and DOHLMAN CH. The role of collagenase in the alkali-burned cornea. *Am J Ophthalmol* **68**: 478, 1969.

23. EISEN AZ, BLOCH KJ and SAKAI T. Inhibition of human skin collagenase by human serum. *J Lab Clin Med* **75**: 258, 1970.

24. SLANSKY HH and DOHLMAN CH. Collagenase and the cornea. *Surv Ophthalmol* **14**: 402, 1970.

25. GUNDERSEN T. Conjunctival flaps in the treatment of corneal disease with reference to a new technique of application. *Arch Ophthalmol* **60**: 880, 1958.

# CLINICAL ASPECTS OF KERATOMALACIA

JOHANNA TEN DOESSCHATE*

Undaan Eye Hospital, Sourabaya, Java, Indonesia

"Conjunctival and corneal xerosis is always seen in weak, badly nourished children who suffer from chronic enteritis. The mothers mention spontaneously that the children at first were not able to see at night; afterward their eyes went bad.

The conjunctiva looks dry, somewhat fatty, with a mother-of-pearl-like sheen, sometimes like fish-scales, and it is covered with a fine foam. The bulbar conjunctiva is thickened and folded in the part which is exposed in the open eye. Tears flow over the abnormal parts without wetting them.

If the child is not treated systemically and if the diet is not corrected, the cornea will often get involved. The tissue loses its luster and becomes opaque. Soon an ulcer is formed which quickly enlarges, until—sometimes in a few days—the whole cornea melts away without signs of inflammation (keratomalacia)."

This description of the clinical unfolding of keratomalacia was published on Java at Bandung, exactly 60 years ago, by Westhoff (1). At that time vitamin A had not yet been discovered, but Westhoff mentions successful treatment with proper feeding and local application of euchinine, tannalbin and Peruvian Balsam to the eye. As far as I can draw on my experience of over 3,000 cases of xerophthalmia in Sourabaya, East Java, this description is still exactly true and xerophthalmia is probably as frequent as it was around 1911.

The first sign of vitamin A deficiency, observed in about 80% of cases, is night blindness: parents have often observed that their child is suddenly no longer able to find its plate of food or to see its cup of tea at dusk. The suddenness of onset indicates that this is not congenital night blindness; and although in very young children exact measurements of dark adaptation are not trustworthy, a check on the child's behavior in the darkroom is always possible and usually tends to confirm the parents' story.

A further reason to attribute this type of night blindness to lack of vitamin A is its very prompt response to treatment with this vitamin (Table 1).

The case history in every case of suspected vitamin A deficiency usually reveals that one or more of the known additional causal factors is (or was) present. The child, generally

TABLE 1. *Recovery from night blindness after treatment*

| Length of treatment (days) | % recovery | |
|---|---|---|
| | Boys (total sample, 48) | Girls (total sample, 31) |
| 4 | 40 | 44 |
| 7 | 90 | 70 |
| 14 | 100 | 100 |

* Present address: Netherlands General Association for the Prevention of Blindness, The Hague, Netherlands.

from a poor family, rarely or never gets either vitamin A or its precursors in his diet. Custom, habits and superstitions play a part in this situation. It is quite possible that a child, on being offered some vegetables or fruit for the first time in his life, will refuse them, with the likely result that such foods will never again be offered, since the parents are convinced that the child does not want them. Traditional child education in Java, which is slowly changing with the spread of general education, is peace-oriented. Excitement, anger and conflicts are to be avoided at any price, and until the age of around four years, a child has the right to refuse anything he does not like, and is appeased at all costs. After the age of four, this permissiveness is changed, and the child will be disciplined. But the result for the younger children is often a very unsatisfactory dietary pattern, especially as long as the child cannot provide himself with side-dishes in addition to the traditional rice diet.

As the general food habits of the adult population in Java make for a diet precarious in vitamin A, as well as in fat and protein, it is probable that many children subsist on a borderline diet after weaning. From the histories of our young patients with night blindness other factors, besides a diet with insufficient vitamin A, have often been detected; for example, the presence of intestinal worms or various acute infections in the recent past, none of which are rare in small children. A child was sometimes "treated" for diarrhea by being given tea or ricewater exclusively, and this therapy was continued for days, even weeks on end, for fear of recurrences. The elucidation of what precisely causes the outbreak of xerophthalmia should be the prime concern of whoever first treats such a child, general practitioner, pediatrician or even ophthalmologist.

Night blindness alone has usually not persisted for more than three weeks before treat-

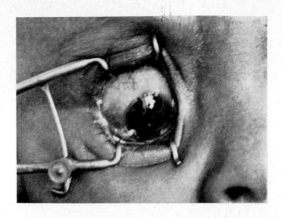

FIG. 1. Xerophthalmia $X_1$; loose foam, dry, pigmented conjunctiva.

ment is sought. In young children under four years of age, it will either heal of itself or progress to a more severe stage. In an older child it can probably be more protracted, but in that case the family is already accustomed to the situation and will not bring the child for treatment.

The next stage in the development of vitamin A deficiency is the complex of signs which gives the disease its name, xerophthalmia, or "dry eye." The exposed part of the conjunctiva, and in later stages also the tarsal conjunctiva, becomes dry. On lateral movements of the eyeball, the bulbar conjunctiva is thrown into folds. Sometimes loose foam floats around, but more often the foam adheres to the classical triangular spot of Bitôt (Fig. 1). The white or yellowish substance which covers the conjunctiva stands out especially clearly in contrast to the greyish background of the pigmented conjunctiva. This pigmentation is typical and is often concentrated in the tarsal folds and on the caruncle. It disappears completely on healing, with a time lag of about two months.

This whole complex of conjunctival xerosis ($X_1$ degree of xerophthalmia) may last for a rather long time even though the parents claim that the child was brought for treat-

**165**

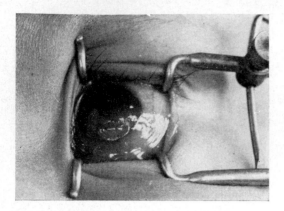

FIG. 2. Xerophthalmia $X_3$; dry, pigmented conjunctiva, corneal ulcer.

ment when the lesion was only a few weeks old. If nothing untoward happens, the $X_1$ stage can last for several months.

Teng Khoen Hing (2–4) at Bandung, West Java, found typical small, whitish flecks in the retina, which he called "fundus xerophthalmicus" in $X_1$ stage cases. I saw some of his cases and detected six at Sourabaya. Bandung is ca. 2,400 feet above sea level while Sourabaya is 30 feet above sea level. Different dietary habits and different climates may contribute an unknown cause for the frequency of the fundus lesion.

In the next phase in developing xerophthalmia the cornea becomes involved. When the eye is kept open for about ten seconds without allowing the child to blink, the cornea may become dry and no longer reflects a sharp image. After blinking, the cornea again seems quite normal but in severe cases it shows gray patches, usually situated in the inferior portions. These may progress to loss of substance, which is traditionally called ulceration, but there is neither inflammation nor redness of the eye. As long as there is no serious ulceration, the cornea can heal without visual loss (Fig. 2).

In children who are rather ill with other signs of malnutrition, ulceration of the cor-

nea can go on to perforation. In this case, one or more adherent leukomas will ensue on healing; in other cases, with alarmingly swift development, the whole cornea will slough away until the entire iris protrudes, sometimes even with extrusion of the lens. In a typical situation the mother may be ill or dead, the child very sick and refusing to open its eyes for fear of the light. In nine out of ten such cases brought to our Outpatients Department, the child was suffering from keratomalacia. The eyes are kept firmly shut. On their being opened with care because of the possibility of corneal perforation, a dry, often gray conjunctiva is revealed with a dry, white or yellowish cornea, showing deep craters or a "fly's head" (an iris knuckle protruding through the perforated cornea). Sometimes the whole cornea is absent, exposing the iris. On occasion, corneal patches and a hypopyon are observed which in these cases does not necessarily mean secondary infection, but can be due to debris from the cornea sloughing off into the anterior chamber. If secondary infection is present, the process usually leads to panophthalmitis, implying loss of the eye (Fig. 3).

Together with the various signs of vitamin A deficiency, there are often other signs of

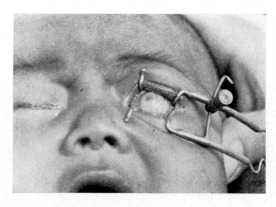

FIG. 3. Xerophthalmia $X_3$; dry, grayish conjunctiva; total corneal ulcer.

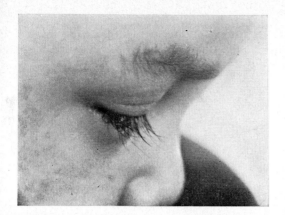

FIG. 4. Very long eyelashes in xerophthalmia.

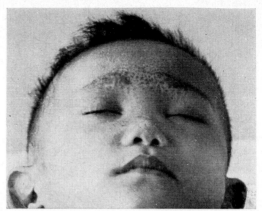

FIG. 6. "Crazy pavement skin" in 3-year-old boy with kwashiorkor and xerophthalmia $X_3$.

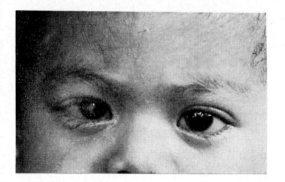

FIG. 5. Lanugo hairs on whole forehead in $2\frac{1}{2}$ year-old child with healed xerophthalmia $X_4$: scar and leukoma adherens right eye.

malnutrition. Thus we rarely saw a healthy child in the $X_3$ group. The signs of malnutrition found around the eyes were:

Eyelashes sometimes very long, sparse or uneven in length (Fig. 4). Lanugo hair on the forehead and in front of the ears, like side-whiskers, even in children too old for remnants of Lanugo hair to be expected (Fig. 5).

Various hair changes of the scalp, as described for kwashiorkor (hair brown, red or even blonde in color, instead of the normal black, also baldness in patches).

Skin lesions: phrynoderma, which probably is specific for vitamin A deficiency; white spectacles in edema and crazy pavement skin, which we found even on the forehead (Fig. 6).

It is important for the oculist to recognize the signs of malnutrition at a glance. These can be found near the eyes, and will lead him to a correct diagnosis of the eye lesion.

With the help of a pediatrician, Mrs. Gondosoebarijo, in a number of cases, the degree of xerophthalmia and the average malnutrition index of Oomen were compared, omitting the score for body length, which was not measured. The degree of xerophthalmia was distinctly parallel to the degree of malnutrition (Table 2).

TABLE 2. *Average malnutrition index (Oomen) in different degrees of xerophthalmia*

| | Boys (total sample, 216) | | | | Girls (total sample, 141) | | | |
|---|---|---|---|---|---|---|---|---|
| | $X_0$ | $X_1$ | $X_2$ | $X_3$ | $X_0$ | $X_1$ | $X_2$ | $X_3$ |
| No. of cases | 14 | 121 | 19 | 62 | 8 | 62 | 20 | 51 |
| Index (average) | 1.3 | 3.6 | 6.6 | 7.4 | 3.4 | 5.7 | 6.0 | 9.0 |

TABLE 3.  *Relationship of serum vitamin A level to degree of xerophthalmia*
*(IU vitamin A/100 ml)*

| | Boys (total sample, 13) | | Girls (total sample, 14) | |
|---|---|---|---|---|
| | $X_1$ | $X_3$ | $X_1$ | $X_3$ |
| Range | 13 to 38 | 14 to 29 | 4 to 26 | 12 to 52 |
| Mean value | 24.6 | 24.5 | 20 | 28.7 |

TABLE 4.  *Relationship of serum protein level (g/ml)*
*to degree of xerophthalmia*

| | Boys (total sample, 12) | | Girls (total sample, 14) | |
|---|---|---|---|---|
| | $X_1$ | $X_3$ | $X_1$ | $X_3$ |
| Range | 4.8 to 7.2 | 5.5 to 8.4 | 5.4 to 8.4 | 6.1 to 8.1 |
| Mean value | 6.2 | 7.1 | 6.6 | 7.1 |

TABLE 5.  *Relationship of A/G ratio to degree of xerophthalmia*

| | Boys (total sample, 12) | | Girls (total sample, 14) | |
|---|---|---|---|---|
| | $X_1$ | $X_3$ | $X_1$ | $X_3$ |
| Range | 0.8 to 1.1 | 0.38 to 1.2 | 0.63 to 1.2 | 0.5 to 2.06 |
| Mean value | 0.97 | 0.87 | 0.93 | 0.88 |

TABLE 6.  *Relationship of body weight to degree of xerophthalmia*
*(compared with normal average)*

| | + % | = % | = to 1 % | 1 to 2 % | 2 to 3 % | 3 % | Weight/standard |
|---|---|---|---|---|---|---|---|
| 415 boys | | | | | | | |
| $X_0X_1$ | 11 | 17 | 43 | 18 | 9 | — | |
| $X_2X_3$ | 2 | 3 | 25 | 26 | 28 | 15 | |
| 243 girls | | | | | | | |
| $X_0X_1$ | 7 | 10 | 47 | 28 | 10 | 5 | |
| $X_2X_3$ | 4 | 5 | 22 | 34 | 22 | 15 | |

Tests could not be done on all patients for levels of vitamin A, proteins and carotenoids in the blood serum, but in the few cases where we were able to estimate these values, they were in the range common for Indonesia, namely: low vitamin A values, low total protein values and a low A/G ratio (Tables 3, 4 and 5).

When body weight alone is taken as an indicator of growth, and probably of the ex-penditure of vitamin A during growth, we find that in the $X_0X_1$ degree of xerophthalmia the girls showed a less favorable body weight compared to normal for their age than the boys. This means that boys will show signs of vitamin A deficiency earlier than girls. This was not found in the $X_3$ group. The same bias is shown by the Oomen index in which all signs of malnutrition are taken into account. Whether keratomalacia is a conse-

TABLE 7. *Recurrence of xerophthalmia within six months of discontinuation of vitamin A therapy*

| Dosage of vitamin A | Number of cases |
|---|---|
| 0 | 1 |
| 50,000 IU | 2 |
| 100,000 IU | 7 |
| 150,000 IU | 5 |
| 200,000 IU | 1 |
| 250,000 IU | – |
| 300,000 IU | 2 |
| $>$ 300,000 IU | 4 |
| Total no. of cases | 22 |

quence only of vitamin A deficiency or also of protein deficiency is not clear (Table 6). A clinical answer to this question requires an unbiased control population, i.e. children without eye lesions. Among the patients in children's wards, very small children were frequently encountered who had probably not grown for several months, but who had completely normal eyes, and who showed no signs of vitamin A deficiency. Further studies on this group could possibly provide the answer. Treatment with vitamin A systemically and orally in the early stages ($X_0X_1$ and $X_2$) is successful if other causal factors are treated at the same time (e.g. intestinal infestations, acute infections, etc.). On the other hand, patients reaching stage $X_3$ will be left with serious corneal scars. In cases of corneal perforation, an adherent leukoma, partial or total, will ensue. In cases of a partial leukoma a dark brown sheet of pigment beginning at the anterior synechia often develops, creeping forward toward the corneal endothelium behind a formerly clear part of the cornea. When this has happened, visual acuity will deteriorate, even long after the cornea has healed. Unfortunately, even the smaller central corneal scars are often not favorable candidates for a corneal transplantation, because the young eye will have become amblyopic. On the other hand, probably because of the regenerative powers of the youthful cornea, a rather large leukoma sometimes became

smaller after an interval of several months. This, however, is rather rare.

Because of the continuously short supply of dietary vitamin A, recurrences are likely in xerophthalmia patients (Table 7). Although xerophthalmia is endemic on most of the larger islands of Indonesia, it is, in a sense, self-limiting as cases of xerophthalmia $X_0X_1$ are rarely seen in persons older than eight years, whereas $X_3$ is virtually nonexistent in older children and adults.

As one becomes vitamin A-minded, one applies this attitude to other corneal diseases. Thus, I give vitamin A systemically and orally in cases of smallpox-keratitis, in Mooren's ulcer and in gonorrheal corneal ulcers.

When an ophthalmologist starts his work in a developing country, he should make certain that the popular diet contains sufficient vitamin A. If he is not certain, then he should look for the various signs of vitamin A deficiency. Often they are found by the alert doctor in a country where xerophthalmia was not known to exist. The examination of young children should not be aggressive: one can learn a great deal just by talking with the mother.

The whole complex of problems, including the factors behind local variations, seasonal peaks and the seemingly erratic behavior of serum vitamin A levels have not yet been elucidated. But the importance of analyzing the clinical aspects of keratomalacia seems to me to be highly important, especially in view of the possibilities of prevention.

REFERENCES

1. WESTHOFF CHA. Eenige opmerkingen omtrent oogziekten op Java. *Feestbundel Geneesk Tijdschr Ned Indie*, 1911, p 141.
2. TENG KHOEN HING. Fundus changes in hypovitaminosis A. *Ophthalmologica* **137**: 81, 1959.
3. TENG KHOEN HING. Perubahan fundus mata pada hypovitaminosis A. Thesis, Djakarta, 1964.
4. TENG KHOEN HING. Serum vitamin and protein levels in fundus xerophthalmicus. *Trop Geogr Med* **17**: 273, 1965.

# G. VENKATASWAMY

Department of Ophthalmology, Madurai Medical College, Madurai, South India

Keratomalacia continues to be a blinding disease in children in many parts of the world. In the Eye Department of Madurai Medical College 250 to 350 keratomalacia cases are seen among 40,000 new patients a year. Although the disease occurs predominantly in preschool children, it is not uncommon in adults. Table 1 shows the age and incidence of 278 cases of keratomalacia treated in our Eye Department in 1970.

*Prevalence of keratomalacia.* A survey in three schools for the blind in South India showed that blindness was due to keratomalacia in about half of the children. A survey of children in public schools in Tamil Nadu State showed that 20 to 25 % had Bitôt's spots, angular stomatitis, xerosis and sequelae of keratomalacia. Of 33,000 school children examined, eight were blind in one eye due to keratomalacia. A similar study carried out in Calcutta in 1960 showed that children in public schools had leukoma-like scars, adherent leukoma and other lesions. In a special survey of physically handicapped children in Madras State in 1961 it was estimated that there were 26,589 totally blind children under four years of age. Only 8,261 of them were born blind; and the rest, 17,328 children, became blind before they were four years old. More than 50 % of the blindness was due to keratomalacia.

In the Eye Camps conducted during the summer of 1971, there were 339 cases of incurable blindness of which 25 (7.37%) were due to keratomalacia (Fig. 1). Of the 278 cases of keratomalacia seen in our Eye Department in 1970 the severe type was found in both eyes of 108 patients, while in 146 patients it was mild in both eyes (Fig. 2). In 24 patients only one eye was involved (Fig. 3). Some patients had corneal xerosis but since they were suffering from severe malnutrition they were first treated in the pediatric ward. In

TABLE 1. *Age and incidence of keratomalacia*

| Age group (years) | Males | Females | Total |
|---|---|---|---|
| 0 to 1 | 6 | 7 | 13 |
| 1 to 2 | 21 | 13 | 34 |
| 2 to 3 | 40 | 51 | 91 |
| 3 to 4 | 31 | 27 | 58 |
| 4 to 10 | 28 | 36 | 64 |
| 10 to 20 | 5 | 4 | 9 |
| > 20 | 9 | 0 | 9 |
| TOTAL | 140 | 138 | 278 |

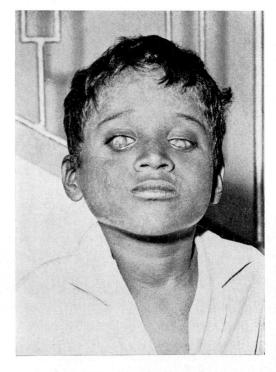

FIG. 1. Total blindness in both eyes due to keratomalacia.

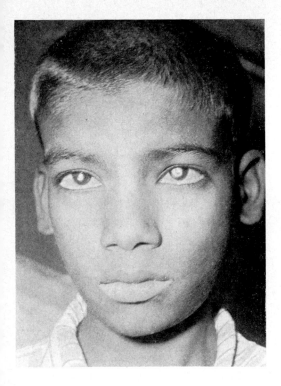

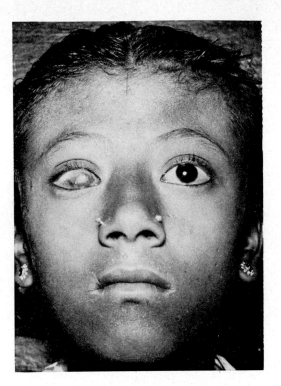

FIG. 2.   Partial blindness in both eyes due to kerato-malacia.

FIG. 3.   Blindness in one eye due to keratomalacia.

some cases the ulceration was superficial, and when the general condition had improved, the ulceration healed leaving a superficial opacity in the cornea. In others, the local necrosis in the lower portion of the cornea sometimes resulted in small iris prolapse. These cases healed with adherent leukomas and some residual vision. In severe cases the entire thickness of the whole cornea was white, and perforation occurred even after treatment.

*Management of keratomalacia cases.* At present, we are unable to admit all kerato-malacia patients to the hospital for necessary treatment. If the child cannot take vitamin A orally, then the vitamin must be injected. In addition a high protein diet is administered in order to improve the general condition of the patients. Early cases of corneal xerosis and early cases of keratomalacia can be cured without much damage to the cornea if the general condition of the patient is improved immediately. If, however, the entire cornea has already started to melt, the prognosis is always grave.

*Mortality in keratomalacia.* Keratomalacia is associated with a high mortality rate. With better care given in the hospitals a large number of patients now survive, but many are totally or partially blind. Some cases develop adherent leukoma; and others, who have corneal ulceration, develop phthisis bulbi, adherent leukoma or anterior staphyloma. Some show Bitôt's spots and xerosis for the rest of their lives.

**171**

# Y. YASSUR, S. YASSUR, S. ZAIFRANI, U. ZACHS and I. BEN-SIRA

Department of Ophthalmology, Hadassah University Hospital, Jerusalem, Israel

Xerophthalmia and keratomalacia, the eye lesions resulting from vitamin A deficiency, occur mainly in association with severe protein and calorie malnutrition. This syndrome is one of the major causes of blindness in many developing countries. Rwanda, in the central highlands near the equator, is the most densely populated area of Central Africa. Dietary studies show a striking deficiency of animal protein and lipids (1). Keratomalacia is considered to be the principal cause of blindness among children in this country. In the present survey we examined the relationship between xerophthalmia, nutritional state, serum vitamin A and serum proteins.

## MATERIAL AND METHODS

The survey was carried out on children aged six months to 16 years, who were divided into four groups:

1) Control group of healthy children without any systemic or ocular disease; 2) children with Bitot's spots without xerophthalmia; 3) children with xerophthalmia without corneal ulcerations; and 4) children with active keratomalacia.

The following parameters were examined in each group: a) Nutritional state was judged by the general physical development of the child, and by signs of malnutrition. The intakes of calories, carbohydrates, proteins, lipids and vitamin A were estimated for each child. b) Dark adaptation was tested on children whose cooperation, age, general physical condition and ocular state permitted a proper examination. The method of testing was that described by McLaren (2). c) Conjunctival biopsies were performed. d) Serum vitamin A was determined according to the Carr-Price method. e) Total serum proteins were measured.

## RESULTS

A summary of the results for all four groups is given in Table 1. All the children in the control group, Group 1, were in a satisfactory nutritional state. They had no dark adaptation disturbances and their conjunctival biopsies were normal. Serum vitamin A and total proteins were within normal limits.

All the subjects in Group 2 were between 13 and 16 years of age. We rarely found Bitôt's spots without xerophthalmia in younger children. Dark adaptation was disturbed in three of nine subjects examined. Conjunctival biopsies were carried out in 10 subjects, all of whom showed pathological changes. However, five of them suffered from solar damage or nonspecific inflammatory changes. Only in five cases were there signs suggestive of hypovitaminosis A: these were hyperkeratosis, loss of goblet cells, basal layer degeneration, edema and degeneration of subepithelial collagen. In spite of this, serum vitamin A and proteins were normal in this group.

Twenty-nine of the 40 children in Group 3 had protein and calorie malnutrition, 28 with kwashiorkor and one with marasmus. The other 11 were in a good to fair nutritional state. Four of these 11 had had some recent acute infection, such as measles, diarrhea or pneumonia. Dark adaptation was disturbed in all of the 12 children examined in this group. All of the conjunctival biopsies revealed changes such as loss of goblet cells, hyperkeratosis, edema, inflammation and collagen degeneration of the subepithelial tissue. Serum vitamin A protein levels were very low in this group.

Seventy-five percent of the children in group 4 were in poor general condition. Twenty-one of the 28 subjects had malnutrition, 20 with kwashiorkor and one with marasmus. Seven children were in a fair nutritional state, but suffered from some acute infection. Only four underwent dark adapta-

TABLE 1. *The prevalence of keratomalacia in 105 children in Rwanda*

| Group | No. of children | Nutritional state (no. of children) | | | Disturbed dark adaptation (no. of children) | Pathological changes in conjunctival biopsies (no. of children) | Serum vitamin A | | Serum protein | |
|---|---|---|---|---|---|---|---|---|---|---|
| | | Good to fair | Kwashiorkor | Marasmus | | | No. of children examined | Mean IU/100 ml (± SD) | No. of children examined | Mean g/100 ml (range) |
| 1 | 25 | 25 | 0 | 0 | — | — | 20 | 51 ± 17 | 20 | 7.2 (6.2 to 7.4) |
| 2 | 12 | 12 | 0 | 0 | 3 (9)a | 10 (10)a | 11 | 52 ± 19 | 11 | 7.1 (6.2 to 7.5) |
| 3 | 40 | 11 (4)b | 28 | 1 | 12 (12)a | 12 (12)a | 21 | 19 ± 6 | 21 | 5.8 (3.6 to 6.2) |
| 4 | 28 | 7 (7)b | 20 | 1 | 4 (4)a | 2 (2)a | 17 | 11 ± 4 | 17 | 4.3 (3.6 to 5.9) |

a No. of children examined indicated within brackets.
b No. of children examined during and after acute infection indicated within brackets.

tion tests; and there was disturbed dark adaptation in all of them. Conjunctival biopsies were taken from only two of the children and both showed the changes described for Group 3. Serum vitamin A and proteins were considerably reduced.

## DISCUSSION

Our survey shows that although the majority of children with xerophthalmia and keratomalacia suffered from kwashiorkor, not all those suffering from this disease develop xerophthalmia. The fact that there was no direct correlation in all cases between xerophthalmia and the decline of serum protein and vitamin A levels may explain this.

Xerophthalmia and keratomalacia were associated with marasmus in only two cases. Kumming (3) also pointed out that keratomalacia was less frequent in children with marasmus than in those with kwashiorkor.

Eleven children in the last two groups had an acute infection which preceded the appearance of xerophthalmia and keratomalacia. The role of acute infection as a trigger for the appearance of keratomalacia has previously been stressed by others (4–6). Sixty percent of Rwandan children are borderline cases from the point of view of protein and calorie intake (2), and it is therefore likely that some of them cannot overcome the superimposed stress.

Scotopic vision was considerably impaired not only when vitamin A levels were low, but also in some cases where these levels were within normal limits. This is in accord with other observations (2, 7).

Conjunctival histological changes similar to those classically associated with vitamin A deficiency (2, 8, 9) were seen not only in children with xerophthalmia and keratomalacia, but also in those with Bitôt's spots, who had normal serum vitamin A levels. They should be regarded, therefore, as nonspecific signs of irritation, which are not exclusively

**173**

pathognomonic of vitamin A deficiency.

There was a concomitant decline in serum vitamin A and protein levels in the last two groups. This decline was more pronounced in the group with keratomalacia than in the xerophthalmia group. There is no animal protein and only limited vegetable protein in the diet of Rwandan children (1). Various authors have already stated that although vitamin A deficiency is the cause of xerophthalmia, serum protein also plays an important role (4, 7, 10, 11). Protein deficiency probably impairs both the absorption of vitamin A from the intestine and its transport in the plasma (10, 12, 13). Oil is also very rare in the Rwandan children's diet (1). Since dietary fat is an important factor in the absorption of vitamin A from the intestine (12–14), the lack of it may be a contributory factor in the pathogenesis of xerophthalmia in Rwanda.

We would like to thank Professor Michaelson for his advice in planning the research. We would like to convey our thanks to Professor Boyde and Dr. Templeton of Makarere University Hospital, Kampala, Uganda, for providing the facilities to carry out the biochemical and pathological investigations.

This research could not have been possible without the help of the team of ISAR-Rubona, Butare, Rwanda and of the ophthalmological staff of the University Hospital in Butare, Rwanda.

## REFERENCES

1. Alimentation et nutrition au Rwanda. *Colloque Fomentro, Giseni, 1966.*
2. McLaren DS. "Malnutrition and the eye." New York, Academic Press, 1963.
3. Kumming BS. The evolution of keratomalacia. *Trans Ophthalmol Soc UK* **87**: 305, 1967.
4. McManus EP. Xerophthalmia in Matabeleland. *Cent Afr J Med* **14**: 166, 1968.
5. McLaren DS, Oomen HAPC and Escapini H. Ocular manifestations of vitamin A deficiency in man. *Bull WHO* **34**: 357, 1966.
6. Oomen HAPC. Clinical epidemiology of xerophthalmia in man. *Am J Clin Nutr* **22**: 1098, 1969.
7. McLaren DS. Nutritional diseases and the eye. *Borden Rev Nutr Res* **25**: 1, 1964.
8. McLaren DS. Bitot's spots. A review of their significance after 100 years. *Br Med J* **2**: 926, 1963.
9. Paton D and McLaren DS. Bitot spots. *Am J Ophthalmol* **50**: 568, 1960.
10. Konmo T, Hansen JDL, Truswell AS, Woold- Walker R and Becker D. Vitamin A deficiency and protein-caloric malnutrition in Cape Town. *S Afr Med J* **42**: 950, 1968.
11. Yap-Kie-Tiong. Protein deficiency in keratomalacia. *Br J Ophthalmol* **40**: 502, 1956.
12. Figueira F, Mendonca S, Rocha J, Azevedo M, Bunce GE and Reynolds JW. Absorption of vitamin A by infants receiving fat-free or fat-containing dried skim milk formulas. *Am J Clin Nutr* **22**: 588, 1969.
13. Manual for Nutrition Survey. Interdepartmental Committee on Nutrition for National Defense. Bethesda Md, National Institutes of Health, 1964, p 124.
14. Roels OA, Debeir D and Trout M. Vitamin A deficiency in Rwanda-Urundi. *Trop Geogr Med* **10**: 77, 1958.

# PREVENTION OF BLINDNESS DUE TO HYPOVITAMINOSIS A

H. A. P. C. OOMEN

Royal Tropical Institute, Amsterdam, the Netherlands

Abnormal keratinization of the eye epithelia, the principal expression of clinical retinol deficiency in man, shows differences in timing and localization. In an infant the onset is usually sudden and the cornea is seriously affected before the typical changes of the conjunctiva are visible. This is keratomalacia *sensu stricto* which so often escapes timely discovery and chance of treatment. In a young child xerosis of the interpalpebral conjunctiva usually precedes affection of the cornea. Very often the typical spots of Bitot are visible and the patient may show, or its mother mention, night blindness. The older the child, the more protracted the course of the disease and the more frequent an isolated xerosis of the conjunctiva. It is then more likely that the condition will be recognized before irreversible corneal damage can occur.

The development of the specific lesions is considerably influenced by intercurrent infectious disease. The little vitamin A there is suddenly appears to become unavailable. Manifestation during postmeasles desquamation or after a period of diarrhea is classical. The appearance of xerophthalmia in Indonesia as a result of various types of infection is illustrated in Table 1.

Protein-calorie malnutrition is a usual partner of the process. Both the kwashiorkor and the marasmus varieties are often accompanied by eye lesions. Here absence of the lipoprotein carrier is a partial explanation. The age-prevalence peak occurs later in the cases of clinical vitamin A deficiency than in protein deficiency without eye affection. The vitamin A deficiency apparently needs more time to develop.

Though no age group is wholly exempt in regions where xerophthalmia is endemic, the victim is preeminently the small child; not so much the infant, who may be protected by the traditional prolonged breastfeeding, but more especially the three- and four-year-olds.

In all prosperous countries and situations, the condition is nowadays extinct. The main reason may be the general availability of cow's milk to the small child and the amounts, even though small, of vitamin A thus obtained. Theoretically, carotene from vegetable sources can supply enough of the vitamin, but the quantity required is about six times that needed of retinol. It is distressing that the carotene abundantly present in the wet green

TABLE 1.  *Xerophthalmia and infection*

| Stage | X1 (%) | X2 to X3 (%) |
|---|---|---|
| Diarrheal | 48 | 30 |
| Tuberculous | 24 | 17 |
| Acute infection | 30 | 50 |

**175**

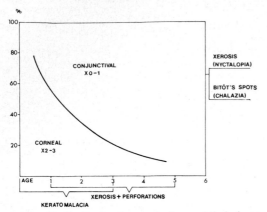

FIG. 1. Stagewise development of xerophthalmia according to age in years.

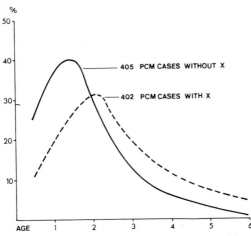

FIG. 2. Age distribution of malnutrition with or without xerophthalmia. PCM = protein calorie malnutrition.

tropics nevertheless often does not reach the rapidly growing small child, whose requirement is relatively the greatest. If such a child is living in the unprotected environment of the city slums of the Far East, or in the poor countryside, or if for some social reason the child does not receive sufficient nutritional care, then the stage is set, not only for malnutrition, but also for its vilest complication: xerophthalmia.

In discussing prevention we have to be aware of the following facts: 1) The sufferer is usually a young child, aged one to four years (Fig. 1 and 2). 2) He is living in a socioeconomically and hygienically under-developed environment where money, transport, nutritional insight and expert medical care are rare. 3) The affection is easily curable, without ophthalmological skills, if discovered in time. 4) The prevalence of conjunctival xerosis, Bitot's spots and night blindness can act as alarm symptoms before the cornea becomes involved. 5) The survivor of the corneal stages, if untreated or if treated too late, will be blind and therefore deprived of the visual aspects of education, thus becoming an intolerable burden to an unprotected society. 6) The cure and the medicine are cheap.

*Curative measures.* The critical corneal stage, like an intestinal perforation, should be considered as an emergency. Any medically trained discoverer of the condition should at once start oral or parenteral treatment with high doses of vitamin A palmitate.

It should be realized that the specific process is painless and often proceeds behind closed lids. Any eye affection in the vulnerable age group should be considered with suspicion.

Cure means that the specter of blindness should definitely be averted. The child should be followed up, even if admission into hospital is impossible, for at least five to seven days, that is, until the effect of vitamin A therapy is visible. This only refers to the prevention of blindness, because much more should be done to cure the accompanying malnutrition, tuberculosis etc. But anyone who has treated a case of xerophthalmia with success should be aware that he cannot treat the environment which produced the patient, and that relapses are not uncommon.

*Preventive measures.* The expert ophthalmologist is too rare a bird in the surroundings where xerophthalmia is endemic. He is usually the last resort when opportunity for appropriate treatment has vanished. He then observes survivors of the catastrophe present-

**176**

ing scarring stages such as phthisis bulbi, leukoma or staphyloma, any of which may have been produced by other causes. If the eye specialist has been trained in Europe or America, chances are slim that he has ever seen a case during his training period.

The pediatrician may have better opportunities of seeing the patient. But he is often so impressed and preoccupied by the malnourished state of the child that he may not pay adequate attention to the critical condition of the cornea.

Any physician who has met cases in practice complains about lost opportunities. Irreversible destruction is often a question of a few days, or even of a single day. The conclusion is that alertness to the problem is essential.

Xerophthalmia is an environmental problem and the cases showing corneal affection are only the tip of the iceberg. Xerosis of the conjunctiva or Bitot's spots may be recognized in a school-age child; but his younger brother, eating from the same pot, may develop the corneal stages after measles or dysentery. Night blindness is often no strange phenomenon to the mothers, as is obvious from the many vernacular terms for it. If the prodromal stages are known to be present in the community, catastrophic development in some young child can be expected.

For the sake of efficiency, alertness to symptoms should be present in the lower echelons of medical care. These workers are often the first to meet the stricken child and much depends on their prompt action. Dosage with vitamin A is a harmless procedure requiring no special skill. This alertness, however, is sometimes lacking even in the highest echelons. In two questionnaires which WHO addressed to all member states, the information given on the role of hypovitaminosis A in blindness was disappointing, even in those areas where sufficient scientific documentation supported the existence of a problem. In Jordan, where the condition was made reportable some years ago, the recording of hundreds of cases per year resulted.

What could be done, medically, to prevent cases occurring? A positive answer was given in the chaotic years in Hong Kong when every small child seen at dispensaries was automatically dosed with vitamin A. This led to a considerable decline in cases of blindness in later years.

Systematic distribution of red palm oil has been practiced in Indonesia, where the oil palm is not a native crop. This is an even more interesting approach. The results are satisfactory but success depends wholly on being able to reach the vulnerable groups.

Recent trials have proved the potential efficacy of protecting the child by periodic repletion of vitamin A stores. For this purpose very small volumes of high-potency liquid preparations are administered orally. Though the prospects are good the details of this preventive technique still have to be worked out. However, it looks as if such a procedure could find a place in immunization schemes employed by child health centers.

*Promotive measures.* The natural pathway by which vitamin A reaches the consumer is by food. This should be considered the most desirable, most universal and safest way of fulfilling requirements. But milk, liver and egg yolks are usually conspicuously absent from the exposed surroundings, so the next best choice is leaf vegetables. Curiously enough, these are highly valued in prosperous societies where retinol sources are not at a premium, but are often neglected where they appear to be the most readily available source. Nutritionally, horticulture is an underdeveloped aspect of many tropical regions, and the blind survivor is often found in the greenest of environments. So long as dependable sources of the preformed vitamin cannot be made available, a better use of provitamin resources by producers and consumers should be advocated.

Even more than animal protein, retinol consumption is a parameter of prosperity. Cow's milk is then a very dependable source of precious protein. But if skimmed milk devoid of vitamin A is given to an infant he may develop xerophthalmia. This deplorable effect has been known for 30 years. It is still necessary to warn the unthinking distributor and consumer again and again, even in this modern era of food technology.

The prevention of child malnutrition does not differ from that of xerophthalmia, once the risk of impending blindness is taken care of. In certain areas, centers to care for the malnourished children, even employing low grade staff, may be very useful in combating hypovitaminosis A before admission to hospital is necessary or possible. In such personnel loving care and alertness to the problem are qualities which in practice may out-weigh the possession of skills or diplomas.

For a variety of reasons, some of which have already been stressed, xerophthalmia has been called the oculist's Cinderella, and I should like to add, the nutritionist's. The subject must belong to the realm of nutritional education. As the fatal effect of xerophthalmia is so easy to demonstrate visually, I should like to advocate the free use of visual aids. Far from sufficient attention has been paid to this scourge in textbooks, health documents, doctors' and nurses' curricula and malnutrition campaigns. As an ophthalmological issue, it vanished from specialist journals several decades ago. This, however, does not preclude the fact that xerophthalmia is yearly the cause of permanent blindness in scores of children in some of the less well endowed areas of the world.

# THE PREVENTION OF CHILDHOOD BLINDNESS BY THE ADMINISTRATION OF MASSIVE DOSES OF VITAMIN A

JAMES A. OLSON

Department of Biochemistry, Faculty of Science, Mahidol University, Bangkok, Thailand

Vitamin A deficiency, particularly when associated with generalized malnutrition, is a major cause of blindness among preschool children in many parts of the world. Since blindness, perhaps more than any other state of reduced physiological function, is socially and psychologically debilitating, its prevention should have a high priority among public health measures. The incidence of nutritional blindness might be reduced in several ways, namely: 1) by improving the overall socio-economic environment, 2) by educating both children and adults in good nutritional practice, 3) by providing better medical care and 4) by using proper food and vitamin supplements.

The first three measures are long-term projects requiring social evolution for effective implementation. In this paper I shall deal only with the fourth approach, and indeed even more narrowly with only one type of vitamin supplement, the administration of massive doses of vitamin A. Although this measure has always been theoretically feasible because of the extensive storage of vitamin A, its slow rate of utilization and its relatively low toxicity, McLaren was, to my knowledge, the first person in recent times to argue forcefully in favor of using massive doses of

vitamin A as a public health measure (1). The National Institute of Nutrition in Hyderabad, India, on the other hand, was the first institution actually to initiate field trials in the use of large doses of vitamin A (2). In the present paper I shall discuss three aspects of this measure: 1) a general biochemical and physiological analysis of the problem; 2) a summary of field results, largely drawn from the Indian group; and 3) a brief discussion of possible ways of improving the effectiveness of the measure.

Major metabolic considerations are depicted in Fig. 1. Of a given amount of vitamin

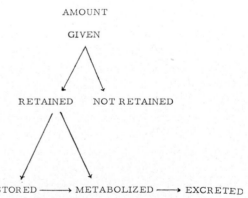

FIG. 1. The metabolic fate of an administered dose of vitamin A.

Administered dose
  Amount
  Chemical form
  Nature of dispersion
  Route of administration
  Frequency of administration
  Accessory compounds
Recipient
  Age
  Sex
  Nutritional state
  Health status
Storage
  Organs involved
  Kinetics of turnover and depletion
  Influencing factors
Other factors
  Cost of vitamin and administration
  Sociocultural acceptance
  Hypervitaminotic symptoms
Evaluation
  Prevention of eye disease
  Reduction in infection
  Stimulation of growth

FIG. 2.    Factors in setting up a public health program.

A or suitable vitamin A-active derivative which is administered, only a certain portion is retained. Of that portion, some is stored and some is immediately metabolized and excreted. Excretion products appear both in the urine and the feces, and consist mainly of glucuronides and of yet unidentified oxidized and partially-degraded metabolites (3). The objective, of course, is to maximize the amount stored from a given administered dose.

Practical factors which should either be controlled or considered in setting up a public health program of this kind are given in Fig. 2. First, the dosing method can be modified in several ways to enhance absorption and storage. The nutritional status and health of the recipient will also affect these parameters. Technical and social factors must also be carefully considered. The incidence of hypervitaminosis A must be minimized, and proper procedures for evaluation must be established. The prevention of nutritional blindness is the major goal, but a reduction in the incidence of infection and possible stim-

ulation of growth might be side benefits of this measure.

In considering various factors individually, we should first inquire what chemical forms might be used. β-carotene is an obvious choice, both because it is the main natural source of vitamin A for a large segment of the human population (4) and because several natural products, such as red palm oil, are rich sources of β-carotene. For example, when red palm oil was administered daily to village children in Indonesia over an appreciable period of time, the incidence of xerophthalmia was reduced (5). However, the use of β-carotene has several major disadvantages. First of all, its absorption is poorer than that of vitamin A and its conversion into vitamin A is relatively slow. Secondly, the relative portion of a dose stored in the liver as vitamin A is inversely proportional to the β-carotene dose. In livestock, β-carotene at low doses is stored about 30% as effectively as retinol (IU/IU) but at high doses the relative effectiveness of β-carotene falls to 12% or less (6, 7). On the other hand, the use of small doses given at weekly or shorter intervals almost certainly requires surveillance. Once the Indonesian study (5) was completed and public health personnel no longer frequented the villages, the practice of using red palm oil declined (A. D. Sediaoetama, personal communication). Finally, the logistics of transport, storage and distribution of relatively large amounts of red palm oil or similar products poses serious organizational and financial problems in developing societies.

Of various forms of vitamin A which could be employed, the esters, such as the acetate and palmitate, are generally preferred to the free forms, such as retinol and retinal, since they are more stable and tend to result both in better storage in the liver when administered orally and in less tissue reaction when injected as compared with retinol (8, 9). In special cases the possibility of using other derivatives of vitamin A such as sterically hindered esters (10) or retinyl methyl ether should be considered.

Vitamin A, in natural oils or in various water-soluble detergent combinations employed as dispersing agents, might be administered either orally or i.m. At the outset the i.m. administration of vitamin A in oil can be discarded, since it is known to be ineffective (11–13). For oral administration, oil is known to enhance vitamin A absorption, probably through its stimulatory effect on bile secretion (14). On the other hand, vitamin A given in a water-soluble detergent is readily absorbed (15) and yields high transient peaks of plasma vitamin A (12). The liver storage of vitamin A, although higher in protein-deficient rats after oral dosing in oil compared with detergents (12), was the same in normal rats when either dispersing agent was employed (16). Retinyl acetate, injected i.m. in a water-soluble detergent, was stored very effectively in rat liver and under some circumstances was even superior to oral dosing in normal animals (9). Intramuscular injections of retinyl acetate in aqueous detergents are not painful, do not produce unpleasant local tissue reactions and are rapidly absorbed from the tissue site (M. Macapinlac and J. A. Olson, unpublished observations).

Of various specific compounds which might aid the absorption and storage of vitamin A, vitamin E is unquestionably the most important. Not only does vitamin E protect vitamin A from oxidation during storage of a pharmaceutical preparation, but it also markedly enhances liver storage of vitamin A in vitamin E-deficient animals (9). Since the vitamin E status of children may well be marginal in generalized malnutrition, vitamin E should routinely be incorporated into vitamin A preparations.

The recipients of vitamin A treatment should be chiefly preschool children, usually from one to six years of age. As might be expected, the child's health and nutritional state critically influence the effectiveness of a given dose of vitamin A. Protein calorie malnutrition, for example, reduces the rate of conversion of β-carotene into vitamin A, the concentration of vitamin A in the plasma and the relative amount stored in the liver (8). In human beings with respiratory infections, the absorption of orally administered vitamin A labeled with tritium was reduced from approximately 80% to as little as 30% (17). Parasitic infestation also markedly affects vitamin A blood levels, probably by reducing carotene and vitamin A absorption (18, 19). In general, therefore, the effectiveness of oral doses of vitamin A is particularly sensitive to the nutritional state and health of the recipient.

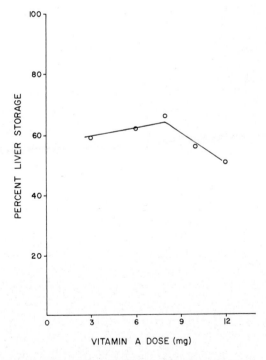

FIG. 3. The relationship between the dose of vitamin A given to rats and the percent stored in the liver. Retinol was administered orally in soybean oil to 100 to 200 g rats and the liver was analyzed 24 hr later for vitamin A (21).

**181**

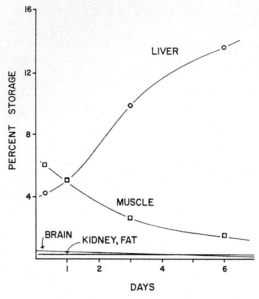

FIG. 4. The dynamics of vitamin A storage in the organs of young rhesus monkeys (1 kg) after the i.m. administration of 100 mg of retinyl acetate in a water-soluble polysorbate detergent. Absorption from the site of injection was rapid, only 3% of the injected dose remaining at 6 hr and 0.3% at 24 hr. Muscle values are calculated from analyses made in samples far from the injection site (W. Watcharakorn, personal communication).

Mammalian liver has an incredible capacity to store vitamin A. In polar bear liver, for example, the vitamin A concentration may be as high as 10 mg/g wet wt of tissue (20). After the feeding of retinol in soybean oil to rats, the percentage of the dose stored in the liver 24 hr after administration remained relatively constant at 60%, with doses up to about 8 mg of retinol (80 mg/kg), and then decreased slightly (21) (Fig. 3). On the other hand, when similar doses (100 mg/kg) were administered i.m. to monkeys in a water-soluble form, storage in the liver reached a maximum value only after several days (W. Watcharakorn, personal communication) (Fig. 4). The possibility that other organs such as muscle store vitamin A, particularly during a transient phase soon after i.m. administration, must

not be overlooked in evaluating the relative effectiveness of various routes of administration. Further studies on the manner in which i.m. and oral doses of vitamin A are handled metabolically in mammals, and particularly in primates, are therefore well worth pursuing. The rate at which vitamin A is mobilized from the liver has been estimated in two kinds of study: depletion experiments and turnover measurements. The results from both kinds of study are essentially the same, namely, that vitamin A leaves the liver at a first order rate at any significant initial level of storage and that the time ($T\frac{1}{2}$) to deplete or replace half of the stores varies from 40 to 80 days: 49 days for steers, 62 days for rats and 27 days for sheep (22). As liver stores of vitamin A dwindle, however, the utilization rate becomes linear (23). We can, therefore, estimate how long a given reserve of vitamin A might last by simply plotting a first order graph, as shown in Fig. 5. Since a one- to

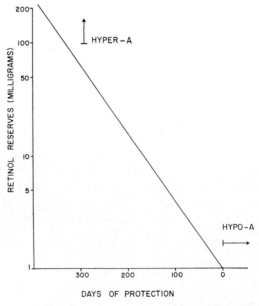

FIG. 5. Estimated relationship between total body reserves of vitamin A and the period of protection against vitamin A deficiency. The $T\frac{1}{2}$ for depletion is assumed to be 50 days.

TABLE 1. *Effect of various doses of vitamin A on the incidence of toxic symptoms and on the period of protection*

| Dose (IU) | Dispersion | Route | Age group | Toxicity | Approximate months protection | Reference |
|---|---|---|---|---|---|---|
| 9,000,000[a] | Liver | Oral | Adult | High | — | 25 |
| 1,250,000 | Aqueous | Parenteral | Adult | None | — | Olson, unpublished observations |
| 600,000 | Aqueous | Oral | Child | None | — | 26 |
| 300,000 | Aqueous | Oral | Preschool | 25%: mild | 6 to 12 | 2 |
| 300,000 | Oil | Oral | Preschool | None | 4 to 5 | 27 |
| 300,000 | Oil | Oral | Preschool | 4%: mild | 6 to 12 | 28 |
| 200,000 | Oil | Oral | Preschool | None? | 6 | 28 |
| 150,000 | Aqueous | Oral | Preschool | 4%: mild | — | 2 |

[a] Estimated amount ingested.

six-year-old child normally requires 20 to 30 μg of vitamin A per kg per day (24), only a fraction of the recommended allowance would be provided by liver stores during the final 50 to 100 days of the protective period. On the other hand, since as little as 6 to 10 μg/kg can either prevent or retard the development of frank symptoms of vitamin A deficiency, and since some vitamin A will unquestionably be ingested during the depletion period, Fig. 5 is probably a roughly valid indicator of the length of the protected period as a function of body reserves.

In practical terms, the size of the dose is limited by the problem of hypervitaminosis A. Early Arctic explorers who suffered from vitamin A toxicity after eating polar bear liver may have ingested as much as 9 million IU or roughly 40 mg/kg body wt (25). However, the i.m. injection of 1.25 million units of vitamin A in an aqueous dispersion to human adult volunteers caused no overt symptoms (J. A. Olson, unpublished observations). In addition, a total of 600,000 IU of water-miscible retinyl palmitate given orally over a six-day period caused no toxicity in one child (26) and 330,000 IU of retinyl palmitate given orally in arachis oil to 27 preschool children was also well tolerated (27). On the other hand, a one-year-old child who received an oral dose of 100,000 IU of water-miscible retinyl palmitate developed bulging of the fontanelle and vomiting (26) and 25% of a relatively large group of preschool children treated orally with 300,000 IU of water-miscible retinyl palmitate developed transient signs of acute toxicity (2, 12). When the same dose was given orally in oil, however, only about 4% of the group was affected (28). A summary of various dosage levels, with the incidence of toxic symptoms and the approximate observed periods of protection is given in Table 1. In view of both the extensive immediate metabolism of administered doses of vitamin A in experimental animals (3, 22, 29) and the relatively high incidence of malnutrition in the field samples, the percentage of the administered dose which is stored in the field trial is probably around 20 to 30% and may even be lower. The observed periods of protection given in Table 2 and the estimated protection for given stores taken from Fig. 4 are in rough agreement.

The effectiveness of the field trial conducted by Swaminathan and his colleagues in Hyderabad (28) in reducing the incidence of xerosis and Bitot's spots is summarized in Table 2. Since 60 to 70% of the children between the ages of one and three were still breast-fed in this sample, the incidence of eye symptoms in the initial one- to two-year-old group is low. After weaning, however, both

**183**

TABLE 2. *Effect of two annual oral doses of 300,000 IU retinyl palmitate in oil on the incidence of xerosis and Bitôt's spots in preschool children*

|  | Age in years | | | | | |
|---|---|---|---|---|---|---|
|  | 1 to 2 | 2 to 3 | 3 to 4 | 4 to 5 | 5 to 6 | 6 to 7 |
| No. of children | 219 | 290 | 288 | 134 | 316 |  |
| Initial % xerosis | 0.9 | 9.0 | 11.8 | 31.1 | 15.5 | — |
| Initial % Bitôt's spots | 0.5 | 5.2 | 6.6 | 9.6 | 9.5 | — |
| Final % xerosis | — | — | 0.5 | 2.8 | 3.8 | 14.2 |
| Final % Bitôt's spots | — | — | 1.4 | 1.7 | 3.8 | 5.9 |
| % expected xerosis |  |  | 4 | 9 | 25 | > 50 ? |
| % expected Bitôt's spots |  |  | 21 | 18 | 40 | > 50 ? |

Data taken from ref. 28.

the incidence of xerosis and Bitot's spots increased markedly to reach a peak in the four- to six-year-old age group. However, after two years of treatment with oral doses of 300,000 IU retinyl palmitate in oil given once a year, the incidence of xerosis and Bitot's spots in all groups was lowered. Vitamin A treatment was most effective when given initially to the one- to two-year-old group and was least effective when given initially to the four- to five-year-olds. Corresponding data on the initial five- to six-year-old group were not given (28). This lack of responsiveness in the older groups is rather puzzling, but may possibly be caused in part by a greater resistance of older eye lesions to therapy, the reduced dosage of vitamin A/kg given to older children and poorer absorption due to more extensive parasitic infestation in older children. No new cases of keratomalacia were encountered during a three-year observation period. Because of this lack of protection in the older age group and the problem of toxicity at doses higher than 300,000 IU, the recommendation was made that 200,000 IU of retinyl palmitate in oil be given orally once every six months (28).

Vitamin A deficiency is best evaluated by the clinical detection of typical eye symptoms. A serum value below 10 µg of retinol/100 ml, which is closely associated with clinical signs of deficiency, is also a useful indicator of actual or impending deficiency. Serum values in the low middle range (10 to 30 µg/100 ml), however, really give very little information about total body stores. For example, no correlation at all was found between serum levels of vitamin A and liver stores in a relatively normal population in New York City that died suddenly or rapidly from unnatural causes (30). Furthermore, after the treatment of children with 100 mg of vitamin A, the steady-state plasma vitamin A concentration was only slightly and apparently not significantly increased in one study (27), although it did rise in another similar study (12). Except for the rather hazardous procedure of liver biopsy, no method now exists for evaluating total body reserves. Unquestionably, the development of such a method would be of enormous utility in selecting suitable populations for preventive treatment, in determining the efficiency of vitamin A storage in human beings under various conditions and in evaluating the length of the protective period.

Although the use of massive doses of vitamin A to prevent nutritional blindness in children is theoretically sound, practically workable and economically feasible (the present cost of a vitamin A preparation which might protect a child for a year is $0.05 to 0.08) the resolution of two major problems would further enhance its attractiveness as a public health measure. First, it would be very helpful if higher doses of vitamin A could be used without causing toxicity symptoms. The possible use of less toxic derivatives of vitamin A or of drugs which offset the toxicity should therefore be explored. Second, attempts should be made to increase the fraction of the dose which is actually stored. If methods could be devised for improving the overall absorption or utilization of the dose and for inhibiting transiently major catabolic pathways, such as glucuronide formation and decarboxylation, the protective period might be significantly increased for a given dose. It is not impossible that a single dose might protect a child for two years if the above problems could be resolved.

But quite apart from possible future technological improvements, the procedure is now successful and has been adopted by several states in India for early implementation. It will be interesting to follow the progress of these public health programs in India and hopefully elsewhere during the next few years.

*Note added to proof:* We have recently found that a large portion of a dose of radioactive retinyl acetate, injected to rats i.m. in oil, remains in extrahepatic tissues as retinyl acetate for relatively long periods. (T. Sueblingvong and J.A. Olson, unpublished observations.) The possible use of i.m. oil dispersions of vitamin A, therefore, should still be considered as a feasible alternative to other methods of administration.

The author, a field staff member of the Rockefeller Foundation, is indebted to Miss Patchari Karnasuta for expert secretarial assistance.

Supported by grants-in-aid from the US Public Health Service, National Institutes of Health (I-ROI-AM-11367–04), the Rockefeller Foundation (GA-BMS-7006), and the Faculty of Graduate Studies, Mahidol University, Bangkok, Thailand.

## REFERENCES

1. McLaren DS. Xerophthalmia: a neglected problem. *Nutr Rev* **22**: 289, 1964.
2. The Nutrition Research Laboratories, Indian Council of Medical Research, Hyderabad, India, Annual report, 1966, p 110.
3. Olson JA. Some aspects of vitamin A metabolism. *Vitam Horm* **26**: 1, 1968.
4. Patwardhan VN. Hypovitaminosis A and epidemiology of xerophthalmia. *Am J Clin Nutr* **22**: 1106, 1969.
5. Gyorgy P. Protein calorie and vitamin A malnutrition in Southeast Asia. *Fed Proc* **27**: 949, 1968.
6. Wellenreiter RH, Ullrey DE and Magee WT. Vitamin A activity of corn carotenes for swine. *J Nutr* **99**: 129, 1969.
7. Faruque O and Walker DM. The relative biological potencies of retinyl palmitate and β-carotene for the milk-fed lamb. *Br J Nutr* **24**: 23, 1970.
8. Ascarelli I. Absorption and transport of vitamin A in chicks. *Am J Clin Nutr* **22**: 913, 1969.
9. Ames SR. Factors affecting absorption transport and storage of vitamin A. *Am J Clin Nutr* **22**: 934, 1969.
10. Forlano AJ, Jarowski CI, Hammer HF and Merritt EG. Sterically hindered esters of vitamin A. II. Vitamin A-α, α-dimethyl palmitate. *J Pharm Sci* **59**: 121, 1970.
11. Pereira SM and Begum A. Studies in the prevention of vitamin A deficiency. *Indian J Med Res* **56**: 362, 1968.
12. Reddy V. Vitamin A deficiency. Decade report of the National Institute of Nutrition, Hyderabad, India, 1970, p 63.
13. Srikantia SG and Reddy V. Effect of a single massive dose of vitamin A on serum and liver levels of the vitamin. *Am J Clin Nutr* **23**: 114, 1970.
14. Gagnon M and Dawson AM. The effect of bile on vitamin A absorption in the rat. *Proc Soc Exp Biol Med* **127**: 99, 1968.
15. Olson JA. The effect of bile and bile salts on the uptake and cleavage of β-carotene into retinol ester (vitamin A ester) by intestinal slices. *J Lipid Res* **5**: 402, 1964.
16. Harris PL. Bioassay of vitamin A compounds. *Vitam Horm* **18**: 341, 1960.
17. Shivkumar B and Reddy V. Absorption of labelled vitamin A in children during infection. *Br J Nutr* **27**: 299, 1972.
18. Migasena S. A study of serum vitamin A levels in patients suffering from parasitic diseases In Thailand. *Proceedings of the First Southeast Asian Seminar on Nutrition, October, 1969,* Djakarta (in press).
19. Kouwenhoven B and Van der Horst CJG. Strongly acid intestinal content and lowered protein, carotene, and vitamin A blood levels in *Eimeria acervulina* infected chickens. *Z Parasitenkd* **32**: 347, 1969.
20. Russell FE. Vitamin A content of polar bear liver. *Toxicon* **5**: 61, 1966.
21. Watcharakorn W. Interaction of vitamin A with natural macromolecules. MSc thesis, Faculty of Graduate Studies, Mahidol University, Bangkok, 1969.
22. Hayes BW, Mitchell GE Jr, Little CO and

SEWELL HB. Turnover of liver vitamin A in steers. *J Anim Sci* **26**: 855, 1967.

23. DOWLING JE and WALD G. Vitamin A deficiency and night blindness. *Proc Natl Acad Sci USA* **44**: 648, 1958.

24. Report of a joint FAO/WHO group on requirements of vitamin A, thiamine, riboflavin and niacin. *WHO Tech Rep Ser* **362**: 1967.

25. MOORE T. Pharmacology and toxicology of vitamin A, in: Sebrell WH Jr and Harris RS (Eds), "The vitamins," 2nd edn. New York, Academic Press, 1967, v 1, p 280.

26. PEREIRA SM, BEGUM A, ISAAC T and DUMM ME. Vitamin A therapy in children with kwashiorkor. *Am J Clin Nutr* **20**: 297, 1967.

27. PEREIRA SM and BEGUM A. Prevention of vitamin A deficiency. *Am J Clin Nutr* **22**: 858, 1969.

28. SWAMINATHAN MC, SUSHEELA TP and THIMMAYAMMA BVS. Field prophylactic trial with a single annual oral massive dose of vitamin A. *Am J Clin Nutr* **23**: 119, 1970.

29. ZACHMAN RD, DUNAGIN PE JR and OLSON JA. Formation and enterohepatic circulation of metabolites of retinol and retinoic acid in bile duct-cannulated rats. *J Lipid Res* **7**: 3, 1966.

30. UNDERWOOD BA, SIEGEL H, WEISELL RC and DOLINSKI M. Liver stores of vitamin A in a normal population dying suddenly or rapidly from unnatural causes in New York City. *Am J Clin Nutr* **23**: 1037, 1970.

# KERATOMALACIA IN HAITI

M. L. SEARS

Department of Ophthalmology, Yale University School of Medicine, New Haven, Connecticut, USA

Estimates of the incidence of chronic vitamin A deficiency in Haiti vary from 8 to 81%. Seasonal variations in the availability of vegetables probably explain the wide range of estimates. However, there is no doubt that vitamin A deficiency, particularly in children who have just been weaned, is an important contributor to the disastrous tissue destruction of the cornea in malnourished children.

Most Haitians have a meager diet. They rely chiefly upon raw sugarcane, maize, rice, sorghum, cassava, beans, yams and plaintains. On very rare occasions, they may eat salted fish, freshly killed goat or pork. Not only is the availability of food a problem but often when food is available, for example in the form of leafy vegetables, the Haitians are not accustomed to including these substances in their diet.

Within the last few years, we have been working in the Artibonite Valley of Haiti, which is a rich and fertile area. We have helped Dr. Larimer Mellon and his wife at the Albert Schweitzer Hospital in Des Chapelles and have been largely responsible for the eye care at this "community hospital."

While we were impressed with the efficacy of the usual doses of vitamin A in the treatment of keratomalacia, we were more impressed by the following observations:

1) Vitamin A deficiency may be a necessary but not sufficient requirement for the condition. 2) There was increased susceptibility at weaning and during the summer months. 3) "Early" signs of keratomalacia are rarely, if ever, present.

Most important of all, we saw that keratomalacia develops not only in weaned babies (age 18 months to two years) but also in somewhat older children, who may otherwise not be suffering acutely from malnutrition. The hazards of superimposed infection in these dry corneas are obvious.

After working in the province of Verret in the Artibonite Valley and developing a feel for the community of several hundred thousand persons, as well as for the community-district hospital, one learns that the "conventional" sources of added vitamin A to the diet of the Haitian are woefully inadequate. We cannot use milk, since cows are only for the wealthy and goats are rarely, if ever, used for this purpose. Carnation evaporated milk is sold in Haiti. A reconstituted quart contains 1,310 units of natural vitamin A, which is less than one-half the daily requirement. Furthermore—and this is the major problem—only 30,000 cases of Carnation milk are sold annually in Haiti.

Prophylaxis programs are recommended by the highly motivated and energetic workers. In some areas these programs may work. Members of our department were very impressed, however, with the nutrition center, developed by members of the staff of the Albert Schweitzer Hospital.

Mothers and children are brought to one of three to six mobile nutrition centers near their homes, where they are instructed over a six to eight-week period in the preparation of a diet from their own native environment. The dietary requirements of calories, protein and vitamins are maintained for as little as $ 0.07 a day. The children are weighed at intervals and the mothers are able to see a weight gain in their children within two months. The circulation and recirculation of these centers are invaluable in any long-range program of nutrition as the population is then able to survive within its own environment from its own natural resources. The incidence of keratomalacia drops each year in the Artibonite as mothers learn to use plaintain, leafy vegetables and oils in the daily preparation of food for their children.

This may seem a tedious and unrewarding process for the impatient worker in a developing country. We merely wanted to report this system to you as one that can be made to work and is working in the Artibonite valley of Haiti. A long range perspective is required. The major problem is one of education. The pediatrician or ophthalmologist gives the best care he can with the acute problems, but without follow-up instruction and long range planning, major medical efforts will be of no avail.

# SURGICAL TREATMENT OF ACTIVE KERATOMALACIA BY "COVERING GRAFT"

I. BEN-SIRA, U. TICHO and Y. YASSUR

Department of Ophthalmology, Hadassah University Hospital, Jerusalem, Israel

### INTRODUCTION

The preventive measures required in kerato-malacia are common knowledge, but little is known about the actual treatment of an acute case. A direct approach to the problem of corneal perforations in keratomalacia has not previously been reported. During the years 1967 to 1970, 256 children with active xeroph-thalmia and keratomalacia were treated in the Queen Elizabeth Central Hospital, Blantyre, Malawi. This report describes a surgical technique, termed the "covering graft" operation, that was performed in 50 of these cases.

### MATERIALS, METHODS OF SURGERY AND POSTOPERATIVE COURSE

One type of lesion commonly found in kerato-malacia is a localized corneal perforation, with an iris prolapse measuring 2 to 4 mm in diameter. This type of lesion was seen in 78 eyes, 50 of which were operated on using the "covering graft" technique.

The conjunctiva adjacent to the corneal perforation was cut at the limbus and reflected to form a fornix-based flap. The corneal wound was cleaned of necrotic tissue and iris. A full thickness cornea, either preserved or fresh, 8 to 12 mm in diameter, was placed over the wound. The graft was adjusted to cover at least 2 mm of corneal tissue around the perforation. The covering graft was secured with several black silk 7–0 sutures to the underlying cornea and sclera as far as possible from the perforation. Suturing of the central recipient cornea was avoided in order to prevent later opacification. Through an oblique corneal incision, air was injected into the anterior chamber, and the iris adhesions on the wound were freed, using an iris spatula.

The conjunctiva was reflected back on top of the graft. Atropine and antibiotics were instilled and both eyes were patched for three to four days. The first postoperative examination was made on the fourth day, under mask anesthesia. If necessary, subsequent dressings were performed in the same way.

The general postoperative treatment consisted of antibiotics, vitamin A injections and other supportive measures as indicated by the general condition of the child.

The postoperative course was uniform. The conjunctival flap retracted in three to five days. The covering graft retained its shape and integrity during the first two postoperative weeks. Thereafter it started to swell, and during the next week or two it became edematous. During the fourth postoperative week the graft disintegrated or became detached from the sutures. At that time, the covering graft or its remnants were removed together with the remaining sutures.

In the first postoperative week, white tissue was observed forming under the covering graft in place of the original perforation. This was edematous for a few days and sometimes contained blood vessels. At the end of the second week this edematous tissue became a leukoma. At the time of removal of the covering graft, in the fourth postoperative week, a stronger scar was already present. No loss of anterior chamber fluid occurred. It was amazing to see how small

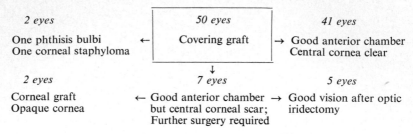

FIG. 1.   Operative procedures in keratomalacia.

scars and clear corneas sometimes followed perforations as large as 3 to 4 mm in diameter.

In the majority of our cases the follow-up period lasted about six months.

### RESULTS

The anterior chamber was permanently restored in 48 out of the 50 operated eyes (Fig. 1). In 41 eyes in which the perforation was eccentric, so that the resulting scar in the cornea was outside the pupillary area, a second operation was not required. In seven eyes the scar in the cornea was central, and a second operation was necessary for visual purposes. An optical iridectomy restored vision in five of these seven eyes; while a corneal transplantation was required in the other two. These two grafts, however, became opaque.

Two eyes developed complications after the covering graft operation: in one, severe secondary glaucoma; and in the other, complete dissolution of the cornea.

### DISCUSSION

Although many surgical procedures are known that can be used for emergency therapeutic keratoplasty, none is suitable for advanced cases of keratomalacia. This is because of the young age of the children, the severity of their corneal involvement and the risk of prolonged anesthesia in these severely debilitated children. The "covering graft" operation, described here for the first time, is a quick, simple and safe procedure. It may also be applied in other cases of acute perforation of the cornea due to viruses, bacteria or fungi.

# DISCUSSION

DR. C. H. DOHLMAN (*USA*): We have heard a great deal about the use of vitamin A in the treatment of keratomalacia, but I feel that the management of active cases should be entirely different and should consist of administration of collagenase inhibitors. It has been established both by Dr. Brown's group and our own that the destruction of the stroma is due to the release of collagenase and other proteolytic enzymes from the damaged epithelium. If these enzyme inhibitors are not effective, then a conjunctival flap should be tried. But even before reaching that stage, I would think that vitamin A applied topically could be of some help unless it has to go through the liver first, perhaps for conversion to an "active" form. What do we actually know at the present time about the topical application of vitamin A in cases of active keratomalacia?

DR. J. A. OLSON (*Thailand*): Our studies have shown that vitamin A applied directly to epithelium, skin and even tumors and other tissue culture preparations has the typical results expected. In contrast to this, the systemic situation is quite different. When vitamin A is given orally or injected, it reaches the corneal epithelium through the basal lamina. We have no idea of how it is transmitted outward into epithelial cells, but this is the normal path of entry into the corneal epithelium. If, on the other hand, you have a deranged tissue and you apply vitamin A topically, it just may not be effective in terms of reaching its site of action. Only in a tissue like skin, which is less sensitive than cornea or conjunctiva, are the effects of locally applied vitamin A indistinguishable from those found after systemic administration.

DR. M. E. LANGHAM (*USA*): I should like to know whether anyone has observed keratinization of the corneal epithelium in vitamin A deficiency. This would be of interest because the corneal epithelial cells are good examples of a cascade type of system. By this I mean that the stratified cell can transform itself into a basal cell under special conditions. If we make a hole in the cornea we can see, within 24 hr, that the new stratified layer slides over and becomes a basal cell layer. We are now studying the mechanism of adhesion between these cells, and find that desmosomes are very scarce in regions where polymeric molecules can be demonstrated. We feel that these substances may play an important role in intercellular adhesion. Now, these observations have been made under carefully controlled experimental conditions but I think similar lines of investigation on vitamin A-deficient corneal epithelial tissue would yield valuable information. Has anyone observed keratinization of the stratified layer in avitaminosis A?

DR. V. RAMBO (*India*): You must consider that keratinization is a chronic condition, and as such is quite different from active keratomalacia which, although it comes on very quickly, can be detected in its preceding stages. These consist first of the "fish-scale" cornea, the prenecrotic stage and then the fingernail-like appearance. A child with either of these prekeratomalacia conditions responds miraculously to an injection of 100,000 units of vitamin A. The cornea clears immediately, but we musn't forget to continue treatment for at least two weeks. Otherwise, the condition returns.

# THE NATURAL HISTORY AND DIAGNOSIS OF HERPES CORNEA

HERBERT E. KAUFMAN

Department of Ophthalmology, College of Medicine, University of Florida, Gainesville, Florida, USA

There is much new information about the mechanism of infection by herpes simplex virus, its pathogenicity and some of the factors causing recurrences.

Whereas for many years herpesvirus was considered to be a single virus type, it is now clear that the large subgroup of herpes includes many different virus antigens falling into two major types. Type 1 herpes causes most infections of the upper body, such as herpes labialis and herpes of the cornea. Type 2 herpes causes most genital infections. A high incidence of positive titers to herpes Type 2 is found in women who develop cervical carcinoma, and aplasia of the cervix has been associated with the virus (1). It can also transform cells to a malignant state in tissue culture, and cause tumors in hamsters (2).

However, Type 2 herpes virus rarely causes ocular infection except in the neonate, who is presumably infected when he passes through the birth canal of a mother harboring herpes. Under these circumstances, it can produce widespread disease infecting the cornea and producing retinitis.

Type 1 herpes infection is the kind commonly seen infecting the cornea. Although clinical disease with this virus, such as herpes labialis and herpes of the cornea, are common, most infections are subclinical. In previous studies in the United States antibodies to herpes were found in 80% of children five years of age. The frequency of subclinical infection is reflected in later clinical disease. Primary infection with herpes is a well recognized entity with vesicles spreading over the skin as well as involving the eye. Most disease is due to secondary rather than to primary herpes, and although clinical manifestations may occur for the first time they apparently occur in people with previous virus exposure.

Herpes infection of the cornea is a common, debilitating and often recurrent disease. The dendritic ulcer represents a rather unique type of virus infection in that its appearance is almost pathognomonic of herpes simplex virus. The pathogenesis of this disease is clear. Virus is present within the cells and moves from cell to cell, killing cells and producing the apparent defect. Hypersensitivity and toxic factors seem minimal, and the disease is a function of virus multiplication alone.

Once an individual has been initially infected with herpes simplex virus he has a 23% chance of getting another infection within two years (2, 3). If he has already had more than one infection his chance of having another infection within two years is approximately 46%. Regardless of the initial treatment, (cauterization, idoxuridine, placebo or even corticosteroids) once the ulcer heals the recurrence rate appears to be about the same (D. Hill, personal communication). These infections can occur despite the presence of high stable neutralizing antibody titers in the bloodstream. These circulating antibodies are not locally protective and do not prevent recurrences.

For many years it was postulated that herpesvirus, like prophage, lived undetected within cells. This virus was felt to produce a latent infection, so that no detectable virus could be found between attacks. Attempts to find "latent" virus between attacks were unsuccessful. These included biopsy of labial skin, which tended to become repeatedly infected, and growth of this skin in tissue culture. They also included irradiation of the skin and other similar techniques.

Our laboratory found that rabbits with recurring ocular herpes simplex (4) often excreted virus in their tears in the absence of clinical signs of infection. The lacrimal gland and conjunctiva of these animals was chronically infected even in the absence of any visible disease and virus multiplication continued with virus being shed into the tears (5). This was confirmed in human patients. In patients subject to labial herpes, very small amounts of virus could be chronically detected in saliva. In patients subject to recurrent corneal herpes, chronic virus excretion was observed in their tears and virus antigen was seen in the lacrimal gland by fluorescent antibody techniques. Even more surprising, some individuals who had never had corneal herpes or herpes labialis chronically excreted virus into their secretions. The question then changed from "Why do recurrences occur?" to "Why don't recurrences constantly occur?"

One possible explanation for this lies in the local system of antibody secretion. Two major types of serum antibodies are responsible for our resistance to infection, IgG antibodies and IgM. On the mucosal surface of the mouth and eye, however, there is another antibody, IgA, which is locally produced in plasma cells immediately under the mucosal surface. A small amount goes into the systemic circulation but must enter the epithelial cells where two molecules are joined by a special secretory protein.

Centifanto and others showed that specific neutralizing IgA antibody to herpes simplex virus was produced in both rabbits and human beings (6, 7). The amount varied from eye to eye and from time to time, but the antibody in tears was a very potent neutralizing antibody which rapidly inactivated virus, and yet its titer appeared relatively independent of the antibody titer in the bloodstream. We showed that this antibody could be stimulated by instillation of dead virus into the cul-de-sac and that an eye so stimulated responded with high IgA neutralizing antibody titers. We were not able to show that the stimulation of IgA antibodies could prevent recurrences of herpes. On the other hand, this is a peculiar animal system employing an exquisitely susceptible host and one of the most virulent virus strains we could obtain. Ample IgA antibody is present with this virulent virus throughout the recurrence period. It is not clear whether the same situation applies in man. In fact, workers at the National Dental Institute have confirmed the chronic excretion of herpesvirus in the saliva (8) and have shown that the only difference between persons with recurrent attacks of labial herpes and those who excrete the virus but who do not get recurrent attacks is that the protected individuals have higher IgA serum antibody titers. This may reflect high local IgA production, also. A further complication is the fact that other antibodies (IgG) may partially coat herpesvirus and protect it from IgA without inactivating it.

Although true recurrences of virus disease occur, it is extremely common to have post-infectious ulcers in which no virus is present

(9). The patient frequently reports having had multiple recurrences within the same month. He will often point out that the attacks began in the middle of the night or on arising in the morning, which is a history typical of a recurrent erosion. Such postinfectious ulcers do not contain virus. Virus can neither be cultured, nor demonstrated with fluorescent antibody stains. Ulcers occur after previous herpes but are not a function of virus multiplication. In these lesions the basement membrane of the epithelium is apparently damaged by the initial infection. The hemidesmosomes which attach epithelium to the underlying layers require considerable time to form. Until the epithelium adheres firmly to the basement membrane, the epithelium is easily rubbed off by the lids or floated off by fluid accumulating under it. We may thus treat postinfection ulcers as we would a recurrent erosion with every expectation of clinical success. In contrast, if the condition is treated as if multiplying virus was there, it usually gets worse.

Stromal disease remains a confusing and frustrating subject as does the problem of herpes iritis. It is clear that herpesvirus can invade the stroma and this has never been a matter of dispute. It is equally clear that this virus can pass through stroma and invade the endothelium. We described this in animals almost 15 years ago (10). It is equally clear, however, that the pathophysiology of corneal herpes cannot be explained simply by the killing of corneal cells by the virus. The severe inflammation and necrosis seen in herpes infection of the stroma cannot be explained by cell death alone, but must implicate either toxic factors or hypersensitivity.

There are three basic types of herpes stromal disease. The first is the dissolution of the stroma by actively invading virus, which may lead to perforation of the globe. Although this severe involvement is particularly common in patients who receive corticosteroids, it was well documented before the advent of corticosteroids and occurs in patients who have never received these agents. This type clearly has virus in the stromal tissue and, in fact, most of the patients studied by Dawson (11), in whom virus was demonstrated in the corneal stroma, were of this type.

The second type of stromal disease presents as a cheesy looking area which is reminiscent of the white superficial stromal lesions under some dendritic lesions. Like the open ulcer in stromal disease, these white infiltrated lesions also contain active multiplying virus. With fluorescent antibody techniques and electron microscopy we have seen virus particles in such lesions. In spite of this, it is likely that hypersensitivity plays some role in the pathogenesis of disease and that simple cell death is not enough to account for the total clinical disease.

The third type of stromal disease is diskiform edema. This is a unique, reversible swelling of the cornea which usually spares an area of cornea in the periphery. It is always accompanied by some anterior chamber inflammation, responds dramatically to antiinflammatory drugs and may disappear with no residue at all. Guinea pigs which have previously been sensitized to herpesvirus (12) can develop a haziness and severe edema when challenged with partially purified dead virus. This is a typical delayed hypersensitivity response. It does, however, produce a reversible edema which is short-lived and is somewhat analogous to diskiform edema. In addition tissue culture has shown that herpesvirus amalgamates with the cell membranes, permanently altering their antigenic composition and favoring a type of antigenic depot which could cause an extremely prolonged hypersensitivity reaction. In clinical terms, diskiform edema responds extremely well to small doses of corticosteroids and disappears completely. It is similar to the hypersensitivity disease seen in animals and is clinically so unlike the direct virus invasion syndromes, that we feel that hypersensitivity plays a major part in its pathogenesis.

Herpes iritis is due to virus invasion, at least in a high proportion of patients. Witmer demonstrated virus particles by electron microscopy in the iris of patients with herpes iritis (13). Patterson demonstrated intracellular antigen by the fluorescent antibody staining of anterior chamber cells (14). We showed that these antibody-containing cells could be helpful in the diagnosis of herpes iritis (16), especially when there was no clear-cut history of dendritic keratitis (15). In addition, Kanai demonstrated free virus particles in the anterior chamber fluid (15). In evaluating these studies (11, 13–15) it is noteworthy that virus could not be cultured from most specimens in which virus was clearly demonstrated by electron microscopy or fluorescent antibody staining. Our present techniques for virus tissue culture are somewhat insensitive, and much virus multiplication occurs within cells. Since virus passes from cell to cell, disease may continue although extracellular antibodies make it impossible to culture the cell-free virus.

Some approaches to therapy, such as the stimulation of local antibodies, are directly suggested by these data. Even rational chemotherapy depends on continued progress in understanding what is actually causing the disease.

## REFERENCES

1. CENTIFANTO YM, HILDERBRANDT RJ, HELD B and KAUFMAN HE. Relationship of herpes simplex genital infection and carcinoma of the cervix: population studies. *Am J Obstet Gynecol* **110**: 690, 1971.
2. NAHMIAS AJ, NAIB ZM, JOSEY WE, MURPHY FA and LUCE CF. Sarcomas after inoculation of newborn hamsters with herpes virus hominis Type 2 strains. *Proc Soc Exp Biol Med* **134**: 1065, 1970.
3. CARROLL JM, MARTOLA E-L, LAIBSON PR and DOHLMAN CH. Recurrence of herpetic keratitis following idoxuridine therapy. *Am J Ophthalmol* **63**: 103, 1967.
4. KAUFMAN HE, BROWN DC and ELLISON ED. Recurrent herpes in rabbits and man. *Science* **156**: 1628, 1967.
5. KAUFMAN HE, BROWN DC and ELLISON ED. Herpes virus in the lacrimal gland, conjunctiva and cornea of man—a chronic infection. *Am J Ophthalmol* **65**: 32, 1968.
6. LITTLE JM, CENTIFANTO YM and KAUFMAN HE. Studies of immunoglobulins in tears. *Am J Ophthalmol* **68**: 898, 1969.
7. CENTIFANTO YM and KAUFMAN HE. Secretory IgA and herpes keratitis. *Infect Immun* **2**: 778, 1970.
8. GREENBERG MS and BRIGHTMAN VJ. Serum immunoglobulins in patients with recurrent intra-oral herpes simplex infections. *J Dent Res* **50**: 781, 1971.
9. KAUFMAN HE. Epithelial erosion syndrome. Metaherpetic keratitis. *Am J Ophthalmol* **57**: 983, 1964.
10. MALONEY ED and KAUFMAN HE. Dissemination of corneal herpes simplex. *Invest Ophthalmol* **4**: 872, 1965.
11. DAWSON C, TONGI B, MOORE TE and COLEMAN V. Herpes virus infection of human mesodermal tissue (cornea) detected by electron microscopy. *Nature (Lond)* **217**: 460, 1968.
12. LAUSCH RN, SAWYERS J and KAUFMAN HE. Delayed hypersensitivity to the herpes simplex virus. *J Immunol* **96**: 981, 1966.
13. WITMER R and INOMATA T. Electron microscopic observation of the iris in herpes uveitis. *Arch Ophthalmol (Kbh)* **79**: 331, 1968.
14. PATTERSON A, SOMERVILLE RG and JONES BR. Herpetic keratouveitis with herpes antigen in the anterior chamber. *Trans Ophthalmol Soc UK* **88**: 243, 1968.
15. KAUFMAN HE, KANAI A and ELLISON ED. Herpetic iritis: Demonstration of virus in the anterior chamber by fluorescent antibody techniques and electron microscopy. *Am J Ophthalmol* **71**: 465, 1971.

# STUDIES ON THE MOLECULAR BIOLOGY OF HERPES SIMPLEX VIRUS

YECHIEL BECKER

Department of Virology, Hebrew University–Hadassah Medical School, Jerusalem, Israel

Herpes simplex virus (HSV) is a DNA virus capable of replicating in cell nuclei. The herpesvirion contains a DNA genome of about $100 \times 10^6$ daltons mol wt (1). About 12% of the DNA genome transcribes messenger RNA (mRNA) which is translated by the host cell ribosomes into virus-specific structural peptides, which assemble into capsids, each composed of 162 hollow cylindrical capsomeres (2). The capsid contains the viral DNA genome and is enveloped by cellular membranes which contain virus-specific glycopeptides (3). Upon infection of sensitive cells the virions adsorb to the cell membrane and penetrate into the cell cytoplasm (4). The herpesvirions uncoat by cellular enzyme action and the DNA genomes are transported to the nuclei, the site of viral DNA replication and transcription. The viral mRNA is transported from the nuclei to the cytoplasm where it interacts with host cell ribosomes to form virus specific polyribosomes, on which viral peptides are synthesized. The viral peptides are responsible for the replication, transcription and coating of the viral DNA by a series of molecular events which are partly viral and partly cellular in nature. The present discussion summarizes recent studies on the replication of HSV performed in our laboratory. This represents a personal viewpoint and not a review of the field of herpesviruses, which may be found in the papers by Roizman (5) and by Kaplan and Ben-Porat (6). I would also like to indicate certain unsolved problems in need of further study.

## THE VIRION OF HERPES SIMPLEX

*Isolation of intact virions.* Electron micrographs of herpesvirions (2) demonstrate the viral ultrastructure as well as the presence of an envelope around the viral capsid. In order to preserve the virions, homogenates of infected cells were centrifuged in 15 to 30% w/w sucrose gradients (7) or in 12 to 52% w/w sucrose gradients (8, 9) permitting the isolation of the mature enveloped virions in a distinct band. Above this two additional bands were obtained: the lower contained naked virions and the upper band, empty capsids. Electron microscopy of stained preparations obtained from the various bands revealed the morphology of the viral particles (9).

*Infectivity of the herpesvirions.* The separation of enveloped from unenveloped virions made possible the study of the role of the envelope in infectivity. Most of the viral infectivity resides in the band of enveloped virions. Electron microscopy of stained preparations demonstrated that a small number of enveloped virions can be found in the band consisting of unenveloped nucleocapsids, a fact which may contribute to the infectivity of the preparation. It was therefore of interest that treatment of enveloped virions with the detergent Nonidet P-40 (9) resulted in complete loss of virus infectivity accompanied by dissolution of the viral envelope. These experiments suggest that the envelope is necessary for virus infectivity (9).

*The DNA genome.* Sodium dodecyl sulfate (SDS) treatment of purified enveloped virions, labeled with radioactive thymidine in the DNA, results in the release of the viral DNA. Centrifugation of the disrupted virions in a sucrose gradient resulted in the isolation of intact DNA molecules which sedimented to the middle of the gradient, while the viral proteins were retained at the top. Cocentrifugation of the herpesvirus DNA with vaccinia virus DNA [$150 \times 10^6$ daltons mol wt (10)] permitted the calculation of the molecular weight of herpesvirus DNA: $100 \times 10^6$ daltons. Electron microscopy of herpes virus DNA confirmed the length of the DNA genomes as being about 50 μm, which corresponds to about $100 \times 10^6$ daltons (1). The density of the viral DNA molecules centrifuged in a CsCl gradient was 1.718 g/ml, which indicates that the $G + C$ content is 68%. The organization of the nucleotides in the DNA molecules is not yet known. Centrifugation of the viral DNA in an alkaline sucrose gradient resulted in the collapse of the DNA, which was distributed over a large portion of the gradient. It is not yet known why the viral DNA molecules were degraded into shorter polynucleotide chains by alkali (M. Gordin, U. Olshevsky and Y. Becker, unpublished results).

*The viral structural peptides.* The various virus bands, unlabeled or labeled with radioactive amino acids, were isolated in sucrose gradients from homogenates of labeled infected cells. Each band was removed and treated with a solution of SDS, urea and 2-mercaptoethanol. This treatment dissolves the viral envelope and capsid and releases the viral peptides, which can be separated by electrophoresis in SDS-containing acrylamide gel. The presence of seven major peptides and two minor ones was thus revealed. The function of the various peptides in the organization of the herpesvirion was determined by a comparison with the peptides present in nucleocapsids and empty capsids. In addition, it was possible to demonstrate that three peptides (designated III, IV and V) are glycopeptides and therefore associated with the viral envelope (3, 11). It was concluded that peptide II, the major component of the viral peptides, has a molecular weight of 110,000 daltons, and is a component of the viral capsomeres. Peptide VIII also seems to be associated with the capsomeres. Peptide VII is rich in arginine as compared to the other peptides, and is thought to be the internal viral basic protein, possibly linked to the DNA. Studies are in progress to isolate and characterize the viral basic proteins.

The viral envelope is composed of three major glycopeptides with molecular weights of 101,000, 85,000 and 58,000 daltons, respectively. The outer layer of the viral envelope was thought to contain mainly glycopeptide III, while the other two glycopeptides make up the inner layers of the envelope (11). It is possible, however, that although the glycopeptides are situated inside the envelope, some of them, or part of each peptide molecule, can also be found on the surface of the envelope. The orientation of the viral glycopeptides in the lipid membrane (the envelope) is not yet known. Treatment of enveloped virions with neuraminidase (J. Levitt-Hadar and Y. Becker, unpublished results) did not remove the radioactively labeled glucosamine from the envelope glycopeptides. However, degradation by neuraminidase was observed after disruption of the envelope with the nonionogenic detergent Nonidet P-40. This result indicated that the glycopeptides, or at least the sugar residues of these peptides, are oriented to the inner side of the lipid membrane which comprises the viral envelope.

*The lipid moiety of the viral envelope.* The lipid composition of the herpesvirion envelope (12) resembles that of the lipid membranes of the host cells. Prelabeling of the host cells with radioactive choline and subsequent infection with herpesvirus yielded a virus progeny labeled in the lipids of the viral envelope, indicating that the host donates the lipid moiety of the envelope, while the glycopeptides are virus specific and their synthesis is controlled by viral genes.

FATE OF HERPESVIRIONS IN THE HOST CELL

*Adsorption.* We studied the interaction of herpesvirions with the host cells ($BSC_1$ cell monolayers originating from green monkey kidney cells). The purified virions were labeled in the DNA and coat proteins. The virions adsorbed gradually to the cell membrane, apparently by an electrostatic interaction. Addition of heparin to infected cultures prevented the attachment of virions and also caused the release of adsorbed virions which were not firmly bound to the cell membrane. It was concluded that the virions are retained on the cell membrane after attachment for a certain period (about 30 min) prior to their penetration into the cell cytoplasm, possibly by cellular processes. During the early attachment stage the virions are sensitive to heparin (4).

*Uncoating.* After 3 hr of incubation, about 50% of the infecting herpesvirions were retained on the surface of the cell membrane in a form which rendered them sensitive to heparin. The second half of the inoculum was found in the cell cytoplasm, partly as virions and partly associated with structures which sedimented to the bottom when centrifuged in sucrose gradients. The uncoating of the viral genomes is thought to take place in these structures, which are membrane-associated.

*Transport of viral DNA to cell nuclei.* The uncoating and transport of viral DNA from the cytoplasm, the site of uncoating, to the nuclei, the site of transcription and replication, was not affected by inhibitors of protein and nucleic acid synthesis (4). A gradual increase in the radioactive viral DNA was noted in the nuclei, while most of the labeled structural proteins were retained in the cytoplasm. Six hr after infection, about 40% of the viral DNA present in the cytoplasm was found in the nuclei. These DNA molecules initiate the growth cycle of the virus.

*Fate of the infecting virus.* It was calculated that 27 herpesvirions constitute one plaque-forming unit (pfu). On the basis of this and the above calculation (that 50% of the infecting virions are retained on the cell membrane and that 40% of the incoming virions migrate to the nuclei) an explanation for the involvement of 27 virions in the formation of one plaque can be obtained. To obtain a one-step growth curve of the virus we infect each cell with 10 pfu of virus (about 270 virions). Only 30% of the virions adsorb to the cell membrane and only half penetrate into the cells (45 virions). Of these, the genomes of only 40% (18 genomes) enter into the nucleus of the infected cell.

REPLICATION OF HERPESVIRUS

*Growth curves in $BSC_1$ and HeLa cells.* We studied the replication of HSV (strain HF) in two cell systems, $BSC_1$ cells in monolayer cultures and HeLa $S_3$ cells in suspension. The growth cycle varies in duration in the two types of cell. In $BSC_1$ cells, the latent period, prior to the formation of the initial infectious progeny, was 6 hr. Virus progeny were gradually synthesized during a period of 12 hr. Afterwards no virions were synthesized. Even at this late stage the virions were intracellular and were not released into the medium (7).

The growth cycle of herpesvirus in HeLa cells was exactly half (9 hr) of that in $BSC_1$

cells. The virus progeny started to appear in the cells as early as 3 hr after initiation of infection and reached a maximum at 9 hr (S. Neuman and Y. Becker, unpublished results).

The reason for the marked difference in the replication of the virus in the two cell-lines is not known.

*Chemical determination of the virus growth cycle.* The progeny of viral DNA which replicates in the nuclei of the infected cells can be found in two forms: completely coated by the viral capsid and therefore resistant to deoxyribonuclease treatment, and partially coated or uncoated and therefore sensitive to deoxyribonuclease. The mature herpesvirions were insensitive to deoxyribonuclease treatment (7). Therefore, the time course of appearance of radioactive DNA resistant to deoxyribonuclease treatment in the nuclei of infected cells was taken as an indication of the formation of mature virions. It was found (7 and S. Neuman and Y. Becker, unpublished results) that the synthesis of herpesvirions, using the determination of deoxyribonuclease-resistant radioactive DNA, resembled the biological determination of herpesvirions by the plaque technique. The radioactivity assay is quick and accurate and takes into account all the mature virions present in the infected cell. We also showed that more virus-specific DNA was synthesized in the infected nuclei than was incorporated into mature virions. About 21 % of the radioactively labeled DNA present in the infected cells was resistant to deoxyribonuclease (13).

*Virus morphogenesis.* Electron microscopy of infected cells revealed empty capsids—mainly nucleocapsids—in the nuclei. Enveloped virions were found mostly in the cytoplasm as well as outside the cells. These observations explained the fact that it is possible to isolate complete and incomplete virions from infected cells.

## SYNTHESIS OF MACROMOLECULES IN THE INFECTED CELLS

*Effect of virus infection on the host cell.* 1) Effect on DNA synthesis: Our studies on $BSC_1$ cells infected with herpesvirus were performed during that period in the cell's growth cycle when DNA synthesis did not take place [presumably G1 phase (14)]. In these cells, host DNA synthesis was initiated 18 hr after replenishment of the medium. As the cells were infected with HSV at the time of change of medium, the virus growth cycle terminated prior to cell DNA synthesis. Indeed, most of the DNA synthesized in the HSV-infected $BSC_1$ cells was viral DNA.

In order to determine the effect of virus infection on the elongation of cell DNA chains in infected HeLa cells, the cells were labeled for 20-min periods at different times after infection and centrifuged in an alkaline sucrose gradient. In the infected cells the synthesis of cell DNA was inhibited, and the elongation of nascent chains prevented.

2) Effect on RNA metabolism: Analysis of the rate of RNA synthesis (the extent of $H^3$-uridine incorporation into RNA) in infected and uninfected HeLa cells revealed that due to virus infection the rate of RNA synthesis markedly decreased. In both $BSC_1$ and HeLa cells the synthesis of host cell RNA was affected within 3 hr after infection. The synthesis of 45S RNA molecules, which are the precursors of the mature cellular ribosomal RNA species, was markedly affected. Thus, in the infected cell the synthesis of new ribosomal subunits is inhibited (J. Levitt-Hadar and Y. Becker, unpublished results; S. Neuman and Y. Becker, unpublished results).

The inhibition of RNA synthesis in the nucleoli of infected cells is associated with the disappearance of the nucleoli. However, the mechanism which inhibits the function of cell DNA-dependent RNA polymerase I is not yet known. It is also not known whether the nucleoplasmic RNA polymerase II is also affected by the virus infection.

3) Effect on cellular protein synthesis: Infection of $BSC_1$ or HeLa cells with herpesvirus resulted in a marked inhibition of cellular protein synthesis. The rate of protein synthesis gradually declined in infected $BSC_1$ cells while in HeLa cells the inhibitory effect of virus infection was more pronounced and occurred immediately after infection (U. Olshevsky and Y. Becker, in preparation; S. Neuman and Y. Becker, unpublished results). This inhibition may have been caused by a direct effect on the cellular polyribosomes or as a secondary effect, due to the inhibition of cellular RNA synthesis. Treatment of HSV infected with cytosine arabinoside did not affect inhibition (S. Neuman and Y. Becker, unpublished results), suggesting that the inhibitory effect was not related to viral DNA replication. This result might indicate that either a component of the viral coat or an early viral function is responsible for the inhibition of cellular nucleic acids and protein synthesis. The latter inhibition seems to be complete, since analysis of cytoplasmic fractions from infected cells by acrylamide gel electrophoresis reveals mainly viral structural peptides, synthesized in the infected cells.

*Transcription of viral mRNA species.* 1) Early viral mRNA: After uncoating, HSV DNA is transported from the cytoplasm to the nuclei, the site of virus formation. Experiments to detect the presence of a DNA-dependent RNA polymerase in the herpesvirions, under assay conditions which revealed the presence of a DNA-dependent RNA polymerase in trachoma elementary bodies (15), failed to demonstrate any enzymatic activity in the virions. Although the herpesvirions may indeed lack a polymerase, it is also possible that the early transcription of the viral DNA molecules is carried out by a nuclear RNA polymerase.

As herpesvirus DNA is continuously synthesized throughout the virus growth cycle, the treatment of infected cells with cytosine arabinoside, which inhibits the replication of viral DNA, might permit the study of the mRNA species synthesized on the parental DNA genomes. In this system a species of 20S mRNA molecules was isolated from the polyribosomes, suggesting that 20S RNA species might be an early mRNA species (S. Neuman and Y. Becker, unpublished results). Analysis of HSV-infected HeLa cells labeled with radioactive uridine revealed the presence of two mRNA species with S values of 10 and 20, 3 hr after infection. The nature of the genetic information encoded in these mRNA species is not yet known.

2) Late viral mRNA: At 5 and 7 hr after infection with HSV, the polyribosomes of infected HeLa cells contain a 35S mRNA species, the content of which gradually increases. Neither this mRNA species nor the 10S mRNA molecules are synthesized in the presence of cytosine arabinoside. It is therefore assumed that both the 10S and the 35S mRNA species are late viral mRNA.

The molecular weights of the three mRNA species in the polyribosomes of HSV-infected cells can be estimated by comparison with cellular ribosomal RNA species ($1.7 \times 10^6$ and $0.7 \times 10^6$ daltons for the 28S and 18S, respectively). The 10S species might be about $0.3 \times 10^6$ daltons; the 20S about $0.7 \times 10^6$ daltons and the 35S about $2.5 \times 10^6$ daltons. Although it is not yet possible to determine which genes of the viral DNA genome are transcribed to the various mRNA species, the genetic information for the viral structural peptides is calculated to be about 12% of the entire genome. Thus, the genetic information for the viral structural peptides is transcribed from one DNA strand with a molecular weight of $6 \times 10^6$ daltons. The largest mRNA species isolated from the polyribosomes, the site of peptide synthesis, was only $2.5 \times 10^6$ daltons, about one half of the total structural genes. This calculation assumes that the viral structural peptides appear only once in the genome (3). A similar analysis suggests that the viral structural peptides with a molecular weight close to 100,000 daltons might be synthesized on either the 20S or the 35S mRNA species. Thus, it is possible that mRNA molecules similar in size might contain genetic information for the synthesis of different peptides.

The nature of the RNA polymerase responsible for the transcription of the late viral mRNA species has not yet been determined.

3) Transport of mRNA molecules from nuclei to cytoplasm and interaction with cytoplasmic ribosomal subunits: The viral mRNA molecules are transported to the cytoplasm, where they interact with ribosomal subunits for functioning ribosomes. Studies carried out in HSV-infected $BSC_1$ cells demonstrated that most of the viral mRNA molecules appear in the cytoplasm as free molecules. Part of this mRNA can also be found in the 100S region prior to its appearance in the polyribosomes (J. Levitt and Y. Becker, unpublished results). Further studies in HSV-infected HEp-2 cells (16) demonstrated that the attachment of viral mRNA to ribosomal subunits took place in the presence of puromycin and the absence of protein synthesis. Three mRNA-ribosome complexes were found: 80S, 105S and 120S. The composition of ribosomal RNA was determined by isopyknic centrifugation of glutaraldehyde-fixed complexes and by the determination of the ribosomal RNA in the complexes. The 80S complex is composed of an mRNA molecule attached to a single ribosome; the 105S complex contains mRNA with one ribosome and one 40S subunit; and the 120S complex contains mRNA and two ribosomes. Thus, ribosomal subunits can interact with mRNA in a region on the mRNA molecule distant from the initiation codon, and the interaction is not dependent on protein synthesis. This provides additional evidence that the ribosomal subunits interact with mRNA, the 40S initially and the 60S subsequently (17).

*Replication of viral DNA.* 1) Time course of DNA replication: A characteristic feature of HSV is the continous synthesis of viral DNA genomes throughout the virus growth cycle. Labeling of infected $BSC_1$ and HeLa cells with radioactive thymidine revealed the synthesis of viral DNA starting about 3 hr after infection. Analysis of the viral DNA, coated by the capsids and resistant to deoxyribonuclease treatment, demonstrated that 2 hr elapse until the newly synthesized DNA molecules are coated (7).

2) Relation between DNA and protein synthesis: Addition of puromycin to the infected cells immediately inhibited the synthesis of viral DNA. It is assumed that the replication of the double stranded DNA by a semiconservative mode requires *de novo* synthesized proteins. The nature of these proteins, as well as the nature of the DNA-dependent DNA polymerase, is still to be studied.

*Synthesis of HSV structural peptides.* 1) Characterization of the viral peptides: Labeling of infected $BSC_1$ cells for 3-hr periods at various intervals after infection and acrylamide gel analysis of the cells demonstrated the nature of the newly synthesized peptides. It was found (U. Olshevsky and Y. Becker, in preparation) that during the period prior to the replication of the viral DNA (3 to 6 hr after infection), the newly synthesized peptides had a profile identical with that of uninfected cells. Later (6 to 9 hr), however, the profile of the peptides isolated from infected cells resembled that of the viral structural peptides, although several peptides (designated VII, VI, V and IV) were found in higher proportions than in mature virions. This suggests that more peptides are synthesized than are used for the formation of mature virions, or else that each band contains several different peptides which have the same molecular weight. It is also possible that certain peptides are synthesized throughout the cycle and others at a specific period in the virus growth cycle.

2) Processing of some viral peptides: Labeling of the infected cells with radioactive amino acids for 5-min periods, followed by a "chase" for an additional 10 min, revealed the presence of radioactive, high molecular weight peptides, which were retained at the top of the acrylamide gel. At this stage the radioactivity in peptide II was quite low. After the 10-min "chase" the large peptide disappeared and the radioactivity increased, instead, in the band of peptide II. Other peptides may also have increased but not to the same extent. It was concluded that peptide II is processed from a precursor (U. Olshevsky and Y. Becker, in preparation).

3) Transport of viral peptides to the nuclei: Due to the replication of the viral DNA in the cell nucleus, the viral structural peptides are transported from the site of synthesis in the cytoplasm to the nuclei. The mechanism of this process is not yet known.

### EFFECT OF ARGININE DEPRIVATION ON HSV REPLICATION

*Effect of lack of arginine on virus replicaton.* Incubation of herpesvirus-infected cells in an arginine-free medium resulted in the inhibition of virus replication and in the prevention of a cytopathic effect.

*Synthesis of macromolecules:* Viral DNA replicated in arginine-deprived cells although virions were not formed (18). Acrylamide gel analysis of the cytoplasmic fractions obtained from arginine-deprived $BSC_1$ cells, labeled with radioactive amino acids, revealed that all the viral structural peptides were synthesized. Nevertheless, these peptides were not transported to the nuclei. The reason for this is not yet known.

*Reversion of the arginine effect:* Addition of arginine to the infected deprived cells resulted in the formation of mature virions. Analysis of the synthesized virions demonstrated that the viral structural peptides synthesized in the absence of arginine in the arginine-free medium were subsequently utilized for virion formation (19).

### ANTIVIRAL DRUGS

*Effect of cytosine arabinoside on HSV replication.* 1) Effect on viral DNA synthesis: Cytosine arabinoside inhibits the synthesis of DNA due to its interference with the *de novo* synthesis of deoxycytidylate (20). When added to herpesvirus-infected cells immediately after infection, cytosine arabinoside immediately and completely inhibits the synthesis of DNA, with the result that virus progeny are entirely absent. However, addition of cytosine arabinoside (20 µg/ml) some time later after the initiation of viral DNA replication, resulted in the complete inhibition of viral DNA synthesis, without any effect on the synthesis of viral proteins or on the formation of herpesvirions. The virions continue to be formed during a period of several hours, although at a slower rate (7). Thus, cytosine arabinoside is effective only when added to the infected cells prior to the synthesis of the viral DNA progeny. Subsequently, the transcription of progeny DNA genomes continues in the presence of the drug, and the coating of the viral DNA molecules occurs.

2) Effect of cytosine arabinoside on the synthesis of viral peptides: Addition of cytosine arabinoside to HSV-infected cells immediately after virus adsorption, under the conditions described above, inhibited the synthesis of several viral structural peptides. This enabled the determination of the viral peptides translated from viral mRNA which were transcribed from the parental DNA genomes (early mRNA) and the mRNA species transcribed from the progeny DNA (late mRNA). Acrylamide gel electrophoretic analysis of

the proteins synthesized in infected cells treated with cytosine arabinoside revealed that peptide VII and some other peptides with similar molecular weights are synthesized in larger quantities than in untreated infected cells. Radioactively labeled peptides with molecular weights resembling the major capsid peptide II and the glycopeptides III and IV can be detected. It is possible that these peptides are not viral structural peptides but peptides with early functions not previously revealed in the infected cells, due to the synthesis of large amounts of the late structural peptides (capsid and glycopeptides) (U. Olshevsky and Y. Becker, in preparation).

*Effect of p-fluorophenylalanine (FPA) on HSV replication.* The addition of FPA to herpesvirus-infected cells prevented the synthesis of virions in the presence of FPA (21). Aggregates of proteins which lacked DNA were detected in a sucrose gradient, but their nature is not yet known. An analogue also affects the replication of viral DNA, indicating possible defects in the viral peptides associated with DNA replication.

*The effect of the antibiotic, Distamycin A, on herpesvirus replication.* The effect of Distamycin on the synthesis of herpesvirus was studied in HeLa infected cells (22). The antibiotic affected virus replication and reduced the yield of infectious virions.

## UNSOLVED PROBLEMS

Within the last decade much information regarding molecular events in the replication of herpesviruses has accumulated [see reviews by Roizman (5) and by Kaplan and Ben-Porat (6)]. However, several major problems have remained unsolved. For example, the nature of the DNA-dependent RNA polymerases which transcribe the viral DNA has not been elucidated; similarly, the DNA-dependent DNA polymerase is still to be isolated and characterized. Very little is known about the organization of the viral DNA genome, the arrangement of the genes in the DNA and the nature of the genetic information for nonstructural viral peptides. Neither is it known how the virus inhibits cellular processes and how the transport mechanism operates in the infected cell in the transfer of mRNA from the nuclei to the cytoplasm and in the transport of peptides to the nuclei.

I wish to express gratitude to my colleagues who helped develop this research on HSV: Dr. Julia Levitt-Hadar, Udy Olshevsky, Haviv Dym, Eynat Weinberg, Shulamit Neuman, Edna Hochberg, Yael Asher and Miriam Adler-Dreifuss.

The author's work with Drs. B. Roizman and E. Kieff at the Department of Microbiology, University of Chicago was aided by a National Science Foundation Senior Foreign Scientist Award.

## REFERENCES

1. BECKER Y, DYM H and SAROV I. Herpes simplex virus DNA. *Virology* 36: 185, 1968.
2. WILDY P and WATSON DH. Electron microscopic studies on the architecture of animal viruses. *Cold Spring Harbor Symp Quant Biol* 27: 25, 1961.
3. OLSHEVSKY U and BECKER Y. Herpes simplex virus coat proteins. *Virology* 40: 948, 1970.
4. HOCHBERG E and BECKER Y. The adsorption, penetration and uncoating of herpes simplex virus in BSC$_1$ cells. *J Gen Virol* 2: 231, 1968.
5. ROIZMAN B. The herpesviruses—a biochemical definition of a group. *Curr Top Microbiol Immunol* 49: 1, 1969.
6. KAPLAN AS and BEN-PORAT T. Metabolism of animal cells infected with nuclear DNA viruses. *Annu Rev Microbiol* 22: 427, 1968.
7. LEVITT J and BECKER Y. The effect of cytosine arabinoside on the replication of herpes simplex virus. *Virology* 31: 129, 1967.
8. AURELIAN L and WAGNER RR. Two populations of herpes virus virions which appear to differ in physical properties and DNA composition. *Proc Natl Acad Sci USA* 56: 902, 1966.
9. BECKER Y, LEVITT-HADAR J, DYM H and OLSHEVSKY U. Effect of the nonionic detergent Nonidet P-40 on herpes simplex virions. *Isr J Med Sci* 7: 656, 1971.
10. BECKER Y and SAROV I. Electron microscopy of vaccinia virus DNA. *J Mol Biol* 34: 655, 1968.
11. BECKER Y and OLSHEVSKY U. Localization of structural peptides in the herpes virion, in: "Oncogenesis and herpes-type viruses, a symposium." Cambridge, 1971 (in press).
12. ASHER Y, HELLER M and BECKER Y. Incorporation of lipids into herpes simplex virions. *J Gen Virol* 4: 65, 1969.
13. OLSHEVSKY U, LEVITT J and BECKER Y. Studies

on the synthesis of herpes simplex virions. *Virology* **33**: 324, 1967.

14. BECKER Y and LEVITT J. Stimulation of macro-molecular processes in BSC$_1$ cells due to medium replenishment. *Exp Cell Res* **51**: 27, 1968.

15. SAROV I and BECKER Y. DNA dependent RNA polymerase activity in purified trachoma elementary bodies: the effect of NaCl on RNA transcription. *J Bacteriol* (in press).

16. KIEFF E, BECKER Y and ROIZMAN B. Synthesis, transport and function of herpes simplex virus (HSV) messenger RNA in the presence of puromycin. *Bacteriol Proc* 1971, p 219.

17. JOKLIK WK and BECKER Y. Studies on the genesis of polyribosomes. II. The association of nascent messenger RNA with the 40S subribosomal particles. *J Mol Biol* **13**: 511, 1965.

18. BECKER Y, OLSHEVSKY U and LEVITT J. The role of arginine in the replication of herpesvirus. *J Gen Virol* **1**: 471, 1967.

19. OLSHEVSKY U and BECKER Y. Synthesis of herpes simplex virus structural proteins in arginine deprived cells. *Nature (Lond)* **226**: 851, 1970.

20. KIM JH and EIDINOFF ML. Action of 1-β-D-arabinofuranosylcytosine on the nucleic acid metabolism and viability of HeLa cells. *Cancer Res* **25**: 698, 1965.

21. DYM H and BECKER Y. Effect of p-fluorophenyl-alanine on the replication of herpes simplex virus. *Isr J Med Sci* **5**: 1083, 1969.

22. BECKER Y, NEUMAN S and LEVITT-HADAR J. The effect of the antibiotic distamycin A and congocidine on the replication of herpesvirus. *Isr J Med Sci* **8**: 1225, 1972.

# THE EFFECT OF THE ANTIBIOTICS DISTAMYCIN A AND CONGOCIDINE ON THE REPLICATION OF HERPES SIMPLEX VIRUS

YECHIEL BECKER, SHULAMIT NEUMAN and JULIA LEVITT-HADAR

Department of Virology, Hebrew University–Hadassah Medical School, Jerusalem, Israel

Studies on the effect of rifampicin on the replication of viruses demonstrated that only poxviruses were inhibited by the antibiotic while herpesviruses and nuclear DNA viruses were not affected (1). The use of other rifamycin SV derivatives demonstrated that the hydrazone sidechain of rifampicin is responsible for the inhibition of replication of Shope fibroma virus (2). To determine whether other antibiotics, which have sidechains different from that of rifampicin, inhibit the replication of herpes simplex virus (HSV), the effect of distamycin A and its derivatives was studied. Distamycin A, a basic oligopeptide extracted from the mycelium of the mold *Streptomyces distallicus* (3), with a chemically known structure (4), was reported to inhibit the replication of both pox- and herpesviruses (5–7). We have investigated the effect of distamycin A and two of its derivatives (Fig. 1), which differ in one of their sidechains, on the replication of HSV in monolayer and suspension cell cultures. We also studied the effect of congocidine (Fig. 1) (which resembles NETROPSIN® and distamycin A) on HSV replication. Both distamycin A and congocidine were found to inhibit the replication of HSV and to prevent the synthesis of the virus progeny.

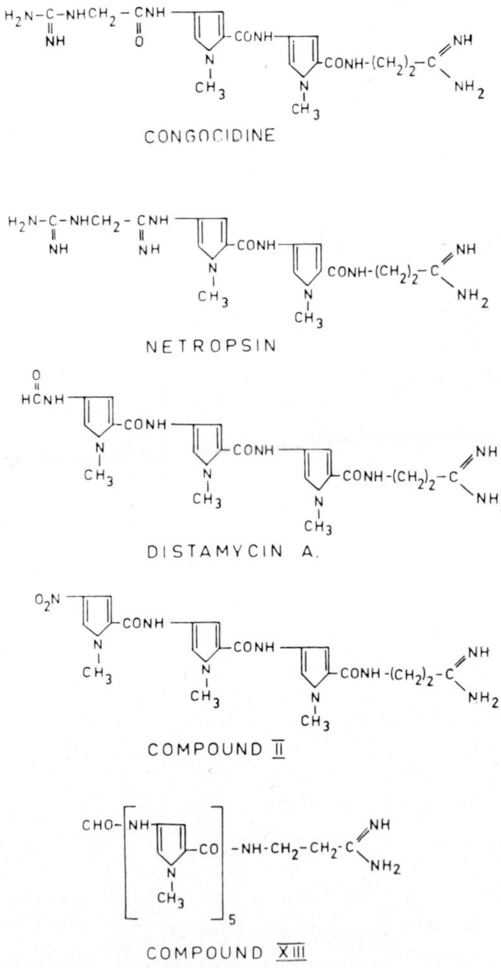

FIG. 1. Molecular composition of the antibiotics.

## MATERIALS AND METHODS

*Cells.* The $BSC_1$ line of monkey kidney cells was

**205**

grown in Eagle's medium containing 10% calf serum. HeLa $S_3$ cells were grown in suspension in Eagle's medium containing either 10% calf serum or 5% fetal calf serum.

*Virus.* The HF strain of HSV was used. Herpesvirus preparations were made by infecting $BSC_1$ cells with HSV and incubating at 37 C for 18 hr. The stock virus was stored at 4 C. The infected cells were subjected to ultrasonic treatment for 60 sec in an MSE ultrasonic disintegrator. The homogenates of the infected cells were used to infect $BSC_1$ monolayers or HeLa $S_3$ cells in suspension at a multiplicity of infection of 10 plaque-forming units (p.f.u.) per cell.

*Plaque assays.* The plaque assays were carried out in $BSC_1$ monolayers grown in plastic Petri dishes (NUNC Co., Denmark) as described by Levitt and Becker (8). After a 72 hr incubation period at 37 C under an agar overlay, the infected cells were stained overnight with neutral red and the plaques were counted.

*Acrylamide gel analysis.* Acrylamide gel electrophoresis was based on the technique of Maizel et al. (9) and has been described in detail by Olshevsky and Becker (10).

*Sucrose gradient analysis of herpesvirions.* Sucrose gradients, 12 to 52% (w/w), were prepared in Tris-buffered saline (TBS) (0.85% NaCl, 0.2 M Tris-HCl, pH 7.3). Virus suspensions were layered onto the gradient and centrifuged for 40 min at 15,000 rev/min at 4 C in the SW 25.1 rotor of the Beckman model L-2 ultracentrifuge (11).

*Isotopes.* $H^3$-thymidine (specific activity 12.4 c/mmole) was obtained from the Nuclear Research Centre, Israel. $C^{14}$-leucine (specific activity 312 mc/mmole) was obtained from the Radiochemical Centre, Amersham, England.

*Antibiotics.* Distamycin A and its derivatives, compounds II and XIII, were received from Farmitalia, Milan, Italy. Congocidine was obtained from Rhône-Poulenc Laboratories, France.

The antibiotics were dissolved in dimethyl formamide (DMF) (BDH, England) in the proportion of 5 mg/0.1 ml DMF. The solution was added to Eagle's medium to a concentration of 1 mg antibiotic/ml. This stock was used for preparing further dilutions of the drug.

## RESULTS

*Effect of distamycin A on the formation of HSV plaques in $BSC_1$ monolayers.* To determine the effect of distamycin A on HSV replication, $BSC_1$ monolayers were infected with

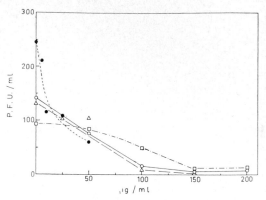

FIG. 2. Effect of different concentrations of distamycin A on plaque formation by HSV. $BSC_1$ cell monolayers in plastic Petri dishes were infected with HSV at a concentration of 100 to 200 p.f.u. per plate in the presence of varying concentrations of distamycin A. After the virus was adsorbed to the cells for 60 to 90 min at 37 C, an agar overlay in Eagle's medium containing the drugs in different concentrations was added to each plate. After 72 hr at 37 C the monolayers were stained with neutral red and the plaques counted.

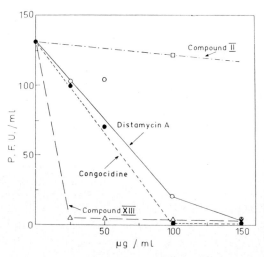

FIG. 3. Effect of different antibiotics on plaque formation by HSV. $BSC_1$ cell monolayers were infected with HSV in the presence of varying concentrations of each antibiotic, which was dissolved in DMF. After the period of virus adsorption at 37 C, different concentrations of the various drugs were added in the agar overlay. After incubation for 72 hr the plates were stained with neutral red and the plaques counted. For explanation of symbols, see Fig. 2.

TABLE 1. *Chemical structure of distamycin A, its derivatives and congocidine*

| Antibiotic[a] | Sidechain | Number of pyrrole groups in the antibiotic |
|---|---|---|
| Distamycin A | HCONH | 3 |
| Compound II | $O_2N$ | 3 |
| Compound XIII | HCONH | 5 |
| Congocidine | $H_2N\text{-}C\text{-}NHCH_2\text{-}CONH$ $\parallel$ $NH$ | 2 |

[a] According to ref. 12.

100 to 200 p.f.u. per plate and treated with varying concentrations of the antibiotic, added to the agar overlay. The results of four experiments are presented in Fig. 2. At 150 µg/ml, distamycin A completely inhibited the formation of HSV plaques. At lower concentrations the inhibitory effect of distamycin A was not complete: the number of plaques was reduced but the residual plaques had a smaller diameter than the untreated plaques.

*The effect of distamycin A, its derivatives and congocidine on HSV plaque development in BSC$_1$ cells.* Treatment of infected BSC$_1$ monolayers with 150 µg/ml of distamycin A completely prevented plaque-formation by HSV (Fig. 2 and 3). Compound XIII (Fig. 1) had a marked inhibitory effect and completely suppressed HSV plaques at a concentration of 25 µg/ml. Congocidine had a completely inhibitory effect at a concentration of 100 µg/ml. In contrast, compound II, which lacks one of the sidechains present in distamycin A, (Table 1) had no effect on the development of HSV plaques (Fig. 3). Since the difference between the various antibiotics is both in the number of pyrrole groups and in the structure of the sidechain, further studies on other distamycin A derivatives are necessary before we can relate the inhibitory effect of the antibiotic to a particular site in the antibiotic molecule.

*Characterization of the viral peptides syn-*thesized in distamycin A-treated BSC$_1$ cells. Studies in our laboratory (U. Olshevsky and Y. Becker, to be published) have demonstrated that it is possible to analyze the radioactively labeled viral peptides of herpes simplex, synthesized in infected cells by means of electrophoresis on acrylamide gel. This is possible because virus infection inhibits the synthesis of host cell proteins within several hours after infection. Labeling of infected cells with radioactive amino acids followed by electrophoresis in acrylamide gels yielded a peptide pattern typical of untreated infected cells (Fig. 4). Peptide II (Fig. 4) was previously (10) characterized as the capsid protein; peptides III, IV and V are glycopeptides of the viral envelope; peptide VI is associated with the viral nucleocapsid and peptide VII is the internal peptide in the viral nucleocapsid (10). However, less radioactivity was incorporated into the viral peptides which were synthesized in the presence of distamycin A, as compared to the untreated infected cells, suggesting that the replication of the viral DNA was markedly affected but not inhibited in the distamycin A-treated infected cells. Under these conditions late viral peptides (e.g. the capsid peptide II) were synthesized. The profile of peptides synthesized in the infected cells in the presence of distamycin A differed from the profile of peptides synthesized in cytosine arabinoside-treated cells

**207**

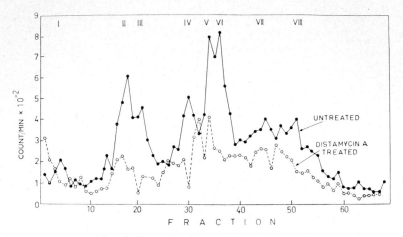

FIG. 4. Acrylamide gel electrophoresis of HSV proteins. $BSC_1$ cells were infected with HSV in the presence or absence of distamycin A (100 µg/ml) and labeled with $C^{14}$-leucine (0.2 µc/ml). After about 20 hr, when the cytopathic effect was complete, the cells were collected into Tris-buffered saline and disrupted by ultrasonic treatment for 60 sec. To a volume of 0.2 ml of each of the cell suspensions, 0.5% (w/v) sodium dodecyl sulfate, 0.5 M urea and 0.1% (v/v) 2-mercaptoethanol made in 0.1 M phosphate buffer pH 7.2 were added for 10 hr at room temperature. The samples were layered on acrylamide gels and electrophoresis was carried out for 10 hr at 6 ma per gel. The gels were sliced and the radioactivity in each slice was determined.

(U. Olshevsky and Y. Becker, to be published), in which the synthesis of peptide VII was markedly increased, indicating that the synthesis of "early" viral peptides was enhanced.

*Effect of distamycin A on HSV replication in suspended cultures of HeLa cells.* HSV replicates in $S_3$ HeLa cells grown in suspension. The effect of varying concentrations of distamycin A on the synthesis of herpesvirions was investigated (Fig. 5). The untreated and distamycin A-treated cells were labeled concomitantly with radioactive thymidine and leucine. The infected cultures were incubated 9 hr, disrupted by ultrasonic treatment and analyzed by centrifugation in sucrose gradients. Two bands, which contained the two isotopes, were resolved in the sucrose gradients (Fig. 5A). The lower band contained the enveloped herpesvirions (11) while the upper contained uncoated DNA molecules and soluble proteins. Treatment of the

infected cells with DMF (final concentration 0.5%) did not affect the formation of the herpesvirions. Treatment of the infected cells with distamycin A at 5 µg/ml slightly diminished the amount of radioactive proteins present in the virus band. However, distamycin A at 10 µg/ml markedly affected the formation of herpesvirions but did not affect the DNA and proteins present in the upper part of the gradient. Treatment of infected cells with 25 µg/ml and 50 µg/ml markedly inhibited the synthesis of DNA and proteins in the infected cells and also prevented the formation of virions. Nevertheless, this inhibitory effect was not complete and radioactive DNA was distributed throughout the sucrose gradients. The effect of distamycin A on the synthesis of herpes simplex virus is dose dependent (Table 2).

A one-step growth cycle analysis of herpesvirus in HeLa cells demonstrates a lag phase of 4 hr and a logarithmic replication period

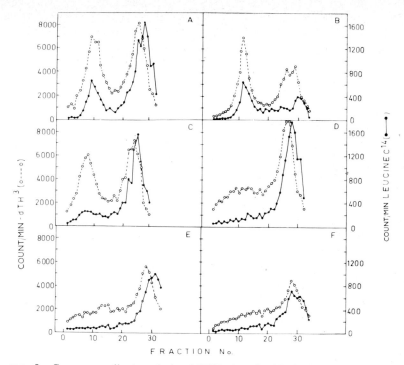

FIG. 5. Sucrose gradient analysis of HSV treated with distamycin A. HeLa S₃ cells were infected with HSV and labeled with H³-thymidine and C¹⁴-leucine (1 μc/ml). The infected cultures were divided into separate cultures containing varying concentrations of distamycin A. One culture remained untreated while another contained DMF at a concentration equal to that used with the highest concentration of distamycin A. Nine hours after infection, the infected cells were washed, disrupted by ultrasonic treatment and centrifuged in 12 to 52% (w/w) sucrose gradients. The gradients were fractionated and the radioactivity in each sample determined. A) HeLa S₃ cells infected with HSV; B) infected cells containing DMF; C–F) infected cells treated with distamycin A; C) 5 μg/ml; D) 10 μg/ml; E) 25 μg/ml and F) 50 μg/ml.

TABLE 2. *Effect of distamycin A on the synthesis of herpes simplex virions in HeLa cells*

| Distamycin A (μg/ml) | % radioactivity in virus band |
|---|---|
| 0 | 100 |
| 5 | 86 |
| 10 | 50 |
| 25 | 35 |
| 50 | 20 |

of 4 hr (Fig. 6). The growth cycle of HSV in HeLa cells takes half the time required for its growth cycle in BSC₁ monolayers (8). Addition of distamycin A (100 μg/ml) to the infected cells resulted in the complete inhibition of virus replication (Fig. 6).

DISCUSSION

Distamycin A and its related antibiotics, compound XIII and congocidine, inhibited the replication of HSV in BSC₁ and HeLa cells, confirming earlier studies (3–7) which demonstrated that distamicin A has antiviral properties. The antibiotics tested in the present study, apart from compound II (12), were inhibitory to HSV. The mode of action of distamycin A was elucidated from *in vitro* studies (13, 14). The antibiotic molecules were

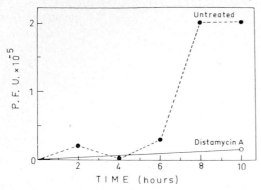

FIG. 6. Effect of distamycin A on the HSV growth cycle in HeLa $S_3$ cells. HeLa $S_3$ cells were infected with HSV and divided into two separate cultures which contained either no antibiotics or distamycin A, 100 µg/ml. Samples taken every 2 hr from the untreated cell culture were titrated in $BSC_1$ cell monolayers for in fectious virus. The infected cultures containing the antibiotics were titrated 10 hr after infection.

found to bind to adenine-thymine-rich DNA (13) and to cause a conformational change in the DNA (14), which interferes with the binding of the DNA-dependent RNA polymerase molecules to the DNA template. This results in the inhibition of RNA transcription. Distamycin A is assumed to inhibit the replication of herpesvirus by a similar mechanism. An inhibitory effect of distamycin A on the synthesis of cellular and viral DNA molecules as well as an inhibitory effect on the synthesis of viral peptides in the infected cells was demonstrated (Fig. 4 and 5, Table 2). Distamycin A also inhibits the replication of Epstein-Barr virus in arginine-deprived Burkitt lymphoblasts (15, 16). Although distamycin A interacts with adenine-thymine-rich DNA (13,14), we have here demonstrated that the antibiotic is capable of inhibiting the synthesis of HSV-DNA, which is rich in guanine + cytidine. Thus, herpesvirus DNA may possibly contain regions rich in adenine + thymine. Studies on the molecular organization of the HSV-DNA genome are in progress.

We wish to thank Prof. M. Ghione and Farmitalia, Milan, Italy for the generous supply of the antibiotics distamycin A compounds II and XIII and congocidine, and for their support. The capable assistance of Mrs. Hava Alkalay is acknowledged.

REFERENCES

1. SUBAK-SHARPE JH, TIMBURY MC and WILLIAMS JF. Rifampicin inhibits the growth of some mammalian viruses. *Nature (Lond)* **222**: 341, 1969.
2. ZAKAY-RONES Z and BECKER Y. Rifampicin—antipoxvirus activity due to the hydrazone side chain. *Nature (Lond)* **226**: 1162, 1970.
3. CASAZZA AM, FIORETTI A, GHIONE M, SOLDATI M and VERINI MA. Distamycin A, a new antiviral antibiotic. *Antimicrob Agents Chemother* 1965, p 593.
4. ARCAMONE F, PENCO S, NICOLELLA V, OREZZI P and PIRELLI AM. Structure and synthesis of distamycin A. *Nature (Lond)* **203**: 1064, 1964.
5. VERINI MA and GHIONE M. Activity of distamycin A on vaccinia virus infection of cell cultures. *Chemotherapia* **9**: 144, 1964.
6. WERNER GH, GANTER P and DE RATULD Y. Studies on the antiviral activity of distamycin A. *Chemotherapia* **9**: 65, 1964.
7. CASAZZA AM and GHIONE M. Therapeutic action of distamycin A on vaccinia virus infections *in vivo*. *Chemotherapia* **9**: 80, 1964.
8. LEVITT J and BECKER Y. The effect of cytosine arabinoside on the replication of herpes simplex virus. *Virology* **31**: 129, 1967.
9. MAIZEL JV, WHITE DO and SCHARFF MD. The polypeptides of adenovirus. II. Soluble proteins, cores, top components and the structure of the virion. *Virology* **36**: 126, 1968.
10. OLSHEVSKY U and BECKER Y. Herpes simplex virus coat proteins. *Virology* **40**: 948, 1970.
11. BECKER Y, LEVITT-HADAR J, DYM H and OLSHEVSKY U. Effect of the nonionogenic detergent Nonidet P-40 on herpes simplex virions. *Isr J Med Sci* **7**: 656, 1971.
12. VERINI MA, CASAZZA AM and FIORETTI A. "Antiviral activity of distamycin A analogues." Milan, Farmitalia, 1969.
13. PUSCHENDORF B and GRUNICKE H. Effect of distamycin A on the template activity of DNA in DNA polymerase system. *FEBS Letters* **4**: 355, 1969.
14. PUSCHENDORF B, PETERSON E, WOLF H, WERCHAN H and GRUNICKE H. Studies on the effect of distamycin A on the DNA dependent RNA polymerase system. *Biochem Biophys Res Commun* **43**: 617, 1971.
15. BECKER Y and WEINBERG A. Distamycin A inhibition of Epstein-Barr virus replication in arginine-deprived Burkitt's lymphoblasts. *Isr J Med Sci* **8**: 75, 1972.
16. BECKER Y and WEINBERG A. Molecular events in the biosynthesis of EB virus in Burkitt lymphoblasts. *Symposium on oncogenesis and herpes-type viruses, Cambridge, 1971.* 1972, p 326.

# MEDICAL TREATMENT OF HERPES

HERBERT E. KAUFMAN

Department of Ophthalmology, College of Medicine, University of Florida, Gainesville, Florida, USA

Idoxuridine (IDU) is safe and effective in the treatment of corneal herpes. It is clear, however, that better drugs are needed. One of the problems has been how to organize the search for such new drugs. This search has been complicated by the fact that once IDU (a prototype drug) was discovered, several other drugs were also shown to have antiviral activity. Testing all these drugs experimentally and clinically presented a tremendous time-consuming task.

The development of quantitative assays of antiviral activity in rabbits helped to provide a guide as to how drugs compared with this initial agent in the treatment of dendritic keratitis (1).

The first additional promising drug was cytosine arabinoside (2), which was much more soluble than the relatively insoluble IDU and could be obtained in much higher effective antiviral concentrations. Unfortunately, its toxicity was also high, so that the potential antiviral activity was of no clinical use.

Two additional drugs have been interesting enough to test in man. One, adenine arabinoside (3), appeared to be at least as active as IDU. It could serve as an alternative to IDU or in the treatment of IDU-resistant cases. Following quantitative animal studies, Langston performed an extensive double-blind study with IDU and adenine arabinoside in patients and found that in the treatment of dendritic keratitis there was no significant difference between these drugs (personal communication). This proved that adenine arabinoside is an equally important alternative agent to IDU, and it validated the predictive ability of the experimental system.

A second promising drug in treating dendritic keratitis was trifluorothymidine. Originally synthesized by Heidelberger (4), its activity was documented in rabbits (5) and it was more potent than IDU and could be obtained in very high concentrations because of high solubility without toxicity. We have recently completed a prospective double-blind study with identical protocols at the University of Florida and at the Moorefields Eye Hospital in London with Professor Barry Jones' group (6). In man, as in animals, trifluorothymidine appears to be significantly superior to IDU as a therapeutic agent. It does not share cross-resistance with IDU and is at present the topical chemotherapeutic agent of choice. It is also superior to IDU in antagonizing the effect of corticosteroids on epithelial herpes.

Interferon has provided an interesting and frustrating approach to herpes therapy. Interferon is a protein made by infected cells or cells exposed to foreign nucleic acid (7), which renders other cells resistant to infection not only by the initial infecting virus but by a broad spectrum of viruses. One of its many peculiarities is that it tends to be most active in a homologous system (e.g. human interferon is most active in human beings and rabbit interferon in rabbits). Because of this, and because of the apparently impossible task of acquiring enough human interferon for practical use, great excitement was caused when synthetic double-stranded RNA [poly-inosinic-polycytidylic acid (poly I:C) in particular] was observed to stimulate cells in a very powerful way to make their own interferon. In rabbits this substance had a weak but definite therapeutic effect (8). More important, however, it effectively prevented infection and prevented recurrences of herpes. The only problem was that in animals the stimulation of interferon waned. Thus, after approximately six weeks (9), protection disappeared in rabbits, even though the interferon stimulator was continued. The hope that this effect would last longer in human beings remained until studies were finally done in man. Our human studies showed that poly I:C induced only a transient and minimal amount of interferon production in tears when administered locally (10). Within about 48 hr, the response disappeared even though the drug was continued. Hill also showed that after systemic administration the same type of brief interferon response to double-stranded RNA was observed in the serum and it was almost impossible to get any interferon after a few days (personal communication).

The development of a new type of interferon of low molecular weight again raised hopes. But this inducer (tilorone) (11), like poly I:C, was extremely effective in mice, partially effective in rabbits and had little or no measurable effect in man (12). We extended these studies with poly I:C to include the nonhuman primates (13), and they, like man, responded with only a negligible interferon response. Moreover, poly I:C did not protect the nonhuman primates against herpes infection. This indicates that the interferon system of primates including man is totally different from that of rodents, and is much less susceptible to interferon stimulation.

The more recent technique of producing human interferon from human leukocyte cultures has brought a resurgence of interest in the system. Although poly I:C produces no protective effect in primates (13), the subconjunctival and topical administration of human interferon does protect monkeys against infection with vaccinia and herpesvirus. We would expect this protection by human interferon to be even more pronounced in human beings. Although it is premature to believe that a drop or two of interferon a day will prevent recurrences of herpes the further study of interferon seems promising.

The treatment of stromal disease is relatively unsatisfactory. The necrotizing lesions which are accompanied by direct virus invasion respond to corticosteroids to some extent, but they clearly respond less well than the diskiform edema and are much more difficult to manage clinically. Once corticosteroids are started in this group, they are often difficult to stop. When any patient with stromal herpes or iritis is treated with corticosteroids then as low a dose as possible should be administered. To control the disease initially we usually give three or four drops of 0.1% dexamethasone per day. The likelihood of epithelial herpes is considerably less when this medication is accompanied by IDU, but some small risk still remains even when modest doses are given. If steroids are given very frequently the risk of epithelial infection is markedly increased, and this should be avoided. If topical corticosteroids given three or four times a day are not adequate to control concurrent cases of herpes iritis and diffuse corneal edema, I prefer to give systemic corticosteroids which affect the iritis and quiet the anterior chamber, while having only a very slight biological effect on the cornea. Brown has shown that dexamethasone acetate

(DECADRON®) diluted about 1,000 times and given three times a day has approximately the same biological effect on the cornea as approximately 80 mg of prednisone a day (14).

These studies were done in rabbits but there are similar differences in man depending on the route of administration. Systemic corticosteroids may be used to minimize the risk to the superficial cornea. It has also become clear that the topical use of large amounts of concentrated steroid can greatly increase the hazards in treating many types of eye disease, without increasing the therapeutic effect. Some diseases such as uveitis require intensive administration of large amounts of corticosteroids. Others, such as vernal conjunctivitis and many cases of stromal herpes, permit a full therapeutic effect with relatively small amounts of less potent steroids. These less potent steroids, although fully effective, carry with them a much reduced glaucoma risk and are less apt to activate or exacerbate herpes infection. In addition, less potent steroids do not inhibit stromal healing.

Although most valuable in the treatment of diskiform edema, corticosteroids are also useful therapy for other types of herpes stromal disease and iritis. However, they are poor agents. They do not cure anything and their use should only spur us on to seek better methods of therapy.

The prevention of recurrences and the treatment of iritis and stromal disease really represent the major problems at present. We have shown that the antimetabolite adenine arabinoside can be given subconjunctivally in animals and can have a significantly beneficial effect when herpesvirus is injected directly into the anterior chamber (3). The eye does not get completely well, but in this double-blind study the iritis is significantly milder than in the controls. This drug is slowly metabolized (15) and its only degradation product is also active as an antiviral agent so that a relatively strong antiviral effect is associated with relatively low toxicity. In addition, the drug is not incorporated into DNA. Although in an open study we treated a number of patients with subconjunctival injections of adenine arabinoside, it is not yet clear how valuable this agent will prove to be.

Another drug of potential value and low toxicity is isoprinosine, an inosine alkylamino alcohol. The mechanism for the antiviral activity of this drug is not clear but under some circumstances it too appears to have a beneficial effect on herpes iritis. There have been problems with the reproducibility of the effect of this drug; and while much remains to be learned about it, the future looks bright.

At present trifluorothymidine is clearly superior to IDU for the treatment of dendritic ulcers and for the antagonism of the steroid effect. Interferon and perhaps further manipulation of the secretory antibody system offer hope for the prevention of recurrences of herpetic infection, while adenine arabinoside and isoprinosine may be of value in treating necrotizing stromal keratitis and iritis.

Supported in part by USPHS Grants EY-00007 and EY-00446 from the National Eye Institute.

## REFERENCES

1. CENTIFANTO YM and KAUFMAN HE. *In vivo* studies of antiviral agents. *Ann NY Acad Sci* (in press).
2. KAUFMAN HE and MALONEY ED. IDU and cytosine arabinoside in experimental herpetic keratitis. *Arch Ophthalmol* **69**: 626, 1963.
3. KAUFMAN HE, ELLISON ED and TOWNSEND WM. Chemotherapy of herpes iritis with adenine arabinoside and cytarbine. *Arch Ophthalmol* **84**: 783, 1970.
4. HEIDELBERG C, PARSONS DG and REMY DC. *J Med Chem* **7**: 1, 1964.
5. KAUFMAN HE and HEIDELBERG C. Therapeutic antiviral action of 5-trifluororomethyl-2′-deoxybridine. *Science* **145**: 585, 1964.
6. WELLINGS PC et al. Clinical evaluation of trifluorothymidine in the treatment of herpes simplex corneal ulcers. *Am J Ophtalmol* (in press).
7. ISAACS A and LENDENMAN J. Virus interferon. I. The interferon. *Proc R Soc Lond [Biol]* **147**: 258.

8. PARK JH and BARON S. Herpetic keratoconjunctivitis: therapy with synthetic double stranded RNA. *Science* **162**: 811, 1968.
9. KAUFMAN HE and GOORHA RM. Interferon and ocular virus disease. *Surv Ophthalmol* **15**: 169, 1970.
10. CENTIFANTO YM, GOORHA RM and KAUFMAN HE. Interferon induction in rabbit and human tears. *Am J Ophthalmol* **70**: 1006, 1970.
11. KRUEGER RG and MAYER GD. Tilorone hydrochloride: An orally active antiviral agent. *Science* **169**: 1213, 1970.
12. KAUFMAN HE, CENTIFANTO YM, ELLISON ED and BROWN DC. Tilorone hydrochloride: human toxicity and interferon stimulation. *Proc Soc Exp Biol Med* **137**: 357, 1971.
13. KAUFMAN HE, KANAI A and ELLISON ED. Herpetic iritis: Demonstration of virus in the anterior chamber by fluorescent antibody techniques and electron microscopy. *Am J Ophthalmol* **71**: 465, 1971.
14. BROWN DC, ELLISON ED and KAUFMAN HE. Quantitative systemic corticosteroid effect on xenograft reaction. *Am J Ophthalmol* **67**: 896, 1969.
15. COHEN SS. Introduction to the biochemistry of D-arabinosyl nucleosides, in: Davidson JN and Cohn WE (Eds), "Progress in nucleic acid research and molecular biology." New York, Academic Press, 1966, v 5, p 2.

# SURGICAL TREATMENT OF HERPES CORNEA

R. STEIN and A. ROMANO

Department of Ophthalmology, Chaim Sheba Medical Center, Tel-Hashomer, Israel

About 20 to 30% of patients with herpetic keratitis fail to respond favorably to medical treatment. The refractory cases do not respond to antiviral therapy for many reason: a) idoxuridine (IDU)-resistant virus is the responsible agent; b) the lesions produce extensive ulcers; or c) superimposed bacterial or fungal infection progresses in spite of all treatment. These cases sometimes develop descemetocele and perforation overnight, especially if steroids have been used. Another group of herpetic affections resistant to antiviral therapy is represented by cases in which the stroma becomes involved, forming a dense opacification known as diskiform keratitis. The more severe forms, in which stromal necrosis dominates the clinical picture, resist nearly all conservative therapeutic attempts. Only after months or years do the eyes become quiescent, with a dense central corneal scar, penetrating nearly all the corneal layers.

Iridocyclitis follows nearly all herpetic corneal affections, and is frequently associated with ocular hypertension. Iridocyclitis may become chronic, probably because of the presence of the virus in the iris, as demonstrated by Kaufman and by Witmer.

Metaherpetic keratitis may follow a dendritic ulcer most often in cases having pronounced corneal hypoesthesia. Small erosions with sinuous or scalloped margins, resembling recurrent corneal erosions, are typical of this state of the disease. In metaherpetic keratitis the original herpetic infection seems to be the responsible factor, but all too often mistreatment by chemical agents may be the real cause.

Not all cases of recalcitrant herpetic, post- and metaherpetic corneal involvements are indications for surgical intervention, and even a deep ulcer and an imminent corneal perforation may benefit from properly managed antiviral treatment. In many of these cases, however, surgical treatment seems to be the optimal method to ameliorate a prolonged and disabling illness.

Though not surgical in the true sense of the word, debridement of diseased tissue may be of help, making medical therapy more effective. This kind of treatment should be tried in early cases of herpes cornea that do not respond to IDU, or in recurrences of the same type. In cases of localized ulcers, in metaherpetic keratitis and in cases where Bowman's membrane is irregular and the overlying epithelium tends to break down, curretage may be beneficial and may considerably improve vision.

Chemical destruction of infected cells, once the mainstay of treatment, should be discontinued since it does not contribute to healing. It may often delay epithelialization, enhance scarring and increase the incidence of metaherpetic keratitis.

**215**

In torpid deep ulcers, a conjunctival flap of the Kuhnt-Gundersen type may relieve the patient and promote healing. We use it only in cases of affections near the limbus, and do not like to cover the whole cornea. Even if anchored well, it retracts when one wishes it to adhere and does not retract when one would like it to do so. It enhances vascularization of the cornea and promotes dense scar formation, rendering later grafting less favorable.

In all cases of extensive localized ulcers that recur, in cases of deep, infected or noninfected ulcers, and particularly in all cases of descemetocele or perforation, therapeutic keratoplasty is strongly indicated. Its effect lies in the replacement of necrotic and infected tissue, thus preventing recurrences and improving vision. In addition to these indications, keratoplasty also has its place in cases of diskiform keratitis which has no tendency to improve. In these instances the eyes improve rapidly after the operation and iritis very quickly subsides.

Whenever possible, a lamellar graft is the preferred one in these active stages of the disease. It is also the only reasonable approach when the lesion involves a very extensive area and approaches the limbus. The dissection should include all infiltrated tissue and, if necessary, should pass as deeply as Descemet's membrane. Puncture of the anterior chamber protects against an undesirable perforation. Lamellar grafting is a safer procedure than a penetrating graft, shortens the stay in hospital and very quickly relieves the patient from pain. It may even be done in the presence of a tiny perforation, and Kaufman's recommendation of filling the chamber with air in order to stop the perforation and keep the bed dry is a device that should be borne in mind.

When the perforation is large, or if it occurs during the dissection, a penetrating graft is unavoidable. If this has to be done as the primary procedure in an active stage of the disease, all diseased tissue must be included, and therefore the indications are rather limited. Lamellar grafts meet the needs in the majority of cases and may even result in a visual acuity of 6/6.

Corneal grafting is not an absolute guarantee for preventing recurrences of the herpetic disease which may occur, particularly if steroids are applied during the postoperative period. If steroids are indicated, they should be used together with an antiviral drug. Recurrences appear more frequently in the host cornea or at the border of the graft, and a lamellar graft that is too thin can be very rapidly destroyed by a virulent herpetic infection. This in fact happened in one of our cases, and early regrafting was necessary. If the case is complicated by a superimposed bacterial or mycotic infection, treatment with specific antibiotics should be continued well after the grafting operation.

Of 340 corneal grafts done in the period under review, 155 (45%) were lamellar, and 195 (55%) were perforating grafts. Of the 155 lamellar grafts, 59 (38%) were done for therapeutic purposes in active inflammation of the cornea, and of these, 31 were active or chronic cases of herpetic keratitis. Of 195 penetrating keratoplasties, 36 were performed for active corneal inflammations. In 1924 instances, there was either a perforation, a large descemetocele or a severe superimposed bacterial infection threatening the existence of the eye. Twelve of these grafts were done in cases of complications resulting from a herpetic infection according to the indications outlined above.

Recurrences occurred after lamellar grafting in 10 eyes (32%), about half of them in the graft and the other half in the surrounding cornea or at the edge of the graft. Relapses were observed after penetrating grafts with almost the same frequency. In two perforating keratoplasties the graft became dystrophic. In six eyes, eight keratoplasties were performed; in two of them twice. Four penetrating keratoplasties were necessary after unsuccessful lamellar grafts. The visual results were on the average the same as in corneal grafting for reasons other than herpes cornea.

# DISCUSSION

DR. H. E. KAUFMAN (*USA*): Can any one throw light on the incidence of herpes cornea among the population affected by trachoma, active or inactive, treated or not?

DR. R. STEIN (*Israel*): Apparently, trachoma does not protect. It may be difficult to diagnose a herpetic lesion in a trachoma patient.

*Question from the floor*: What is the role of cryo-freezing in dendritic lesions?

DR. STEIN: It acts as a slight debridement.

DR. KAUFMAN: I agree with this opinion. There is no doubt that it helps clinically.

I would like to comment about herpes of the cornea after the introduction of foreign bodies. This may be a medicolegal problem and the association is well-documented in the literature over the years. It also concerns the use of contact lenses. I think that the damage to the cornea can make the tissue more susceptible to virus infection, just as Friedenwald showed in vaccinia in rabbits, if there is virus in the tears and the cornea is scarified.

*Question from the floor*: What is the rationale of smallpox treatment?

DR. KAUFMAN: The persons who get recurrent herpes have high titers of circulating antibodies but there is little cross reactivity with smallpox. There is, in my opinion, no real evidence that smallpox vaccine or any other kind of vaccine is of any help in preventing recurrence of herpes.

# MOBILE EYE CLINICS

## THE CHALLENGE

VICTOR C. RAMBO

530 L Model Town, Ludhiana, Punjab, India

Dear Fellow Ophthalmologists,

Do not carry lightly in your hearts the plight of the curable blind in developing nations. The Chatterjee/Rambo PL 480 India Research has shown that most of the blind villagers in the vast populations of developing countries are curable.

In the so-called "developed countries" the curable are largely cured. In the so-called "developing countries" they are not cured and live in misery in their world. Until death they do not see. Why? Because ophthalmology does not reach them.

"What have I to do with the village blind?" asked a noted surgeon with a great central eye institute and hospital in a developing country. "It is the job of the Public Health Department!" he said.

There are congresses, academies, institutes, eye departments and private practitioners. Each does some special supporting work to make it easier to reach more curable blind people with sight, but the responsibility is upon us as ophthalmologists.

Ophthalmologists, you are responsible for giving the incentive to those societies and governmental agencies which must be challenged to support mobile eye hospitals, coming from the eye departments of medical colleges in developed countries, to go out to the uncured curable blind of the world—into every village—in every developing nation. No village is beyond three or four days travel by jet and helicopter from any place on earth.

I repeat, fellow ophthalmologists, do not carry lightly in your hearts the plight of the millions of curable blind—each one is a challenge to an ophthalmologist's professional ability and his heart. There is inexpressable joy and satisfaction, which nothing can excel, in reaching the curable blind.

# MOBILE EYE HOSPITALS AND CATARACT SURGERY IN INDIA

ARIN CHATTERJEE

Eye Department, Christian Medical College, Ludhiana, Punjab, India

The problems of blindness which involve the prevention and treatment of eye disease and rehabilitation are especially pressing in developing countries. In India 80% of the population are villagers. Because of poverty, environmental factors, poor sanitation, illiteracy, ignorance, superstition, taboos, malnutrition, inadequacy of facilities for treatment and quackery, the incidence of eye disease and blindness is high.

A survey of the extent of visual disability and the pattern of eye disease is essential for assessing the type of treatment required. In the states of Punjab and Himachal Pradesh in northwestern India, the average diet is comparatively better than in the rest of India; hence nutritional deficiencies do not play an important role in causing blindness. In this area, the leading causes are geriatric conditions such as cataract and glaucoma, and trachoma with its sequelae of secondary infection and corneal opacity.

Our survey revealed that most of the blindness is curable or preventable, provided that the necessary measures are available. Large-scale ophthalmic facilities are required, but unfortunately the financial condition of both the population and the government is inadequate to support these. Furthermore, there is a lack of well trained personnel in ophthalmology. In USA and U.K., there is one eye doctor for every 22,000 people; in India there is one for every 3 million. Considering the population explosion and the number of ophthalmic personnel trained every year, this ratio is not likely to improve.

We have demonstrated that some of these needs may be met through mobile eye hospitals which cover the same area every year at the same season. These move from one site to another, but distances are kept to a minimum so that patients from previous stations may return if there are any complications. In other words, one mobile eye hospital is the temporary replacement of 10 or even 20 permanent ones. Another advantage is that it brings both clinic and surgery into the patients' own area and environment, thus providing treatment with a minimum of alteration of their way of life in the villages.

Sight restoration is possible when either corneal opacity or cataract is involved. In mobile eye hospitals, optical iridectomy and autograft remain the operations of choice for corneal opacity because of nonavailability of donor material, a difficulty occurring even in established hospitals. Public education in this direction is the only solution.

Cataract is a major problem in India. The early onset of senile cataract has existed here for thousands of years. Sushruta, the ancient Indian surgeon, described the couching technique in his Somhita, a surgical manual. The itinerant coucher of ancient times was the forerunner of today's eye camp. He still practises today, although illegally and furtively. There are also quacks and unqualified self-styled "eye specialists" who operate eye camps using out-of-date methods and giving little or no postoperative care. On the other hand, there are eye camps sponsored by philanthropic organizations in which surgery is done by competent qualified ophthalmologists. Most of these, however, are occasional, do not have a continuing program, and their work is limited to only a few conditions such as cataract and entropion of the eyelids. We appreciate all sincere efforts to meet the problem of rural eye care but regret the limitations. Because of substandard eye camps and their poor results, the term "Eye Camp" carries the implication of quackery.

We, therefore, use the name "Mobile Eye Hospital" to describe our units, and every effort is made to provide a well rounded program of diagnosis, medical and surgical treatment, and refraction at a standard equivalent to those of medical colleges. A few principles and guidelines, from some 45 years of the experience of Dr. Victor C. Rambo in India, may be helpful: 1) Every mobile unit should have the eye department of a hospital as its base, to which patients needing special treatment may be referred, and from which extra

TABLE 1. *Combined statistics of two mobile eye hospital units sponsored by the Christian Medical College Hospital and "Sight for Curable Blind" (Regd.), Ludhiana, Punjab, India 1965–70*

| | Year | | | | | | Total |
|---|---|---|---|---|---|---|---|
| | 1965 | 1966 | 1967 | 1968 | 1969 | 1970 | |
| No. of locations | 9 | 17 | 21 | 21 | 27 | 32 | 127[a] |
| Total no. of patients attending clinics | 8,346 | 11,825 | 16,314 | 21,089 | 20,844 | 26,259 | 104,677 |
| Total no. of operations performed | 1,151 | 1,803 | 2,671 | 2,887 | 2,866 | 3,329 | 14,707 |
| No. of cataract operations performed | 610 | 853 | 1,541 | 1,499 | 1,659 | 1,723 | 7,885 |
| Refractions | 2,790 | 2,281 | 5,644 | 10,624 | 6,399 | 6,095 | 33,833[b] |

[a] Majority in Punjab State, others in Himachal Pradesh, Haryana, and Jammu and Kashmir.
[b] Nearly two-thirds of the patients received glasses.

doctors and nurses may be drawn when needed. 2) Basic minimum personnel for the unit should include: surgeon, trained ophthalmic nurse, surgical technician and optometrist. There might also be an advance publicity man, a part-time social worker, a driver-mechanic, a cook and an orderly. 3) A full complement of diagnostic and surgical instruments should be carried, including a slit lamp biomicroscope. Unless working close to the base, a portable autoclave is essential. 4) In selecting locations for work, one should consider the needs of the area, cooperation from local leaders, availability of suitable accomodation for clinics, surgery, wards and staff quarters. 5) The schedule should be planned to allow an adequate period for postoperative care before discharge. 6) The optometrist should be able to supply glasses to cataract patients, and should also have available simple prescriptions such as for presbyopia. 7) Careful records should be kept, both to insure proper care of the patients and to provide material for study and research. 8) A program for educating village people in the care of the eye and the prevention of blindness should be an integral part of the service. 9) One must continually strive to combine economy, simplicity and elimination of unnecessary "frills" with the highest standards of professional skills and service.

Table 1 summarizes the work done over a period of six years by two mobile eye hospital units, one under the Christian Medical College Hospital and the other under Sight for Curable Blind (Regd.), an organization founded by Dr. Rambo in Ludhiana.

Although the same technique is followed for cataract surgery in the established hospitals in India as in any advanced country, the procedure must be modified in mobile eye hospitals. A surgeon can meet the challenge of quantity as well as of quality only if he has well trained paramedical staff.

Patients receive premedication and preoperative preparation outside the operating room. Local anesthesia, that is the retrobulbar and facial block are given by the ophthalmic nurse. The surgeon performs incisions, sutures, iridectomies, extraction of the cataractous lens and closure of wound.

Patients are discharged on the 10th day following surgery, with temporary aphakic glasses of +10 spherical diopters, a green shade, necessary medicines and instructions to attend the follow-up clinic a month later. Any patients having complications are kept under observation.

It is important to select patients as well as operating rooms carefully. In the surgical procedure a strict "no touch" technique is observed as a result of which a good rate of success has been achieved in spite of the primitive working conditions. Our handling

TABLE 2. *Type of surgery performed and extent of cataract surgery*
*(Mobile Eye Hospital: Statistics from eight months in 1968)*

| | Surgery performed | |
| Diseases | Type | No. |
| --- | --- | --- |
| Sight restorative surgery | | |
| Cataract | Cataract extraction | 428 |
| | Cataract needling | 12 |
| | Capsulectomy | 9 |
| Corneal opacity | Optical iridectomy | 21 |
| Preventive measures | | |
| Pterygium | Pterygium surgery | 65 |
| Glaucoma | Filtration surgery | 16 |
| Lid | Entropion correction | 80 |
| | Ectropion correction | 3 |
| | Tarsorrhaphy | 4 |
| | Others | 6 |
| Strabismus | Squint correction (cosmetic) | 1 |
| Chronic dacryocystitis | Dacryocystorhinostomy | 21 |
| Injury | Foreign body eye | 3 |
| | Cornea and globe repair | 5 |
| | Lid repair | 1 |
| Miscellaneous | | 10 |
| Painful blind eye | Destructive surgery | 12 |
| | TOTAL | 697 |

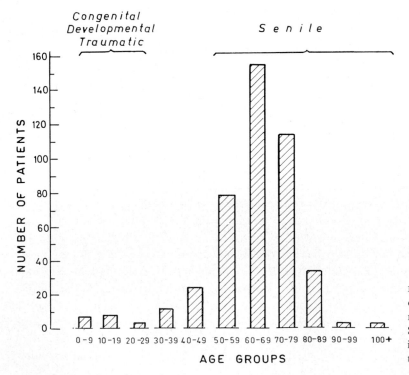

FIG. 1. Age group of patients operated on for cataracts by mobile eye hospital units. Statistics are for eight months in 1968. (The bars represent the number of patients.)

and exposure of ocular tissue are kept to a minimum in order to avoid infection.

Statistical analysis of an eight-month period shows that over 63% of all types of surgery was for cataract, chiefly for senile cataract which appears at an unusually early age in India (Table 2 and Fig. 1). Useful vision was restored to the majority of patients after surgery although some had anisometropia. A contact lens, though desirable, is usually not feasible for financial reasons.

Both the mobile eye hospitals and the eye camps reach only a small fraction of the huge number of India's blind and visually handicapped. The problem is enormous, yet in our time, when spaceships travel to the moon, surely something more can be done to restore sight to the 70% of the blind who are curable. This would be true rehabilitation. The farmer after cataract operation goes back to tilling his land and the village carpenter and shoemaker, wearing cataract glasses, go back to their crafts. Just as important, they are no longer dependent on family and friends.

# THE FUNCTION OF A MOBILE EYE CLINIC

S. FRANKEN*

University Eye Clinic, Groningen, the Netherlands

The idea of extending ophthalmic care and even ophthalmic surgery beyond the hospital walls is not new. In Indonesia, Tyssen initiated mobile rural eye work, while in India "eye camps," especially those which call themselves "free," enjoy tremendous popularity. The quality of the work in many of these camps ranges from poor to very poor. Unfortunately, there are untrained or poorly-trained people who assume the title of "Doctor" and by clever advertising deceive ordinary people. They pose as experienced surgeons and lure blind people to entrust themselves to them. The day surgery is completed, they disappear, leaving postoperative care to someone who will be blamed for bad results, while the patient finds peace in the thought that it was all written in the stars.

Little wonder, therefore, that most medical colleges have voiced opposition to "eye camp" work and many ophthalmologists have made active propaganda against them. They were right to protest against what they regarded as dangerous quackery.

Dr. V. C. Rambo took up the idea of going out to serve the needy, and modified the eye camp principle into a procedure which was to him, as a trained eye surgeon, acceptable. He did this while working in Central India, in Madhya Pradesh at the Mungeli Mission Hospital. Later, he introduced his methods into two medical colleges, Vellore and Ludhiana, linking a mobile eye clinic to the administration of the college and its eye department.

One can describe the functions of the mobile units as follows: a) extending ophthalmic care to areas where it is not available at an acceptable standard; b) promoting the concept of good eye care and elementary hygiene; c) training medical students in prac-

* Former member of the Eye Department of the Christian Medical College, Ludhiana, Punjab, India.

223

tical aspects of village life and making them familiar with village ideas; d) training residents in ophthalmology; e) opening the eyes of staff and students to the fact that modern medical facilities have to be made available to the poor and underprivileged in remote areas, thus counteracting the tendency of medical collges to limit their immediate influence to the campus area.

The work is carried out by a regular team to which other staff members of the eye department are attached for each session. An area is chosen, and the organizer visits the proposed center to establish contact with the authorities and to search for a suitable building. This might be a school building attached to a temple, a factory or similar structure. The organizer has the interior cleaned and whitewashed. Then, after deciding on the clinic hours, he advertises them by handbills and by posters on shutters and houses, to make the camp known within a radius that depends on local transportation. Nevertheless, people sometimes walk for two days across the mountains to avail themselves of the opportunity to receive treatment for their eyes.

Two days before the clinic opens, team members arrive, pitch tents if necessary, unpack their equipment and set up all that is needed to run the clinic. The day after, doctors and students arrive. Of the doctors who run the clinic, one is always a qualified surgeon and the others are residents. Students attend and present cases. When patients arrive, a team member makes them sit in line and takes their name and village or whatever other particulars are needed. Each patient keeps his own slip. The complaints are recorded and the patient has his visual acuity checked. The doctor sees the patient with relevant data on the slips. He examines him by using a battery-run slit lamp and an ophthalmoscope and decides whether the patient needs medicine, refraction and glasses, or surgery. We use a refractionist who works on his own time schedule and gives further appointments on that basis.

Two days of surgery follow two days of clinical examination. Each team member has his own task. Nurses give premedication and facial block, handle the instruments, cut eyelashes, dress the eyes and organize the stretcher bearers. The latter are usually volunteers who carry patients to their beds outside. The patient, on his own bed, is further transported. Relatives take care of the nursing. The doctor and nurse take care of the dressing on alternate days. The team remains with one doctor for 10 days after surgery. The total duration depends on the need for surgery. Any type of nonroutine surgery will be scrutinized for its safety. With the "no-touch" technique, infection rates are often as low as 1/800. I believe Dr. Chatterjee holds the record with 1,400 cases of intraocular surgery without any bad effects in the form of intraocular infection.

On the ninth day eyes are seen through the slit lamp, aphakia correction lenses are given and complicated cases are referred to the hospital. School examinations are also carried out. In many places, talks by medical students on elementary hygiene are given. Students take care of the general checkups as well. In the later days of such a session, the advertising man is again on his way to announce the next camp. In the hot summer season, the Rural Eye Service carries out its work in mountain areas such as Kangra, Kulu, Simla, Baderwah and Kashmir. In the colder winter season, the team works in the open plains of the Punjab. Of a total of 11,000 patients seen in 1970, 1,400 had surgery and 2,500 had refraction. Many students became convinced that village life could be enjoyable after all. The eyes of many of the village blind were opened and students began to see that there was a need for their contribution in such areas.

The Rural Eye Service puts into practice what I found in King's book (1):

"Patients should be treated as close to their home as possible in the smallest, cheapest, most humbly staffed and most simply equipped unit that is capable of looking after them adequately. The quality of medical care must never be judged from the splendor or otherwise of the building in which it is undertaken."

REFERENCE

1. KING JH JR. "Medical care in developing countries." London, Oxford University Press, 1966.

# MOBILE EYE UNITS IN KENYA

G. G. BISLEY

Department of Ophthalmology, Kenyatta National Hospital, Nairobi, Kenya

It is well to remind ourselves at the outset of some of the more important problems that face all developing countries. Failure to do this will result in a lack of proper perspective and therefore a wrong approach to our subject.

1) There is an acute shortage of skilled manpower. There is about one doctor per 10,000 people in Kenya today and about one ophthalmologist per 900,000. Coupled with this ratio is a very high population growth of 3.5% per annum. This means that despite intensive medical training programs, the doctor-patient ratio will not improve, and we must, therefore, lean increasingly on the use of paramedical personnel to fill the many gaps. This will most certainly apply to the staffing of our mobile eye units.

2) The population is widely scattered. A real difficulty is posed in bringing aid to remote districts, particularly if the inhabitants are nomadic. Furthermore, whereas 90% of the doctors live in towns, and chiefly in Nairobi, 90% of the people live in the country.

3) Communications are difficult. Main trunk roads are now good, but country roads leave much to be desired. This raises problems of vehicle maintenance, difficulties arising in rainy weather, physical fatigue of the staff etc.

4) Limited finances pose a chronic problem. At present, about one-half of the national budget of Kenya is allocated to education. Medical requirements compete for the remaining half, with many other pressing priorities.

We should like to pay warm tribute to the many and various agencies which most generously supply supplementary aid. We are extremely grateful for all that our host country, Israel, has done and is doing towards supplying technical expertise and ophthalmic training in various parts of Africa; and also, for the direction and encouragement so enthusiastically given by our very dear friend Dr. Isaac Michaelson. We also thank the American Foundation for the Overseas Blind and the Professor Weve Foundation in Holland. As to local agencies, we think of the Rotary and the Lions' clubs, and most of all the Kenya Society for the Blind. Last, but not least, we recall the British Royal Common-

* Author's address: P.O. Box 30024, Nairobi, Kenya.

wealth Society for the Blind, with its immense humanitarian effort focused in the person of Mr. John Wilson. It is true to say that none of the achievements of the Kenya Ophthalmic Program would have been possible without the generous aid and continual encouragement of all these agencies.

One of our great English authors once wrote: "you must employ the material which lies closest to your hand: you must contrive your story out of the simplest everyday matters as a small bird builds its nest from the mosses and twigs of the trees it lives in."

These immortal words of Jane Austen have highlighted for us in Kenya an important principle, with both material and personal applications. It has been our aim, whenever possible, to use local materials and talent; to build slowly and wisely, rather than to start big and end in failure.

*The vehicle of the mobile eye unit.* In its early days the mobile eye unit consisted of a man and a motor bicycle. The experience gained was invaluable in the planning of the next stage when, in 1963, the first long wheel base (l.w.b.) Land Rover was put on the road with a staff of three medical auxiliaries. We chose the Land Rover because it was readily available, and we knew it could go almost anywhere. Strong wooden boxes were made to hold the instruments and camp equipment: an important detail. The contents are kept dustproof, and careful packing avoids not only much waste of time, but also the breakages and losses which are inevitable if built-in cupboards are used.

In our experience, the large, cumbersome, highly sophisticated vehicle should be avoided at all costs. It is very costly to maintain and run, it cannot negotiate the rough terrain of the remote areas and is easily bogged down in the rain. We use the standard Land Rover with perhaps the addition of a roof rack: in fact the simpler the better. We have also used the Renault Roho, a much lighter vehicle,

cheaper to buy and to run, but it carries less equipment and is less durable.

*The staff.* As already mentioned, the shortage of doctors entails making the maximum use of paramedical personnel. All of our mobile units, of which there are five at present, are run entirely by such men. They are not however, left, "to go it alone." It is absolutely essential that the ophthalmologist himself take a personal interest in all the activities of each unit. He must be prepared to pay regular visits and to join in with the field work, and he must also have the time and the patience to deal with the day-to-day problems which may arise; and to find solutions, as far as possible, on the spot.

Happy personal relationships between doctor and staff are vital. Without these, good team work is impossible. Success also depends on a very careful selection of staff, and in this, character is as important as clinical acumen, energy, resourcefulness and the ability to get along with people.

The most valuable member of the team is the medical assistant. He will already have completed a four-year paramedical training course at the Government Medical Training Center, and will also have proved his worth for at least a year in a District Hospital or Health Center. If selected for ophthalmic training, he will have done this under the supervision of the Senior Ophthalmologist at the Kenyatta National Hospital. At present, ophthalmic training lasts for one year, and during this time, the trainee spends periods in the field attached to a mobile unit, thus gaining valuable practical experience.

The medical assistant is in charge of the unit, plans its visits, and is responsible for the welfare of his assistants, usually an enrolled male nurse and a driver. He is always consulted in the selection of the other two members, as it is extremely important for them to be able to work well together with the minimum of supervision.

The driver is regarded as a vital member of the team. Normally, drivers work to very rigid rules in Africa and confine their activities to driving and nothing else. Our men not only drive, but have to be willing to undertake many other duties as well, such as helping with simple eye treatments, care of camping equipment, cooking for the team and, when necessary, helping in operating sessions by performing such tasks as holding the operating lamp.

In Kenya we are fortunate in having the invaluable services of a non-government ophthalmologist, who devotes all his time, in a semihonorary capacity, to the supervision of our mobile units. It is very largely due to his dedicated help that these units run so smoothly and happily. Such supervision could never be given by a busy Government ophthalmologist. Any country considering a similar scheme would do well seriously to consider this aspect of administration.

We have left the kingpin to the last. He is the lay administrator. In our case, this is the Executive Officer of the Kenya Society for the Blind. A happy family needs a wise and sympathetic father, and this epitomizes the major function of the good lay administrator. Not only does he look after the cash and arrange for the purchase and care of vehicles and equipment, but he also spends considerable time sorting out the personal affairs of the mobile teams and generally ensuring that things run smoothly, and are done decently and in order.

A clear but simple plan of working, with well-defined aims and objectives, is a first essential. In Africa, ophthalmic needs are so great and resources are so small, that it is vital that we first define the major problems and then decide what can be undertaken with the available resources. A useful guiding principle is to grasp only as much as you can get your arms comfortably around and no more.

*Aims and objectives.* We have confined the activities of our mobile units to the prevention and treatment of the major causes of blindness in this country. These are: senile cataract (43.6%) and infections (36.9%).

The infections from purulent organisms or from trachoma virus occur mainly in children, while their later complications of leukoma and entropion are to be found in somewhat older groups.

Our objectives are therefore: 1) visits to primary schools to help prevent and treat conjunctivitis and trachoma. Briefly, this involves the teaching of simple ocular hygiene and treatment with antibiotics and sulfa drugs; 2) Surgical treatment of entropion, leukoma and senile cataract.

*Working methods.* Mobile unit work is exacting and exhausting work, and we have found from experience that the best results are achieved only if the staff are given adequate periods of rest and, if possible, some time for working in the main eye center in order to maintain steady interest. On an average, therefore, one week per month is spent at the home base. This also allows for a period off-duty for each member, and time for servicing and replenishing the vehicle. In addition, each unit is given one-month's annual leave.

The mobile unit is the ideal method for bringing skilled ophthalmic help to country districts, particularly where the people are responsive and where basic facilities already exist in district hospitals, health centers and dispensaries. This is our most successful working area, because the eye unit can attach itself temporarily to such an institution, make use of its beds and medical staff, and thereby accomplish a very great deal of useful work in a very short time. But the visit must be well publicized beforehand by every available means, including, when possible, announcements in churches on the preceding Sundays.

The usual period of stay is about three days in any one center. The first day is spent in

TABLE 1. *Capital and recurrent expenditure of the new mobile eye unit sponsored by the Kenya Society for the Blind in 1971*

| | Kenya £ |
|---|---|
| Capital costs | |
| l.w.b. Land Rover | 1,509 |
| Registration, licence, medical and safari equipment | 143 |
| TOTAL | 1,652 |
| | |
| Recurrent costs | |
| Insurance, petrol, maintenance, driver's wages and allowances | 770 |
| Drugs and dressings | 200 |
| TOTAL | 970 |

TABLE 2. *Results of the Kenya Mobile Unit Program, 1970*

| | | |
|---|---|---|
| Units in operation | | 5 |
| School visits | | |
| Pupils examined | | 2,957 |
| Pupils treated (mainly trachoma) | | 554 (18.1%) |
| Hospital and other visits | | |
| Patients examined | | 82,499 |
| Operations | | |
| Cataract | 460 | |
| Entropion | 1,414 | |
| Miscellaneous | 899 | 2,773 (3.3%) |

seeing patients, the second in operations, and the third in preparing first eye dressings, after which the team moves on to the next center. In the meantime, the local staff have been instructed in postoperative care, which is normally minimal. Whenever possible, the unit visits the center again within a week, and at this time the cataract patients are examined and discharged.

*Surgery.* All our medical assistants and enrolled nurses are trained to perform entropion operations under local anesthesia. We regard this operation as vital for the prevention of blindness. In general, optical iridectomy for suitable cases of leukoma and lens extraction are carried out by the ophthalmologist. Should suitable paramedical personnel be permitted to perform such operations in the country at the present time? Our answer is emphatically "yes," provided that the operator is very experienced, responsible and thoroughly trustworthy. After six years of extensive experience, we have had no cause to regret this decision, as a result of which hundreds of elderly cataract patients, who otherwise would never have had the chance of surgery, have had their sight restored and are now living in happy independence. We have been impressed, on a return visit, by the large numbers of patients who turn up at the center for the second eye to be treated, and by the excellence of the surgical result in the first eye. Some failures are inevitable, but the auxiliaries' results are usually as good as or even better than the ophthalmologist's.

*The nomadic peoples.* We have been disappointed in our efforts to reach the nomadic peoples by means of mobile units. Immense expenditure of energy and time is required, and the response is poor. Such peoples are very conservative and accept blindness as an essential part of the common lot. It would seem that we must continue patiently with our endeavors until education and other forces produce a desire for change and social betterment. It has been our experience that very often the most needy people are the most difficult to help. At present, the health of the cow is more important than the health of man.

*Costs.* This is an important matter but of greater interest to the administrator than the doctor. Table 1 summarizes costs, both capital and recurrent, for one mobile eye unit operating in Kenya for one year.

RESULTS

These are shown in detail for the year 1970 in Table 2. No further comment is necessary to show the very considerable contribution that mobile eye units can make in the relief of suffering and in the restoration of sight to those in the greatest need, namely, the "Wananchi," the people of the country.

228

I am grateful to my colleagues in the Kenyan Ministry of Health for granting leave of absence and permission to read this paper, and to Dr. I. C. Michaelson of the Hadassah Medical Organization, for inviting me to attend. Also to Mr. Alex MacKay, Executive Officer to the Kenya Society for the Blind for permission to use, and for supplying, the medical and financial statistics for this paper.

## REFERENCES

1. BISLEY GG. Some aspects in the prevention and treatment of blindness in Kenya. *Trans Ophthalmol Soc UK* **84**: 55, 1964.
2. CALCOTT RD. "Blindness in Kenya." London, British Empire Society for the Blind, 1956.

# EYE CAMPS

## CATARACT EXTRACTIONS
## IN A PAKISTANI VILLAGE HOSPITAL
### Organization, Techniques and Results

NORVAL E. CHRISTY

Christian Hospital, Taxila, Pakistan

The surgical removal of cataracts is generally considered to be curative rather than preventive ophthalmology. But in some developing countries where there are large numbers of patients with cataracts and where the number of ophthalmologists who are ready and able to remove these cataracts is small, many patients may become blind as a result. In such situations the removal of cataracts can be considered prophylactic. In rural areas of Pakistan this is the case.

Pakistan has a population of about 125 million people and about 10,000 physicians—a ratio of 1:10,500. The incidence of blindness from all causes in West Pakistan, tabulated in the 1961 census, was 15.5 per 10,000 persons. Of the physicians in Pakistan, perhaps 250 are ophthalmologists and there are also a number of other surgeons who perform eye surgery as well as general surgery. However, as in so many other developing countries, and indeed in almost all countries, the distribution of physicians is not at all uniform and the rural areas have very few doctors.

My experience has been in a village hospital in West Pakistan which has been in operation for about 50 years, the Christian Hospital, Taxila, Pakistan. Our eye department, which has only two ophthalmologists, faces the problem of handling 35,000 outpatients and a surgical load of 9,000 cases including 7,000 cataract extractions per year. This load has grown gradually, and over the years some methods of handling it have been developed. Sharing information about this experience may be of value to others facing similar situations in developing countries.

In the rural areas of Pakistan eye surgery is very seasonal. The reasons for this are 1) climatological—the weather is very hot in the summer and in northern Pakistan it is quite chilly in the winter; 2) agricultural—at harvest times most able-bodied men are needed in the fields and are not free to accompany their blind or infirm relatives to the hospital; and 3) traditional—over the centuries the belief has grown up that eye surgery can be successfully performed only during the so-called "eye seasons." These "eye seasons" last for three or four months in the spring and about three months in the fall. During these two periods almost all of the eye surgery in our hospital, and most of the eye surgery in Pakistan and northern India, is carried out.

In our hospital we try to bring modern eye care to patients under conditions which our poor village people can accept, in which they will feel comfortable and secure, and at a cost which they will be able to pay. Except for the salary of one doctor and one nurse, the hospital receives no subsidy from outside sources. As is usual in Pakistan and in some other countries, patients who come to our hospital are required to bring their own bedding, their own food, and a relative or friend to help with their care. Naturally, this system raises many problems, but it also helps to solve some others both for the hospital administration and for the patient. The advantages to the patient are psychological, social and financial. Many of our patients are elderly, blind, uneducated villagers, some of whom have never previously left their own village. To make a journey to a hospital which may be 50, 100 or even 200 miles away is a great event in their lives: a great and frightening event. The fact that a patient may bring along a friend or relative; that he may, while in the hospital, eat the food to which he is accustomed; and that he may sleep in the type of bedding to which he is accustomed gives him a sense of security and encourages him to go home and tell his neighbors to come to such a hospital.

Many of our patients are farmers who do not have a cash crop. It is simpler and cheaper for them to bring a sack of wheat to the hospital than it would be for them to bring cash. This system offers several advantages to the hospital. We are able to carry on without having an extensive hospital kitchen; we are able to care for large numbers of patients without having to maintain a large inventory of linen and the staff necessary for cleaning, repairing and safeguarding this linen.

The greatest advantage, however, is that we are able to operate a hospital with a relatively small permanent staff. The seasonal nature of our work means that our hospital, which at times contains 100 patients, may at other times of the year contain 1,000 to 1,200 patients. The number of trained nurses in Pakistan is relatively small and there is no pool of available trained medical workers on which we can draw, so it is not realistic for us to maintain an adequate staff to care for 100 for part of the year and for 1,000 at other times. By depending on the patients' relatives and friends to care for their feeding, bathing and toilet needs we are able to carry on our work with approximately 25 registered nurses.

The financial savings of this system are passed on to the patients. The patient pays the hospital for admission, a cataract extraction, routine medicines and eight days' stay, a total of about 25 rupees, equivalent to US $ 5.25. To an unskilled laborer this represents about 10 days' wages.

Patients are seen in our outpatient department six days a week and surgery is performed six days a week. An effort is made to see patients in the order in which they arrive and are registered at the clinic. For initial screening patients are seated on a long bench in a darkened corridor, and the ophthalmologist, using flashlight illumination and an ophthalmoscope, is able to diagnose and prescribe for patients having simple or external diseases; to sort out those needing further examination, refraction, dilatation of the pupils, slit lamp examination, measurement of intraocular pressure, laboratory tests etc.; and to separate those who require admission for treatment, further investigation or surgery. For this initial screening we find that it is much more efficient to move the sighted doctor than the blind patients.

Patients for cataract surgery have their intraocular pressure measured, the integrity of their lachrymal drainage apparatus tested with fluorescein, their blood pressure checked and a sugar urinalysis done. The patients are given 750 mg/day of chloramphenicol for four days starting on the afternoon before surgery. Their faces are washed with soap and water; eye lashes are clipped; an anti-

**231**

biotic ointment is applied to the eye which is covered with a sterile pad, removed the following morning at the time of surgery. If at that time there is excessive or purulent discharge on the pad or if the eye is inflamed, the patient's surgery is postponed and the patient is started on local antibiotics or, in some cases, on systemic antibiotics. Routine preoperative medication consists of one and a half grains of phenobarbital and 25 mg of chlorpromazine 1 hr before the operation. Pupils are dilated using 10% phenylephrine (NEOSYNEPHRINE®) and homatropine. In our operating room, we have three tables and the surgeon moves from table to table. As soon as an operation is completed on one table the surgeon moves to the next table where the patient has been prepared and draped for operation. Only seconds are spent between operations. The first patient is quickly bandaged, removed from the table and replaced by another whose eye is then washed and draped. Preparation includes a modified Van Lint type of facial nerve block using 2% procaine and a retrobulbar injection using 2% lignocaine containing hyaluronidase and adrenalin. These injections are given before the patient is put on the operating table. The skin of the lids is washed with sterile water and the conjunctival sac is irrigated with sterile water after a von Graefe speculum has been placed in the eye. A sterile cloth drape about 12 × 18 inches and having a small hole in the center is applied.

The surgical technique includes the following: A 180° incision is made at the limbus with a von Graefe knife. One small peripheral iridectomy is performed in most cases. The corneoscleral sutures are then placed. Preferably three sutures are used, although when we are rushed we use two or even only one corneoscleral suture. Virgin silk, threaded and tied on a Jameson Evans type needle and with a loop tied at the end, is used as the suture material. The lens is then delivered using capsule forceps. Usually the lens is tumbled but other techniques are used as indicated. The iris is reposited as necessary and the sutures are tied. At the end of the operation 4% pilocarpine and an antibiotic solution are placed in the eye. A sterile pad is placed on the operated eye and the eye is bandaged using a gauze roller bandage and including a protective shield made from used X-ray film. In cases having two cataracts the second operation is performed four days after the first, provided that the first eye appears to be progressing normally. The instruments, including all sharp instruments, are sterilized by steam autoclaving. Four small, speed autoclaves are used and 14 sets of instruments are rotated through the operating theater, an ultrasonic cleaner and the autoclaves. Small stainless steel trays have been devised to hold the instruments so that all of the instruments from a single operation can be picked up at one time and placed in the cleaner and the autoclaves.

At the end of the operation the patient, who has walked to the operating theater, is assisted down from the operating table, led to the door of the theater, and returned to the care of his relative who has accompanied him to the operating block. He then walks back to his bed. We have done studies on the rates of postoperative complications and find that this degree of postoperative ambulation does not increase them. This system has been used for the past 50,000 cataract cases in our hospital.

With these methods and with a team of 10 persons in the operation and preparation rooms, including only one ophthalmic surgeon, we are able to perform cataract extractions very quickly and are able, when called upon to do so, to perform 100 or more cataract operations per morning. Our outpatient clinic is scheduled for 10 AM, so we aim to have eye surgery finished by that time. In order to get this much work done by 10 AM it is fairly routine for us to commence eye surgery in our busy seasons at 4 AM.

When the hospital is not crowded postoperative dressings are done daily on all patients. When the hospital has more than about 200 patients these dressings are done every other day: on the first, third, fifth and seventh postoperative days. For patients having bilateral aphakia or unilateral aphakia in their only useful eye, + 10 diopter spherical lenses are prescribed at the time of discharge as temporary glasses. These are prescribed for about 30% of the patients. Those who are not fully satisfied with their temporary lenses or who wish to have glasses for near sight are advised to return for refraction in six to eight weeks. The fact that many of our patients have come from long distances and the fact that only 15% of our patients are literate are factors contributing to the fact that many of our patients do not return for refraction and permanent glasses.

We have developed a simplified system for recording information at the time of operation and postoperatively on rounds, so that very little writing is required. From the recorded data we are able to collect statistics on patients and results.

Approximately 35,000 patients were seen in eye clinics last year. About 1,300 minor eye operations were performed and approximately 7,700 major eye operations, including 6,975 cataract extractions. Of the patients on whom cataract surgery was performed, 55% were males and 45% were females. The average age of the males was 62.5 years and of the females 57.2 years. The age range in both cases was from 3 to 100 years. The distribution of cataract types was as follows: juvenile, 1.5%; immature, 6.2%; intumescent, 16.3%; mature senile, 70.4%; hypermature, 4.2% and morgagnian, 1.2%. The condition of the patient's other eye was as follows: normal, 2.3%, eye absent or having no light perception, 8%; immature cataract, 52%;

mature cataract, 14.1% and aphakic, 23.6%. One half of one percent of the patients with cataracts had acute glaucoma in this eye at the time they came to the hospital; and 1.8% had sugar in their urine at the time of admission.

Among 10,000 cases operated upon by one surgeon in the past three-and-a-half years the following techniques were used for lens removal; capsulotomy, 0.3%; linear extraction, 1.6% and intracapsular extraction, 98.1%. In these intracapsular extractions the following techniques were used: Arruga technique with lens tumbled, 82.5%; Smith Indian technique using only external pressure, 3.2%; a combination of the Arruga and Smith techniques, 9.7%; sliding technique, 1.4%; vectis or lens loop extraction, 0.8% and cryophake extraction, 0.5%.

α-chymotrypsin was used in 1.1% of the cases, generally in patients between the ages of 20 and 40. In 0.2% a reverse cyclodialysis was performed at the time of cataract extraction because of preexisting open-angle glaucoma. The capsule was burst at some point during the lens extraction in 8.9% of the cases. A peripheral iridectomy was performed in 89.5% of the cases; a basal or sector iridectomy was done in 8%; and in 2.5% no iridectomy was performed. In 1.5% of the cases no corneoscleral sutures were used; these were the cases which had linear extractions. In 73.4%, one suture was used; in 17.9%, two sutures were used; and in 7.2%, three sutures were used.

In these 10,000 cases the following complications were seen. A retrobulbar hemorrhage occurred at the time of the original retrobulbar injection in 1.5% of the cases; vitreous was lost in 0.95% of the cases; blood was seen in the anterior chamber at some time during the postoperative course in 5.3%; striate keratitis was noted in 14.4%; lens cortex was visible to the naked eye in the anterior chamber in 2.6%; lens capsule was visible

**233**

in 4.1%; the anterior chamber was flat at some time in the postoperative course in 6.9%; it was flat on the eighth postoperative day in 0.5%; an iris prolapse was seen in 3.0%; infection occurred in 0.5%; there was an expulsive choroidal hemorrhage in 0.1%; a cellular and exudative reaction in the vitreous which, for want of a more accurate description, was called posterior uveitis, was seen in 0.9%; needling for blood was done in 0.3% and for cortex in 0.1%; a secondary suturing of the wound was done in 0.3%; secondary air injection was done in 0.5%; iris prolapse was excised in 1.4% and reposited in 1.0%; at the time of discharge 8.4% of the patients had U-shaped or key-hole-shaped pupils and 91.6% had round pupils.

The follow-up of our patients is admittedly very poor. Although it is very difficult to get an exact measurement of the visual acuity of our patients because of the rush of work, lack of staff, and the illiteracy and low degree of cooperation of many of our patients, the following postoperative visual results were noted at the time of the patients' discharge. On the seventh or eighth postoperative day

96% of the patients were able to count fingers promptly and accurately; 0.9% of the patients counted fingers with some difficulty; 1.6% recognized only hand movements; 0.8% had light perception only; and 0.7% had no light perception. It is recognized that this is an area in which we need to refine our observations.

These data have been presented to point out that even in a simple hospital it is possible to keep accurate and fairly complete records, to collect useful data, to practice acceptable modern ophthalmology despite certain required adaptations in technique and in the handling of patients, and to obtain acceptable results from surgery despite handicaps and despite the fact that extremely large numbers of patients may have to be handled.

I would plead with those who are preventing blindness by the removal of cataracts even under rather primitive conditions to examine their techniques to see what adaptations can be made without the loss of any vital parts of the operations, to maintain as high a level of ophthalmology and ophthalmic surgery as possible, to keep accurate records and to review their results from time to time.

# EYE CAMPS IN INDIA

## G. VENKATASWAMY

Department of Ophthalmology, Madurai Medical College, Madurai, S. India

In India the prevalence of blindness (vision less than 3/60) due to cataract is about 2% in areas where there are eye hospitals. In Madurai, nearly 80% of all blindness is due to cataract. The number of eye doctors available in Tamil Nadu State (population nearly 41 million) is less than 200, and they are found

in large cities such as Madras and Madurai. The number of ophthalmic beds available in government hospitals and mission hospitals is less than 700 and the number of persons who are unilaterally or bilaterally blind due to cataract is nearly 0.8 million. No more than 40,000 people are operated on every year. All the others remain blind, with considerable suffering to themselves and to their families.

About 30 years ago, many eye camps were conducted by private agencies jointly with private doctors. However, this has been discontinued. In 1961 the Government of Tamil Nadu initiated two mobile ophthalmic units, one for Madras and the other for Madurai. Each had a budget of Rs 5,000 (Rs, rupee; 1 rupee = $ 0.12); each had a medical officer, an optician and a van with equipment, and was expected to conduct four camps a year. We tried to reach high standards by carefully selecting the cases and minimizing the complications as far as possible. By improving the administration, we reach the maximum number of patients possible and give them the best treatment available.

*Selection of site.* At present we are conducting eye camps only in buildings such as schools, colleges, halls and public buildings. The public within a radius of 20 miles is informed of the date and time during which the camp will be open. Publicity is conducted free of charge through the government radio stations. In addition, we use newspapers and loudspeakers attached to the van as it passes through the village. However, in spite of all our efforts, communications are still very

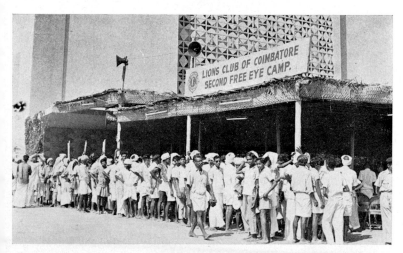

FIG. 1. Patients lining up to attend the eye camp.

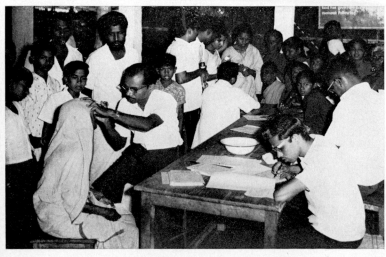

FIG. 2. Initial medical examination.

poor. The message does not spread easily. The blind person is usually confined to his home and the information, even if it reaches him, does not always help unless he can find some money and be brought to the camp. In a recent survey in two villages within two miles of the camp, we found that nearly half of the people were unaware of the existence of the eye camp. Another discouraging factor is that people may think they are too old for an operation and accept blindness as a part of old age.

Our camps usually start on a Saturday when we examine all people and select the cases for operation (Fig. 1 and 2). On the first day patients are registered and those who can tolerate it have their tension tested by opticians with a Schiøtz tonometer. (Cases with obvious eye infections are excluded from glaucoma screening.) Afterwards, the anterior segment is examined with a torch and loupe. Patients with cataract or leukoma are easily diagnosed. Others who have no obvious pathology are referred for refraction.

All cases of cataract and immature cataract with visual acuities of less than three meters in the better eye are admitted for surgery. They are given a separate cataract card and are sent for testing the patency of the ducts and for preparation of the eye for surgery, provided that they have no obvious infection of the lachrymal sac or other external infections.

After the lachrymal duct is found to be patent, the eyelashes are cut, the face is washed with soap and water, the eye is cleaned with normal saline, and a sterile pad and bandage are applied. We call this a trial bandage. Patients are then admitted as inpatients and the blood pressure is taken, usually by medical students.

Cases with fundus pathology such as papilledema, optic atrophy or detachment are sent to the nearest eye hospital where facilities for treatment are available. A separate glaucoma clinic is run in these camps and all suspected cases are examined by doctors and a qualified optician.

We discuss all cases of incurable blindness and try to find the etiology. Some of the people between the ages of 18 and 40 years are admitted to the Blind Rehabilitation Center, Madurai. Totally blind children of school age are sent to the School for Blind Children run by the National Association for Prevention of Blindness. In some camps the nutritionist of our department runs a separate section for eye diseases resulting from malnutrition. Patients with Bitôt's spots, xerosis, keratomalacia and angular stomatitis are interviewed and the mothers are told about proper diets for their children. Small exhibitions are arranged in the camp to explain diseases such as glaucoma, nutritional eye diseases and squint.

*Operation day.* Cataract operations are performed on the second day. The patients are awakened early in the morning and the doctors examine their trial bandage. When they show discharge, the patients are not operated on, but advised to apply antibiotic ointment

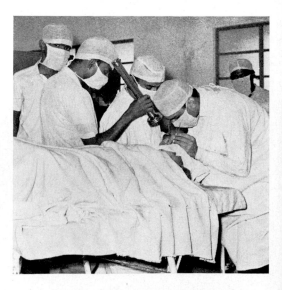

FIG. 3. A cataract operation.

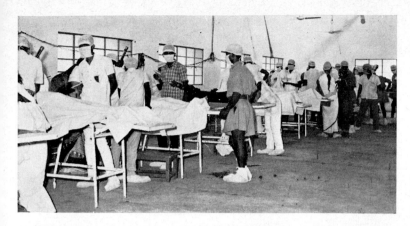

FIG. 4. Operating theater where seven surgeons can operate simultaneously.

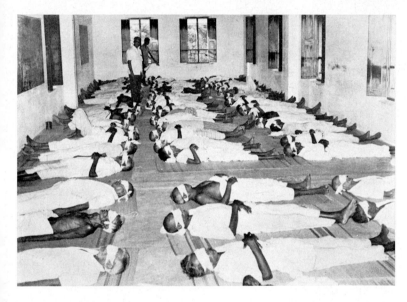

FIG. 5. Postoperative ward in an eye camp.

and to come to the hospital or to another eye camp at a later date. Those who have no discharge are given breakfast and their eyes are washed and made ready for operation. The medical officers, nurses and other staff and volunteers are prepared for the operating theater before 6 AM.

*Anesthesia and premedication.* Patients usually receive one tablet of chlorpromazine (LARGACTIL®) and one tablet of acetazolamide (DIAMOX®). Two or three doctors give facial and ciliary block. The pupils are dilated with Drosyn drops and anesthetic. Procaine (NOVOCAINE®), 4%, is then administered.

*Operating theater.* The facial and ciliary block are given outside the theater. Depending upon the number of cases to be operated, 10 to 14 operating tables are arranged. Blunt instruments such as speculum and fixation forceps are sterilized by boiling and are kept inside the theater while sharp ones are sterilized in Dettol or carbolic acid. A bright torch is used for lighting (Fig. 3). Every surgeon has two tables and is assisted by a nurse (Fig. 4).

The lids and conjunctival sacs are washed again, a small sterile sheet is placed over the face and a speculum is applied. After passing

237

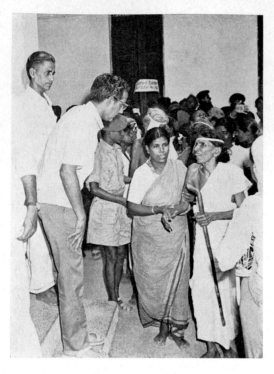

FIG. 6.   Going home after operation.

On the average six or seven surgeons operating at a time will be able to operate on 60 or 70 cases an hour.

*Postoperative care.* For the first 24 hr both eyes are bandaged and the patients are attended to in their beds (Fig. 5). Volunteers work in shifts. At the end of 24 hr an eye surgeon examines the eyes, applies the necessary antibiotic drops or ointments and bandages on the operated eye. The patient is allowed to sit up and move about and, 24 hr after the operation, is given two good meals and one breakfast. At the end of the seventh day the bandage is removed and the patient is sent home if all has gone well (Fig. 6).

The postoperative complications are mainly shallow anterior chamber, infections or ex-

TABLE 1.   *Complications in 389 cases operated on in the T. Kalluppatti camp in 1971*

| Complication | No. of cases |
| --- | --- |
| Blood in anterior chamber | 19 |
| Shallow anterior chamber | 24 |
| Keratitis | 7 |
| Expulsive hemorrhage | 1 |
| Endophthalmitis | 5 |
| Panophthalmitis | 1 |
| Iris prolapse | 1 |
| TOTAL | 58 |

a superior rectus suture an *ab externo* incision is made with a von Graefe knife. After the section, a corneoscleral stitch is placed under the conjunctival flap using 6/0 braided silk. Total or peripheral iridectomy is performed and the lens is extracted intracapsularly by forceps or by erysiphake. The corneoscleral stitch is tied, penicillin drops are applied and both of the patient's eyes are bandaged. By the time this operation is finished, another patient is ready on a second table. Operations for glaucoma such as trephining and iridectomy are also carried out on the same day.

Operations are performed continuously from 6 AM until all the work is over. We have conducted a maximum of 808 operations in one day. There are about 16 surgeons available during two to four operating days. This year we performed 1,131 cataract operations in two operating days. The operation time for each case varies from 5 to 10 min.

TABLE 2.   *Cost of treating a cataract patient*

| Material | Cost (Rs*) |
| --- | --- |
| Medicines and dressings | 5.00 |
| Food for seven days | 12.00 |
| Sanitation, water supply and electricity | 1.50 |
| Volunteer expenses | 2.00 |
| Publicity | 2.00 |
| Construction of additional sheds | 2.50 |
| Travel expenses for medical and other staff and equipment, e.g. knives and needles | 10.00 |
| TOTAL | 35.00 |

*   1 Rs = $ 0.12

pulsive hemorrhage, although the incidence is minimal (Table 1). With improvement in our techniques we hope to further minimize these complications.

Voluntary organizations usually provide a free supply of +10 spherical glasses at the time of discharge or when the patient returns after six weeks. Those who can afford to buy glasses themselves go to opticians.

*Minor operations.* The incidence of dacryocystitis is high in many places. Dacryocystectomies and excision for pterygium are carried out from the third day until the camp moves on. Patients requiring such treatment are dealt with as outpatients.

*Examination of eye defects in schoolchildren.* In some camps large scale examinations of schoolchildren are conducted by the doctors and refractionists. In one camp at Sivakasi, all the elementary and high school teachers were provided with pamphlets containing instructions on how to examine the children, 35,000 in all in this area. Every school was given a Snellen's chart. Of the 35,000 children examined, nearly 4,000 were found to have defective vision and were subsequently examined by the staff.

*Costs.* The cost of treating a cataract patient are shown in Table 2.

# REGIONAL ORGANIZATION
# OF OPHTHALMIC SERVICES IN MALAWI

E. AVIEL, I. BEN-SIRA, U. TICHO and R. DAVID

Department of Ophthalmology, Hadassah University Hospital, Jerusalem, Israel

Malawi has a population of 4.5 million within an area of 45,747 square miles, roughly one-fifth of which is occupied by Lake Malawi. The Republic of Malawi, formerly Nyasaland, attained independence in 1964.

Most of the country is well above sea level except for the southernmost part, the valley of the Lower Shire, which has a very damp and hot climate. The rest of the country enjoys a temperate climate with a moderate degree of humidity. The flat expanses of land are savannah, whereas the hilly areas are densely wooded. There are many streams throughout the country. The lake provides a plentiful supply of edible fish. The population is largely rural. There are only a few urban centers, of which Blantyre is the largest with a population of about 100,000.

Schistosomiasis, leprosy and tuberculosis are highly prevalent in the country. The main ophthalmic problems are cataract, glaucoma and traumatic conditions of the eye. In the last group, damage to the conjunctiva and cornea from the application of traditional medicine to the eye is an important cause of blindness in the country. Idiopathic retinal detachment is practically absent: the occasional cases encountered, nine in one year, were all traumatic except for one case with a myopia of –25 diopters.

Ophthalmic services in Malawi are centered in its only eye department at the Queen Elizabeth Central Hospital in Blantyre. The hospital has about 500 beds and is the largest and best-equipped medical center in the country. The eye department has 54 beds and is staffed by two ophthalmologists, one ward nurse, one theater nurse and five medical assistants. The department maintains its own operating theater, and this enables the eye surgeons to operate without having to depend on the facilities of the main theater serving the other surgical wards.

During a one-year period starting 1 April 1970, there were 1,132 admissions to the ward, and 1,549 operations were performed during this period (Table 1). The ophthalmic out-

TABLE 1. *Diagnoses of 1,132 patients admitted to the eye ward of Queen Elizabeth Central Hospital, Blantyre 1 April 1970 to 31 March 1971*

| Diagnosis | No. of patients |
|---|---|
| Cataract | 325 |
| Diseases of cornea | 185 |
| Glaucoma | 116 |
| Ocular perforations | 92 |
| Uveitis | 71 |
| Retinal detachment | 9 |
| Diseases of conjunctiva | 45 |
| Diseases of lachrymal apparatus | 21 |
| Panophthalmitis | 19 |
| Orbital cellulitis | 7 |
| Mucocoele of paranasal sinuses | 8 |
| Squint | 3 |
| Others, ill-defined | 112 |

patient department, which is operated by the eye ward staff, had an attendance rate of 40,000 during the same year.

Until 1969 there was no provision for ophthalmic services outside Blantyre District. Now there are several smaller peripheral hospitals of 100 to 150 beds each in the different districts. These hospitals are staffed by one medical officer and a varying number of medical assistants and nurses. The medical assistants are trained in government and mission hospitals. Matriculation certificates are not a prerequisite for admission to the course for medical assistants, which lasts for three or four years and includes training in all branches of medicine and surgery. The candidates are trained both to diagnose and treat patients. In distant areas where no medical officer is available, the medical assistants perform urgent operations such as cesarean sections and relief of strangulated hernias. They are thus paramedical personnel capable of acting without the supervision of qualified doctors.

The small number of young Malawian doctors barely suffices to man the central and district hospitals. None were available for formal training in ophthalmology. In an effort to expand ophthalmic services it was decided to institute a course for ophthalmic medical assistants in the central hospital in Blantyre. The trainees were recruited from among young medical assistants who had completed a four-year training period in medicine and surgery in government or mission hospitals. Applications to join the course were voluntary and the candidates were interviewed by the ophthalmologists before admission to the course, which lasted for one year and included theoretical as well as practical training in the clinic and in the ward. Ophthalmology was taught in some detail. Basic extraocular surgical procedures were taught and the trainees each performed a number of these procedures in the ward

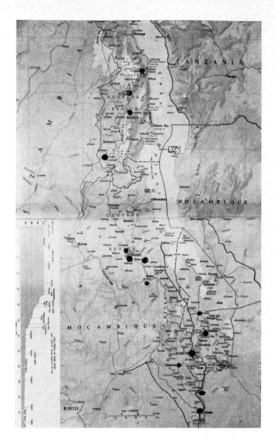

FIG. 1. The distribution of the static eye units in Malawi.

theater under the surgeon's supervision.

At the end of the course, seven ophthalmic medical assistants were posted to different peripheral hospitals where they set up small static units for eye care. Four medical assistants were retained as permanent staff at the central hospital. One was assigned to a mobile eye unit operated by the Royal Commonwealth Society for the Blind in the southernmost part of Malawi. In the following year a new course was instituted and six additional ophthalmic medical assistants were trained. At the completion of the course in June 1971, they were assigned to six other peripheral hospitals, thus bringing the total number of ophthalmic medical assistants

**241**

TABLE 2. *Yearly outpatient attendance and types of operation performed in three static eye units in outlying areas*

|  | Lilongwe Hospital | Rumphi Hospital | Zomba Hospital |
|---|---|---|---|
| Period of survey | 1 April 1970 to 31 March 1971 | 1 May 1970 to 30 April 1971 | 1 January 1970 to 31 December 1970 |
| Yearly outpatient attendance | 3,746 | 3,057 | 12,000 |
| No. of operations performed: |  |  |  |
| Trichiasis | 35 | 18 | 21 |
| Chalazion | 60 | 6 | 18 |
| Conjunctival tumors | 10 | 18 | 12 |
| Enucleations | 9 | 6 | 4 |
| Eviscerations | — | 4 | 15 |
| Repair of lids | — | 7 | — |
| Tarsorrhaphy | 1 | — | — |
| Pterygium | — | 3 | — |
| TOTAL | 115 | 62 | 70 |

operating outside Blantyre to 14 (Fig. 1). One of these medical assistants manned the mobile unit.

In the outlying units, most ophthalmic medical assistants are allowed the use of a room which is set up as an eye clinic. The room can be darkened when necessary. Visual testing charts are available. In one hospital in the south where little room space is available, patients have to be examined in the open. When an ophthalmoscopic examination is required, the patients are led into one of the wards. In all hospitals the ophthalmic medical assistants can make use of the hospital beds for urgent cases: mainly purulent conjunctivitis damage from the application of traditional medicines and cases requiring operation.

The ophthalmic medical assistants are not engaged in full-time ophthalmic work. Usually one-half of their time is spent in treating other general medical and surgical cases. Any case presenting with an eye complaint is referred to them for treatment. They are allowed time in the operating theater for their own surgery and general anesthesia is available.

The amount and type of work performed in some of the more efficient peripheral eye units is summarized in Table 2.

It takes considerable cooperation from the hospital authorities to make these ophthalmic activities possible. The work load in peripheral hospitals is usually very heavy, and there is always a tendency to assign the ophthalmic medical assistants to routine medical and surgical duties in spite of their training in eye diseases. Nonetheless, good cooperation is usually achieved.

The supervising ophthalmologist travels from Blantyre to the outlying eye units once every three months. During his visits, he helps to solve such problems as may have arisen between the ophthalmic medical assistants and the hospital authorities. He also examines selected ophthalmic cases and discusses them with the ophthalmic medical assistant on the spot. The ophthalmologist also sees to it that a regular supply of drugs is dispatched to the eye units from the central hospital in Blantyre.

The activities of the ophthalmic medical assistants (Fig. 2–4) in the peripheral units

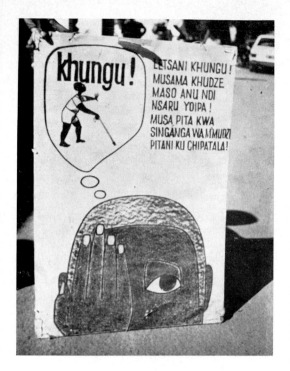

FIG. 2. A poster used by the ophthalmic medical assistants. "Prevent blindness by keeping the eyes clean, do not go to the traditional healers to seek treatment for the eyes, go to the hospital."

consist primarily in diagnosis, treatment, referral of patients and health education and preventive measures.

Cataract represents by far the most common cause of blindness in Malawi. Although it is difficult to assess accurately the patient's age in rural areas, the onset of the lens opacity is probably much earlier than one is accustomed to see in Europeans. The medical assistants have no difficulty in diagnosing the condition under mydriasis. The indication for operation is decided by them, reliance being placed on light perception and projection and the two-candle test. Cataract patients are referred to Blantyre for surgery when both eyes are blind or when one eye is blind and there is progressive cataract in the other eye. This group is sent for operation in order to avoid even a short period of blindness and the ensuing severe disability.

Once the decision to operate has been reached, the patients are sent directly to Blantyre for admission. Unless a large number of patients is sent at one time, five or more, there is no need for the medical assistant to obtain the ophthalmologist's prior approval.

Glaucoma is a far more difficult problem for early diagnosis. Primary closed-angle glaucoma is notably absent among the African population. Most patients come for examination at advanced stages of optic nerve damage although a small group of educated patients seeks help at early stages because of transient blurring of vision. When a diagnosis of glaucoma is made in this category of patients, in many instances the medical assistant initiates

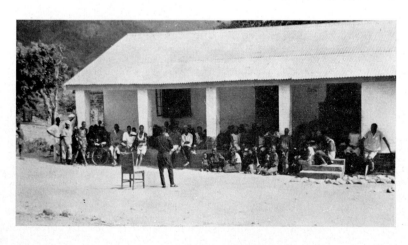

FIG. 3. An ophthalmic medical assistant gives a lecture on the hygiene of the eyes to the rural population in Nsanje District in the south of Malawi.

**243**

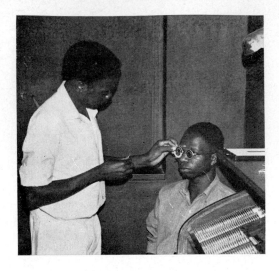

FIG. 4. An ophthalmic medical assistant performs refraction on a patient in the eye clinic in Blantyre.

treatment with miotics and acetazolamide (DIAMOX®) if necessary. If the tension is thus brought under control, the medical assistant performs a visual field examination every three months and uses the Bjerrum tangent screen. During his visits to the outlying stations, the ophthalmologist examines those cases which are controlled medically and decides on the indication for surgery. Most cases eventually undergo filtering procedures at the central hospital in Blantyre. Very few patients remain under miotic treatment over prolonged periods of time.

Damage due to the application of traditional medicines is treated by the medical assistant in all cases in which corneal perforation has not occurred. The traumatizing substance is washed out of the conjunctival sac and local antibiotic ointments and atropine are applied. Cases with corneal perforation are immediately referred to the central hospital in Blantyre where a tectonic corneal graft is usually employed.

End results of the application of traditional medicines consist mainly of corneal scarring and trichiasis. The latter is treated surgically on the spot by the ophthalmic medical assistant, usually by performing a modification of the Jasche-Arlt procedure on the upper lid. With the correction of the entropion, there is often a dramatic improvement in the visual acuity, the discomfort and tearing caused by the inturned lashes rubbing on the cornea disappear, and the patients are then quite fit to return to their agricultural work with a reduced visual acuity in the range of 6/60 to 6/24. When more severe impairments of visual acuity are present, patients are referred to the central hospital for corneal grafting.

Conjunctivitis is always readily diagnosed and treated on the spot by the medical assistant. Severe cases are hospitalized locally, especially when associated with measles.

In the field of health education and local preventive action, the availability of local ophthalmic care is probably the most effective measure since it deters the rural population from resorting to the medications of traditional healers. The ophthalmic medical assistant assembles the outpatients waiting to be examined and gives them short talks on eye health. Particular stress is placed on the dangers inherent in the use of traditional medicine in the eyes. The causal role of malnutrition in the development of keratomalacia is illustrated with picture posters. Attendance at such lectures is usually high.

The ophthalmic activities of the medical assistant play an important role in the prevention of severe blinding conditions. Periodic examinations of school children for visual acuity are being initiated but have not as yet reached any degree of regularity. The ophthalmic medical assistant sends monthly reports of cases examined and treated at the outlying stations to the ophthalmologist in Blantyre.

A description of ophthalmic services in a developing African country would be incomplete without considering the response of the local population to conventional medical and surgical treatment. In the early stages, one

244

had to overcome the accepted practice of seeking help from traditional healers. Conventional care as provided by the hospital was regarded as an unknown and possibly hazardous course of action. This belief is gradually being overcome as medical services expand, but in many rural areas the traditional healer is still regarded as the man who gives the best and "strongest" medicine. The great numbers of blind cataract patients who return sighted to their villages after successful surgery provide convincing proof that good treatment can be had at the hospital. However, this has not as yet appreciably reduced the reliance on traditional healers, who enjoy a high social standing in the tribal community. At the central hospital in Blantyre at least 20 of the 54 beds in the eye department are occupied by patients with severe corneal damage from applications of traditional medicine to the eyes; and this is an indication of the magnitude of the challenge facing the ophthalmologist and his medical assistants in the field of health education.

The scheme of training ophthalmic medical assistants to work in peripheral eye units has proved efficient in extending ophthalmic services to large segments of the rural population. For years to come, and until health services reach the stage at which a sufficient number of eye specialists is available, the scheme will constitute a significant step in the eradication of preventable blindness in Malawi.

# PREVENTION OF
# VITREOUS CONTACT WITH CORNEA IN APHAKIA

M. L. SEARS

Department of Ophthalmology, Yale University School of Medicine, New Haven, Connecticut, USA

There are certain differences in the aims and methodology of the cataract surgeon in a developing environment compared with an already developed one. In both instances, however, when a quiet healing eye is obtained after cataract surgery one key postoperative problem remains: namely, the forward movement of the vitreous. Dire consequences of this anterior dislocation of the vitreous face result from attachment of the vitreous to the cornea, iris and corneoscleral wound or to all three (1, 2).

We know of no drug that selectively influences the movement of the vitreous gel. An observation in one aphakic patient after the use of topical cocaine prompted us to explore again the use of this compound in order to learn its effects upon the position of the anterior hyaloid face. The suggestion (3) that, in the absence of a leaking wound, in some patients (in whom conservative measures are indicated or expedient) topical application of cocaine, ADRENALINE® (epinephrine) or both may usefully influence the position of the anterior hyaloid face after surgery, was investigated further.

Over the past two years, patients who had recent cataract extraction and who were found to have had their vitreous face in contact with the corneal endothelium, were treated with topical cocaine in order to determine the effect of the drug on corneo-vitreal contact. The treated eyes were part of a group of 262 operated on by the authors (3). Eleven eyes (4.2%) in this group developed a shallow to flat anterior chamber at some time during the postoperative period. All eyes were suspected of an occult wound or suture leakage; however, Seidel testing confirmed only two cases of leak from the operative wound. Two eyes developed a shallow anterior chamber in the immediate postoperative period; in the remaining nine eyes, the onset of the development of shallow anterior chamber occurred 10 to 20 days after cataract surgery. Cataract of the anterior hyaloid face to the endothelium of the cornea was noted 11 to 25 days after surgery. Prior to the instillation of cocaine, maximal mydriasis and cycloplegia was achieved with phenylephrine, MIDRIACYL®(tropicamide), homatropine, scopolamine and atropine used individually or in combination. If a response to cocaine was found, the drug was subsequently used alone. Although the changes could easily be observed with the slit lamp, comparisons of the depth of the anterior chamber for quantitative purposes, i.e. distance between the endothelium of the cornea and anterior hyaloid, were made by the photographic method of Bleeker previously reported for phakic eyes (4).

In the two of 11 eyes that had definite

wound leaks, watchful waiting, including maximum mydriasis and pressure patching, appeared to solve the clinical problem, and these patients are not included in the present study. Two other patients developed a shallow anterior chamber. Corneovitreal adherence did not appear in the first and was rapidly relieved by maximal mydriasis in the second. These four patients will not be described in this paper. The remaining seven patients will be described in detail.

The surgical technique was similar in each case although the operations were performed by several different senior house staff. Neither air nor saline injections were used. Chemical zonulolysis was not used.

Elschnig (5) is credited with the original detailed report (1925) describing the tendency of the intact anterior hyaloid face to herniate through the pupil after cataract extraction. He specifically noted that it could occasionally approximate the posterior cornea. This was considered a complication by Vannas (3, 6) in 1932, who later stated that correction of the postoperative lesion to the cornea was a more difficult procedure than the cataract extraction itself. The basis of concern lies in the observation that persistent contact between the anterior hyaloid face and the corneal endothelium leads to permanent adhesion, compromise of the endothelium, widespread corneal edema accompanied by intraocular inflammation and a corneal scar (1, 2) and, finally, bullous keratopathy. Chandler (7) has commented that no cornea will tolerate the intact hyaloid adhesion and if edema develops it never resolves spontaneously.

The syndrome of corneovitreal adherence has been well described by Vannas (6), de-Roett (8), Goar (9) and Leahey (10) among others. The respective incidence in their series was 9, 2.4, 4 and 13%. The incidence in the present series was 4.2%. Leahey (10) suggests a figure of 0.5% for the further development of chronic corneal edema secondary to vitre-

ous adherence in his series of cataract extractions. In our experience it is rare to see this occurrence in eyes with iritis after surgery, but it appears to be more prevalent in the quiet eye where the vitreous face is without inflammation.

Flat or shallow anterior chambers after cataract surgery are generally divided into two groups: early and late. The early cases appear to be most often related to a demonstrable wound leak. In the late occurrences a demonstrable wound leak is often not found. Conservative management usually succeeds. Whether hyposecretion caused by ciliary body detachment is a primary or a secondary event is debatable (11). Most are agreed, however, that once hypotony supervenes, a degree of pupillary block encourages the development of a flat chamber (12, 13). For this reason, it is generally agreed that extreme or maximum mydriasis should constitute the initial therapeutic approach to reformation of a shallow anterior chamber. Some surgeons report success after binocular patching alone (14). Repeated treatment with hyperosmolar agents to dehydrate the vitreous has been used. A variety of other medical and surgical procedures have been recommended to restore the anterior chamber (15–19). The injection of air or drainage of vitreous from within the vitreous cavity or both or supraciliary drainage of the ciliary body detachment through a posterior sclerotomy have been used in various combinations. Once contact becomes more persistent, opening the anterior chamber may be necessary to peel or pull the vitreous back from the cornea (1). This procedure is difficult and chronic corneal edema may result at this late stage.

Weisel and Swan and others have mentioned the use of topical cocaine or epinephrine or both (20–22). Improvement in their patients was attributed to relief of pupillary block by extreme mydriasis.

This explanation did not appear to apply

to our patients in whom the cocaine instillations relieved the contact of the anterior hyaloid face with the corneal endothelium. (In several patients with loose vitreous and broken hyaloid face, cocaine was, however, without effect.) The hyaloid face regressed markedly within 15 to 20 min after a few drops of topical 5% cocaine were given, and stayed so in some instances for as long as 1 to 2 hr; subsequent recurrences responded similarly to further cocaine instillations. The use of several instillations of sterile 5% cocaine for preventative purposes is feasible in postoperative aphakia until such time as the vitreous finally assumes a more posterior position, usually after a few days.

The mechanism of action of cocaine in causing retraction of the hyaloid face after cataract surgery is not known. Cocaine action on the iris and ciliary body apparently does not cause posterior movement of the vitreous since in all cases maximal mydriasis was achieved before the cocaine instillations. A second possibility might be some increase in the formation of aqueous humor, but the rapidity with which the effect occurred rules out this possibility. Third, intense vascular constriction might reduce the volume of the posterior segment of the eye, allowing more room for the vitreous posteriorly. But in these instances the use of phenylephrine, a potent vasoconstrictor drug, in many instances after three or four dosages, preceded the instillation of cocaine; this makes it unlikely that a reduction in vascular volume could be the explanation. It is plausible that in some instances cocaine, which blocks the axonal uptake of adrenergic antagonists, may act so as to place these compounds in higher concentration at receptor sites. Whether the receptors involved lie in the iris, in the vasculature of the eye or elsewhere in the eye is not certain. In many instances cocaine alone was effective, indicating possible potentiation of endogenous norepinephrine present within uveal axonal storage sites. Whether cocaine has a direct effect on the hyaloid structure itself, changing its elasticity, or whether water is actually expressed from the vitreous as a result of the action of this drug on the binding of water by the vitreous, is doubtful, but remains a question that needs further exploration.

## REFERENCES

1. MAUMENEE AE. Postoperative cataract complications. Symposium, part III. *Trans Am Acad Ophthalmol Otolaryngol* **61**: 51, 1957.
2. REESE AB. Herniation of the anterior hyaloid membrane following uncomplicated cataract extraction. *Trans Am Ophthalmol Soc* **46**: 73, 1948.
3. SEARS ML, MCLEAN EB and BELLOWS AR. Drug-induced retraction of the vitreous face after cataract extraction. *Trans Am Acad Ophthalmol Otolaryngol* (in press).
4. BLEEKER GM. Serial recordings of the depth of the anterior chamber. *Arch Ophthalmol* **63**: 821, 1960.
5. ELSCHNIG A. Extraction of senile cataract in the capsule. *Am J Ophthalmol* **8**: 355, 1925.
6. VANNAS M. Klinische und experimentelle Untersuchungen über die vorderen Teile des Glaskörpers, insbesondere nach intrakapsularen Lisenextraktionen. *Klin Monatsbl Augenheilkd* **89**: 318, 1932.
7. CHANDLER PA. New York Society for Clinical Ophthalmology, March 31, 1958. *Am J Ophthalmol* **47**: 244, 1959.
8. DEROETT AF. The vitreous face following intracapsular extraction. *Am J Ophthalmol* **45**: 59, 1958.
9. GOAR EL. Postoperative hyaloid adhesions to the cornea. *Am J Ophthalmol* **45**: 99, 1958.
10. LEAHEY BD. Bullous keratitis from vitreous contact. *Arch Ophthalmol* **46**: 22, 1951.
11. CAPPER SA and LEOPOLD IH. Mechanism of serous choroidal detachment. *Arch Ophthalmol* **55**: 101, 1956.
12. BOYD BF. Management of complications following cataract surgery, in: "Symposium on cataracts." St Louis, CV Mosby, 1965, p 173.
13. CHANDLER PA and JOHNSON CC. A neglected cause of secondary glaucoma in eyes in which the lens is absent or subluxated. *Arch Ophthalmol* **37**: 740, 1947.
14. WELSH RC. Late flat anterior chambers after cataract surgery. *Ann Ophthalmol* **3**: 765, 1971.
15. BELLOWS J, LIEBERMAN H and ABRAHAMSON I. Flattened anterior chamber. *Arch Ophthalmol* **54**: 170, 1955.
16. DUNNINGTON JH. Hypotony after cataract extractions. *Am J Ophthalmol* **40**: 30, 1956.
17. FINE LM. Acetazolamide in the treatment of postoperative absent anterior chamber. *Arch Ophthalmol* **73**: 19, 1965.
18. MEISEKOTHEN WE and ALLEN JC. Treatment of

pupillary block caused by aqueous pooling in the vitreous. *Am J Ophthalmol* **65**: 877, 1968.

19. VILLASECA A. Late emptying of the anterior chamber and choroidal detachment in cataract operations. *Arch Ophthalmol* **52**: 250, 1954.

20. CHRISTENSEN L. Postoperative shallowing of the anterior chamber. *Am J Ophthalmol* **64**: 600, 1967.

21. KRONFELD PC. Delayed restoration of the anterior chamber. *Am J Ophthalmol* **38**: 453, 1954.

22. WEISEL J and SWAN K. Mydriatic treatment of shallow anterior chamber after cataract extraction. *Arch Ophthalmol* **58**: 126, 1957.

# A SURVEY OF
# COMBINED GLAUCOMA AND CATARACT OPERATION

P. PROTONOTARIOS, P. TSIBIDAS and J. VASSILIADES

Department of Ophthalmology, Hippokration General Hospital, Athens, Greece

The coexistence of glaucoma and cataract is more common today than previously because of increased life expectancy in general, and better medical care as a result of earlier diagnosis of glaucoma in particular. Consequently we have today a large group of elderly patients in whom defective visual acuity is the result of lens opacities rather than of glaucoma. In addition, the use of strong miotics such as echothiopate iodide (PHOSPHOLINE IODIDE®) may accelerate the formation of cataracts. Moreover, especially with central lens opacities, the deterioration of visual acuity after the use of miotics is not proportional to the actual lens changes.

There is considerable controversy today regarding the surgical management of these cases. The most commonly used procedures are:

*Routine cataract extraction.* This is performed in cases where the intraocular pressure has been well controlled by conservative treatment. Normal intraocular pressures are anticipated postoperatively either with or without the use of miotics. In cases not well controlled postoperatively, an operation for glaucoma on the aphakic eye is indicated. The disadvantage of this method is that a fistulizing operation cannot be performed on an aphakic eye because of the scarring of the previously dissected conjunctival flap. There

is, in addition, always a risk of vitreous prolapse into the bleb.

*Initial glaucoma surgery and extraction of the lens at a later stage.* This has been the method of choice in patients with cataract and glaucoma not well controlled by conservative treatment. Nevertheless the disadvantages of this approach are considerable, mainly because of technical difficulties in extracting the lens while at the same time keeping the filtering bleb intact. Apart from this, the loss of glaucoma control in successfully fistulized eyes is a great problem. In this two-step procedure, closure of the bleb has been estimated to occur in nearly half of the cases.

*Combined glaucoma-lens extraction operation.* In theory this method has many advantages over others. For example, an elderly patient needs only one operation, which is a great saving, both physically and financially. Moreover, there are now many glaucoma procedures available for a combined operation. These include: sclerectomy, iridencleisis, sclerectomy with iridencleisis, trephination, cautery, cyclodialysis and reverse cyclodialysis.

An extensive survey was recently made on 840 cataracts extracted from patients with open-angle glaucoma. Three types of surgery were performed: a) cataract extraction alone, b) uncomplicated cataract extraction after a

250

previous filtering operation and c) uncomplicated filtering cautery-sclerotomy and cataract extraction.

The following conclusions were reached: 1) Cataract extraction alone in cases of open angle glaucoma was unquestionably of benefit where mild or moderate medical therapy had been sufficient to maintain normal intraocular pressure preoperatively. Cases where strong or maximum medical therapy was needed preoperatively should undergo the combined operation because in any case so many of them require cyclodialysis at a later stage. 2) In cases in which a cataract extraction was performed after a previous filtering operation, nearly 50% of the previously functioning blebs closed. 3) The combined operation (filtering cautery-sclerotomy and cataract extraction) was successful in 75% of the cases where the intraocular pressure had been medically controlled with mild or moderately strong therapy.

The availability of new and improved techniques greatly facilitate the performance of the combined operation. Although many ophthalmologists have in the past objected to the combined glaucoma-cataract operation, it is nevertheless now becoming more popular and in many cases is the operation of choice.

### MATERIAL AND METHODS

One hundred and ten eyes of 86 patients have been operated on according to the method

TABLE 1.  *Types of glaucoma in 110 cases*

| Coexisting glaucoma | No. of cases |
|---|---|
| Open angle glaucoma | 92 |
| Closed angle glaucoma | 8 |
| Unsuccessful glaucoma operation (filtering) with peripheral iridectomy | 7 |
| Secondary glaucoma | 3 |
| TOTAL | 110 |

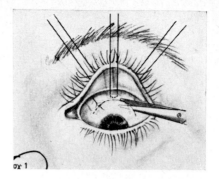

FIG. 1.   Preparation of conjunctival flap.

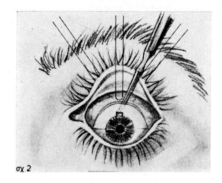

FIG. 2.   Preparation of scleral flap.

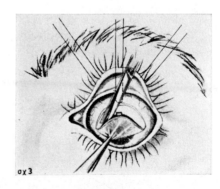

FIG. 3.   Enlargement of the incision.

described below. The average age was 73.5 years. The postoperative follow-up period was one to four years These were usually elderly patients whose general health did not permit two successive operations, or patients unwilling or unable to follow the prescribed conservat-

251

tive traetment. The local indications were: a) glaucoma with lens opacities that reduced the visual acuity to 2/10 or less, uncontrolled by medication or controlled only by strong miotics or acetazolamide b) patients allergic to miotcs; c) lens opacities following unsuccessful glaucoma filtering operation with peripheral iridectomy and d) fixed pupil following the prolonged use of miotics. The various types of coexisting glaucoma in our patients are listed in Table 1.

*Operation.* Traction sutures are placed in the upper and lower lids and in the superior rectus. Lateral canthotomy is effected and a conjunctival flap is raised between 3 and 9 o'clock (Fig. 1).

A scleral flap measuring 1.5 × 3 mm is prepared at the 12 o'clock position according to Stallard's method. The incision on either side is enlarged, and four virgin silk 9.0 sutures are placed at 2, 1, 11 and 10 o'clock (Fig. 2 and 3).

The iris is picked up near the pupillary margin and two parallel basal iridotomies are performed. The isolated portion of the iris is inverted and let down onto the sclera so that its pigment epithelium is in contact with the scleral and conjunctival flaps (Fig. 4 and 5).

Enzymatic zonulolysis is performed with α-chymotrypsin 1:10,000, which is afterward washed out with saline. The cataract is extracted with the aid of either Arruga forceps, suction cup, pressure or cryosurgery (Fig. 6). The sutures are closed and air is introduced into the anterior chamber. Occasionally two or more scleroscleral sutures are placed. Finally, the conjunctiva and Tenon's capsule are sutured in one layer (Fig. 7). Pilocarpine (2%) and neostigmine (3%) are instilled. Atropine and local steroids with anti-

biotics are given twice daily from the day following the operation.

## RESULTS

Good filtering results, with normal intra-ocular pressure, were achieved in 95 eyes

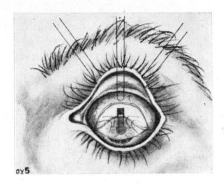

FIG. 5. Inversion and apposition of the iris flap onto the sclera.

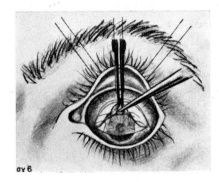

FIG. 6. Extraction of lens.

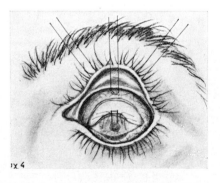

FIG. 4. Performance of two parallel basal iridotomies.

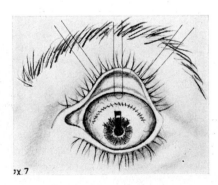

FIG. 7. Suturing of conjunctiva and Tenon's capsule.

TABLE 2. *Results of combined cataract-glaucoma surgery*

| Intraocular pressure (mm Hg) | No. of patients before surgery | | No. of patients after surgery | | |
|---|---|---|---|---|---|
| | Untreated | Treated | Untreated | Treated | After cyclodialysis |
| 10 to 20 | | 35 | | | |
| 20 to 30 | 25 | 62 | 95 | 9 | 4 |
| 30 to 40 | 72 | 11 | 9 | 5 | |
| 40 to 50 | 8 | 2 | 6 | 1 | |
| 50 | 5 | | | | |

TABLE 3. *Complications following combined cataract-glaucoma surgery*

| Complications | No. of cases |
|---|---|
| During the operation | |
| Rupture of the lens capsule | 6 |
| Vitreous loss | 4 |
| Hole or tearing of the conjunctival flap | 2 |
| Iris wound (iridodialysis) | 3 |
| Early postoperative complications | |
| Vitreous prolapse into the filtering bleb | 3 |
| Early hyphema (2 to 3 mm) | 32 |
| Persistent hemorrhage of the anterior chamber | 4 |
| Choroidal detachment with delayed reformation of flat anterior chamber | 16 |
| Flat anterior chamber restored after cyclodialysis | 2 |
| Late postoperative complications | |
| Retinal detachment | 3 |
| Anterior vitreous synechiae | 1 |
| TOTAL | 76 |

(86.3%), but in 15 eyes (13.7%) there were high intraocular pressures (Table 2). Of these, nine (8.1%) were controlled with mild miotics, and in four of the remaining six eyes with intraocular pressures exceeding 30 mm Hg, with maximum medical treatment, cyclodialysis was performed with good results. The other two patients refused further surgery.

The average intraocular pressure in the 110 eyes was 35 mm Hg preoperatively and 16.8 mm Hg postoperatively. In the 15 eyes with high intraocular pressures after surgery, the rise occurred either immediately following the operation or within the first postoperative month. In contrast, the eyes with good filtering results had no remarkable fluctuations of pressure even six months after the operation.

The complications (Table 3) were not serious. The number of cases with slight hyphema and choroidal detachment appeared to be somewhat greater than is usually found in simple cataract extractions. However, this quickly disappeared without influencing the final results.

More serious were three cases of vitreous prolapse into the filtering bleb. This required reopening of the conjunctival flap, incision of the prolapsing vitreous and iris, and suturing of the scleral flap. These complications appeared to be due to extraneous causes. The intraocular pressure was later controlled with conservative treatment.

In two cases of postoperative angle closure glaucoma with persistent flat anterior chamber, normal chambers were restored by posterior sclerectomy with drainage of the suprachoroidal fluid and the injection of air.

Finally, three cases of retinal detachment occurred not immediately but 3, 7 and 18 months after surgery.

In one case of angle closure glaucoma, a dystrophic keratitis developed as a result of anterior vitreous synechiae which cyclodialysis failed to break.

Visual acuity improved in all cases, the extent of improvement depending on the previous glaucomatous changes present, the visual field defects and the presence or absence of senile changes at the posterior pole.

# CORNEAL GRAFTING IN DEVELOPING NATIONS

## J. H. KING, Jr.

International Eye Foundation, Sibley Memorial Hospital, Washington, D.C., USA

Blindness and impending blindness due to chronic opacities of the cornea and to active corneal disease are often of major importance in developing countries. Some cases are curable and others are inoperable. Corneal surgery may be a curative means or a preventive measure in many instances.

The causes of corneal blindness are more numerous and varied in the developing nations than they are in the so-called developed countries. In addition to involvement of the cornea due to keratoconus, dystrophies, herpetic virus and trauma, there are special conditions commonly found in certain climatic areas. Economic circumstances also play a role. Avitaminosis A, trachoma, secondary infections from childhood diseases (especially measles), pterygium and particular occupational injuries uncommon in developed countries (such as those caused by the machete in sugar cane countries) usually constitute the major causes of corneal blindness in developing nations. Although nonsurgical preventive measures are most important, keratoplasty must be considered by the ophthalmologist for both prevention and cure. Many cases are less favorable for obtaining improvement from operation than in the United States.

When a keratoplasty program is begun and an eye bank is organized in a developing nation several considerations are important.

First, the ophthalmic surgeon must receive special training in grafting techniques. He should learn the organization of an eye bank and he must have proper instrumentation. It is essential to operate first upon the most favorable cases in order to obtain the support and confidence of the lay public and the government. A series of initial failures does much to discourage potential donors as well as patients.

Most cases require penetrating keratoplasty to offer any hope of restoring the best vision. Few of these operations are possible because of the scarcity of fresh donor eyes in most developing countries. Lamellar grafting often prevents blindness by acting as a treatment for progressive corneal disease. Under some conditions, visual improvement can be obtained by the lamellar technique. Donor corneas not suitable for penetrating grafting and preserved donor corneas may be available for lamellar keratoplasty.

Total corneal opacification resulting from active or inactive keratomalacia offers a poor prognosis for any type of keratoplasty. Corneas with clouding due to active trachoma, leprosy and other indigenous diseases do not give favorable results with grafting. Corneal scarring with synechiae to the area of old perforation (adherent leukoma) presents a problem. Cataract and secondary glaucoma complicate many of these cases. Extensive corneal vascularization offers a poor prognosis for any type of corneal grafting.

Central corneal scars, involving all layers of the cornea and surrounded by fairly clear and healthy cornea, present the best prognosis for penetrating grafting. A central descemetocele offers a good prognosis. Moderate keratoconus with the cone confined to 7.5 to 8 mm is a prime indication for penetrating grafting. A thin cone extending beyond 8 mm is best treated by the lamellar technique as a primary surgical procedure.

When the prognosis is good and suitable donor material is available the technique of penetrating keratoplasty does not differ from that being done regularly in other countries. Lamellar grafting without penetrating the anterior chamber is a safer procedure than a penetrating graft. The technique is often more difficult. Hospitalization and recovery time is shorter, and it would be a rarity to lose an eye following a lamellar graft. It is the procedure of choice when improvement can be expected.

The lamellar graft may be applied as a therapeutic measure in chronic recurrent and recalcitrant corneal ulceration not amenable to medical therapy. This type of graft is useful in recurrent pterygiums to prevent further recurrence and possible vision loss. Massive pterygiums, with diminished vision, can be treated with a total lamellar graft after excision of the growths. A peripheral ulceration or degeneration can be repaired by using a horseshoe donor graft of cornea or of cornea and sclera.

Glycerine-preserved corneas heal well. Smaller patch grafts of various sizes and shapes will benefit many marginal corneal diseases or injuries. Eyes can sometimes be saved when Mooren's ulceration and scleromalacia are repaired by patch grafts or total crown grafts of cornea and sclera.

Opacification of the cornea that appears to be deep, even by slit-lamp examination, may "funnel in" from the surface and not be too extensive in the deeper layers. The surgeon can begin the operation with a deep lamellar dissection (diameter up to 8 mm) and then decide upon one of the following courses: 1) If there is relatively clear cornea in the deep layers, a lamellar graft with fresh or glycerine-preserved donor tissue is applied. Useful vision can be expected in many of these cases. 2) If deep scarring remains centrally, it is often possible to obtain a clearer area directly over the pupillary space by creating a descemetocele. The rounded edge of a knife-blade (Bard-Parker No. 15) is used to gently and repeatedly scrape the central area. A lamellar donor graft is then applied. 3) If the deep central layers remain opaque and the periphery is much clearer, a lamellar graft can be used, to be followed by performing an optical iridectomy through a small cornea-scleral incision not connected with the graft. Travel-vision can often be obtained by this method. 4) If the opacification involves the thin inner corneal layers to such an extent that the entire pupillary area remains occluded after excision of the outer layer, the operation can be continued as a penetrating transplant. Fresh donor material must be available.

When one of the techniques of lamellar grafting can be applied and a cataract is present, a combined operation may be done. The graft is first completed in the usual manner and this is followed by the cataract extraction from above using the surgeon's routine technique.

The success of a lamellar graft usually depends upon many factors. The careful execution of technical details is most important. The dissection must be deep and smoothly done staying in a lamellar plane. The bed must be left meticulously clean with no blood or foreign materials. Suturing of the donor graft must be exact leaving no dehiscences. With a large graft, a paracentesis may be required for good apposition. A firm pressure dressing is maintained for several weeks. If vascularization was present then the steroid methylprednisolone acetate (DEPOMEDRAL®) should be injected beneath the conjunctiva. Systemic steroid therapy and β-irradiation may be advisable during the postoperative course.

In conclusion, much blindness can be prevented and cured by keratoplasty. A penetrating graft is usually required to obtain the best vision. However, donor materials are often unavailable in developing countries. Lamellar grafting is a useful tool in prevention and cure of selected cases of corneal diseases. The success of a keratoplasty operation is not measured by the Snellen chart since many patients are illiterate; and any degree of improvement is usually worthwhile. A patient who obtains 20/100 vision or, even better, travel vision, can often become self-supporting rather than remaining a burden on society. The lamellar graft, with variations, can often effect visual rehabilitation in difficult cases.

# COMBINED
# CORNEAL GRAFT AND CATARACT SURGERY

P. D. TREVOR-ROPER

Eye Department, Westminster Hospital and Moorfields Eye Hospital, London, England

No country in the world is without its own sad catalogue of the various causes of blindness and poor sight. But whereas in the developed temperate countries cataract, glaucoma and macular dystrophies vie for first place, in most tropical and developing countries corneal scarring is predominant, and among children, even in nontrachomatous areas, it normally heads the list. And while those other causes of blindness normally affect the aging, with their active and economically useful life behind them, corneal scarring generally occurs in the young, who must face a normal lifespan as an afflicted appendage of society, a burden to their families and their states. Hence the importance of corneal grafting and the need for improved supply of donor eyes, for simplification of technique and for training of more surgeons.

The trouble is, of course, that grafting away the scarred cornea is not the whole answer, for these eyes nearly always have coincident troubles that confound the result. The childhood measles or nutritional ulcers that are sufficient to leave a scar worth grafting, have usually perforated and damaged the lens, or the prolonged coincident uveitis has left such a deposit that an anterior polar cataract is found as soon as the corneal disk is lifted off. In our own series of 44 cases that we grafted in Ethiopia ten years ago, about half had lens opacities which materially impaired vision, and similar experience has been noted by others. According to the accepted procedure, after an interval of not less than six months, one removes the cataract. But whereas this is only a temporary disappointment and embarrassment in Western Europe, in Africa it generally means that the disenchanted patient returns to his village and is never seen again. Even if he does turn up again, and it happens that the surgeon and his team are still available the following year, the personal and economic disadvantage of this long wait are considerable, not forgetting that some grafts of poor viability become opaque after the further trauma of the extraction.

This traditional regime of leaving a long interval between operations is occasioned by the poor results of attempting to remove the cataract at the same time, because of the difficulties of exact suturing, the difficulties of expressing the lens from a collapsed eyeball and the almost inevitable vitreous synechiae to the back of the graft. But in the last decade many things have changed, and nowadays the problem is quite different. The opaque lens can readily be lifted out of the collapsed eyeball by a cryoprobe without any expression. The vitreous can be retracted so that it presents a concave face after extraction with little inclination to adhere to the edges of the graft. Effective i.v. administration of osmotic agents may be aided if necessary by a vitrectomy, and, indeed, a good anesthetist can now, by suddenly lowering the blood pressure, still further retract a vitreous that tends to bulge. Finally, the use of a Flieringe ring, (sewn to the limbus and not to the equator) supported by sutures, which are held by an assistant, will usually obviate that buckled oval hole so difficult to suture exactly.

In short, if one suspects that an opaque cornea hides an underlying cataract, one must always be prepared to do a combined operation, and therefore to use an 8 mm trephine, and give preoperative mannitol or urea.

Glaucoma is a common problem after such operations, and it is often unrecognized, since estimations of intraocular pressure are then so difficult. Sometimes glaucoma comes as a transient episode, possibly from a postoperative trabeculitis associated with the large graft. Sometimes it derives from the steroid treatment, and we usually give copious drops and prednisolone tablets after the sixth day. Therefore, acetazolamide (DIAMOX®) is normally prescribed as a prophylactic.

The operating microscope, which is so valuable in lamellar grafting and in removing sutures, is often a disadvantage when the cataract is being removed, and a wide field is desirable.

Our standard practice of using four direct 8.0 silk sutures, and then a continuous 10.0 Perlon suture has proved particularly satisfactory in underdeveloped countries, where follow-up is difficult, since the Perlon can be left indefinitely without causing problems.

Some surgeons, who have done this combined operation, prefer an "open-skies technique," removing the cataract before the donor disk is attached; but our objection to this is that the vitreous often herniates through the trephine opening; however, it can then usually be coaxed back into the anterior chamber by pressing down the preplaced graft with a brush.

My colleague at the British National Eye-Bank, Tom Casey, who has himself done an impressive series of 110 of these combined procedures, quotes an 80% success rate. Keeping in mind that these are by definition eyes with multiple disorders, that figure is very satisfactory.

Professor Michaelson did well to remind us some months ago that, in talking about our eye treatments, we must not ignore the factor of their cost—as we are so apt to do in Western countries, where we are a prey to the ruthless commercial enterprise of the drug houses and instrument makers. This is particularly relevant in dealing with those developing countries in which every clinic is crowded with cases deserving treatment, and finances are often so slender. As he said, we must constantly reexamine our priorities. Absolute sterility is not so essential, if this means less time or money available, resulting in fewer patients treated. We must constantly strive for simplification. A single silk-threaded needle is ample for all the sutures we may need for each cataract operation, with an extra Perlon-threaded one or two for each graft. Where one operation will take the place of two, as in the technique I have described, this in itself is a further recommendation.

# THE ROLE OF TOTAL KERATOPLASTY IN UNFAVORABLE CASES

U. TICHO and I. BEN SIRA

Department of Ophthalmology, Hadassah University Hospital, Jerusalem, Israel

Corneal transplantation has been successful in a large percentage of favorable cases. Unfortunately, however, a great number of eyes, especially in developing countries, belong to the unfavorable category. There is a high prevalence of infective and nutritional diseases, a delay in treatment and, in many cases, maltreatment with native medicines (Fig. 1) in developing countries. In these eyes, the corneas are densely vascularized and have extensive opacities; the anterior chamber is nearly absent due to anterior synechiae. Ectasia of the cornea and symblepharon may be present, and cataract with secondary glaucoma is also common.

To improve the surgical chances for eyes with poor prognosis, the only procedure possible is a transplantation of the whole cornea together with removal of the lens and atrophic iris; and, if necessary, anterior vitrectomy. Several surgeons, notably Filatov (1, 2), Elschnig (3), Schimanowski (4) and others (5–15), have attempted this procedure with poor results; hence the operation has generally been abandoned.

We here report on 14 patients on whom total keratoplasty was performed. Seven of them underwent further partial penetrating keratoplasty or keratoprosthesis.

## MATERIAL AND METHODS

Fourteen patients (11 males, 3 females) underwent total keratoplasty in Malawi during the years 1968–69. Some had a single good eye and others had a fellow eye with very poor vision. The corneal pathologies were of various origins (Table 1).

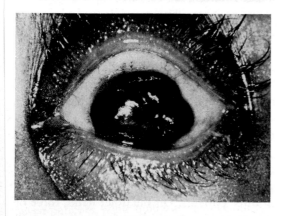

FIG. 1. Total corneal loss after the application of native medicine.

TABLE 1. *Etiological factors involved in the cases of 14 patients undergoing keratoplasty*

| Cause of corneal damage | No. of patients |
| --- | --- |
| Native medicines | 5 |
| Traumatic perforation | 2 |
| Herpetic keratitis | 1 |
| Smallpox | 1 |
| Keratomalacia | 1 |
| Undetermined | 4 |
| TOTAL | 14 |

261

the secondary glaucoma caused by creeping of the iris root toward the wound, resulting in closure of the angle. This complication can be prevented by excision of the entire iris, and by the use of a button of donor's cornea larger than the recipient's bed. Systemic steroids and cytotoxic drugs postpone, but do not prevent, clouding of the graft.

This major procedure is, therefore, indicated and justified only in desperate cases, either as an optical operation (should the graft remain clear) or as preliminary constructive surgery before final partial keratoplasty or keratoprosthesis.

### REFERENCES

1. FILATOV VP. Concerning problems of complete corneal transplantation. *Vestn Oftal* **30**: 534, 1913.
2. FILATOV VP. Transplantation of the cornea. *Arch Ophthalmol* **13**: 321, 1935.
3. ELSCHNIG A. Keratoplasty. *Arch Ophthalmol* **4**: 165, 1930.
4. SCHIMANOWSKI A. Transplantation des vorderen Augenabschnittes. *Vestn Oftal* **29**: 712, 1912.
5. BURKE JW. Total keratoplasty. *Arch Ophthalmol* **50**: 147, 1921.
6. KEY BW. Report of a case of transplantation of the human cornea. *Trans Am Ophthalmol Soc* **28**: 29, 1930.
7. ASCHER KW. Zur Keratoplastikfrage. II. Überpflanzung der ganzen Hornhaut. *Arch Ophthalmol (Paris)* **107**: 241, 1922.
8. CASTROVIEJO R. Total penetrating keratoplasty. *J Int Coll Surg* **21**: 761, 1954.
9. VANNAS S. Experiences on large penetrating corneal grafts. *Acta Ophthalmol (Kbh)* **42**: 329, 1964.
10. MORTADA A. Nine-mm penetrating keratoplasty for total anterior staphylomata. *Arch Soc Am Oftal Optom* **6**: 199, 1967.
11. RYCROFT BW. The scope of corneal grafting. *Br J Ophthalmol* **38**: 1, 1954.
12. STALARD HR. "Eye surgery," 4th edn. Baltimore, Williams and Wilkins, 1965, p 429.
13. SHERSHEVSKAYA I. Some observations on total penetrating keratoplasty with scleral rim performed for replacement and reconstruction. *Oftal Zh* **23**: 355, 1968.
14. MAUMENEE AE. Penetrating autokeratoplasty of the entire cornea. *Am J Ophthalmol* **47**: 125, 1959.
15. BARRAQUER J. Total penetrating keratoplasty. *Proc R Soc Med* **54**: 1116, 1961.
16. MAUMENEE AE. Clinical aspects of the corneal homograft reaction. *Invest Ophthalmol* **1**: 244, 1962.
17. NELKEN E, NELKEN D, MICHAELSON IC and GUREVITCH H. Late clouding of experimental corneal grafts. *Arch Ophthalmol* **65**: 584, 1961.

# THE PRESENT STATUS OF KERATOPROSTHESIS

D. P. CHOYCE*

Hospital for Tropical Diseases, University College Hospital, London, England

KERATOPROSTHESIS

(INTRACORNEAL ACRYLIC IMPLANT)

*Nonperforating keratoprosthesis*

*Bullous keratopathy.* Acrylic corneal inlays were first used by us in 1963 as a mechanical barrier to the movement of aqueous through the cornea from endothelium to epithelium (1). It is an effective method of controlling bullous keratopathy and rendering painful, watering eyes comfortable and tolerable. Unfortunately the visual results are not likely to be much better than 6/36. The inlays must be inserted fairly deep in the cornea, as near to Descemet's membrane as possible without entering the anterior chamber. Greyish white opacification of the central part of the cornea superficial to the inlay tended to form after a year or so in some cases. It was considered that this was most probably nutritional and for the last 30 cases out of 80 treated by us, "calculated leak" inlays were used with 12 perforations 0.33 mm in diameter surrounding the central 4 mm. This arrangement has certainly lessened the subsequent opacification of the overlying stroma without allowing sufficient aqueous to pass through to invalidate the purpose of the operation. Colored, opaque, haptic inlays can also be provided should the condition of the iris within the eye necessitate this modification.

*Albinism, aniridia and traumatic mydriasis.* These colored haptic inlays can, of course, be used in annular form, with a hole 4 mm in diameter in the middle (polomint inlays) when the iris is deficient, as in these conditions. Only small numbers have been treated. The results are quite encouraging.

*Economics*

| | | |
|---|---|---|
| Cost of inlays | = | £30 |
| Seven-day stay in hospital at £10 per day | = | £70 |
| TOTAL | | £100 |

*Perforating keratoprosthesis*

Intracameral implants and completely buried corneal inlays seem to bear out our experience, that implants fashioned from completely inert materials and completely enclosed within the body's integuments are tolerated and accepted by the tissues for many years, often for the rest of the patient's natural life. Perforating keratoprostheses, on the other hand, are an exception to this general rule, and the body's reaction seems to represent an attempt either to extrude or to encapsulate such a foreign body, so that the main difficulties to be overcome are: a) corneal breakdown

---

* Author's address: 9 Drake Road, Westcliff-on-Sea, Essex, England

TABLE 1. *Perforating keratoprostheses*

| Type of prosthesis | Date of introduction |
|---|---|
| Osteo-chondro-odonto, Strampelli | 1963 |
| Choyce Mark II two-piece | 1967 |
| Cardona—bolt and nut | 1968 |

TABLE 3. *Indications for keratoprosthesis*

| | | |
|---|---|---|
| Aphakic keratopathy | 21 | 50% of these |
| Aphakic keratopathy + Mark I | | patients were |
| anterior chamber implant | 13 | diabetics |
| Old trachoma | 3 | |
| Old injuries | 5 | |
| Herpetic keratopathy and uveitis | 4 | |
| Mustard gas keratitis | 1 | |
| Fuchs's dystrophy | 1 | |
| Old interstitial keratitis | 2 | |
| | 50 | |

TABLE 4. *Surgical routine at two- to three-month intervals*

1. Complete iridectomy
   Separation of synechiae
   Lens extraction
2. Tectonic keratoplasty
3. Insertion of flush-fitting two-piece Mark II perforating keratoprosthesis
4. Trephination of central 4 or 5 mm of cornea
   Replacement of flush-fitting central cylinder with externally-projecting cylinder

leading to leakage, resulting in intraocular infection or extrusion of the prosthesis; b) the formation of a retroprosthetic membrane; c) uveitis and glaucoma.

We know that there are many cases of corneal blindness where orthodox keratoplasty has repeatedly failed or was never practicable in the first place. For example, grossly opaque, densely vascularized corneas of uneven thickness, associated with dense anterior and posterior synechiae, shallow or flat anterior chamber and cataract or aphakia. There is general agreement that patients in these categories can be helped only by effecting a reasonably lasting bond between living tissue and nonliving plastic. Table 1 lists three implant techniques available to accomplish this, and these are compared in Table 2.

I have no experience of either Strampelli's method (2) or of Cardona's bolt and nut prosthesis (3). However, after seven to eight years of clinical trials I introduced in 1967 the Mark II two-piece perforating keratoprosthesis (4) and I can now report on 50 cases treated since then. This prosthesis is modified from a design of Stone's used by him on rabbits in the early 1960s (5). It is currently available in two sizes: 8 mm diameter flange and 3.5 mm diameter central cylinder for the smaller eye (which provides about 70% field of vision) and 9 mm diameter flange and 4.5 mm diameter cylinder providing 90% field of vision for the larger eye. The 36 small perforations in the flange have been replaced by eight radial slits. This design is sturdier, is cosmetically more acceptable and there is a surgical advantage, as I will explain later.

Table 3 gives the indications for using our keratoprosthesis.

Table 4 shows the routine followed since 1967, which should not be departed from if the best results are to be obtained.

TABLE 2. *Central cylinder comparison*

| | Osteo-chondro-odonto | Choyce two-piece | Cardona bolt and nut |
|---|---|---|---|
| Diameter of optic | 1.5 mm | 3.5 to 4.5 mm | 2.5 mm |
| Possible visual acuity | 6/6 | 6/6 | 6/6 |
| Field | 30% | 70 to 90% | 50% |
| Removable and replaceable | No | Yes | No |
| Operative procedures | 1 | 3 | 1 |

This means three operations, six to eight weeks apart, four if the eye is phakic, to allow for lens extraction. I cannot understand the reluctance of many colleagues to follow this routine when one considers that plastic surgeons are prepared to undertake 10 or more procedures to rebuild a badly burnt face.

Experience has shown the importance of the following points:

1) When the lens is extracted a complete or sector iridectomy should be performed above and a sphincterotomy below. Anterior synechiae should be divided if present.

2) Both partial and full thickness tectonic grafts have been used and both have proved satisfactory. If a full thickness intralamellar graft is used, four to six months should elapse before insertion of the keratoprosthesis as it takes twice as long to be properly assimilated as a lamellar disk. Grafts 8 mm in diameter are used for the smaller eye, 9 mm and occasionally 10 mm for the larger. There have been no complications following preliminary tectonic keratoplasty. Of the 50 cases, one received an onlay lamellar graft, four received full-thickness intralamellar grafts and 45 received partial thickness intralamellar grafts.

3) Insertion of the two-piece keratoprosthesis with flush-fitting central cylinder is the essence of this method. If all goes well final success is very likely. Proper centering and fixation are vital, particularly when the posterior layer of cornea is of uneven thickness and liable to tear when the central disk is trephined. A special centering device has been made, the trephine being operated through the central aperture. After trephining out the central disk of posterior cornea, instruments should be passed into the anterior chamber to clear away residual lens remnants, synechiae, etc. Some vitreous may escape at this stage, but this has to be accepted and, provided the loss is not excessive, does not invalidate the final result. The other very important part of this operation is not to

screw the flush-fitting cylinder too tightly into the tunnel, otherwise unscrewing it at the last operation may be unexpectedly difficult.

A double-ended virgin silk suture, passed through one of the radial slits, both ends being brought out through the cornea just above the limbus at 6 o'clock, can be used both to fix and center the keratoprosthesis. Additional sutures can be used at 3, 9 and 12 o'clock if necessary; when the double layer of cornea is resutured these are covered.

Postoperative reaction is variable and has been controlled by oral prednisolone, the dosage varying between 5 and 30 mg daily, according to individual requirements.

Postoperative infection has occurred once. The cornea overlying the central cylinder started to slough, and it was decided to bring forward the timing of the last operation, which went smoothly. However, about a month later a lower-half retinal detachment developed which is still present despite scleral resection and cryotherapy. There is an excellent view of the fundus, no retinal tear or hole is visible, just a large detachment. Another promising result has been impaired by the development of a lower half detachment (no hole seen). Encircling operation was performed.

4) At the final operation the centering device is again used to ensure that the disk of strengthened cornea which is removed is exactly over the flush-fitting central cylinder. Providing this was not too tightly screwed in to begin with, unscrewing it with the special "screwdriver" should be fairly easy. Having removed it, some retroprosthetic membrane will usually be found to have partially occluded the inner opening of the tunnel. This can be fairly easily removed with instruments passed down the tunnel until pulsation of the heartbeat is seen in the fluid of the tunnel. The final step before screwing in the externally projecting cylinder is to irrigate the anterior chamber through the tunnel with a solution of

**267**

TABLE 5. *Management of complications*

| Complication | Treatment |
|---|---|
| Refractive error Insufficient or excessive anterior projection | Change cylinder |
| Retroprosthetic deposit or membrane | Remove and clean cylinder Incise membrane Replace cylinder |
| Extrusion threatened | Free scleral graft |

TABLE 6. *Central cylinder removed and replaced; 50 cases (1967–71)*

| Reason | No. of cases |
|---|---|
| For optical reasons | 3 |
| To adjust external projection | 4 |
| To deal with retroprosthetic membrane | 3 |

TABLE 7. *Summary as of August 1971 of results with Choyce two-piece keratoprosthesis; 50 cases (1967–71)*

| | No. of cases |
|---|---|
| Eyes lost | 0 |
| Anatomically and functionally satisfactory | 38 |
| Functionally disappointing due to posterior segment pathology | 7 |
| Threatened extrusions | 5 |
| Retained by scleral grafts | 3 |
| Replaced by corneal grafts | 2 |

framycetin (SOFRAMYCIN®). The final cylinder can and should be screwed in fairly tightly.

At first dressing the patient can usually see splendidly and there is great rejoicing. Thereafter a low-grade uveitis, with formation of vitreous opacities and consequent temporary reduction of vision, may set in. To avoid disappointment, the patient should be warned in advance of this possibility, and that it may last several weeks. A combination of prednisolone, 5 mg daily, with oxyphen butazone (TANDERIL®), one tablet daily, for several weeks is efficacious in shortening this stage. After this initial phase ocular function slowly im-

proves and continues to do so for the next 6 to 12 months.

MANAGEMENT OF COMPLICATIONS

Certain complications may be expected when such an elaborate routine is used in such difficult cases. Table 5 summarizes them.

Most complications can be dealt with by taking advantage of the removable nature of the central cylinder (Table 6), which demonstrates how the two-piece principle justifies itself in practice.

RESULTS

It must be stressed that this can still only be regarded as a short-term progress report. The results are given in Table 7.

Cold statistics never really convey an accurate impression, and I think these results are truly promising. Most of the patients have been elderly and frail and have healed poorly. The younger the patient, the better the result.

Of the seven cases with posterior segment pathology, four had retinal detachments—one secondary to retinitis proliferans (no treatment offered), one subtotal (treatment refused), two lower half only (one treated unsuccessfully, already referred to and the other very recent). Of the five threatened by extrusion, the two replaced by corneal grafts were treated thus because they were functionally disappointing (disseminated choroiditis and old glaucomatous optic atrophy, respectively).

ECONOMICS OF TWO-PIECE PERFORATING KERATOPROSTHESIS

The two-piece implants are expensive. The cost of posterior perforating component plus flush-fitting cylinder, plus externally projecting cylinder plus screwdriver for the individual case = £80, to which must be added the cost of repeated stays in hospital, say 30 days at £10 a day = £300; a total of £380, which does not include the surgeon's or anesthetist's fees. These figures relate only to the author's hospital in England.

## CONCLUSIONS

The use of a two-piece perforating kerato-prosthesis by a three or four stage technique is costly and elaborate but almost certainly better than less elaborate one-stage operations. Multistage procedures involving repeated visits to hospital are undesirable when dealing with primitive communities, but it is difficult to visualize any short cut which would not lead to an unacceptably high rate of kerato-prosthesis rejection. The problem of the successful insertion of a keratoprosthesis into a

pathologically dry eye has not yet been solved.

## REFERENCES

1. CHOYCE DP. Management of endothelial corneal dystrophy with acrylic corneal inlays. *Br J Ophthalmol* **49**: 432, 1965.
2. STRAMPELLI B. Osteo-odonto-keratoprostheses. *Ann Ottalmol Clin Ocul* **89**: 1039, 1963.
3. CARDONA H. Mushroom transcorneal kerato-prosthesis (bolt and nut). *Am J Ophthalmol* **68**: 604, 1969.
4. CHOYCE DP. The present status of intra-cameral and intra-corneal implants. *Can J Ophthalmol* **3**: 295, 1968.
5. STONE W JR. The plastic artificial cornea (an 18-year study): Basic principles and preliminary clinical report. Removable insert implants. Corneo-plastic surgery. *Proc 2nd Int Corneo-Plastic Conf London, 1967*, p 375.

# A. B. RIZZUTI

Corneal Service, New York Medical College, New York, New York, USA

Prosthokeratoplasty is a surgical procedure in which a keratoprosthesis, usually a special type of plastic material, is inserted in an eye to replace a diseased and scarred cornea. The materials used consist of methyl methacrylate or silicon rubber. In addition to these, Strampelli has added osteo-odonto material.

Since the first clinical evaluation reported by Cardona in 1962 (1) in which methyl methacrylate was used for the construction of a keratoprosthesis, many advances have been made in this special type of eye surgery. In view of the promising results subsequently reported with a variety of Cardona prostheses (1–6), the writer was encouraged to use them in a series of patients who presented very difficult problems for conventional keratoplasty (7–9). The following report is a condensed analysis of the results obtained in 85 human eyes in which three different types of Cardona keratoprostheses were used.

The indications for prosthokeratoplasty

are: 1) eyes with unsuccessful keratoplasties; 2) advanced bullous keratopathy; 3) severe chemical burns of the cornea.

The following prerequisites for a prostho-keratoplasty procedure are mandatory: 1) The eye must present proper light perception and projection in the cardinal fields. 2) The eye must not be hypotonic. 3) The etiology of secondary glaucoma should be investigated, including ultrasonography and X-ray studies, to rule out the possible presence of a neoplasm. 4) Ocular hypertension must be controlled by one or multiple cyclodiathermy procedures. 5) The thickness of the corneal stroma should not be less than 1.3 mm.

TYPES OF KERATOPROSTHESES–PRESENT MODELS

*Type I.* This implant (Fig. 1) consists of a threaded through-and-through central cylinder measuring 2.3 mm in diameter and 3.8 to 4.5 mm in height, with a supporting inter-lamellar plate 4.5 mm in diameter with three

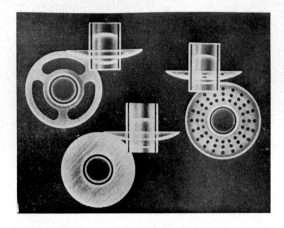

FIG. 1. Keratoprosthesis models Types I and II (courtesy Dr. H. Cardona).

threaded through-and-through central cylinder measuring 2.5 mm in diameter and 5.5 mm in height, with an anterior circular disk 8.5 mm in diameter. The disk is painted to match the color of the iris of the fellow eye. The posterior threaded supporting plate consists of siliconized Teflon. It is 5.5 mm in diameter and approximately 1.0 mm in thickness.

SURGICAL TECHNIQUES

1) For Type I and Type II, either an interlamellar pocket dissection of the recipient cornea or a full thickness fresh or preserved donor graft on a deeply dissected recipient corneal bed can be used.

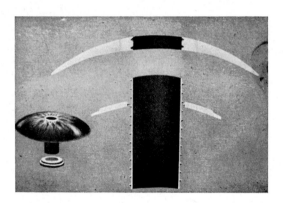

FIG. 2. Keratoprosthesis model Type III (courtesy Dr. H. Cardona).

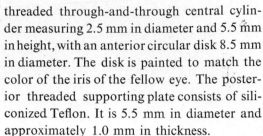

FIG. 3. Severe eye burn of cornea and conjunctiva with marked symblepharon and absence of lower cul-de-sac.

fenestrations for free interchange of fluid. The central optical cylinder contains lenses with a dioptric power of +56.00.

*Type II.* This model (Fig. 1) consists of a through-and-through central cylinder measuring 2.3 mm in diameter and 3.8 to 4.5 mm in height and a siliconized Teflon meshwork skirt measuring 5.5 mm in diameter. The wall of the optical cylinder is black to prevent light scatter. The dioptric power is +56.00.

*Type III.* This implant, shown in Fig. 2, is called the anterior mushroom keratoprosthesis or the "nut and bolt," and consists of a

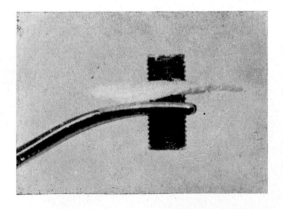

FIG. 4. View showing screw mechanism of Cardona keratoprosthesis with siliconized Teflon skirt.

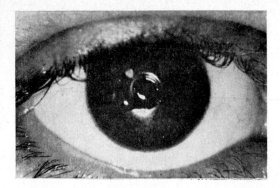

FIG. 5.  Cosmetic thin-painted corneal shell with central opening fitted over Cardona-imbedded keratoprosthesis.

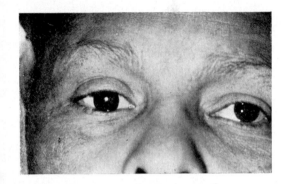

FIG. 6.  Final results of patient shown in Fig. 3 with corneal lye burn of the left eye; final visual results, 20/70.

2) In severe chemical burns of the cornea, a Type II (siliconized Teflon) prosthesis is preferred (Fig. 3 and 4). A special technique

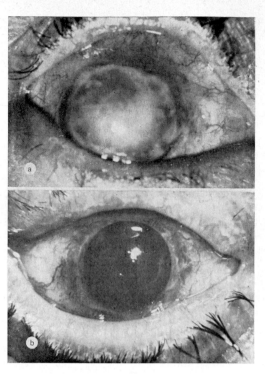

FIG. 7a and b.  Patient with Type III "nut and bolt" keratoprosthesis.

is used consisting of a superficial keratectomy and an overlay of a scleral graft from a donor eye. A sliding conjunctival graft or a free buccal mucous membrane graft is then used to cover the sclera and the embedded keratoprosthesis. After a waiting period of approximately two months, the central portion of the mucous

TABLE 1.  *Results of implantation of Cardona keratoprosthesis, Types I, II and III*

| | No. of eyes | |
| --- | --- | --- |
| Clinical outcome | Types I and II | Type III |
| Vitreous hemorrhage | — | 1 |
| Eye lost to phthisis bulbi | 1 | 2 |
| Extruded implant | 4 | 3 |
| Partial aseptic necrosis around optical cylinder | 6 | — |
| Secondary glaucoma (controlled by cyclodiathermies) | — | 2 |
| Retroprosthetic membranes (detected by loss of fundus reflex) | — | 2 |
| Haziness on posterior surface of optical cylinder | 7 | — |
| Vision improved from counting fingers to 20/20 | 4 | 5 |
| Vision improved from counting fingers to between 20/30 and 20/200 | 18 | 25 |
| No improvement in visual acuity | — | 5 |
| TOTAL | 40 | 45 |

membrane covering the optical cylinder is excised with sharp scissors (Fig. 5 and 6).

3) The surgical techniques for the Type III consist of a central 2.5 mm trephination followed by a corneoscleral incision. The posterior plate is introduced into the anterior chamber, held in place behind the cornea and screwed to the stem of the anterior plate. If the lens is present it must be extracted whether it is cataractous or not. A motion picture showing the surgical highlights of the use of the "nut and bolt" keratoprosthesis was presented (Fig. 7a and b).

The results of Cardona prosthokeratoplasty are summarized in Table 1.

REFERENCES

1. CARDONA H. Keratoprosthesis. *Am J Ophthalmol* **54**: 284, 1962.

2. CARDONA H, CASTROVIEJO R and DEVOE AG. The Cardona keratoprosthesis: first clinical evaluation. *XIX Acta Concilium Ophthalmologicum* **2**: 1211, 1962.

3. CARDONA H. Anterior and posterior mushroom keratoprosthesis. *Am J Ophthalmol* **61**: 498, 1966.

4. CARDONA H, CASTROVIEJO R and DEVOE AG. Techniques of prosthokeratoplasty: evaluation of results with the Cardona keratoprosthesis. Presented at the *XX Int Cong Ophthalmol, Munich, 1966*.

5. CARDONA H. Keratoprosthesis with a plastic fiber meshwork supporting plate. *Am J Ophthalmol* **64**: 228, 1967.

6. CASTROVIEJO R, CARDONA H and DEVOE AG. Present status of prosthokeratoplasty. *Am J Ophthalmol* **68**: 613, 1969.

7. RIZZUTI AB. Treatment of bullous keratopathy using the Cardona implant. *Ann Inst Barraquer* **9**: 436, 1969.

8. RIZZUTI AB. Management of bullous keratopathy. I. Review of medical and surgical techniques. *J Ophthalmol Surg* **1**: 26, 1970.

9. RIZZUTI AB. Management of bullous keratopathy. II. Clinical evaluation of the Cardona keratoprosthesis. *J Ophthalmol Surg* **1**: 1970.

# EYE BANKS AND THE AVAILABILITY OF CORNEAS

J. H. KING, Jr.

International Eye Foundation, Sibley Memorial Hospital, Washington, D.C., USA

The first organized eye banks in the United States were established in the middle 1940s. The need for eye banks was recognized although it is estimated that only about 15 ophthalmologists in the United States were capable of performing cornea grafts at that time. The need for more grafting operations was apparent. It was determined that some 20% of all blindness was due to the cornea.

There are now about 80 recognized eye banks which serve most sections of the United States. The majority are members of a national organization, the Eye Bank Association of America (EBAA), whose main purpose is to standardize procedures and to maintain ethics conforming to those established by the American Academy of Ophthalmology and Otolaryngology. Eye tissues are also procured by individuals or groups of surgeons from the pathology laboratories of their hospitals or from university centers. An eye bank is not usually required unless it serves an area where there is a need, and in which a number of surgeons are performing keratoplasty. As in other facets of ophthalmic surgery, not every ophthalmologist performs keratoplasty. Unless a surgeon does more than an occasional operation, it is advisable to refer the patient to someone who does grafting regularly.

The number of grafts has increased markedly during the past 20 years and an accurate figure is not available. The demand for donor tissues is known to exceed the supply. No generally acceptable criteria have been established regarding donor age, time of use after enucleation or storage procedures. Most eye banks are "banks" in name only and act as collecting and distributing agencies.

Even though there are shortages of eyes in some areas of the United States, there are times when some tissues cannot be used for grafting because of the age of the donor, cause of death, unavailability of a patient and prolonged time elapsing since enucleation. Many of these eyes are assigned to research laboratories and some are sent to the International Eye Bank branch of the International Eye Foundation from which they are transshipped to other countries.

England, most of the European continent, the USSR and many of its satellites have no problems in obtaining donor material and the organization of eye banks is unimportant. Eyes are removed as needed as long as no prior objections have been registered. Donor tissues are usually ideal, as many are from young persons suffering accidental death.

Paradoxically, those countries with large numbers of corneal blind are unable to obtain eyes for grafting because of custom, religion, or in some instances, legal obstacles. Eye banks are nonexistent or are present in name only.

Despite numerous difficulties in obtaining donor tissues, it may be advisable to organize an eye bank in a developing country where the need exists. It affords the local ophthalmologists a liaison with laymen who are interested in the dramatic and emotional impacts accompanying a successful cornea transplant operation. Lay support can be stimulated and the funds derived can be used to educate the public and to perform eye research in problems peculiar to the area. With continuing effort, time and patience most of the obstacles involving the procurement of corneas can be slowly overcome.

This is one of the most urgent areas in world ophthalmology where the "have" countries can help the "have not" nations to prevent and cure more blindness not only due to corneal disease but in all other categories of eye surgery. Excess donor tissues must be sent from countries with active eye banks to support a newly established bank in a developing nation until it becomes self-sufficient. Well-publicized successful results are an impetus to the activities of a new eye bank. Therefore, it is most important in the early stages to operate only upon those cases with the best prognosis.

EVALUATION OF DONOR MATERIAL

The criteria for selecting eye donor tissue vary from country to country and depend upon need. The greater the need, the less rigid the rules. In the United States the following requirements are generally accepted:

The past and current history of the condition of the donor's eye are considered important in determining the suitability of the corneas for transplantation.

Eyes are rejected if the deceased suffered from certain eye diseases such as acute or chronic glaucoma, with questionable control or uncontrolled tension. These do not usually constitute the best tissue for grafting. Corneal edema or clouding is a definite reason for rejection. Absolute glaucoma and hemorrhagic glaucoma jeopardize the health of the cornea and such eyes are best rejected. If glaucoma is well controlled, with a clear cornea, the corneas may be considered for grafting.

A soft and degenerated phthisical eye that has suffered from chronic ocular disease should not be used. A prolonged history of eye disease such as chronic keratitis, recurrent viral keratitis, pemphigus, frequently recurring acute or chronic uveitis, may be causes for rejection. Acute or chronic ocular infection, trachoma, purulent conjunctivitis, corneal ulceration, corneal scarring and other obvious local conditions render the eye unsuitable for grafting because of the danger of infection, as well as an unhealthy cornea.

Corneas from eyes with malignant tumors of the sclera or cornea and melanoma of the anterior segment (anterior chamber) should not be used. If a well confined posterior segment melanoma is present with a normal anterior segment, the corneas are acceptable by most surgeons. Because of the danger of seeding of the tumor cells, the presence of retinoblastoma makes the eyes undesirable in the opinion of most surgeons.

If a donor suffers from certain systemic diseases, these may also preclude the use of the eyes for grafting. The eyes of a person who has a positive serologic test for lues are not to be used for grafting—mainly from the medical-legal standpoint. Interstitial keratitis is a definite reason for rejection. Acute hepatitis of viral etiology is cause for not using the eyes. Patients with chronic hepatitis or patients with icterus may or may not have jaundice of the eyes. Intense ocular jaundice may also involve the cornea and these eyes should not be used. Diseases such as septicemia, meningitis and similar systemic conditions of the donor which could involve the eyes make them undesirable for grafting.

Generalized cancer suspected of being viral

in etiology poses a medical-legal decision in some areas of the United States. However, no definite evidence of transmission by cornea grafting is known.

Death following a debilitating illness makes the use of the corneas doubtful. A high percentage of the endothelial cells is often found to be degenerated or nonviable even in a young person suffering prolonged illness and malnutrition.

If the eye history and the cause of death are acceptable, the surgeon must then consider other pertinent factors. The majority of surgeons feel that the best eye tissue is that obtained from a young person suffering sudden death. The age of the donor is unrelated to the success of a penetrating graft (1) and corneas from older donors are even preferable to those from younger donors. Kaufman and his group (2) found guttate keratopathy in 18% of normal eyes over 50 years of age. Most agree that corneas from donors over the age of 60 are not as suitable as from younger persons. They must be carefully evaluated because of potential endothelial deficiency.

The host cornea itself plays an important role in the surgeon's decision to use an eye from a certain age group. If the host cornea is markedly deficient and degenerated as in advanced Fuchs' dystrophy it is ideal to use the youngest and healthiest donor cornea. If the surrounding host cornea endothelium is in good condition as in moderate keratoconus or scarring from trauma, a more aged donor cornea will do well.

In lamellar grafting a donor cornea from any age, young or old, is suitable. In penetrating grafting, stillborn corneas are not good as they are too soft and malleable. A donor of any age below 10 years must be carefully evaluated. It is recommended that the donor cornea for a graft on a child should be matched in age as nearly as possible. The ideal age span for donor eyes can generally be listed as between 10 years and the late 50s.

The donor eye should be removed as soon as possible after death—immediate transfer from donor to host would be ideal. With few exceptions, the time between death and enucleation should not exceed 6 to 8 hr. The body should be refrigerated as soon as possible after death.

Removal of the eyes should be performed under conditions as sterile as circumstances permit. When the eyeballs are removed, gauze is packed in the orbits and a conformer is placed in the conjunctival sac to maintain a normal appearance. The corpse must not be disfigured in any way and close cooperation is necessary between the eye bank and the mortician.

The enucleated eyes should be thoroughly flushed with a mixture of antibiotic solutions (neosporin) and then placed in a sterile jar. Most eye bank vials are of glass approximately 60 ml in size, with an aluminum rack for supporting the eyeball so that the cornea is erect. It is held secure by a sterile pin placed through the optic nerve. Cotton, moistened with sterile saline covers the bottom of the vial to maintain a moist chamber since the eye must not be immersed in saline. It is stored in its closed bottle on the bottom shelf of a refrigerator at 4 C (not in or near the freezing compartment).

Eyes are transported to and from the eye bank in a special insulated container. The container used by the International Eye Bank is made of heavy cardboard and is reasonable in cost. It is lined with polyurethane and is designed to hold four eyes and nine pounds of ice in a plastic bag. Extensive testing has been done which shows that a temperature of below 40 F is maintained for 72 hr. Its light weight is an advantage for long distance and international shipping.

The sooner after enucleation the cornea is used for grafting, the better. Some surgeons will not use a cornea stored for more than

12 hr, whereas most will use the tissue up to 48 hr following donor death especially if the donor was young. At the recent Society of Eye Surgeons Congress, Saleeby reported excellent results using corneas grafted from older age groups 72 hr or more after enucleation.

The evaluation of donor material is most important. The eye is inspected grossly for firmness and corneal clarity. A soft eye with a hazy or wrinkled cornea probably should be rejected without further examination.

Every cornea should be critically examined with the slit-lamp biomicroscope before it is accepted for a penetrating graft. It should not be viewed through the glass bottle but should be removed and held by a sterile clamp.

Critical evaluation of the endothelium must be made in donor eyes from persons 50 years of age or older. Kaufman found that 15% of the eyes from this age group which were initially considered normal after examination with a slit-lamp biomicroscope showed significant endothelial changes when stained with dye.

The eye should be rejected if the endothelium is diseased, scarred or is the site of keratitic precipitates.

### PRESERVATION OF DONOR TISSUES

*Lamellar grafting.* Preservation for short periods includes 1) immersing the eyeball or the excised cornea in liquid paraffin and storing it in a refrigerator at 4 C. The cornea is generally used after four to six weeks. 2) The cornea can be frozen in a deepfreeze at –40 C or at –80 C and can be used for up to two months (–100 C is required for prolonged cell preservation). 3) Immersion in glycerine without refrigeration will also preserve the cornea for several months. With any of these methods, the cornea undergoes autolysis after prolonged storage.

Long-term preservation for lamellar grafting by lyophilization in glycerine and sealing in a vacuum was first introduced by McNair and King in 1955 (3). In 1959 Payrau and Pouliquen (4) introduced lyophilization of corneas by chemical means with silica gel. These corneas are brittle, dry and difficult to work with.

The first successful clinically applicable method of long-term preservation utilizing glycerine dehydration was devised by King in 1956 (5). It was further simplified by our group by dehydration in glycerine with molecular sieve, a physical adsorbent, resulting in immersion in anhydrous glycerine, and storage for prolonged periods at room temperature. This method is an office procedure.

*Penetrating grafting.* Short term methods of preservation include immersion in liquid paraffin, storing in the recipient's serum and replacement of the aqueous with polyvinylpyrrolidone 25% solution. These methods extend the usefulness of a fresh eye up to 7 to 10 days.

Long-term preservation requires the use of a freezing technique and maintaining the tissue in this state until it is thawed for grafting. Kaufman et al. (2) refined and further developed freezing in liquid nitrogen and report results equal to those obtained using fresh corneas. This method has been proven successful by many surgeons and should be in use in every active eye bank to maintain a constant supply of "fresh" corneas. It is not at present suitable for long distance shipping.

A true eye bank receiving tissues on a regular basis should employ some method of preservation. To relegate every eye beyond 24 or 48 hr after enucleation to research denies an operation to a blind person who is on the waiting list of many other eye banks.

In conclusion, the surgeon performing grafting must make the sole decision concerning the use of a donor eye and each eye must be individually assessed. It should not be arbitrarily used if it is fresh and from a young healthy donor nor should it be rejected only because it is from an older person.

Donor corneas not needed by an eye bank within 72 hr from enucleation should be offered to other banks in the same country. If there is no demand for tissues at a certain time, one should share this precious tissue with his neighbors. The training of some eye surgeons in keratoplasty and the establishment of eye banks in developing nations with a high incidence of corneal blindness is an urgent need. It is the responsibility of ophthalmologists in the self-sufficient countries to give every possible help to their confreres in the devloping nations so that they may reach many more curable blind.

## REFERENCES

1. Fine M. Therapeutic keratopathy in Fuchs' dystrophy. *Am J Ophthalmol* **57**: 371, 1964.
2. Kaufman HE, Escapini H, Capella JA, Robbins JE and Kaplan M. Living preserved corneal tissue for penetrating keratoplasty. *Arch Ophthalmol* **76**: 471, 1966.
3. McNair JN and King JH Jr. Preservation of cornea by dehydration. *Arch Ophthalmol* **53**: 519, 1955.
4. Payrau MM and Pouliquen Y. A practical process of conservation of corneas and scleras. *Bull Soc Ophtalmol Fr* **3**: 209, 1959.
5. King JH Jr. Keratoplasty. Experimental studies with corneas preserved by dehydration. *Trans Am Ophthalmol Soc* **54**: 567, 1956.

# PROGNOSIS OF KERATOPLASTY IN PHAKIC AND APHAKIC PATIENTS AND THE USE OF CRYOPRESERVED DONOR TISSUE

JOSEPH A. CAPELLA, HERBERT E. KAUFMAN and FRANK M. POLACK

Department of Ophthalmology, College of Medicine, University of Florida, Gainesville, Florida, USA

This communication presents a series of 585 penetrating keratoplasties, analyzes the prognosis for different types of corneal disease and examines some of the factors which seem responsible for graft success or failure. Results of cases using cryopreserved donor tissue are compared with those using refrigerated tissue, and both short- and long-term results are discussed.

### METHODS AND MATERIALS

Five hundred and eighty-five consecutive keratoplasties done at the University of Florida Teaching Hospital were analyzed in terms of disease categories, results and donor tissue. This paper reports the results of several surgeons; many keratoplasties were performed by the authors (H.E.K. and F.M.P.) but a number were carried out by residents and fellows.

In the categories of Fuchs' dystrophy and bullous keratopathy, disease was far advanced in virtually all cases, the vast majority being limbus-to-limbus bullous keratopathy. At no time during this series were keratoplasties done for early bullous keratopathy with the hope of obtaining better results. In almost all cases surgery was performed because of advanced disease and severe visual handicap.

The University of Florida is a referral center. Many patients came from various areas of the United States, as well as other countries, so that complete follow-up was sometimes impossible. Every effort was made, however, to locate all patients or contact their referring physicians and to report the total follow-up. Nearly all grafts were between 7.0 and 8.0 mm in size. All were done under the microscope, and 8–0 silk was used for many, but 10–0 nylon was used in later cases. In all aphakic grafts and all combined grafts and cataract extractions, a double Flieringa ring was used to give the anterior segment greater rigidity.

In the severe corneal edema category, there were basically two types of patient. Some were diagnosed specifically as having Fuchs' dystrophy when the endothelial and epithelial changes were typical. This provides a generally similar group of patients with advanced corneal disease. The bullous keratopathy category was much more heterogeneous, however, and these patients had severe corneal edema for reasons that were not always certain. Some almost certainly had Fuchs' dystrophy which had advanced after surgery. Others had markedly severe trauma during cataract surgery, with updrawn pupils, vitreous contact, glaucoma before surgery or absent anterior chambers.

In this study, it was impossible to measure the intraocular pressure in patients with corneal edema. The MacKay-Marg tonometer was not recognized at the time as being the only reliable way to measure raised intraocular pressure in eyes with corneal edema. Therefore, the presence or absence of glaucoma could not be accurately ascertained before surgery.

Twelve patients with interstitial keratitis underwent keratoplasty. All were graded on the basis of the severity of vascularization before surgery on a subjective 1 to 4 basis, with 4+ being severe vascularization with deep vessels clearly carrying blood. Postoperative complications were closely monitored in these patients and are described.

Thirty-one patients with keratoconus and sixteen with bacterial ulcers required keratoplasties. Some categories, such as the regrafts and post-traumatic grafts, often had extensive and varied intraocular damage and glaucoma; these were difficult to analyze.

The choice of refrigerated or cryopreserved tissue (1) was generally random and made after examination and evaluation. If refrigerated tissue from eyes that were carefully examined and appeared excellent was available, it was used. In no case was tissue used more than 48 hr after death of the donor; the majority of eyes were less than 24 hr old. It was unusual for eyes from a donor more than 60 years of age to be used. It was felt that it was safer for the patient to receive cryopreserved tissue rather than tissue from an older donor more than 24 hr after death. When, on rare occasions, such tissue was used, the endothelium of the second eye was stained and examined as a guide to the suitability of the tissue from the donor.

No graft was considered clear unless it was crystal clear and edema free. Eyes with improved vision but with partially swollen grafts were classified as cloudy.

## RESULTS

Patients with severe Fuchs' dystrophy had grafts with randomly chosen refrigerated or cryopreserved tissue; the results are tabulated in Table 1. Seventy-four percent of grafts done with refrigerated tissue were clear at three months. With cryopreserved tissue, 77% of the Fuchs' dystrophy category were clear. Of those clear at three months, 84% of the refrigerated and all of the cryopreserved grafts were clear at six months.

In patients with Fuchs' dystrophy, the results with cryopreserved tissue were not significantly worse than with the refrigerated tissue, although in both categories the patients with combined procedures seemed to do less well than either the simple phakic or aphakic keratoplasties. The results of combined Fuchs' dystrophy and bullous keratopathy are shown in Table 2. There was no significant difference in any of these categories between the refrigerated and the cryopreserved tissue. The overall results indicate a

TABLE 1.  *Penetrating keratoplasty in Fuchs' dystrophy (results after three months)*

| | No. of cases | | | | | |
|---|---|---|---|---|---|---|
| | Refrigerated | | Corneal tissue clear (%) | Cryopreserved | | Corneal tissue clear (%) | Total clear (%) |
| | Clear | Cloudy | | Clear | Cloudy | | |
| Phakic | 13 | 5 | 72 | 7 | 0 | 100 | 80 |
| Aphakic | 14 | 4 | 78 | 8 | 0 | 100 | 85 |
| Graft and cataract | 5 | 2 | 71 | 8 | 7 | 53 | 59 |
| TOTAL | 32 | 11 | 74 | 23 | 7 | 77 | 75 |

TABLE 2.  *Penetrating keratoplasty in all types of bullous keratopathy*

| | No. of cases | | | | | |
|---|---|---|---|---|---|---|
| | Refrigerated | | Corneal tissue clear (%) | Cryopreserved | | Corneal tissue clear (%) | Total clear (%) |
| | Clear | Cloudy | | Clear | Cloudy | | |
| Phakic | 14 | 5 | 74 | 10 | 0 | 100 | 83 |
| Aphakic | 41 | 10 | 80 | 29 | 10 | 74 | 78 |
| Graft and cataract | 8 | 5 | 62 | 13 | 10 | 57 | 58 |
| TOTAL | 63 | 20 | 76 | 52 | 20 | 72 | 74 |

TABLE 3. *Comparison of survival time using cryopreserved and refrigerated tissue*

| Total no. of grafts after six months | % remaining clear at | | | |
|---|---|---|---|---|
| | *1 year* | *2 years* | *3 years* | *4 years* |
| Cryopreserved grafts | | | | |
| 1 | | | | → 100 (1/1) |
| 4 | | | → 100 (4/4) | |
| 9 | | → 88.8 (8/9) | | |
| 18 | 94.4 (17/18) | | | |
| Refrigerated grafts | | | | |
| 8 | | | | → 62.5 (5/8) |
| 11 | | | → 63.6 (7/11) | |
| 15 | | → 66.7 (10/15) | | |
| 27 | 81.4 (22/27) | | | |

reasonably favorable prognosis for this category of disease. It seemed important at this point, having done a preliminary analysis of acute disease, to determine the long-term prognosis of keratoplasty in these patients and how the different types of tissue survived with time. As many patients as possible who had clear grafts at six months were followed up to determine the fate of the graft with time. It was found (Table 3) that a graft's survival was good for at least three years, and that during this time, cryopreserved tissue was no worse than refrigerated tissue.

Given a reasonable prognosis for a graft's survival once clear, it appeared important to review the cause for graft failure and to compare the refrigerated and cryopreserved tissue (Table 4). In this group there were obvious causes of graft failure in the majority of patients. Only those which are listed as unknown could not be put into a category of definite homograft reaction as opposed to inadequate donor material or persistent iritis which was difficult to detect. We found only a minority of cases which we could attribute to failure due to the homograft reaction and

no difference in complications which could be related to tissue type.

In the group of patients with Fuchs' dystrophy and bullous keratopathy, we also studied the effect of vitreous aspiration through the pupil or pars plana using a No. 22 needle (Table 5). When aspiration was done through

TABLE 4. *Causes of failure in bullous keratopathy*

| | Refrigerated corneal tissue | Preserved corneal tissue |
|---|---|---|
| Glaucoma | 4 | 1 |
| Bacterial ulcer | 1 | 0 |
| Vitreous contact | 3 | 3 |
| Synechia | 2 | 1 |
| Suture abcess | 2 | 1 |
| Bleeding | 0 | 1 |
| Wound leak | 2 | 2 |
| Homograft | 1 | 1 |
| Unknown | 7 | 4 |

TABLE 5. *Effect of vitreous aspiration in bullous keratopathy*

| | No. of cases | | Clear (%) |
|---|---|---|---|
| Site of aspiration | Clear | Cloudy | |
| Pars plana | 36 | 7 | 84 |
| Pupil | 16 | 4 | 80 |

TABLE 6. *Graft totals*

| | No. of cases | | | | |
|---|---|---|---|---|---|
| | Refrigerated corneal tissue | | Preserved corneal tissue | | Total |
| | Clear | Cloudy | Clear | Cloudy | Clear (%) |
| Keratoconus | 13 | 2 | 15 | 1 | 90 |
| Bacterial ulcer | 3 | 2 | 8 | 3 | 69 |
| Interstitial keratitis | 6 | 0 | 6 | 0 | 100 |

the pupil, the needle was inserted through the center of the pupil and liquid vitreous was aspirated. The excision of solid vitreous through the pupil was considered as aspiration through the pupil, but through much of this series, cellulose sponges were not used to remove solid vitreous. Only later in the series was the excision of solid vitreous combined with aspiration of liquid vitreous to clear the wound and the anterior segment thoroughly of vitreous. There was no significant difference in results with the different types of vitreous aspiration.

Figures on the excision of solid vitreous are not adequate for analysis, but this technique seems to have further improved results. However, when vitreous remains intact and is not loose in the anterior chamber or incarcerated in the wound, we prefer not to aspirate vitreous or to excise solid vitreous. The reason for this is that complications such as retinal detachments, vitreous opacities and, in some cases, hemorrhage seem to be minimized if it is not necessary to manipulate the vitreous body.

Thirty-two grafts were performed for keratoconus. Thirteen of the 15 with refrigerated tissue and 16 of the 17 with preserved tissue remained clear (Table 6). The eyes that received fresh tissue were phakic. One developed a bacterial endophthalmitis, a second clouded after a severe iritis and possible homograft reaction. Fifteen of the eyes re-

ceiving the cryopreserved tissue were phakic. Two, however, were subjected to combined grafts and cataract extractions. One of these receiving the combined procedure with vitreous aspirated through the pars plana remained clear. A second, however, developed endophthalmitis at a time when the cryoextractor used for the lens extraction came from the factory with imperfect packaging and was presumably contaminated. After the operation, one of the refrigerated eyes developed a severe iritis but remained clear. Three of the cryopreserved eyes developed a severe iritis but remained clear. In this category, no grafts which were clear at three months clouded during the next two years.

Twelve grafts were done for interstitial keratitis (Table 6). Nine of these 12 had significant vascularization. All of the grafts remained clear, although two refrigerated and three preserved developed a moderately severe iritis after surgery. The clarity was independent of the vascularization, even where there was deep 4+ severe vascularization. No clouding was seen in this series during subsequent follow-up.

Sixteen grafts were performed for bacterial ulcers (Table 6). Of these, five were performed in eyes that were severely and acutely inflamed at the time of surgery and had massive corneal necrosis. In this series, five were aphakic, or were subjected to cataract extraction at the time of surgery. Because of the acute nature of their disease, four of the severely inflamed eyes received preserved corneas since the grafts were done as an emergency. There was no unusual operative trauma in the group receiving preserved corneas that remained clear; one eye had vitreous in the wound at the time of surgery and a second, extensive synechiae which required traumatic and extensive lysis at the time of surgery. Of the three receiving cryopreserved corneas that became cloudy, one had vitreous in the wound.

**281**

DISCUSSION

The generally favorable prognosis of keratoplasty in patients with bullous keratopathy appears due to the recognition of several basic principles. 1) The abandonment of the old teaching that all diseased tissue should be excised. Even in cases of limbus-to-limbus bullous keratopathy, clear grafts can be obtained with donor buttons of between 7 and 8 mm. Grafts more than 8 mm in diameter carry a poor prognosis because of peripheral synechiae to the iris and vitreous and the glaucoma that frequently supervenes. 2) Although the grafts must not be too large, they must be large enough to contribute enough normal endothelium. A 7-mm graft contains twice as much endothelium as a 5-mm graft, and when the endothelial damage which occurs at the graft edges from excision of the button or crushing with scissors is considered, this difference is further accentuated. Perhaps with time, patients with small transplants will have excessive endothelial leakage in the recipient which dissects through the corneal lamellae and causes edema in the donor. 3) The third concept in this series was that elaborated by Fine and others, that whether vitreous remains in the eye or not is less important for graft clarity than being certain that vitreous does not remain in the wound. Vitreous aspirations were done from the beginning of this study; it seemed to make little difference whether they were done through the pupil or through the pars plana. Newer techniques of managing vitreous loss, utilizing cellulose sponges, may further improve these results. The finding that vitreous removal through the pupil is not an additional hazard may make it possible to do grafts on aphakic patients without the routine removal of vitreous, but only manipulation of the vitreous, in those patients who require it.

A major factor in graft failure in the patients with corneal edema was glaucoma. At the time this study was done, there was no satisfactory way to measure the intraocular pressure in patients with corneal edema or corneal scarring. Similarly, the pressure soon after keratoplasty could not be measured. Toward the end of the study, however, various research workers (2, 3) showed that the MacKay-Marg applanation tonometer could measure the intraocular pressure and permit the detection and control of glaucoma in these patients. The finding of pressures of 70 mm Hg or higher in many of the combined procedure group for a significant period of time after surgery might well influence the prognosis, and control of this factor may improve the results significantly. Similarly, the finding that cryosurgery of the ciliary body can be used in keratoplasty patients after grafting with reasonable success and little chance of causing the graft to cloud, further indicates that glaucoma, a significant contributor to our graft failures, may well be minimized and controlled in the future.

The effect that measurement of intraocular pressure and the ability to control it in eyes before and after surgery will have on the final prognosis is not yet clear. However, we believe that the ability to detect and control elevated intraocular pressure will be of special importance in patients with combined keratoplasties and cataract extractions. Even without this, however, Paton (4) reported that 19% of clear grafts clouded at the time of cataract extraction and Lemp et al. (5) found that 20% of clear grafts clouded with cataract extractions so that the combined procedure seems to offer no significant hazard over doing the transplant first and the keratoplasty later.

In this series vascularization of the cornea seemed to play a relatively small role in the long-term prognosis. In our experience, no cornea with extensive chemical burns, on which we have done a keratoplasty, remained clear. In the past, it has been assumed that the reason grafts failed in chemical burns was because of extensive vascularization and a homograft reaction. This is certainly not established and we believe that there are other reasons. If the patients with chemical burns are omitted, then even eyes with severe vascularization do extremely well after keratoplasty and the prognosis is not significantly different from that in cases without vascularization. This does not imply that vascularization has no influence on the incidence of homograft reaction, but may indicate that patients with severely vascularized corneas were managed with anti-inflammatory drugs quite differently from those without vascularization. In avascular corneas, especially in older people with bullous keratopathy, healing of the graft is a problem. Several grafts showed dehiscence at the time of suture removal, three or four months after placement of 10–0 nylon sutures. We used steroids in this group only with the greatest of caution and with a specific indication. On the other hand, corneas with severe vascularization healed much more rapidly and rarely showed problems of wound dehiscence. Corticosteroids were used in this group with little risk.

There are different pharmacological effects of corticosteroids which can be utilized. The one usually employed after keratoplasty is a nonspecific anti-inflammatory effect. This decreases iritis, which can damage a graft, even without a specific immune reaction, and by its nonspecific anti-inflammatory effect can suppress immune reactions after they have begun. There is another effect of corticosteroids, however, which is similar to that commonly employed with the immunosuppressive agents. When corticosteroids are given in significant doses from the time of surgery, or the time of antigen appearance, and minimize recognition by the tissues that a foreign substance has been implanted, they can prevent sensitization. This depends on the use of systemic corticosteroids from the time of surgery and was employed only in people with very marked vascularization and generally with deep vascularization. Doses of about 80 mg of prednisone were usually given and elevated doses maintained for about 7 to 10 days, at which time gradual tapering off of the steroid dosage was begun over a period of several weeks. Topical steroids several times a day were employed throughout the postoperative course in these patients, and, in patients with heavily vascularized corneas, small doses of topical steroids were frequently continued for months, or occasionally for an indefinite period, in eyes that tended to get inflamed when steroids were stopped. This maintenance dose of as little as a drop of topical corticosteroid a day seemed extremely important in some patients prone to recurrent inflammation. It became clear that when drugs were used in this way, although immune reactions might have a greater tendency to develop in patients with heavily vascularized corneas, the number of grafts lost to immune reactions were exceedingly small. The reactions, if they occurred, could usually be controlled. These good results in vascularized corneas (excluding chemical burns) raise serious questions as to whether the use of highly toxic drugs, such as immunosuppressive agents which may have long-term deleterious effects on genetic make-up, with the production of late cancers and other systemic side effects, is justifiable in these patients. A careful, simultaneously controlled study must be done to establish if there is a sufficient beneficial effect to justify their use.

Under carefully controlled clinical conditions, the use of cryopreserved corneas has been shown to be safe and effective, and to have no apparent disadvantage over refrigerated corneas. The ability to perform surgery when the patient and the doctor are ready for such surgery and the operative team can be optimally mobilized is a great advantage, and one which may improve the results. On the other hand, the cryopreserved tissue is partially dehydrated and somewhat thinner than normal corneal tissue. To properly appose it, especially when grafting into severely edematous, thickened corneas with limbus-to-limbus bullous keratopathy, we place our corneal suture deep—slightly above Descemet's membrane both in the donor and the recipient, thus "lining up Descemet's membrane and the endothelium" as much as possible. In addition, this tissue handles like young very fresh donor tissue, in being somewhat flexible and requiring meticulous apposition with multiple sutures.

Schultz (6) has reported that partial hydration of the tissue with a balanced salt solution makes the tissue easier to handle and may wash out some additional dimethylsulfoxide. Since the safety of this procedure has not yet been clearly demonstrated, even though it may ultimately be desirable, we have not used it. In our hands, the present procedure has been adequate. Cryopreserved tissue, like most donor tissue, is extremely sensitive to endothelial damage. The endothelium should never be touched with an instrument or placed on any object. It is not necessary or desirable to wash the endothelium with any fluid since the albumin solution is more than adequate to prevent it from drying out. Most antibiotic solutions which contain cytotoxic preservatives should be avoided, as should rubbing the endothelial surface to the graft back and forth on the iris and lens.

The principles of keratoplasty employed in this series are not greatly different from those outlined in the work of Fine and others, and confirm that the prognosis of aphakic keratoplasty has greatly improved. We feel strongly that the good results in this type of surgery are not a function of unique surgical skill, but are similar to those documented in other series by experienced corneal surgeons such as Brown and Fine (7) and depend, to be sure, on continuing experience with keratoplasty, but also on the appreciation of the basic considerations outlined above. In cases

of Fuchs' dystrophy and bullous keratopathy, no significant difference is seen between the different types of tissue. This seems especially important since in very favorable cases in which the host cornea is healthy, healing of the endothelium could take place by migration of host cells. It is extremely unlikely that such could occur in severe Fuchs' dystrophy or extensive bullous keratopathies.

Even more interesting than acute clarity is the survival of the graft for a period of time after surgery. In this series, graft clarity persists better in the cryopreserved donor than in those receiving the usual refrigerated tissue. It is tempting to speculate that the improved survival of cryopreserved tissue may be due to the fact that it was taken from significantly younger donors and preserved soon after death, whereas the refrigerated tissue was taken from somewhat older donors and was used later. Kanai's electron microscopic studies (8) of corneal endothelium in donor eyes after death would suggest that this is a likely possibility; other factors may also have been involved, however.

Supported in part by USPHS Grants EY–00226 and EY–00446 from the National Eye Institute.

## REFERENCES

1. CAPELLA JA, KAUFMAN HE and ROBBINS JE. Preservation of viable corneal tissue. *Arch Ophthalmol* **74**: 669, 1965.
2. IRVINE AR and KAUFMAN HE. Intraocular pressure following penetrating keratoplasty. *Am J Ophthalmol* **68**: 835, 1969.
3. WIND CA and KAUFMAN HE. Validity of MacKay-Marg applanation tonometry following penetrating keratoplasty in man. *Am J Ophthalmol* **72**: 117, 1971.
4. PATON RT. "Keratoplasty." New York, Blakiston, 1955.
5. LEMP MA, PFISTER RR and DOHLMAN CH. Effect of intraocular surgery on clear corneal grafts. *Am J Ophthalmol* **70**: 719, 1970.
6. EDELHAUSER HF, VAN HORN DL, GALLUN AB and SCHULTZ RO. Experimental rehydration of cryopreserved corneal tissue. *Invest Ophthalmol* **10**: 100, 1971.
7. FINE M. Corneal grafts and aphakia, in: "Cor-

neo-plastic surgery." *Proc Second Int Corneo-plastic Conf London, 1967.* New York, Pergamon Press, 1969.

8. KANAI A, VALENT JG and KAUFMAN HE. Ultra-structural studies of cryopreserved corneal endothelium in corneal preservation, in: "Clinical and laboratory evaluation of current methods." Springfield, Ill CC. Thomas (in press).

# DISCUSSION

DR. A. B. RIZZUTI (*USA*): There are a number of cases, 10 to 12, who had erosions of the cornea due to the keratoprosthesis. The number of erosions is now being reduced, since we prevent drying of the cornea. Keratoprothesis is still an experimental tool, but it has a great future. We have some patients who have had useful vision for six years.

DR. C. H. DOHLMAN (*USA*): The problem of availability of graft material could be helped considerably by persuading our governments to adopt more sensible legislation. There are countries in Europe that permit an autopsy on anyone who dies in a hospital without the specific permission of the next of kin. In this way all donor problems are solved.

DR. H. E. KAUFMAN (*USA*): I couldn't agree more with Dr. Dohlman. We do about 250 keratoplasties a year on patients coming great distances. Our autopsy forms indicate that tissues, including the eye, may be examined or removed for therapeutic purposes. If this stipulation is not specifically deleted, we can take out the eyes without going to the next of kin. Dr. Frank Pollak has been running an educational program teaching morticians in Florida how to remove the eyes; this has been very satisfactory.

DR. J. H. KING, JR. (*USA*): I would like to emphasize one point. In a developing nation, the cases with the best prognosis are the ones that should be done first. For example, cases with central corneal opacities surrounded by healthy corneal tissue should precede highly vascularized corneas, where chances are very poor. When the results are not so good, the government and patients become discouraged, and the enterprise fails.

MR. P. D. TREVOR-ROPER (*UK*): Dr. Kaufman has made a good point. In England the doctor himself must remove the eye; this is clinically and economically tiresome. How lucky they are in those countries in Europe where they are able to take what they need. We have had no occasion to use deep-frozen eyes because we are now getting fresh material without many problems. I have been involved in starting a number of eye banks in different developing countries, particularly in Africa. The real function of an eye bank is to serve as a quick distribution center. Its success depends on the imagination and the enthusiasm of the actual doctor who runs it.

DR. KAUFMAN: As far as developing countries are concerned, our experience in Salvador is a beautiful example. There was an excellent corneal surgeon, plenty of people with corneal disease, but no corneal tissue. It was a perfect kind of setup for someone to go in with a supply of preserved eyes, and really to be able to help the population.

DR. DOHLMAN: I was impressed by Dr. Ticho's paper illustrating the difficulties with total corneal grafts, in which edema appeared after a while, presumably due to an immune reaction. This is a good series for stressing this point. However, I do not think this procedure is something we should do lightheartedly. Of course, if the cornea has melted away and the iris is exposed, then we have no choice. We should realize that the chances of getting a clear graft are not very good. Optically, we need a central 5 or 6 mm, and there should be no temptation to do a larger graft than we actually have to do. Our average case requires about 8 mm, and when we get up to 9 mm, success is less assured.

DR. KAUFMAN: Dr. Dohlman has shown that the risk of a graft becoming cloudy after a cataract retraction is significant, around 20%. A combined graft and cataract procedure did not increase the risk of graft opacification, but has the advantage of saving the patient from another operation. Following the combined operation we found very high pressures even without the use of α-chymotrypsin or steroids. The elevated pressure, which lasts for about three weeks, is about 70 to 80 mm Hg.

DR. DOHLMAN: The problems with keratoprosthesis are not mechanical, optical or material; nor do they involve the surgical technique to any great extent. The problem is biological and is probably due to the release of proteolytic enzymes from damaged epithelium.

A keratoprosthesis may give fair results in cases where the epithelium is essentially normal to start with. In these cases regular keratoplasties are usually satisfactory. We really need keratoprosthesis mainly in chemical burns and in the dry eye, where the results are often not good. The field is a good one and it is important that many groups be engaged in it. However, keratoprosthesis cannot be distributed on any mass basis to any country.

CLINICAL PROBLEMS IN DEVELOPED COUNTRIES

# NATURAL HISTORY OF DIABETIC RETINOPATHY

MORTON F. GOLDBERG

Department of Ophthalmology, University of Illinois Eye and Ear Infirmary, Chicago, Illinois, USA

If diabetes is diagnosed at the age of 20, the risk of blindness at age 30 is only 0.1%, and it increases to 3.5% at the age of 50 (a 35-fold increase) (1). For the general population, by comparison, the risk of blindness from all causes at age 30 is 0.09% and at age 50 is only 0.15% (a 1.6-fold increase). At the age of 50, therefore, the diabetic is about 23 times more likely to be blind than his nondiabetic counterpart. Furthermore, the numerical magnitude of diabetic blindness is underscored by the observation that as many as 11 to 12% of the United States blind population owes its visual deficiencies to diabetes (2). In other countries such as Denmark the percentage has been as high as 23% (1). Visual disability in diabetes can be caused by cataract, retinopathy, refractive change, rubeosis iridis (with secondary glaucoma) or by a combination of these diseases. Of these, diabetic retinopathy and secondary glaucoma are the major causes of blindness.

*Development of diabetic retinopathy.* Most cases of diabetes are inherited; that is, they are in a sense primary. One of the most common late sequelae is diabetic retinopathy, a term encompassing all pathologic phenomena in the retina. Diabetic retinopathy has also been observed in patients with a variety of other diseases which in turn lead to carbohydrate intolerance as a secondary manifestation. These include the following: chronic pancreatitis, pancreatectomy, hemochromatosis, Cushing's syndrome, acromegaly and Werner's syndrome. Surprisingly, patients with diabetes secondary to pheochromocytoma have not yet been observed to suffer from retinopathy (3) perhaps because the patient with the primary disease does not have the disease sufficiently long.

The preponderance of evidence suggests, therefore, that a chemical aberration in carbohydrate metabolism is the common etiologic forerunner of diabetic retinopathy. The intervening pathogenesis responsible for the conversion of carbohydrate intolerance to diabetic retinopathy remains somewhat obscure, but certain conclusions regarding the natural history of this serious retinal disease can be drawn. Regardless of basic etiology, approximately 2% of all diabetics become blind from retinopathy alone. This prevalence is approximately 10 times greater than that of blindness from all causes in the general population (3).

What factors are related to the development of diabetic retinopathy? Duration of diabetes appears to be the primary factor affecting the frequency of retinopathy. If diabetes is diagnosed before the age of 30, for example, and lasts for five to nine years, approximately 10% or less of the affected individuals will have retinopathy (3). When the diabetes is diagnosed before the age of 30 and lasts for 15 years, however, approximately 50% of the individuals will have observable retinopathy. When the diabetes is diagnosed before the age of 30 and then lasts for more than 25 years, 80 to 90% of individuals are found to have retinopathy. These figures may be contrasted to those obtained from the preinsulin era of 1921, when the life expectancy of the juvenile diabetic was considerably lower and only about 8% of living diabetics had retinopathy (4).

The principle that the development of retinopathy is related to duration of the underlying diabetic state is modified slightly by the age of the patient. For example, when diabetes is diagnosed before the age of 30 and lasts five years or less, the risk of retinopathy developing is about 2% per year (3). When, however, the diabetes is diagnosed after the age of 30 and lasts for a similar period, the risk of retinopathy is about 7% per year. Presumably, therefore, aging makes the retinal vasculature more vulnerable to the diabetic process whatever it may be, and makes the older patient more likely than his younger counterpart to develop retinopathy within a given period of time.

In addition to duration of the systemic disease, metabolic control may affect certain forms of retinopathy. Caird (5) and Knowles (6) have summarized evidence that the frequency of retinopathy may be reduced and the age of onset raised if regulation of diabetes is particularly strict during the first five years following discovery of the systemic disease. However, once most retinal lesions are established, metabolic control has little, if any, influence on the retinopathy. This point is controversial, and retinal venous irregularities, such as dilatation, tortuosity, beading, etc., may be reversible with appropriate therapeutic management via diet, insulin, etc. Other more permanent lesions such as neovascular and fibrovascular proliferations appear to be minimally influenced by systemic effects of dietary management or metabolic control. Intervention in the natural course of diabetic retinopathy by other metabolic means, such as by pituitary ablation appears to be able to minimize or reverse many forms of the retinal disease (7). Carefully controlled and documented studies, however, are remarkably few in number.

*Local factors in the development of diabetic retinopathy.* Although the exact pathogenesis of early diabetic retinopathy is unknown evidence from a variety of techniques suggests that initial vascular changes in the diabetie retina occur in the capillary bed. The most widespread change is a thickening of the capillary basement membrane, which is associated with increased permeability. Its pathogenic significance, however, is not known. Cogan and Kuwabara used trypsin digestion and histologic techniques in investigating whole mounts of diabetic retinas (8, 9). They showed that diabetic microaneurysms developed at the sites of degenerated mural cells (intramural pericytes) in the capillary wall. It was postulated that loss of the mural cells caused loss of capillary tone, and that this, in turn, resulted in channeling of blood into a few distended capillaries. These vessels presumably became in effect shunt vessels or arteriolar-venular anastomoses. The bypassed capillaries were then thought to undergo occlusion, accounting for the well-known microinfarctions and cotton-wool spots of the diabetic retina.

Kohner, Dollery and others have utilized careful fluorescein angiography to study capillary closure *in vivo* (10, 11). Their evidence suggests that capillary closure and microaneurysm formation precede rather than follow shunt vessel formation. Possibly both sequences may occur in a given retina. If, indeed, capillary closure is the primary event its pathogenesis also remains obscure. Ashton has postulated that the capillaries may be squeezed shut by edematous surrounding retinal tissue or that the arteriolar perfusion

292

pressure become reduced as the result of arteriolar hyalinization or other factors (12, 13). Both mechanisms may apply. Alternatively, intrinsic capillary disease may cause closure *sui generis* as from endothelial swelling or proliferation. The initial pathologic event, however, is still unknown.

That the shunt vessels may represent preexisting capillaries and not newly formed tissue is supported by the observation that they do not leak significant amounts of intravascular fluorescein into the vitreous whereas true neovascular tissue does. Similar observations have been made in proliferative sickle retinopathy where arteriolovenular anastomoses do not leak fluorescein either (14).

Regardless of the precise initial sequence of events retinal capillary closure certainly occurs early in the natural history of diabetic retinopathy (11) and probably has a fundamental effect on subsequent phenomena. The induced ischemia and tissue hypoxia can be demonstrated by laboratory techniques such as trypsin digestion and flat mounting and by clinical techniques such as perimetry and fluorescein angiography (3). With trypsin digestion of whole, flat mounts of diabetic retinas, zones of ischemic, acellular capillaries that are surrounded by clusters of microaneurysms are easily demonstrated. Perimetry shows small scotomas up to one-fourth disk diameter in the central visual field, and as many as 50% of diabetics have such scotomas even in the absence of ophthalmoscopically visible retinopathy (3). Fluorescein angiography readily reveals zones of nonperfusion. Finally, simple observation shows silver wire arterioles and cotton-wool spots which are both signs of retinal ischemia.

At some critical point in time capillary endothelium begins to proliferate, to the point that true neovascularization can be said to have occurred. Early theories that hemorrhages were required to induce neovascularization have not been substantiated (15).

The precise factors responsible for this proliferative phase of diabetic retinopathy are unknown, but the onset of a proliferative phase heralds the onset of a particularly dangerous period for the eye.

Even with onset of neovascularization ischemia is often found to play a role, because early patches of neovascular tissue appear to grow into or towards a zone of retinal hypoxia seemingly in an attempt to revascularize this area. It is possible, therefore, that hypoxic zones of retinal tissue liberate some vasoproliferative substance such as a chemotactic factor which induces budding of retinal capillary endothelium (16, 17).

Although proliferative diabetic retinopathy may create an apparently haphazard jungle of newly formed tissue its pattern and course are not wholly undecipherable. Taylor and Dobree and others have shown that neovascular tissue arises most commonly on retinal venules in the posterior pole of the eye (18). The next most common location is immediately on the optic disk. Proliferative lesions are rarely found directly in the macular area. The distribution of lesions on major retinal venules is as follows: most commonly on the superotemporal vein, next on the inferotemporal vein, then on the supernasal vein and least commonly on the inferonasal vein (18). This quadrantic predilection interestingly is identical to that observed in proliferative retinopathy of sickle cell diseases (19) and is similar to that observed in retrolental fibroplasia.

The proliferative lesions in the temporal quadrants were found by Taylor and Dobree to be on the average 3.36 disk diameters from the disk, and those in the nasal quadrants to be 2.35 disk diameters from the disk (18). Nearly all of the proliferative lesions were associated anatomically with an arteriovenous crossing.

Dobree's classification of proliferative diabetic retinopathy is useful in outlining the

**293**

course of this disease. Proliferative lesions passed through three well-defined stages: 1) a collection of fine, naked vessels; 2) a stage of vascular proliferation with connective tissue formation; and 3) a stage of regression of vessels and contraction of connective tissue (15). The first two stages may take one and a half to three and a half years to evolve during which small and large hemorrhages may occur.

That a useful distinction exists between nonproliferative and proliferative diabetic retinopathy is underscored by data relating to visual prognosis. If, for example, diabetes is diagnosed before the age of 60 only 3% of patients on the average will be blind in the ensuing five years when nonproliferative retinopathy alone existed at the beginning of the five-year period (3). Obviously, an attempt at therapy during this stage of retinopathy will have to show a remarkably high rate of preservation of vision in order to compare favorably with the natural course of the disease. The presence of proliferative changes, such as neovascularization, signifies a considerably worse prognosis. For juvenile diabetics below the age of 20, for example, 30 to 40% on the average will be blind within five years if proliferative diabetic retinopathy had been present at the beginning of the five-year period (3).

Davis (20) and Tolentino et al. (21) have shown that once neovascularization has taken place on the surface of the retina, subsequent loss of vision leading to the aforementioned grim statistics depends largely on changes in the vitreous. Changes in the vessels themselves are frequently less conspicuous than the profound effect on vision would suggest. As new vessels grow on the surface of the retina adherence to the posterior surface of the vitreous gel takes place. Whether or not this adherence or the subsequent massive outpouring of fluid, protein, salts, etc. that occurs from the neovascular tissue into the vitreous causes or

accentuates the otherwise natural process of vitreous detachment is problematic, but it is the vitreous detachment which tugs on the adherent retinal vessels and drags them forward (not into the vitreous gel itself but into the space between the detached posterior vitreous face and the anterior surface of the retina). In the process, tearing of fragile, newly formed blood vessels occurs and hemorrhages ensue such as preretinal and intravitreal. Tugging on the retina may also lead to localized retinal detachment with or without holes but, as in all forms of diabetic retinopathy, even the retinal detachments usually remain confined to the area posterior to the equator. In the process of gradual, intermittent vitreous contraction with its series of induced hemorrhages and retinal detachments a variety of visual symptoms and deficits occur. Davis observed the entire process to require months or years to reach completion (20).

When the process of vitreous contraction terminates, the recurrent hemorrhagic episodes are either significantly reduced or are altogether stopped. In this relatively quiescent stage, the retina is left with no or many local detachments, with or without a functioning macula and with or without a significant amount of blood or fibrous opacities in the visual axis. In addition, the remaining retina shows marked reduction in caliber and number of its vessels. Many silver wire arterioles appear, and the retina presents an overall appearance of ischemia. Davis has used the word "remission" to describe this late "burned out" phase (20).

Another phenomenon, "regression," has been observed in approximately 10% of patients having neovascular tissue but no vitreous contraction (20). Instead of following the course of episodic vitreous contractions (and associated hemorrhages), neovascular tissue in these patients simply regresses and atrophies, so that major vascular extravasations are rare. The factors responsible for this phenomenon are currently unknown, but are obviously important in devising successful treatment of diabetic retinopathy.

Interference with vision occurs in both the proliferative phase of diabetic retinopathy and in its nonproliferative phase. Although most therapeutic attempts center around the neovascular tissue with its hemorrhagic propensities and its tendency to eventuate in macular detachment, edema and exudates in the macula account for a high proportion of cases of reduced visual acuity. Myers et al. (22) found that macular edema primarily occurring in eyes with nonproliferative retinopathy was the third most common cause of visual loss in a series of 200 diabetic eyes. (Vitreous hemorrhage and macular detachment were the most common causes.) Additional controlled studies are required in order to learn if, when and how the nonproliferative diabetic retina should be treated.

## REFERENCES

1. CAIRD FI. Diabetic retinopathy as a cause of visual impairment, in: Goldberg MF and Fine SL (Eds), "Symposium on the treatment of diabetic retinopathy." Washington DC, PHS Pub no 1890, Superintendent of Documents, 1969, chap 3.
2. HATFIELD EM. "Estimated statistics on blindness and vision problems." New York, National Society for the Prevention of Blindness, Inc.
3. CAIRD FI, PIRIE A and RAMSELL TG. "Diabetes and the eye." Oxford, Blackwell Scientific Publications, 1969.
4. DUKE-ELDER S and DOBREE JH. "Diseases of the retina." London, Henry Kimpton, 1967, p 412.
5. CAIRD FI. Control of diabetes and diabetic retinopathy, in: Goldberg MF and Fine SL (Eds), "Symposium on the treatment of diabetic retinopathy." Washington DC, PHS Pub no 1890, Superintendent of Documents, 1969, chap 11.
6. KNOWLES HC JR. The control of diabetes mellitus and the progression of retinopathy, in: Goldberg MF and Fine SL (Eds), "Symposium on the treatment of diabetic retinopathy." Washington DC, PHS Pub no 1890, Superintendent of Documents, 1969, chap 12.
7. LUNDBAEK K, MALMROS R, ANDERSEN HC, RASMUSSEN JH, BRUNTSE E, MADSEN PH and JENSEN VA. Hypophysectomy for diabetic angiopathy: A controlled clinical trial, in: Goldberg MF and Fine SL (Eds), "Symposium on the treatment of diabetic retinopathy." Washington DC, PHS Pub no 1890, Superintendent of Documents, 1969, chap 25.
8. COGAN DG and KUWABARA T. Capillary shunts in the pathogenesis of diabetic retinopathy. Diabetes 12: 293, 1963.
9. COGAN DG, TOUSSAINT D and KUWABARA T. Retinal vascular patterns; IV. Diabetic retinopathy. Arch Ophthalmol 66: 366, 1961.
10. KOHNER EM and DOLLERY CT. The natural history of diabetic retinopathy, in: Goldberg MF and Fine SL (Eds), "Symposium on the treatment of diabetic retinopathy." Washington DC, PHS Pub no 1890, Superintendent of Documents, 1969, chap 6.
11. KOHNER EM and DOLLERY CT. Fluorescein angiography of the fundus in diabetic retinopathy. Br Med Bull 26: 166, 1970.
12. ASHTON N. Pathophysiology of retinal cotton-wool spots. Br Med Bull 26: 143, 1970.
13. GARNER A. Pathology of diabetic retinopathy. Br Med Bull 26: 137, 1970.
14. GOLDBERG MF. Natural history of untreated proliferative sickle retinopathy. Arch Ophthalmol 85: 428, 1971.
15. DOBREE JH. Proliferative diabetic retinopathy. Evolution of the retinal lesions. Br J Ophthalmol 48: 637, 1964.
16. ASHTON N. Studies of the retinal capillaries in relation to diabetic and other retinopathies. Br J Ophthalmol 47: 521, 1963.
17. ASHTON N. Oxygen and the growth and development of retinal vessels, in: Kimura S and Caygill WM (Eds), "Vascular complications of diabetes mellitus." St Louis, CV Mosby Co, 1967, chap 1.
18. TAYLOR E and DOBREE JH. Proliferative diabetic retinopathy. Site and size of initial lesions. Br J Ophthalmol 54: 11, 1970.
19. GOLDBERG MF. Proliferative sickle retinopathy. Classification and pathogenesis. Am J Ophthalmol 71: 649, 1971.
20. DAVIS MD. Vitreous contraction in proliferative diabetic retinopathy. Arch Ophthalmol 74: 741, 1965.
21. TOLENTINO II, LEE PF and SCHEPENS CL. Biomicroscopic study of vitreous cavity in diabetic retinopathy. Arch Ophthalmol 75: 238, 1966.
22. MYERS FL, DAVIS MD and MAGLI YL. The natural course of diabetic retinopathy: A clinical study of 321 eyes followed one year or more, in: Goldberg MF and Fine SL (Eds), "Symposium on the treatment of diabetic retinopathy." Washington DC, PHS Pub no 1890, Public Health Service, 1969, chap 7.

# CAPILLARY MICROANEURISMS AND SHUNT VESSELS IN DIABETIC RETINOPATHY

## A Hypothesis on Pathogenesis and Prevention

ABRAHAM L. KORNZWEIG

Department of Ophthalmology and Ophthalmic Research, Jewish Home and Hospital for the Aged, and Mount Sinai School of Medicine of the City University of New York, New York, USA

Diabetic retinopathy is now one of the major complications of longstanding diabetes mellitus. The subject has been dealt with exhaustively in many publications and symposia. Lately, emphasis has been on different methods of treatment and prevention of loss of vision.

This paper is mainly a study of the retinal circulation in postmortem human eyes. The subjects studied were residents of the Jewish Home and Hospital for the Aged, New York City. The clinical course of the diabetes was observed during the stay at the institution, lasting from six months to many years. In many instances postmortem examinations were made, particularly of the eyes. The retinal vasculature was isolated using the trypsin digestion technique of Kuwabara and Cogan (1). Routine histological sections were also prepared from many of these eyes. A total of 130 patients were thus studied clinically and pathologically.

The clinical features of this group of patients are as follows: Their ages ranged from 70 to 93 years, most of them being in the late 70s and early 80s. Females exceeded males by a ratio of 3:2. In all these patients the diagnosis of diabetes mellitus was confirmed by repeated blood glucose and urine analyses. Many, but not all, patients suffered from changes in the retina due to diabetic retinopathy. These included all the known retinopathic findings, such as hard and soft exudates, retinal hemorrhages, microaneurisms, proliferating retinopathy and vitreous hemorrhages. Emphasis in this presentation will be placed upon the circulatory changes noted in postmortem eyes and upon a hypothesis on pathogenesis and possible prevention.

The pathological findings are well known, the most striking being capillary microaneurisms. These are occasional in mild cases and very numerous in advanced cases (Fig. 1 and 2). They range in size from 10 to 15 μm in the early stage to 75 and 150 μm in the late stage, and generally consist of lateral protrusions or sacculations from the affected capillary and occasionally fusiform dilatations. The large ones may contain many blood and endothelial cells, the small ones an occasional endothelial cell. I have never seen ruptured capillary microaneurisms on pathological specimens, though this may happen clinically. Also, old hyalinized microaneurisms are present, especially in longstanding cases (Fig. 3).

Another interesting finding is the presence

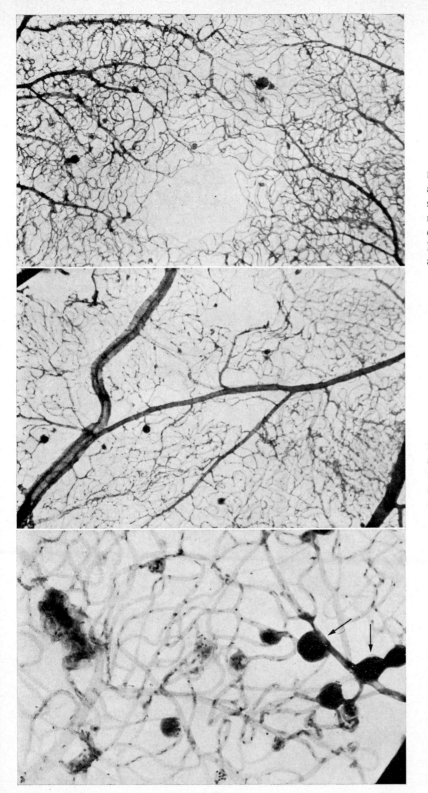

FIG. 1. Diabetic retinopathy showing numerous small and large capillary microaneurisms in macular area around fovea. Periodic acid-schiff (PAS) and Giemsa. × 21.

FIG. 2. Diabetic retinopathy in early case, showing occasional microaneurism. Midperipheral area. PAS and Giemsa. × 21.

FIG. 3. Old hyalinized capillary microaneurisms (arrows) are present in this advanced case of diabetic retinopathy. Some newly formed microaneurisms containing epithelial cells and blood cells are also shown. PAS and Giemsa. × 85.

297

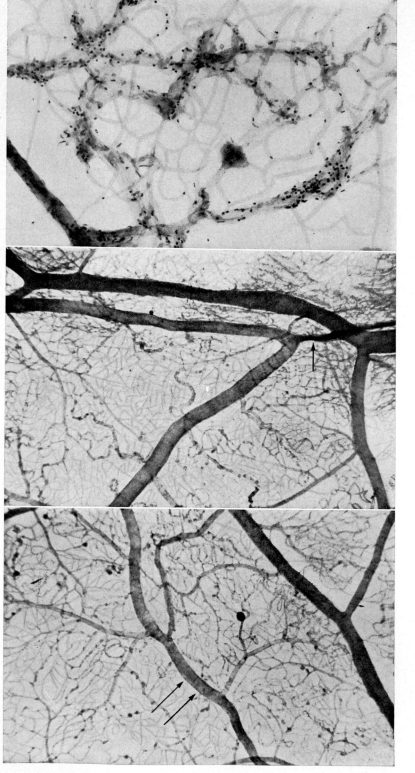

FIG. 4. Shunt vessels in advanced case of diabetic retinopathy. Bypassed atrophic capillaries are visible in background. PAS and Giemsa. × 85.

FIG. 5. Occlusion of branch of central retinal vein (arrow). Numerous shunt vessels and some capillary microaneurisms are also seen. PAS and Giemsa. × 21.

FIG. 6. Occlusion of branch of central retinal vein. Numerous capillary microaneurisms and shunt vessels can be seen surrounding occluded vein (arrow). PAS and Giemsa. × 21.

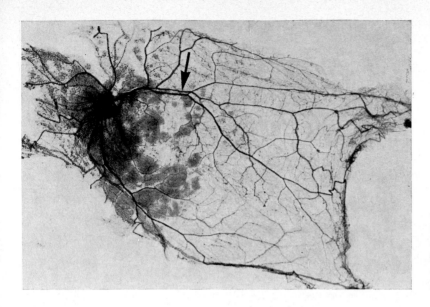

FIG. 7. Low-power view of occluded branch of central retinal vein (arrow). Capillary microaneurisms and shunt vessels are limited to area drained by occluded vein. PAS and Giemsa. × 4.2.

of shunt vessels. These are irregularly shaped, enlarged capillaries that appear in moderately advanced and in advanced cases of diabetic retinopathy. They are not newly formed capillaries as in proliferating retinopathy, but regular capillaries enlarged and dilated in order to maintain an overburdened capillary circulation. An accompanying result of shunting is atrophy of bypassed capillaries. These can be seen wherever shunt vessels are present, even as isolated occurrences (Fig. 4).

In the course of studying the retinal vasculature of the eyes in old age, a number of specimens were obtained exhibiting occlusions of retinal veins and arteries. Among these were four specimens with branch occlusions of the central retinal vein and one specimen with total occlusion of the central retinal vein. In the latter the capillary structure was almost completely replaced by shunt vessels. In the other four cases of branch vein occlusions, numerous shunt vessels and many capillary microaneurisms were seen (2). A recent case not previously described is shown here. The site of occlusion of the venous branch is seen near the disk where it is crossed by a retinal artery. The narrowed retinal vein is distinc-

tive (Fig. 5). As the vein is followed to its branches, numerous capillary microaneurisms are seen, clustered around these venules, and many shunt vessels appear in a widening sector approaching the periphery (Fig. 6). Surrounding the shunt vessels are numerous atrophic capillaries. The remainder of the retinal circulation is the relatively normal circulation of the aged eye, showing no microaneurisms, no shunt vessels and relatively few atrophic capillaries, as is common in old eyes (Fig. 7). The similarity of the appearance of the retinal circulation in these two conditions, diabetic retinopathy and venous occlusion, is striking and would seem to indicate that the basic pathologic factors are also similar.

At this point it may be possible to reconstruct the pathogenesis of diabetic retinopathy. Much work has been done on this phase of the problem (3). Much is known from clinical, pathological and physiological studies. The electron microscope has contributed important information on changes in the basement membrane of the capillaries and other ultramicroscopic structures.

Clinicians since Mackenzie and Nettleship in the 1870s (4) all agree that the initial indication of vascular change in the retinal circulation of the diabetic is a venous engorgement. The usual ratio of artery to vein of 2:3 is changed to 2:4 or more. This condition may last several years. The first sign of retinopathy is the appearance of small punctate hemorrhages, usually around the posterior pole on the temporal side. The duration of the diabetes appears to be a more important factor in the onset of retinopathy than the severity of the condition. There is no evidence of retinopathy in several patients seen clinically with severe, so-called brittle diabetes, with marked fluctuations in blood sugar from very high to very low, and several incidents of acidosis and insulin reaction. The onset of pinpoint hemorrhages is usually followed by the appearance of small gray-white exudates indicating a beginning vascular decompensation caused by venous obstruction initially involving the smaller branches. In addition, pathologic changes occur in the basement membranes of the capillaries in these areas. This is a fundamental condition; whether it results from decompensated capillary circulation and partial anoxia, or is a direct result of toxemia due to the diabetes, is not known. In any event, the basement membrane undergoes thickening and vacuolization, especially that portion between the mural cell and the outer border of the capillary (5, 6). The mural cell, also called intramural pericyte, undergoes eosinophilic degeneration (7), ultimately becoming so-called ghost cells (8). This rather selective degeneration may in turn be partly dependent on degeneration of adjacent glial and retinal cells, also considered to be concomitant with vascular decompensation, or a direct result of the metabolic toxemia of the diabetes. This area of the capillary wall is weakened and gives way under intracapillary blood pressure, leading to the sacculated outpouching seen ophthalmoscopically as minute pinpoint hemorrhages or capillary microaneurisms. The latter vary in size depending upon tissue strength, intracapillary blood pressure and the degree of venous obstruction.

Serum and blood cells exude through weakened capillary walls and lipid substances are deposited in the retina. Since circulation is poor, these substances remain as retinal exudates and hemorrhages.

Another drastic change takes place as a result of venous obstruction, whether localized to branch occlusion or to central vein occlusion. This is the formation of shunt vessels, which are dilated capillaries, not necessarily newly formed vessels, which attempt to take over the decompensated circulation to more patent veins nearby. In the process of shunt formation, surrounding capillaries are bypassed and undergo capillary atrophy. This is indicated by the narrowing of the capillary, loss of staining capacity, and loss of endothelial as well as mural cells.

Still another and more malignant phase of diabetic retinopathy is the formation of new vessels, usually at the disk margins and also in the retina proper. These new vessels are an attempt to reestablish the circulation in areas of venous obstruction and to compensate for the anoxia of the retinal tissue. Here a vasoformative factor postulated by Michaelson in 1954 (9), called the X-factor, may stimulate new vessel formation in the retina proper and such vessel formation may also extend into the vitreous. These thin-walled, newly formed capillaries bleed easily in the retina, and also as a result of vitreous traction when they extend into the vitreous. This was beautifully demonstrated by Davis (10). Eventually, recurrent vitreous hemorrhages and the formation of bands of fibrous tissue adhesions between vitreous and retina will result in retinal detachment and complete loss of vision. In an article by Beetham quoted by Davis (10), eyesight was lost in over 50% of eyes with proliferative retinopathy in a group of 351 patients studied over a period of 1 to 13 years. There is some comfort in the fact that

35 to 55% of these patients with proliferative retinopathy retained vision of 20/40 or better for prolonged periods of time.

There is a definite relationship of vein occlusion to arteriosclerosis of the central retinal artery and its branches in many cases of diabetic retinopathy with capillary microaneurisms and small and large hard exudates to an arteriovenous crossing nearby. This has been demonstrated (11) in three non-diabetic patients with so-called venous occlusion. These cases showed capillaropathy, diminution of endothelial and mural cells, and microaneurismal formation with pericapillary edema. Taylor and Dobree (12) studied 103 diabetic patients with proliferative retinopathy by serial fundus photography in 86 eyes. They found a high degree of correlation between the size and site of the lesion and the nearness of the arteriovenous crossing.

Apart from diabetic retinopathy and venous obstruction, microaneurisms have been seen in the eyes of old people, in macroglobulinemia, in eyes removed due to absolute glaucoma, and in sickle cell retinopathy. In the eyes of old people microaneurisms are usually found in the periphery, where the circulation is poor and cystic degeneration frequent. They are usually small, fusiform in shape, and several occur on the same capillary, forming capillary beading. In eyes removed due to absolute hemorrhagic glaucoma, the underlying cause is frequently venous obstruction of the central retinal vein. In macroglobulinemia and sickle-cell retinopathy, vascular decompensation may also be an underlying pathologic cause. While I have not had the opportunity to examine such eyes, they have been reported by others (13, 14).

Diabetes mellitus is a chronic condition requiring constant supervision and observation from the time of known onset and for the remainder of the patient's life. Methods of control and treatment have to be checked frequently. The control of hyperglycemia and glycosuria is a basic requirement in the management of the diabetic patient and in minimizing the ravages of diabetic retinopathy. This has been clearly shown by Balodimos et al. (15). We hereby suggest that current methods for the control of venous occlusion be included in such management. They should be started early, perhaps even at the time when treatment for diabetes is started. Patients with retinal vein obstruction treated with anticoagulants have shown much improvement, especially in branch occlusion. The danger in anticoagulant therapy is the possibility of an increased bleeding tendency. This has been pointed out by several investigators, particularly in the late stages of retinopathy. It should, however, be possible to control anticoagulant therapy at a safe prothrombin level and to maintain it for prolonged periods of time. In one study of a small group of cases on the use of oral heparin for a six-month period, improvement in diabetic exudative retinopathy was noted (16). The control of the blood lipids is also helpful in the total management of the diabetic patient. This may help to decrease atherosclerosis leading to venous obstruction at the arteriovenous crossing in the retina. When the diabetic is hypertensive, antihypertensive medication should be included in the regimen. The burden is on those physicians who specialize in the total care of the diabetic patient. These methods are certainly preferable to pituitary ablation and perhaps even to the use of photocoagulation after the onset and progression of diabetic retinopathy. Photocoagulation is useful where localized areas of newly-formed blood vessels and proliferative retinopathy can be seen and treated. Secondary bleeding may also occur in these cases. Such methods of treatment are late attempts to control a potentially malignant process.

A vigorous all-inclusive management of the

diabetic patient is suggested in the hope of preventing or ameliorating diabetic retinopathy, and perhaps other late sequelae of diabetes mellitus.

Thanks are due to Drs. M. Feldstein, J. Schneider, I. Eliasoph and A. S. Haft for the clinical histories, to Raymond Rivera for laboratory work and to Mrs. Ann Johnston for secretarial assistance.

Supported in part by Research Grant 2 R01 EY00533–04, from the National Eye Institute of the National Institutes of Health, Bethesda, the Medical Research Fund of NIH and the Fanton Foundation.

## REFERENCES

1. KUWABARA T and COGAN DG. Studies of retinal vascular patterns. I. Normal architecture. *Arch Ophthalmol* **64**: 904, 1960.
2. KORNZWEIG AL, ELIASOPH I and FELDSTEIN M. Occlusive disease of retinal vasculature. *Arch Ophthalmol* **71**: 542, 1964.
3. KIMURA SJ and CAYGILL WM (Eds), "Vascular complications of diabetes mellitus, with special reference to retinal angiopathy." St Louis, CV Mosby Co, 1967.
4. MACKENZIE S and NETTLESHIP E. A case of glycosuric retinitis, with comments, cited in: Duke-Elder S and Dobree JH. "System of ophthalmology." St Louis, CV Mosby Co, 1969, v 10, p 410.
5. BLOODWORTH JMB JR. Diabetic retinopathy. *Diabetes* **11**: 1, 1962.
6. BLOODWORTH JMB JR. Fine structure of retina in human and canine diabetes mellitus, in: Kimura SJ and Caygill WM (Eds), "Vascular complications of diabetes mellitus, with special reference to retinal angiopathy." St Louis, CV Mosby Co, 1967, p 73.
7. ADDISON DJ, GARNER A and ASHTON N. Degeneration of intramural pericytes in diabetic retinopathy. *Br Med J* **1**: 264, 1970.
8. COGAN DJ, TOUSSAINT D and KUWABARA T. Retinal vascular patterns. IV. Diabetic retinopathy. *Arch Ophthalmol* **66**: 366, 1961.
9. MICHAELSON IC. "Retinal circulation in man and animals." Springfield Ill, Charles C Thomas, 1954.
10. DAVIS MT. Natural course of diabetic retinopathy, in: Kimura SJ and Caygill WM (Eds), "Vascular complications of diabetes mellitus." St Louis, CV Mosby Co, 1967, chap 10.
11. RABINOVICZ IM, LITMAN S and MICHAELSON IC. Branch vein thrombosis—a pathologic report. *Trans Ophthalmol Soc UK* **88**: 191, 1968.
12. TAYLOR E and DOBREE JH. Proliferative diabetic retinopathy: site and size of initial lesions. *Br J Ophthalmol* **54**: 11, 1970.
13. ASHTON N, KOK D'A and FOULDS WS. Ocular pathology in macroglobulinemia. *J Pathol Bacteriol* **86**: 453, 1963.
14. KUWABARA T, CARROL JM and COGAN DJ. Retinal vascular patterns. III. Age, hypertension, absolute glaucoma, injury. *Arch Ophthalmol* **65**: 708, 1961.
15. BALODIMOS MC, AIELLO LM, GLEASON RE and MARBLE A. Retinopathy in mild diabetes of long standing. *Arch Ophthalmol* **81**: 660, 1969.
16. FINLEY JK and WEAVER HS. The use of heparin in the treatment of diabetic retinopathy. *Am J Ophthalmol* **50**: 483, 1960.

# RETINAL MICROCIRCULATION IN AREAS TREATED WITH PHOTOCOAGULATION

W. LEMMINGSON

Universitäts-Augenklinik, Tuebingen, German Federal Republic

There is considerable evidence suggesting that photocoagulation can be very effective in the treatment of diabetic retinopathy (1). However, in spite of all the experimental work done in this field, the mechanism leading to a vascular effect remains unknown. Changes in the large vessels (2) and atrophy of the capillaries (3) after photocoagulation have been demonstrated. Other investigations (4) have shown that xenon-arc coagulation may cause alterations in the permeability of the retinal vessels. In all of these studies, one point has never been examined, namely the effect of photocoagulation on the microcirculation of the treated areas. The present report describes some preliminary findings on this problem.

### MATERIAL AND METHODS

The pigmented eyes of 13 anesthetized cats were treated with a Zeiss photocoagulator. No more than four lesions were applied to the area of the tapetum nigrum with intensities I and II, diaphragm 0 and aperture 3°. The area of the tapetum lucidum was treated in the same manner in two cats. Microcirculation was studied by the incident-light technique using a Leitz vital microscope. The vessels were studied immediately after coagulation as well as one, three and seven days later. The vital microscopic examinations were complemented by fluorescein angiography at 3 frames/sec.

### RESULTS

The vital microscopic aspect of the capillary network about half an hour after photocoagulation with intensity I is illustrated in Fig. 1. Increased permeability of the deep capillary loops is characterized by exudation into the retinal tissue. Small arteriolar branches crossing the coagulated area showed segmental constrictions without thickening of the walls. The main arteries and veins were unaffected and capillary flow in the coagulated as well as in the surrounding areas was not appreciably altered. A slight plasma-skimming was found in some of the capillary loops adjacent to the center of the coagulated area. This suggests that the irregularities in the capillary network of the treated area may be stimulated by the so-called "plasma-skimming." Although neither stasis nor red cell aggregation were observed, there was a slight reduction in flow rate.

The effect of photocoagulation can be observed particularly well in the area of the tapetum lucidum (Fig. 2). The irregularities in the circulatory pattern of the capillary network are in this case caused by plasma-skimming.

Fluorescein angiography gave no evidence at all of capillary constriction. On the contrary, the capillary bed in the treated areas as well as in the surrounding zone showed marked dilatation. During the early arteriovenous phase additional capillaries became visible within the lesion, and a few seconds

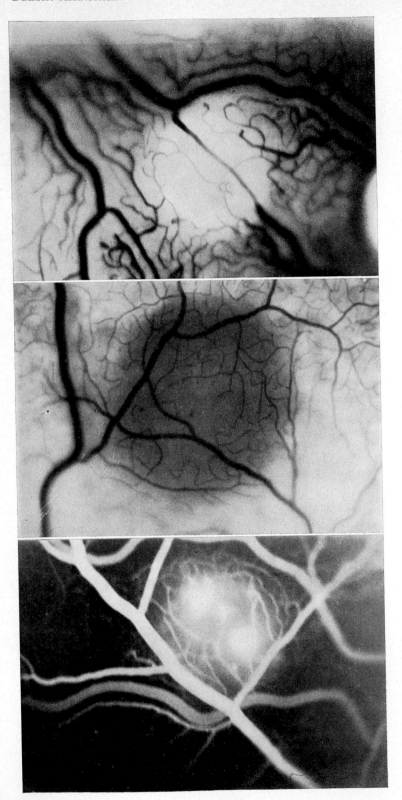

FIG. 1. Capillary network in cat's retina approximately half an hour after photocoagulation with intensity I. Vital microscopic observation.

FIG. 2. Photocoagulation with the same intensity in the area of the tapetum lucidum.

FIG. 3. The effect of photocoagulation one day later. Note the irregularities in the capillary network during fluorescein passage.

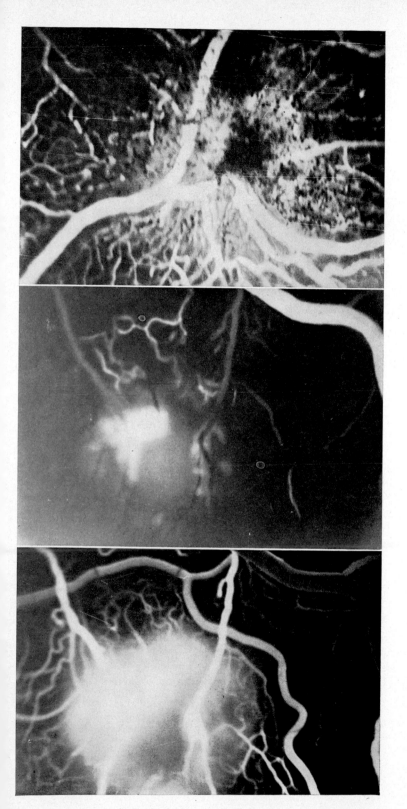

FIG. 4. Capillary pattern outside the pigmented scar seven days after photocoagulation with intensity I.

FIG. 5. Fluorescein angiogram one day after photocoagulation with intensity II. Extensive leakage from choriocapillaris.

FIG. 6. Circulatory bypass during capillary inflow. Arterial phase of fluorescein angiography.

305

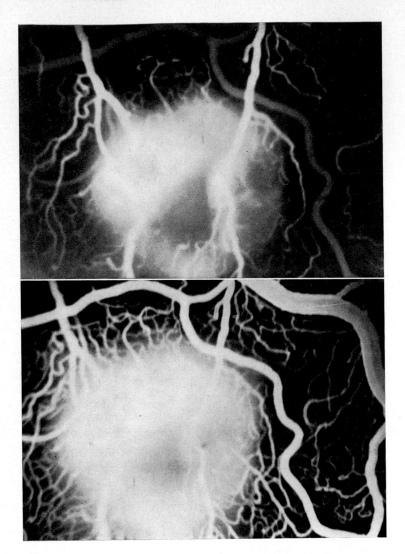

FIG. 7. Venous phase of fluorescein angiography.

FIG. 8. Complete filling of capillary network at the margin of necrotic area during serial angiogram.

later the coagulated area was covered by a dense cloud of leaking fluorescein.

Fig. 3 illustrates the changes observed one day after photocoagulation. Considerable dilatation of the capillary bed was still evident. Immediately after the injection of fluorescein, during the arterial phase of angiography, multiple but more or less circumscribed fluorescein clouds appeared and spread rapidly. Irregularities in the capillary network at the border of the leakage are consistent with recent obliteration. A pronounced dilatation of capillaries outside the irregular network was a frequent finding.

On the third day after photocoagulation the first ingrowth of pigment into the coagulated area became visible. Outside the lesion, the circulatory pattern showed a normal architecture and an intact flow. At the border of the coagulated area the capillary bed was still dilated but no alteration of capillary flow was visible. Capillary circulation was absent from the central part of the lesion.

Seven days after treatment, there was no

longer any exudation. Considerable pigment migration into the lesion had occurred. The capillary network in the central part of the coagulated area was completely replaced by pigmented scar tissue (Fig. 4). A dense capillary network showing no leakage of fluorescein surrounded this pigmented area.

A series of microphotographs taken during the fluorescein passage demonstrates the effect of intensity II photocoagulation one day after treatment. As early as in the choroidal phase multiple and rapidly extending fluorescent spots appeared in the coagulated area (Fig. 5). They were not located exactly in the area of central necrosis but more towards the margin. The inflow of fluorescein dye into the capillary bed of the treated area as well as into the adjacent zone was markedly delayed and the dye reached the capillaries only in the venous phase. The majority of the vessels were bypassed, suggesting that pronounced filling of the precapillary arterioles was followed by rapid outflow through the dilated postcapillary venules as illustrated in Fig. 6 and 7. Later in the course of fluorescein passage, complete filling of the intact capillary network at the margin of the necrotic area took place (Fig. 8). The central part of the coagulated area was still devoid of fluorescein although there was well-marked leakage. In the late venous phase some venous branches crossing the treated area showed a flow of fluorescein without any signs of intravascular thrombosis.

### DISCUSSION

Since photocoagulation is a circumscribed thermal injury, its primary effect is a disturbed permeability in both the choriocapillaris and deep retinal capillary loops. A well marked dilatation of the capillary bed occurs secondarily in the affected areas although there is neither red cell aggregation nor intravascular stasis. A slight plasma-skimming immediately

after coagulation exaggerates the reduction of the capillary pattern.

When intensities higher than I were used immediate damage to the capillary bed in the coagulated areas was observed. Contrary to the histopathological changes found by Wood and Watzke (3), the first obliterative signs in the cat's retina started as early as 24 hr after coagulation. Due to the rapid migration of pigment into the coagulated area visible on the third day after treatment it was difficult to follow any further changes in the capillary bed. The capillary bed surrounding the coagulated area was unaffected.

The delayed inflow of fluorescein into the coagulated areas and the bypass during the venous phase are particularly interesting. The bypassing of the affected capillaries may explain why no hemorrhages occurred. As previously discussed by Rosan et al. (5) the photographs taken during dye passage show that both the vascular supply and flow dynamics are altered.

Since the capillary obliteration produced by low and medium xenon-arc intensities is gradual, the microcirculation is able to adapt itself so that an acute breakdown of capillary circulation in both coagulated and adjoining areas does not occur. This may explain the normalizing effect of photocoagulation in vascular disorders of the retina.

Supported by Deutsche Forschungsgemeinschaft.

### REFERENCES

1. MEYER-SCHWICKERATH G. "Light coagulation." St Louis, CV Mosby Co, 1960.
2. MILES DR and RUIZ RS. The effects of photocoagulation on the large retinal vessels of the rabbit eye. Am J Ophthalmol 64: 1089, 1967.
3. WOOD LW and WATZKE RC. The effects of photo- and laser coagulation on the retinal vasculature. Arch Ophthalmol 82: 499, 1969.
4. WESSING A, in: "Fluoresszenzangiographie der Retina." Stuttgart, G Thieme, 1968.
5. ROSAN RC, FLOCKS M, VASSILIADIS A, ROSE HW, PEABODY RR and HAMMOND A. Pathology of monkey retina following irradiation with argon laser. Arch Ophthalmol 81: 84, 1969.

# TREATMENT OF PROLIFERATIVE DIABETIC RETINOPATHY BY REPEATED LIGHT COAGULATION, OPERATIONS AND REST

J. H. DOBREE

St. Bartholomew's Hospital, London, England

The treatment of proliferative diabetic retinopathy by destruction of potential bleeding points using direct photocoagulation or laser beams is now generally accepted to be of value in certain cases, particularly where an active bleeding site can be identified and eradicated. This communication reports a large number of cases which have been treated for more than six years on principles based on a knowledge of the natural evolution of the condition, in which all possible bleeding areas have been systematically eradicated as and when they occur; and the bleeding tendency of other groups has been minimized by restricting certain forms of physical activity.

*Natural evolution.* The formation of new vessels on the disk or on the course of the main retinal vessels starts as arcades of capillaries without supporting connective tissue (Stage I). After a year or so when these arcades enlarge, connective tissue mantles surround them (Stage II). After a further period varying from one to three years, the new vessels, having reached their greatest development, then regress. At the same time the connective tissue surrounding them becomes denser, until finally the new vessel formations are entirely replaced by connective tissue. This is Stage III or the cicatricial stage.

All groups of new vessels pass through these stages, and different groups in the same eye are often found at different stages of development. During Stage I and II the new vessels are likely to bleed, and in Stage III the bleeding tendency decreases, but the contracting connective tissue carries with it the danger of retinoschisis or retinal detachment.

*Rationale of treatment.* The new vessels themselves are directly attacked by light coagulation with two overriding exceptions: 1) new vessels on the disk are not directly coagulated and 2) if they are progressing to the natural cicatricial stage (Stage III), not only is coagulation unnecessary, but it may cause sudden contraction of connective tissue and precipitate a schisis or detachment.

Light coagulation has three distinct roles in treatment. The first role is direct coagulation to eradicate as many as possible of the new vessel groupings which often number some 10 to 20 in a single eye. The tendency to hemorrhage is thereby considerably reduced. The second is indirect treatment of disk vessels by multiple coagulation of normal retina, as advocated by Aiello (1). These vessels often show marked regression or rapid evolution to the cicatricial stage. Finally, the coagulation of new vessel groupings along the retinal vessels when they are at an early stage prevents the formation of connective tissue, with its attendant evils of schisis, detachment and dragging on the normal vessels.

*Clinical material.* One hundred and sixty-four eyes of 122 patients were treated by light coagulation and restriction of physical activity. These were compared with 59 controls which have already been described (2). The cases were observed for seven years or more, and the controls for longer. Eleven of the eyes in the treated series were observed for over five years, and 17 of the control eyes for a similar period.

*Preliminary assessment.* The general diabetic state and the state of the heart, peripheral circulation, kidneys and peripheral nerves were carefully assessed by a physician specializing in diabetes.

*The ocular assessment.* The corrected visual acuity was determined, and the media explored for evidence of cataract. New vessel formations and connective tissue bands were carefully mapped. Pathology in the veins and arterioles and the state of the posterior poles with regard to hard and soft exudates, microaneurysms and hemorrhages were noted. Particular care was taken to identify the source of bleeding responsible for any subhyaloid or vitreous hemorrhages. Finally, the fundus was carefully photographed to include the disk and macula, the main vessel groupings as far as the equator, and any other peripheral pathological features that may be present. Only after this assessment was treatment started.

*Initial treatment.* Depending on the extent of the new vessel formations, from 10 to 100 coagulations were applied in a single session. It was rarely necessary to exceed a total of 150 initial coagulations in all. The 4.5 aperture was used with the Green II setting.

Thereafter cases were reviewed at intervals of four months or in exceptional circum-stances six months. Very rarely—in the case of overseas patients—review was done once a year. At follow-up the fundus was carefully explored for further new vessels, especially if there had been symptoms indicating hemorrhage. If any retinal new vessels were present the patient was readmitted for further coagulation. In these cases the coagulations required were much fewer in number, usually from about 10 to 20. On the average, four coagulation operations were spread over a five-year period and the greatest number was 11.

Details of treatment and technique are fully described in ref. 2 and 4. All types of retinal new vessel formation were tackled, including those well forward from the retina. Disk vessels and vessels with much connective tissue in their direct vicinity were left strictly alone.

Disk vessels sometimes completely or partially regressed as shown by the "pattern bombing" method of Aiello (1). We are still undecided whether it is better to "bomb" the retina in the vicinity of the main vessel groupings or towards the periphery. However, we have found that regression or rapid cicatrization is liable to occur in eyes which have had over 100 coagulations. The 4.5 aperture is normally used and the destruction of about one-sixth of the normal retina was calculated to occur. Six of the cases in the present series in which regression occurred were reported earlier (3).

*General measures.* Complete bed rest is mandatory if a hemorrhage occurs between observations. If the hemorrhage is large, patients are hospitalized. Remarkable clearing of hemorrhages which had been present for months occurred with two or three weeks of complete bed rest. We observed the patients daily and attempted to determine the source of bleeding. In heavy bleeding from disk vessels it was often possible to reduce the bleeding tendency by waiting for a clearing to take place at the periphery and pattern bombing there. Perhaps the most important measure was constantly to stress the importance of living with considerably reduced physical activity. Stooping, lifting and straining at coughing or at stool should always be avoided, and if the hemorrhagic phase of the first three or four years can be safely passed without extensive hemorrhages the long-term prognosis is immeasurably better.

### RESULTS

This is a complete and continuous series of patients with photographic observations extending over 10 years, who were treated by photocoagulation for more than seven years. Only three cases were discarded from the series because of failure in follow-up. Thus the failures in treatment previously reported by Dobree (2) and Dobree and Taylor (4) were still included. Despite this our series includes 164 eyes from 122 patients which, we think, were of at least average severity, since most were referred from other clinics. It is possible to compare the parameter of "retention of visual acuity" in cases and controls as was done in the figures of the Airlie House Symposium (1). The figures for the controls were taken directly from the data already published in the proceedings of that meeting. Of the 59 control eyes, 23 (38.9%) retained the same visual acuity during the whole period of observation. Of 164 treated eyes observed from a comparable period, 100 (60.9%) retained the same vision as they had before the first light coagulation. A comparison of cases followed for three, four and over five years is more meaningful. After three years, 8 of 29 eyes in the control group retained the same visual acuity (27.6%) whereas in the treated group, 25 of 50 eyes retained the same visual acuity (50%). In the four-year group, 6 of 25 (24.0%) eyes from the control group and 8 of 19 (42.1%) treated eyes retained vision. The trend for the few

TABLE 1.   *Retention of visual acuity cases*

| Years under observation | No. retaining original vision | No. of controls retaining original vision |
|:---:|:---:|:---:|
| 5+ | 6/11 | 4/17 |
| 4 to 5 | 2/ 8 | 2/ 8 |
| 3 to 4 | 17/31 | 2/ 4 |
| 2 to 3 | 27/38 | 2/ 9 |
| 1 to 2 | 17/34 | 9/15 |
| 0 to 1 | 31/42 | 4/ 6 |
| TOTAL | 100/164 | 23/59 |

eyes surviving over five years is the same: with 4 of 17 in the control group (23.5%) and 6 of 11 in the treated group (54.5%) retaining the same visual acuity. See Table 1.

It is thus possible to enable patients to retain good vision for many years longer than was supposed some years ago. In terms of the economics of treatment this is undoubtedly expensive since light coagulators, lasers and hospitalization and the training of staff in the use of coagulators are all costly. However, since diabetes is an increasing world problem, money for education, research and treatment would be well expended on this group of patients, usually at the prime of life and the peak of their working capacity.

### REFERENCES

1. AIELLO L, BEETHAM WP, BALODIMOS MC, CHAZAN BI and BRADEY RF. Ruby laser photocoagulation in treatment of diabetic proliferative retinopathy: Preliminary report, in: Goldberg MF and Fine SL (Eds), "Symposium on the Treatment of Diabetic Retinopathy." Public Health Service Pub No 1890, Washington, DC, Government Printing Office, 1968, p 437.
2. DOBREE JH, in: Goldberg MF and Fine SL (Eds), "Symposium on the treatment of diabetic retinopathy." Public Health Service Pub No 1890, Washington DC, Government Printing Office, 1968, pp 479, 775.
3. TAYLOR E. Proliferative diabetic retinopathy. Regression of optic disc neovascularization after retinal photocoagulation. *Br J Ophthalmol* **54**: 535, 1970.
4. DOBREE JH and TAYLOR E. Treatment of proliferative diabetic retinopathy by light coagulation. *Trans Ophthalmol Soc UK* **88**: 313, 1968.

# TREATMENT OF
# DIABETIC RETINOPATHY BY PHOTOCOAGULATION

TH. N. WAUBKE

Augenklinik der Ruhr-Universität, Bochum 43 Essen, German Federal Republic

Diabetic retinopathy represents one of the major causes of blindness in adults. The many attempts to influence the progress of the angiopathy either by drugs or by neurosurgical intervention reflect the magnitude of the problem.

Photocoagulation made possible the treatment of the process in the eye itself (1–9). In 1959 Meyer-Schwickerath (10) reported the use of photocoagulation in five patients with diabetic retinopathy. Four of them, being in the proliferative stage of the disease, could not be helped; while one patient, with only microaneurysms and hard exudates, showed a marked improvement. This treatment was cautiously continued by us in the following years. Our aim was to prevent the recurrent hemorrhages arising from microaneurysms and newly formed vessels, and at the same time to prevent retinal detachment by multiple coagulations. In spite of some very impressive results, we remained sceptical for a long time. However, a review of our material in 1964 revealed the efficacy of photocoagulation. It was mainly the early stages that seemed to show obvious improvement, both anatomically and functionally.

Meanwhile other authors also reported the treatment of diabetic retinopathy by photocoagulation. At a symposium of the U.S. Public Health Service held in Warrenton, Virginia (11), all available treated cases were thoroughly discussed. This included a total of 1,635 proliferative and 159 nonproliferative cases. Although the effectiveness of photocoagulation seemed limited in advanced stages of the disease, in other cases blocking the progress of the disease and even improvement could be achieved by means of photocoagulation. Furthermore, the possibility of combining hypophysectomy with photocoagulation and the use of laser coagulators instead of the conventional xenon apparatus were discussed.

We here present our technique of photocoagulation as well as the results of this treatment.

### METHODS

Most of the photocoagulations were performed with the Zeiss xenon-arc coagulator. We usually coagulate microaneurysms and newly formed vessels at the level of the retina, and small early proliferations in the vitreous if they are present. The diameter of each area of coagulation is between 1.5 and 3 degrees. The intensity is chosen in such a way that a slight whitish discoloration of the retina becomes visible within 0.5 to 1.0 sec. We usually remain approximately two disk diameters away from the macular area.

If the diabetic changes are not too extensive, the whole area is coagulated in one session. The number of coagulations may range from 100 to 350. If the changes are rather advanced and extensive, we prefer to perform the coagulation in two or sometimes three sessions. Most of the treatments are performed as outpatient procedures. Only in difficult cases is the patient admitted to hospital for treatment.

Complications are extremely rare if the treatment is undertaken in the early stages. Any hemorrhages which may occur are usually small. However, in those cases in which proliferation is present in the vitreous, the danger of postcoagulation hemorrhages is great. A further complication is the occurrence of an exudative retinal detachment in those cases in which many coagulations are performed. However, this exudative detachment usually disappears within a few days.

As far as optical conditions permit, all outpatients are photographed before and after coagulation. The material was studied case by case and the fundus photographs, which often had been taken at intervals of several years, were compared and evaluated.

## RESULTS

The principal results of this study are the following: 1) Microaneurysms, dilated capillaries and rete mirabile formations at the retinal level are obliterated and disappear after photocoagulation. 2) The vascular changes recede even when affected areas have not been directly hit by the light beam. 3) The volume of the veins decreases. 4) Edema of the retina, which practically always occurs in diabetic retinopathy, disappears after coagulation. The pattern of the choroid, previously obscured by the retinal opacity, becomes visible again. 5) Waxy hard exudates regress. Depending on how long they last, they leave behind either a functioning retina or a scar. 6) In juvenile diabetics the regression of the pathological changes takes place much faster than in patients over the age of 50. 7) Photocoagulation is able to prevent the proliferation of vessels into the vitreous body. 8) In cases where vitreal proliferations are already present, photocoagulation becomes difficult. In our experience, only initial proliferations can be controlled. Because of the danger of shrinkage, fibrotic areas should not be coagulated.

TABLE 1. *Results of treatment of 189 eyes by photocoagulation*

| Classification | No. of patients | | |
| --- | --- | --- | --- |
| | Improve- ment | No change | Pro- gression |
| Group B: background retinopathy | 81 | 39 | 9 |
| Group N: retinopathy with new vessel formation and fibrous proliferation | 12 | 34 | 14 |

Over the last years we have treated several thousand patients with diabetic retinopathy. However, prior to the end of 1967, we had treated only 127. Of these patients, 44 were male and 83 were female. Twenty-four were under 40 years of age and 103 were older. Altogether, 189 eyes were treated. These cases are grouped according to the O'Hare classification. We have put the proliferative cases in group N of this classification. The period of observation was between nine months and seven years, with an average of 2.6 years.

Table 1 shows the results of treatment as judged by ophthalmoscopic findings. The results in group B, i.e. cases having a pure background retinopathy and little blurring by hemorrhage, are very favorable. Eighty-one of 129 eyes in group B showed regression of diabetic changes, especially a disappearance of microaneurysms and yellowish exudates, as well as of retinal edema. In 39 eyes, diabetic changes with some microaneurysms and exudates still remained. These effects were, however, less severe than before treatment. In only nine cases did we find an increase in diabetic changes and the occurrence of new hemorrhages.

In group N (proliferative retinopathy), the results are quite different, and much less favorable. Only 12 of 60 eyes improved, and 14 eyes became blind.

If we analyze only those cases observed

TABLE 2. *Results of treatment by photocoagulation after three years (48 eyes)*

| | No. of cases | | |
| | Improve-ment | No change | Pro-gression |
|---|---|---|---|
| Classification | | | |
| Group B: | | | |
| background retinopathy | 25 | 9 | 4 |
| Group N: | | | |
| retinopathy with new vessel formation and fibrous proliferation | 1 | 7 | 2 |

for three years or more (Table 2), an increasing discrepancy between the results of treatment in pure background cases and in the proliferative cases is observed.

The same is shown by analyzing the visual acuity in the nonproliferative cases. In group B, the overall visual acuity remained unchanged before and after treatment. There are some patients with loss of visual acuity and others with marked improvement. In contrast, in group N there is a marked trend toward impairment of visual acuity, and, in many cases the final result is, practically, blindness. This is true for the diabetic retinopathy of both young and old patients.

Complications are rare in group B, but are more frequent in group N. In 129 cases of nonproliferating diabetic retinopathy, there were only six patients with hemorrhage after photocoagulation. In group N, however, 22 hemorrhages occurred among 80 treated patients. Furthermore, there were four cases of secondary glaucoma, three of exudative detachment and two of optic atrophy.

It is remarkable that most of our patients did not realize the defects in the visual field which occur after photocoagulation, even in those cases in which several hundred coagulations had been performed. Recording of the visual field by the Goldman perimeter generally showed a small and irregular restriction. Also, when a small and circumscribed coagulation had been performed close to the disk and the macula, large field defects did not occur. Coagulation in the area of the papillomacular bundle damaged neither central vision nor nerve fibers, if it were performed with a small diameter and with low intensity.

DISCUSSION

The evaluation of the results of any attempt to treat diabetic retinopathy raises some fundamental difficulties. Currently, little is known about its natural course. Periods of rapid progression and cessation alternate; and spontaneous remission may occur. Even advanced cases of retinopathy can come to a standstill and to a stage of relative healing. For the determination of these phenomena and of the therapeutic effect of treatment, measurement of central vision is by no means sufficient: on the one hand, minimal changes in the macula can lead to a severe loss of vision, while on the other hand, in the periphery, advanced proliferation of vessels into the vitreous can, for a time, remain without a distinct decrease in visual acuity.

Therapeutic results can, therefore, best be interpreted by considering the morphologic details. Here, comparative fundus photography is our most useful method, since we can analyze microstructural changes over a long period of time.

When photocoagulation is applied before the stage of vessel proliferation, the symptoms of diabetic retinopathy are almost always reversible. By treatment in the early stage, late sequelae with proliferations, hemorrhages and retinal detachment can be prevented. If, however, vessel proliferation and fibrous changes are already present at the time treatment is begun, photocoagulation is too late to prevent the progression of the disease.

The way in which photocoagulation acts on diabetic angiopathy of the retina is unknown. It has been suggested that changes in intravascular pressure or an improvement in the oxygen supply to the remaining undestroyed retina may play an important role. Fluorescein studies performed by us in the past three years have shown that after photocoagulation, marked changes occur in the capillary pattern, and these fall into one of two types:

1) *Improvement in the disturbed permeability.* Return of capillary disorders to normal may occur at some distance from the area of photocoagulation. The angiogram before coagulation shows the typical changes of diabetic angiopathy: dilatation of capillaries and microaneurysms. It also shows that at the margin of the disk there is severe impairment of permeability, a sign of early formation of new capillaries. In the arteriovenous phase, fluorescein passes through the wall, and in the venous phase the disk and its surrounding area are hidden by a dense cloud of fluorescein. The control photograph a year after photocoagulation shows that all of this has disappeared. The margin of the disk can be clearly seen during the different phases of the angiogram, and there is no sign of fluorescein leakage from the vessel.

This regression of the impaired permeability indicates that after photocoagulation, a functioning blood tissue barrier may be reestablished.

2) *Occurrence of a new capillary pattern.* The angiogram before coagulation shows typical findings: capillary dilatation, microaneurysms, hemorrhages and leakage of dye. In contrast, a pattern of rather large capillaries extending quite regularly over the whole posterior fundus is seen in the angiogram taken a year after photocoagulation. Some of the microaneurysms are still visible, but the leakage of fluorescein into the tissue has been considerably reduced. This new pattern is not a temporary effect of the treatment, but a long-lasting change in the whole capillary network. This was made clear by many follow-up control examinations over a period of more than one and a half years. In untreated eyes we never observed this typical alteration of the capillaries which extends so regularly over the whole fundus. The newly formed capillary pattern which develops after photocoagulation seems to demonstrate new adaptations in both the hemodynamics and the metabolism of the retina.

### CONCLUSION

We cannot explain how photocoagulation acts in diabetic retinopathy. It is doubtful whether direct coagulation of microaneurysms and newly formed vessels is essential for regression of the symptoms. As we have seen, abnormal vessels and microaneurysms disappear even if no coagulation treatment is given. It is well established (12–17) that diabetic retinopathy may be either prevented or caused to regress in the presence of high myopia, optic atrophy, disseminated choroiditis or extensive diathermy scars. It may be concluded that the effect of photocoagulation is due to the destruction of retinal tissue, thereby causing an improvement in the oxygen supply of the remaining retina. Hickham and Fraser (17) have shown by fluorescein angiography that there is a marked decrease in the blood flow in diabetic retinopathy.

Photocoagulation is certainly a destructive and symptomatic treatment of diabetic retinopathy. We recommend it in the early stages when the risk of this treatment is low.

### REFERENCES

1. GUILLAUMAT L. Indications et limites de la photocoagulation dans le traitement de la retinopathie diabetique. *Bibl Ophthalmol* **76**: 154, 1968.
2. GUILLAUMAT L and ESTA A. Indications et limites de la photocoagulation dans le traitement de la retinopathie diabetique. *Ann Ocul (Paris)* **201**: 516, 1968.
3. MOURA-BRAZIL N and DE-REZENDE J. Le role de la photocoagulation en ophthalmologie. *Bull Soc Ophthalmol Fr* **74**: 699, 1961.
4. THORNFELDT PR. Treatment of retinitis proliferans by photocoagulation. *Excerpta Med (Amst)* Sect XII **74**: 35, 1964.

5. THORNFELDT P. Treatment of retinitis proliferans by photocoagulation. *Northwest Med* **64**: 928, 1965.
6. WETZIG PC and JEPSON CN. Treatment of diabetic retinopathy by light coagulation. *Am J Ophthalmol* **62**: 449, 1966.
7. WETZIG PC and JEPSON CN. Further observations on the treatment of diabetic retinopathy by light-coagulation. *Trans Am Acad Ophthalmol* **71**: 902, 1967.
8. WETZIG PC and JEPSON CN. The intravenous use of fluorescein as an adjunct in light-coagulation. *Mod Probl Ophthalmol (Basel)* **7**: 276, 1968.
9. WETZIG PC and WORLTON JP. Treatment of diabetic retinopathy by light-coagulation. *Br J Ophthalmol* **47**: 539, 1963.
10. MEYER-SCHWICKERATH G. Lichtkoagulation. *Klin Monatsbl Augenheilkd* **33**: 1959.
11. GOLDBERG MF and FINE SC. "Symposium on the treatment of diabetic retinopathy." PHS Pub No 1890, Public Health Service, Washington, 1968.
12. AMALRIC P. Nouvelles considerations concernant l'evolution et le traitement de la retinopathie diabetique. *Ophthalmologica* **154**: 151, 1967.
13. AMALRIC P and BIAU C. La diathermiecoagulation et la photocoagulation dans le traitement de la retinopathie diabetique. *Arch Ophthalmol (Paris)* **27**: 553, 1967.
14. OKUN E. The effectiveness of photocoagulation in the therapy of proliferative diabetic retinopathy *Trans Am Acad Ophthalmol Otolaryngol* **72**: 246, 1968.
15. OKUN E and CIBIS FA. The role of photocoagulation in the therapy of proliferative diabetic retinopathy. *Arch Ophthalmol* **75**: 337, 1966.
16. MEYER-SCHWICKERATH G. Photocoagulation in diabetic retinopathy. *Am J Ophthalmol* **66**: 597, 1968.
17. HICKHAM JB and FRASER R. Studies of the retinal circulation in man. Observations on vessel diameter, arteriovenous oxygen difference and mean circulation time. *Circulation* **33**: 302, 1966.

# RUBY LASER PHOTOCOAGULATION IN DIABETIC RETINOPATHY

LLOYD M. AIELLO

Department of Ophthalmology, New England Deaconess Hospital, Boston, Massachusetts, USA

Xenon arc photocoagulation has been successfully used to destroy patches of neovascularization. However, when used extensively and diffusely, it may produce serious visual field defects, active hemorrhages, an increase in fibrous tissue with resulting traction and secondary retinal detachment. A strikingly similar retinal picture is observed in the few arrested cases of diabetic retinopathy because of either spontaneous remission, pituitary ablation or xenon arc photocoagulation as well as in those diabetic eyes with chorioretinitis scarring, optic atrophy or high myopia. In the spontaneously arrested cases, there is much less venous distention; the arterial tree becomes smaller and attenuated; the patches of neovascularization appear to shrink and disappear; the fibrous tissue becomes thin, lace-like and reticulated; the optic disk is often pale, suggesting mild atrophy; hemorrhages and microaneurisms become scarce or absent. A similar diminution in retinal vascular activity occurs in patients successfully treated by pituitary ablation. The eyes of diabetics with nonspecific disseminated chorioretinitis show not only an absence of visual field disturbance, but also relatively small retinal arteries and veins and pale optic nerve heads with no evidence of diabetic retinal vascular disease.

It has been suggested (1) that a reduction of the vascular activity in the posterior pole of patients with diabetic retinopathy might be accomplished by producing or creating numerous small, relatively harmless scars in the retina and choroid by ruby laser photocoagulation. A technique of modified chorioretinal suppression might thus be possible without producing the large sector field defects seen after treatment with the xenon arc photocoagulator. Modified chorioretinal suppression, by inducing hemodynamic and metabolic changes which could alter the natural course of the disease at an early stage, may prevent the severe and irreversible changes that occur at later stages.

## MATERIALS AND METHODS

Using the American Optical Co. ruby laser photocoagulator, 200 to 300 applications of $2.5°$ (0.75 mm) Grade II ruby laser lesions are made during each of three or four sittings: a total of 600 to 1,000 lesions. Care is taken to avoid the maculopapular bundle, disk and macula. Neither retrobulbar nor any other anesthesia is necessary and each treatment takes 20 to 30 min. The patients experience no discomfort other than the slight irritation of having to keep their eyes open without blinking for intervals of 2 to 3 min. Once the lesions are properly placed, no complications from the treatment ensue. As with any photocoagulation technique, excess energy input may cause immediate preretinal or vitreous hemorrhage.

## RESULTS

Since February 1967, 500 patients have had one of their eyes treated by the circumferential ruby laser coagulation technique. A three-year follow-up was carried out on 115 of the patients. Twenty-three of these died and 12 failed to appear for follow-up study.

Among 80 patients, there was a definite reduction in the neovascular and background angiopathy in 78% of the treated eyes, compared to 3% of the untreated eyes. Although 55% of the untreated eyes became worse, 42% did not progress in their degree of neovascularization. These findings suggest that a longer follow-up period is necessary.

Of greater significance is a group of 99 "control" patients who were followed up for two years. These were divided into three groups: Group 1, 36 patients having neovascularization at the retinal level but not involving the disk; Group 2, 36 patients showing very early neovascularization of the disk with or without neovascularization elsewhere flat on the retina; Group 3, 27 patients showing advanced neovascularization of both the retina and the disk.

In all the patients in the above groups, both eyes were equal in both type and degree of diabetic proliferating retinopathy before treatment. Only one of the eyes was treated in each patient and the other served as a control. Ophthalmoscopy, color retinal photography and fluorescein angiography were used to determine the similarity of the disease in both eyes.

In Group 1, 32 of the 36 treated eyes showed a reduction in the degree of neovascularization whereas in the untreated eyes, none showed any improvement. Of the latter group, 27 remained unchanged. In Group 2, improvement in the neovascularization stage occurred in 26 of 36 eyes in the treated group. There was no improvement in any of the eyes in the untreated group, although 24 of them remained unchanged over the follow-up period of two years. Considering Groups 1 and 2 together, 80% of the treated eyes showed definite improvement towards a lesser stage of neovascular retinopathy, while 54% showed a complete disappearance of neovascularization. The condition of all the untreated controls either remained unchanged or worsened; none of them improved. In Group 3, 20 out of 27 (74%) of the treated eyes showed a stabilization of both vision and angiopathy for two years following treatment, as compared with only 26% of the patients in the untreated group.

In patients with severe fibrous proliferation and neovascularization, ruby laser treatment appeared to have a beneficial effect only on the neovascular component. Frequently, however, secondary retinal detachment followed some months later. The laser scars thus did not prevent the development of secondary retinal detachment. On the other hand, the ruby light itself decreased the hazards to the media at the low energy level used in these studies. Postoperative vitreous traction was not related to treatment per se, and delayed postoperative hemorrhage could not be attributed to the ruby laser treatment technique.

## DISCUSSION

The results of these studies suggest the interesting and exciting hypothesis that the progress of diabetic neovascular proliferating retinopathy can be altered by reducing the amount of functioning retina. The retinochoroidal metabolic or hemodynamic balance can be altered by producing numerous small harmless nonfunctioning chorioretinal scars with a ruby laser photocoagulator. This is now being tested on a large group of patients with proliferating diabetic retinopathy. The short-term results have been encouraging and suggest that this treatment causes a regression of certain manifestations of diabetic retinopathy. However, only long-term observations can enable us to assess accurately the efficacy of ruby laser photocoagulation.

We are currently in great need of a common classification of controlled groups of patients and of long-term observations of both treated and untreated eyes. The latter requires that the degree of retinal pathology be equal in both eyes of a given patient before any of the photocoagulation techniques are tried. Such prospective control studies are important (especially in view of the new methods becoming available) in order 1) to verify short- and long-term results and complications and 2) to control our eagerness to photocoagulate every eye of all diabetics without taking into consideration the natural history and complexities of this disease process, the mechanisms by which treatment may be effective and finally both the short- and long-term hazards of this therapeutic tool.

REFERENCE

1. BEETHAM WP, AIELLO LM, BALODIMOS MC and KONCZ L. Ruby laser photocoagulation of early diabetic neovascular retinopathy. *Arch Ophthalmol* **83**: 261, 1970.

# ARGON LASER PHOTOCOAGULATION IN DIABETIC RETINOPATHY

ARNALL PATZ

Wilmer Institute, Johns Hopkins Hospital, Baltimore, Maryland, USA

The introduction of the argon laser by L'Esperance (1–4) introduced a new dimension to photocoagulation therapy. The precise focusing capabilities, the high energy density and the high absorption of the energy by hemoglobin make the argon laser especially useful in the treatment of several retinal vascular diseases, and particularly in proliferative diabetic retinopathy.

### PROLIFERATIVE DIABETIC RETINOPATHY

The management of advanced cases of proliferative diabetic retinopathy, especially those involving neovascularization at the disk, has presented a special problem in technique. Routine argon laser photocoagulation, without concern for the vascular flow characteristics of the neovascularization, can result in a significant incidence of hemorrhage at treatment or during the first few days after therapy. Some of these hemorrhages are of such severity as to result in severe visual impairment. Following these major hemorrhages, a significant fibrous proliferation and further neovascularization may ensue. The minor hemorrhages of less than 1/10 the disk diameter, which seem to result from extrusion of the trapped blood in the tips of the neovascular tuft during coagulation, are of no major concern, and are usually absorbed within a day of treatment.

Behrendt et al. (5) first advocated the use of fluorescein angiography to identify the characteristics of arterial and venous flow, as a guide to therapy. This has proven especially useful in our hands in selected cases. However, in the majority of patients, the distinct arterial feeder to the tuft has not been identified. Furthermore, when a distinct pattern is identified, it is frequently difficult to translate the high contrast vascular landmarks of the fluorescein photograph to the intact fundus. We have found the technique useful in about one-third of 100 consecutive disk neovascularization cases.

In those cases without a specific arterial-venous flow pattern, one can reduce the frequency of hemorrhage by adhering to the following plan. The smaller, usually brighter pink vessels, which tend to be on the arterial side, are treated with repeated subthreshold coagulation, gradually building up power until the blood column fragments. After such fragmentation in these vessels, energy is gently applied to the remaining part of the tuft, treating the larger vessels last. The energy is reduced on these larger, usually darker, venous vessels and the spot size is increased to at least twice the size of the vessel. Multiple applications of subthreshold power are then directed at these larger vessels until fragmentation of the blood column results, and treatment is stopped. Continuous application of the laser energy, especially if the power is increased, will result in a significant incidence of hemorrhage. Occasionally, it is useful to direct a mild photocoagulation reaction at the larger "venous" side of the tuft to cause a backflow of blood into the smaller feeding components. The arterial feeders can then be treated.

Frequently, the entire vascular tuft will appear obliterated after treatment is completed. On reexamination of the patient, in a few hours, it is apparent that a large portion of the tuft was closed by spasm, and as much as 60 to 80% of the vasculature was still patent. A repeat application of energy—carefully avoiding excess power—to the patent vessels may be done after 4 to 6 hr. The patient is then reexamined on the following day and, if any residual patent vessels are observed, a final treatment is given. Therapy may therefore frequently involve three or even four separate treatments within a 30-hr period.

If a low-vacuum contact lens is used so that no retrobulbar anesthetic is required, there is no need to hesitate in performing repeated therapy at these short intervals.

In our hands, the management of disk neovascularization has resulted in a significant reduction in the hemorrhagic complications encountered when treatment with much higher energies attempts complete obliteration in one sitting (6).

### MACULAR EDEMA AND LIPID DEPOSITION

The argon laser is especially useful in treating cases of macular edema and lipid deposition in the diabetic patient because it produces small discrete coagulations. The ability to place coagulation spots as small as 50 μm permits treatment in the paramacular area without significant risk to the foveal area. Patients with macular edema or lipid deposition may experience a significant impairment in visual acuity. When long-standing macular edema is present some degree of cystoid degenerative changes may frequently be observed in the neuroepithelium.

In treating 54 patients with macular edema, improvement in vision resulted in approximately 90%. In those instances in which improvement in vision did not result, the patients had evidence of long-standing changes. The lipid resolution that followed photocoagulation in the paramacular area was quite dramatic. The visual improvement, however, in those patients with heavy lipid deposition was much less striking and, indeed, lipid clearing was often unaccompanied by improvement in vision, as only about 50% of those treated showed significant visual improvement.

In a careful evaluation of the macular cases, it was apparent that no instance of macular pucker resulted from therapy. No other complications of treatment in the posterior pole and in the paramacular area were noted.

### REFERENCES

1. L'ESPERANCE FA JR.   An ophthalmic argon laser photocoagulation system: Design, construction and laboratory investigations. *Trans Am Ophthalmol Soc* **66**: 827, 1968.
2. L'ESPERANCE FA JR.   The treatment of ophthalmic vascular disease by argon laser photocoagulation. *Trans Am Acad Ophthalmol Otolaryngol* **73**: 1077, 1969.
3. LITTLE HL, ZWENG HC and PEABODY RR.   Argon laser slit-lamp retinal photocoagulation. *Trans Am Acad Ophthalmol Otolaryngol* **74**: 85, 1970.
4. ZWENG HC, LITTLE HL and PEABODY RR. "Laser photocoagulation and retinal angiography." St. Louis, CV Mosby, 1969.
5. BEHRENDT T, RAYMOND RD and DUANE T. Evaluation of microlesions in diabetic retinopathy. *Am J Ophthalmol* **64**: 721, 1967.
6. PATZ A, MAUMENEE AE and RYAN SJ.   Argon laser photocoagulation—advantages and limitations. *Trans Am Ophthalmol Soc* **75**: 569, 1971.

# DIABETIC MACULOPATHY IN MATURITY ONSET DIABETICS

HAROLD F. SPALTER, M.D.

Institute of Ophthalmology, Columbia Presbyterian Medical Center, New York, New York, USA

"Simple" diabetic retinopathy is characterized by hard, also called lipid or waxy, exudates. One characteristic form taken by the exudates is that of a ring, partial or complete, of varying size. Typically the ring is in a D-shaped configuration, temporal above or below the macula. Rarely the complex is nasal to the macula. The circinate complex consists of a central area of edematous retina with enlarged capillaries, large microaneurysms and occasional hemorrhages.

Fluorescein studies have revealed that the retina enclosed by the cluster of hard exudates is abnormally permeable to the dye. There is gradual late leakage increasing with time. Visual function is compromised as the edema invades the macular area.

The natural history of these lipid complexes is not precisely known, but Dobree's recent elegant studies have greatly assisted our interpretation (1). It is estimated that the ring form may require up to several years to disappear spontaneously. The smaller isolated clusters of deposits may regress in a period of several months. However, these dense, central, yellow plaques of large size, may take years to resolve, resulting in irreversible macular damage. Low-fat diets and cholesterol-lowering drugs may hasten the absorption of the exudates but not necessarily affect visual improvement.

Analysis of the epidemiological statistics of patients with diabetic retinopathy dominated by these circinate complexes compared to the patient population without such complexes reveals interesting differences (Table 1). A group of 85 positive patients are compared with 85 persons without circinate exudates. All of the patients had visual symptoms attributable to diabetic retinopathy and all were being considered as candidates for photocoagulation therapy. These data emphasize the later onset of the diabetes and the much shorter duration of the disease before visual symptoms develop in the circinate group. The key reporting feature was age of onset of subjective visual symptoms, not objective funduscopic changes which may antedate the symptoms by years.

Other interesting features found in com-

TABLE 1. *Comparison of 85 patients with and 85 patients without circinate maculopathy present with symptomatic diabetic retinopathy who are candidates for photocoagulation*

|  | Circinate maculopathy | Without circinate maculopathy |
| --- | --- | --- |
| Average age of onset (years) | 44 | 26 |
| Average age when first seen (years) | 59 | 46 |
| Average duration of diabetes (years) | 15 | 20 |

**321**

TABLE 2. *Comparison of other manifestations of diabetic retinopathy in 85 patients with 85 patients without circinate maculopathy*

| | Circinate maculopathy (%) | Without circinate maculopathy (%) |
|---|---|---|
| Venous abnormalities | 32 | 51 |
| Neovascularization | 18 | 51 |
| Fibrous proliferation | 16 | 47 |
| Vitreous hemorrhage | 14 | 35 |

paring the two groups are the differences in incidence of the other manifestations of diabetic retinopathy (Table 2). In the patient with circinate complexes there is a relative lack of neovascularization and proliferative disease. As a consequence, the risk of vitreous hemorrhage, surely an ominous complication, is decreased significantly in this population. These data suggest that the visual morbidity attending circinate maculopathy is primarily dependent on the macular changes. The high incidence of this type of pathology in persons with maturity-onset diabetes often as the only manifestation of their retinopathy threatening vision makes an effective therapeutic program especially desirable. This inverse relationship of maculopathy and proliferative disease makes the successful therapy of the macular lesions even more rewarding, since the threat of diabetic blindness from the other causes

of neovascularization, *retinitis proliferans*, vitreous hemorrhage and retinal detachment is minimized.

Closure of the vascular leakage sites revealed by the fluorescein should prevent further retinal edema and reduce visual loss. The diagram in Fig. 1 illustrates a hypothesis that elimination of the microaneurysms and incompetent vessels should reverse the pathogenetic sequence of increased permeability, edema and exudates. Ideally such therapy would be prophylactic, that is, before macular damage occurs. This concept has been our rationale for early and direct photocoagulation therapy to the center of the circinate lipid complexes. Work by Meyer-Schwickerath and Schott (2), Welch (3), Spalter (4) and Dobree (1) have supported such a theoretical consideration.

At first conservatism and timidity dominated our clinical trials. Peripheral ring complexes in nonvital areas were treated to test our hypothesis. The rapid resolution of the surrounding exudates encouraged bolder approaches to the macular and perimacular complexes. The xenon arc coagulator made by Zeiss, West Germany was used throughout. The smaller focal sizes of 3° and 1.5° were utilized whenever possible. The lower energy settings of Green I and Green II were usually satisfactory although if the retina was

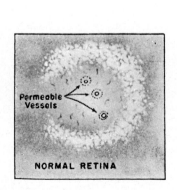
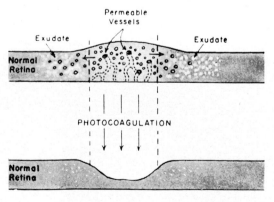

FIG. 1. Diagrammatic schema of rationale of photocoagulation for diabetic maculopathy.

TABLE 3. *Results of therapy in 49 patients having diabetic retinopathy with circinate maculopathy with follow-up of six to forty-five months*

|  | Treated |
|---|---|
| Exudate decreased | 41 |
| Exudate increased | 2 |
| Exudate same | 6 |
| Vision improved | 20 |
| Vision same | 19 |
| Vision worse | 10 |

particularly edematous increased energy was required to obtain a visible reaction. Retrobulbar injection of xylocaine 2% was used throughout to obtain absolute ocular immobility. When photocoagulating in the macular zone, absence of eye movements is mandatory to avoid inadvertent treatment of the fovea or papillomacular bundle. Adequate spacing of the coagulations was required to allow free venous drainage from the macular region. No macular hemorrhages or macular striae have resulted from the treatments. The edematous retina seems to act somewhat as a sponge, absorbing and dissipating the photocoagulation energy without mechanical deformation of the tissue such as may follow treatment of a retina of normal thickness.

The results to date in the treated patients have been moderately encouraging (Table 3) with over two-thirds of the 49 treated patients maintaining or showing improvement in visual acuity. The number of treated patients and the longest follow-up of 45 months are as yet inadequate to draw any firm conclusions. A small group of untreated contralateral "control" eyes had a much higher percentage of continued deterioration.

One must anticipate, in any event, that the persistence of the diabetic microvascular problem throughout the lifetime of the individual would tend to limit long-term effectiveness of photocoagulation. However, the diminished life span of the diabetic with vascular complications makes the short-term effectiveness of any program to preserve sight relatively more important in such a subject.

In conclusion, this preliminary study has encouraged us to continue evaluating photocoagulation therapy for this particular macular manifestation of diabetic retinopathy which is so threatening to the visual life span of the maturity onset diabetic.

## REFERENCES

1. DOBREE JH. Treatment of simple diabetic retinopathy by light coagulation. Preliminary report, presented at Oxford Ophthalmological Congress 1970.
2. MEYER-SCHWICKERATH G and SCHOTT K. Diabetic retinopathy and photocoagulation. *Am J Ophthalmol* **66**: 597, 1968.
3. WELCH RB. The treatment of diabetic retinopathy, in: Golberg MD and Fine SL (Eds), "Symposium on the Treatment of Diabetic Retinopathy." PHS Pub No 1890, Washington DC, Public Health Service, 1969, p 563.
4. SPALTER HF. Photocoagulation of macular lesions in diabetic retinopathy. *21st Int Cong Ophthalmol, Mexico City 1970* (in press).

# PHOTOCOAGULATION THERAPY

## INVITED DISCUSSION

### C. KUPFER

National Eye Institute, National Institutes of Health, Bethesda, Maryland, USA

It is apparent from the preceding papers that diabetes is rapidly becoming a major public health problem in many nations of the world. At the present time, diabetic retinopathy is the second leading cause of new adult blindness in the United States. There is every reason to believe that within the next five to ten years, it will be the leading cause of new adult blindness not only in the United States but in many of the countries of Europe. Because of the seriousness of this public health problem, it is appropriate for the National Eye Institute to play an active role in the support of research directed towards the prevention and treatment of diabetic retinopathy. Towards this end, a cooperative study among 10 participating hospitals will soon begin to test the hypothesis that photocoagulation can affect the clinical course of diabetic retinopathy in a beneficial manner. Since this disease is so erratic in its natural history, which is characterized by exacerbations and remissions, a large number of patients is necessary in such a study. It is estimated that this cooperative study will enroll between 1,200 and 1,500 patients during an initial three-year period. In addition, patients coming into this study will be randomly assigned to either a treatment group or to a control group. Following the initial three-year period of accession of cases, it is planned to study the patients for an additional five-year period. If this study is successful, it will be the first long-term controlled series assessing the effects of photocoagulation on the course of diabetic retinopathy. Of particular importance is the need to assess the success or failure of treatment not in the appearance of the retinopathy but in terms of the visual acuity of the patient. This criterion is surely the most important for us in our role as clinical ophthalmologists, certainly more than the waxing and waning of vessels on the retina or exudates near the macula. It is my hope that other studies in which therapy is being assessed would also attempt to assess visual acuity.

The ability to conduct a cooperative study in assessing the effect of photocoagulation on the course of diabetic retinopathy is complicated by several factors. First, many practicing ophthalmologists are already convinced that photocoagulation is beneficial. Therefore, patients will not be referred by this group of clinicians for inclusion in a controlled study. Secondly, it is possible for a patient who is being followed in the study, but who is not satisfied with the level of his visual acuity, to leave the study and seek ophthalmological care elsewhere, where similar photocoagulation equipment is available. Finally, all studies relying on the cooperation of a large number of institutions suffer from the difficulties of varying criteria in the selection of patients and of varying techniques in the assessment of retinopathy and its subsequent treatment. No matter how well the protocol is described, these variations tend to be present.

There is a unique opportunity for emerging nations to play an important role in clinical studies, such as on the efficacy of photocoagulation in the treatment of diabetic retinopathy. Several countries could arrange to make joint use of a xenon arc photocoagulator located in one specific clinical facility, so that a large number of patients could come to this one locus for diagnosis and treatment. Inasmuch as no other treatment facility would be available to them, it would then be much easier to standardize treatment, and simpler to maintain and follow up the patients in the study. In addition, it may be possible for high risk patients, such as diabetics who have already lost vision in one eye due to retinopathy, to be randomized for treatment or no treatment with respect to the other eye. The answer as to efficacy of treatment could be forthcoming in perhaps three years. Such unique opportunities for international cooperation in clinical research are particularly likely to receive support from the National Eye Institute.

## M. L. SEARS

Department of Ophthalmology, Yale University School of Medicine, New Haven, Connecticut, USA

Several highly skilled and eminent ophthalmologists have pioneered in the investigations of the natural history of diabetic retinopathy. Studies of the evolution, progression and, in some instances, regression of the disease have called to our attention the need for a careful evaluation of any protocol for treatment. Furthermore, the report of complications as a result of therapy supports the need for caution. Several years ago hypophysectomy was heralded as an important therapy for some forms of diabetic retinopathy. When it became evident that the improvement was not commensurate with the degree of ablation of the pituitary functions, doubt was cast upon this form of therapy. In short, neither the successes nor the failures could be explained in terms of the rationale for treatment.

Now in the case of photocoagulation as treatment for retinopathy, the conventional arguments for controls can be made but are difficult to sustain because it has been demonstrated that light coagulation can be very effective in destroying individual bleeding sites. It is difficult for the doctor not to apply his knowledge of these impressive demonstrations to help his patient. The pressures upon the patient and upon his physician will at times be awesome. In spite of these terrible pressures there will be a need for a controlled evaluation of the effects of light coagulation in the treatment of retinopathy of diabetic origin.

To this end a small series of 17 eyes were treated alternately by xenon arc. Twenty patients, five of whom were classified as one-eyed, had proliferative retinopathy in all phases, but mostly in the early phases. The treatment with the xenon arc varied its intensity. The duration of application was less than 0.5 sec with an aperture of 3°. All treatable proliferative areas were treated. Evaluation of therapy was based on the best corrected visual acuity after diagnostic examination, which included indirect and direct ophthalmoscopy, five area photos of the retina, contact lens examination and fluorescein angiography.

The results can be briefly summarized: of 17 eyes alternately selected for xenon treatment follow-ups were possible in some for up to seven years. Others have been followed for only one to two years. Six of these seventeen eyes were considered, by the criterion of visual acuity, to have been improved. It is too early to draw definite conclusions, but the results thus far do not indicate a clear-cut benefit from light coagulation. We hope to continue this study of one of the most difficult clinical problems in ophthalmology. Thanks to this conference we shall be able to draw upon the experience and expertise of the acknowledged pioneers and leaders in the field.

# DISCUSSION

DR. R. STEIN (*Israel*): There is a time course in the development of diabetic retinopathy. There are relatively numerous cases with good vision and only a few nicks on the disk. In half a year a proliferating retinopathy develops which reaches such a state that you cannot do anything more. This is opposed to taking a 7% progression rate which may be general and not for the specific case.

DR. M. GOLDBERG (*USA*): I think the observations of a worsening of proliferative changes is certainly valid; we have all observed such changes. The factors responsible are very unclear. Perhaps the sudden increase in proliferative changes in a given diabetic individual is due to many factors. One may be the effect of the vitreous on the blood vessels since contraction and detachment of the vitreous may occur very suddenly in any individual patient, this leads to either increased visibility of the abnormal vessels or to increased growth of the neovascular tissue. In any given patient, I would therefore agree that at some unpredictable period, a very rapid increase may occur. The precise factors responsible in a specific patient are frequently hard to decipher. The figures presented to you in the lecture reflect average values for large populations of patients.

DR. A. L. KORNZWEIG (*USA*): I had in mind the fact that at the time when there is an ischemic phenomenon in the retina resulting either from the closure of the arterial blood vessel or from decompensation due to venous occlusion, there seems to be a stimulating factor in the retina which will cause neovascularization. This was described originally as a hypothesis by Dr. Michaelson in his book on retinal circulation in man and animals (1954). Dr. Michaelson mentions this factor as the "X" factor which is responsible for vasoproliferation in the area of retinal ischemia. I think that the sudden proliferation around the retina probably results from the need for additional circulation because of the ischemia, and that this is probably responsible for the marked proliferation in this area in a short period of time.

DR. G. GORIN (*USA*): Dr. Kornzweig, you made a very interesting attempt to give us a unified concept of the lesions in central retinal vein thrombosis and in diabetes. I would like to know whether you could explain why both conditions develop rubeosis iridis, and whether the increased venous pressure could not be the initiating factor in this.

DR. KORNZWEIG: In my concept of diabetic retinopathy, the primary underlying pathology may be venous obstruction. However, it is too much to assume that this is the only pathological basis for everything that happens, and how this causes rubeosis iridis, I cannot say.

DR. M. L. SEARS (*USA*): How do you explain the frequent occurrence of neovascularization on the disk?

DR. GOLDBERG: Perhaps I could comment briefly on the frequency distribution of neovascular lesions on the disk before Dr. Kornzweig answers your question. Dobree and Taylor have shown that the most common location of neovascular lesions is on the major vessels within only a few disk diameters of the disk. This is therefore a posterior polar phenomenon except that the macula is almost never involved. After the most common location, on the major vessels as they leave the disk, the second most common location of true neovascularization is the disk itself.

DR. KORNZWEIG: There seems to be a difference in the type of circulation around the disk as compared with that in other parts of the retina. There seems to be some involvement with choroidal circulation as well as with retinal circulation in this area, so that this type of neovascularization may also be an indication of an attempt on the part of the choroidal circulation to participate in and to help the retinal circulation. This is purely hypothesis on my part.

MR. J. DOBREE (*U.K.*): We have given a lot of thought to this question of why new vessels occur at the disk and why they occur at crossings. Now it may be that at the disk, there is a close proximity of arteries and veins and what is simply happening is that the blood is going round the easier way.

DR. STEIN: I cannot understand your explanation if we assume that the proliferation of the vessels is due to the need of some metabolic requirements.

MR. M. KLEIN (*U.K.*): Dr. Kornzweig mentioned sluggishness of the circulation in the development of diabetic complications of the retina and the use of anticoagulants. Could you give us some practical information about the use of anticoagulants?

DR. KORNZWEIG: So far we have had only a few cases that have been treated with anticoagulants in diabetic retinopathy. I have spoken to a number of my colleagues at Mt. Sinai Hospital who are specialists in diabetes and asked them to treat some of our common patients with anticoagulants. The objective was not to allow the anticoagulant to make the prothrombin time too prolonged in order to avoid secondary hemorrhage. The number of cases is very low. The results were poor, possibly because these were very advanced cases. I felt that we should start the treatment at a much earlier period if it is going to have any effect.

DR. A. PATZ (*USA*): I thought I might talk about Dr. Aiello's approach to scattered treatment with the ruby laser. He spares the papulomacular bundle area and avoids the immediate area of the disk. His technique has been used in his own department on approximately 500 patients. According to his communication to me, which he said could be quoted, he does not feel that he has found a significant change in disk neovascularization in patients treated by this scattered or peripheral barrage, although the few cases of early disk neovascularization that disappeared after treatment were encouraging. He now treats neovascularization on the disk with the argon laser first and then applies his scattered treatment to the periphery.

DR. M. SHUSTERMAN (*Canada*): I would like to ask Dr. Patz how many of these vessels that are treated at the disk will later reopen? How long has the study been going on?

DR. PATZ: The average disk neovascularization patient is treated four times in our present series of about ninety patients. We do not use a retrobulbar anesthetic. Frequently, we will send the treated patient out for lunch and bring him back four to five hours later. At this time what looked like 100% obliteration or fragmentation of the blood column in a vascular tuft will now show only about 20% occlusion. The changes noted after treatment were presumably spasm. We treat the patient again on the same day. At the time of treatment, either the blood column will segment or the vessels will appear obliterated but the actual percentage of vessels that are occluded is usually less than 50%; and so repeat treatment is required.

With regard to arterial feeders of neovascularization and the diagnostic use of fluorescein, only about one-fourth of patients with disk neovascularization show a clear arteriovenous pattern by fluorescein and only in 10 to 15% of patients can one recognize the arterial feeder.

DR. G. THEODOSSIADIS (*Greece*): Dr. Waubke said that he obtained good results in cases with neovascularization in the macular area by using light coagulation not directly on the affected vessels but in the normal periphery. We are very happy to hear about his observation because whenever we tried it, we failed. We think that in the particular case, we can directly destroy the vessels in the area of the macula which create the leakage and exudation. Otherwise the results are not favorable.

DR. M. L. SEARS: There has been much evidence that low fat diets or cholesterol-lowering drugs reduce exudates in diabetic retinopathy.

DR. H. F. SPALTER (*USA*): The circinate exudates indicate that an active pathogenic mechanism is going on in the macular area. They are the end result of serum lipid seepage. Therefore, the cholesterol-lowering drugs, when they reduce lipids, also clear up the pattern of the macula but do not necessarily change the fluorescein leakage pattern. I have seen this many times. However, the time required for these lipid-lowering diets or drugs to work is too long to protect the macula. By the time they work, which is usually 12 to 16 months, the macula may be irreversibly damaged.

MR. J. DOBREE: As for the specific question about maculopathy, our experience has been exactly similar to Dr. Spalter's in that the exudates go quite rapidly in a matter of weeks.
Though our experience is not as large as his, we also found that the recovery of vision takes a very long time in some patients. Many have taken over 18 months to obtain their best vision after photocoagulation.

DR. H. LINCOFF (*USA*): For the past seven or eight years we have been using at Cornell only total elimination of all neovascularization as our standard criterion for success. We try to eliminate all of the neovascularization in the first months and we subsequently treat any recurrence at four- or six-month intervals. In order to obtain this we have found, chiefly with juvenile diabetics, that we have to give somewhere between 1,000 and 1,200 applications during the first four or six months at one-month intervals. This is considerably more than Dr. Waubke was suggesting. Our series runs over five years, some cases have lasted as long as seven and we have some patients, who although they have had up to 1,700 applications in a single eye, were not protected from neovascularization.

# THE NATURAL HISTORY OF
# PRIMARY OPEN-ANGLE GLAUCOMA

ALLAN E. KOLKER

Glaucoma Center, Department of Ophthalmology and Oscar Johnson Institute, Washington University School of Medicine, St. Louis, Missouri, USA

Understanding the natural history of primary open-angle glaucoma ultimately involves elucidation of the many factors responsible for the development of visual damage in patients with this disease. Since many of these factors are unknown and most are incompletely understood, our knowledge of the natural history of glaucoma is incomplete. This is unfortunate since the eventual aim in glaucoma management is the prevention of visual loss before it occurs. The ability to predict accurately the development of glaucoma in the individual patient before field loss has occurred is perhaps the major problem in glaucoma detection at the present time.

In the light of presently available information, it seems reasonable to consider the following stages in the disease. 1) Preglaucoma begins with the genetic predilection, develops (in most instances) through the phase of ocular hypertension and concludes with the first evidence of optic nerve damage. 2) Overt glaucoma starts with early field loss where treatment may reverse the damage, passes through the stage of progressive damage where therapy will usually stabilize the condition and ends with absolute glaucoma and blindness.

### THE PREGLAUCOMA STAGE

*Genetic predilection.* Primary open-angle glau-coma has been demonstrated repeatedly to be a familial and hereditary disorder. Numerous pedigrees have been published showing transmission through several generations, thus suggesting an autosomal dominant mode of transmission. However, a large number of patients with proved primary open-angle glaucoma failed to give a family history of glaucoma and the results of all tests were normal in their parents and siblings.

Studies with topical corticosteroids have led to the consideration of autosomal recessive inheritance for primary open-angle glaucoma (1). Volunteer subjects can be divided into three groups on the basis of their intraocular pressures after six weeks of treatment with topical dexamethasone. The genotypes nn, ng and gg have been suggested for the three categories of response (Table 1). Findings in volunteers suggest that the responder gene is quite prevalent in the United States population (0.2 to 0.25), with about 35%

TABLE 1. *Classification of corticosteroid response[a]*

| Genotype | Intraocular pressure (mm Hg) |
|----------|------------------------------|
| nn | < 20 |
| ng | 20 to 31 |
| gg | > 31 |

[a] Dexamethasone treatment 0.1% four times daily for six weeks.

**330**

TABLE 2.  *Topical corticosteroid test*

| Category | Sample no. | Applanation pressure response after dexamethasone treatment[a] | | |
|---|---|---|---|---|
| | | < 20 mm Hg (%) | 20 to 31 mm Hg (%) | > 31 mm Hg (%) |
| Volunteers | 300 | 58 | 36 | 6 |
| Primary open-angle glaucoma patients | 50 | 0 | 8 | 92 |
| Offspring of glaucoma patients | 120 | 6 | 70 | 24 |
| Siblings of glaucoma patients | 70 | 19 | 50 | 31 |

[a]  Dexamethasone treatment, 0.1% four times daily for six weeks.

TABLE 3.  *Topical corticosteroid test*

| | Corticosteroid response | | | Glaucoma (field loss) (%) |
|---|---|---|---|---|
| | nn (%) | ng (%) | gg (%) | |
| Water provocative test $P_0/C > 100$ | 6 | 32 | 92 | 94 |
| PTC nontasters | 25 | 35 | 50 | 51 |
| PBI < 5.5 mg/100 ml | 8 | 12 | 34 | 34 |
| Diabetes (positive GTT) | 2 | 4 | 17 | 22 |
| Cup/disk diameter > 0.3 | 15 | 20 | 52 | 81 |
| | | | | Opposite eye 60 |

PTC = phenylthiocarbamide.    PBI = protein-bound iodine.    GTT = glucose tolerance test.

intermediate and 5% high steroid responders (Table 2). In patients with primary open-angle glaucoma, however, about 90% were found to fit into the high steroid response category, with pressures > 31 mm Hg after six weeks of treatment with topical dexamethasone (0.1% four times daily). The hypothesis was therefore proposed that the gene determining corticosteroid responses and primary open-angle glaucoma are intimately related and perhaps identical. The hypothesis suggested that this type of glaucoma was recessively inherited and that the glaucomatous individual was homozygous. All offspring of glaucomatous patients should then be gg responders, have glaucoma or be carriers of the gene. Findings in such offspring approached this prediction. Studies in siblings of glaucoma patients also closely fitted the predicted response.

The ultimate validation of the above hypothesis will require prolonged study. There is, however, considerable evidence supporting the closeness of the relationship between the homozygous high steroid responders (gg) and patients with primary open-angle glaucoma (Table 3). Thus, a $P_0/C$ ratio > 100 after drinking a liter of water is found in over 90% of glaucomatous eyes and in over 90% of high steroid responders (gg) (2). This finding, however, is seen in only 32% of the intermediate (ng) and 6% of poor (nn) steroid responders. When tested for ability to taste phenylthiocarbamide (PTC) (3), 51% of patients with primary open-angle and 50% of gg responders are nontasters. In the nn and ng groups, the percentages are 25% and 35%, respectively. Serum protein-bound iodine (PBI) values less than 5.5 mg/100 ml are found in 34% of glaucoma patients and gg responders, but in only 8% of the nn and 12% of the ng groups (4). Positive glucose tolerance tests (GTT) (plasma glucose total over 0, 1, 2 and 3 hr $> 600$ mg/100 ml) occurs in 22% of glaucoma patients and 17% of the gg population (5). However, only 2% of the nn population and 4% of the ng population have positive tests. A cup/disk diameter (2) ratio over 0.3 is found in over 80% of eyes with glaucomatous field loss. A cup/disk ratio over 0.3 is found in the opposite eyes of 60% of glaucoma patients with unilateral field loss. Ratios over 0.3 are found in 52% of high steroid responders (gg), but in only 15% of eyes of poor steroid responders and 20% of eyes of intermediate responders. In all of these parameters the gg responders closely resemble patients with primary open-angle glaucoma and differ markedly from the nn and ng groups.

It should be emphasized that most patients in the homozygous high steroid response category do not have sustained elevated intraocular pressures when not subjected to corticosteroid administration. On close follow-up intermittent pressure elevations may occur and outflow facility is often abnormal, but pressures are usually maintained at normal levels for many years, either because of the intermittency of expression of the outflow defect or by hyposecretion of aqueous. However, in the vast majority of cases that develop visual damage, ocular hypertension precedes the damage. The factors responsible for this change are not known, but one can postulate progressive outflow impairment and/or inability to maintain hyposecretion. Iatrogenic factors such as prolonged corticosteroid administration (topically and/or systemically) may also be important in some instances. Similarly, aging, diabetes mellitus, trauma, intraocular pigmentary disturbance with pigment deposition in the angle and pseudoexfoliation of the lens capsule may contribute to the glaucomatous process.

*Impaired outflow facility.* As noted, high steroid responders frequently have impaired outflow facilities. Such outflow impairment can occur at a very young age (teens or younger) and may represent the earliest manifestation of the glaucomatous process. Studies in relatives of glaucoma patients demonstrate that with even moderate outflow abnormality, intraocular pressure may remain normal for many years presumably because of hyposecretion of aqueous. In some cases the outflow abnormality appears to improve spontaneously with the return of aqueous dynamics to normal. In other instances a progressive decrease in outflow facility develops. Water provocative testing at this stage may show marked elevation of pressure even though undisturbed pressures may be relatively normal or only intermittently elevated. Further outflow impairment, however, leads to a gradual rise in intraocular pressure and persistent ocular hypertension.

*Ocular hypertension.* There is little doubt that elevated intraocular pressure is associated with primary open-angle glaucoma and is the chief factor in the development of visual damage. Some investigators [e.g., Leydhecker (6)] have suggested that most patients with ocular hypertension will develop field loss; 52% of eyes with pressures $> 20$ mm Hg and normal fields developed field defects within seven years. Most other studies, however, indicate that this is not the case. Linnér and Strömberg (7) followed 152 patients with ocular hypertension ($P_0$, 21.7 to 25.9 mm Hg) for five years and three patients developed field loss. Armaly (8) followed 3,936 initially nonglaucomatous individuals for nine years. Only four developed glaucomatous field loss, 1,123 eyes had initial applanation pressures $> 20$ mm Hg and two of the four who developed visual loss had initial pressures $< 200$ mm Hg.

The Collaborative Glaucoma Study, with up to 10 years of follow-up of several thousand ocular hypertensives and close relatives of glaucoma patients, has seen remarkably few patients develop visual damage. The bulk of evidence, therefore, indicates that, while almost all cases of glaucoma have ocular hypertension, most patients with ocular hypertension do not have visual loss and many quite possibly will never develop damage in their lifetimes.

It is obvious, therefore, that while elevated intraocular pressure is an extremely important factor in the natural history of primary open-angle glaucoma, other factors also influence the development of optic nerve damage. Unfortunately, our knowledge of these other factors is extremely limited. Even less well understood is how they alter the susceptibility of the optic nerve to pressure damage.

There is general agreement that the nerve destruction which results from glaucoma is based upon vascular insufficiency to the nerve. The relationship between intraocular pressure and ophthalmic artery blood pressure is thus of extreme importance. Fluorescein angiography has demonstrated delayed filling of retinal and choroidal blood vessels at high intraocular pressures. Choroidal filling appears to be more delayed than filling of the central retinal vessels especially in patients with field loss (9). The predictive value of these changes in patients without field loss has not been proven.

Eyes with large cup/disk diameter ratios which have been shown to be genetically determined are more susceptible to glaucomatous damage. As noted previously, some 60% of the opposite eyes of patients with unilateral glaucomatous field loss have cup/disk ratios $> 0.3$ (Table 3). Thus, the large cup often precedes the development of visual damage.

In normal individuals, circulating plasma levels of cortisol are markedly suppressed by a small oral dose of dexamethasone. Pretreatment with diphenylthydantoin (DPH) (DILANTIN®) for one week blocks this effect of oral dexamethasone in most instances. These

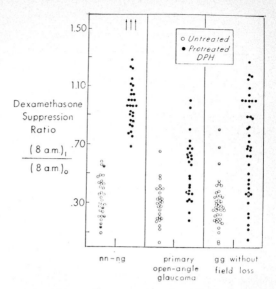

FIG. 1. Dexamethasone suppression of plasma cortisol in untreated and diphenylhydantoin pretreated patients (10).

TABLE 4. *Plasma cortisol suppression after DPH[a]*

| Classification | Plasma cortisol[b] $> 25\%$ suppression | |
| --- | --- | --- |
| | *No. of patients* | *%* |
| nn and ng | 2 of 31 | 6 |
| Open-angle glaucoma | 24 of 27 | 89 |
| gg | 22 of 40 | 55 |

[a]  DPH 100 mg three times daily for one week.
[b]  Dexamethasone 9-hr suppression test.

expected responses are demonstrated in the nn and ng steroid populations (10). In patients with primary open-angle glaucoma, however, DPH fails to block the cortisol suppression response (Fig. 1). High steroid responders (gg) without field loss divide into two almost equal groups, one resembling the nn-ng individuals and the other the glaucomatous patients (Table 4). This has led to the speculation that those members of the gg population who demonstrate poor dexamethasone suppression of plasma cortisol may be resistant to field loss.

The presence of diabetes mellitus has been shown to be associated with increased susceptibility of the optic nerve to glaucomatous damage (5). In one series in which intraocular pressures were elevated with topical dexamethasone, 8 of 12 diabetic subjects developed reversible field changes, while such changes were found in only 1 of 12 nondiabetics. In glaucoma patients matched for degree of field loss, comparable damage was found at lower pressures in those with diabetes than in those without.

While the vast majority of eyes with chronic simple glaucoma have ocular hypertension, a few patients may develop visual damage at normal levels of intraocular pressure (low-tension glaucoma). Such patients often have a history of episodes of severe blood loss, marked systemic hypotension, carotid insufficiency or other evidence of vascular disease. Interestingly, most of these patients are high responders when tested with topical corticosteroids even though their visual loss occurs at normal intraocular pressures, thus emphasizing the importance of the genetic predilection.

*Optic nerve damage.* The usual method of assessing glaucomatous damage to the optic nerve is by evaluation of the visual fields. Leydhecker (6) has stated that "field defects always develop before any disk changes are visible." While this is no doubt true in most instances, exceptions do occur and have been documented photographically. Cupping of the disk tends to occur rapidly in the eyes of young patients when pressure is increased and may reverse within a short period with normalization of the intraocular pressure. Such changes in the disk may develop without alteration in the visual field. Whether demonstrated by progressive cupping or by the development of early field loss, the presence of optic nerve damage concludes the stage of preglaucoma and establishes the diagnosis. Such a change in classification is important.

It illustrates that the eye is no longer able to tolerate the level of intraocular pressure present and active steps are needed to prevent further damage. While opinions vary as to when or if ocular hypertension should be treated while visual function is normal, there is complete agreement that therapy is mandatory in the stage of overt glaucoma.

## THE OVERT GLAUCOMA STAGE

*Early field loss.* The definition of early glaucomatous field loss has undergone considerable change in recent years with the development of new techniques and instruments for examination of visual fields. Aulhorn and Harms (11), in particular, demonstrated that the isolated paracentral scotoma represents the earliest specific field defect in chronic simple glaucoma. These scotomas can only be demonstrated by careful perimetry using small stimuli and testing in the appropriate areas of the field. They are often found on the nasal side of fixation, frequently just a few degrees from fixation. Baring of the blind spot, enlargement of the blind spot and generalized contraction of the peripheral field are found in glaucoma, but also in many other conditions and are not specific as early signs of glaucomatous field loss.

The establishment of the paracentral scotoma as an early field defect is an important step in the natural history of glaucoma. Equally important is the demonstration that such changes may often disappear with early treatment and normalization of the intraocular pressure. The concept that glaucomatous damage, once present, is permanent and irreversible can no longer be held especially in the early stages of field loss. Occasionally even more advanced changes may disappear with proper therapy.

*Progressive damage.* Just as ocular hypertension is the major factor in the development of field loss, so is it the primary factor in the progression of the damage. Such damage

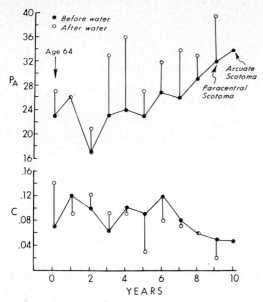

FIG. 2. Patient 1. Intraocular pressure (above) and outflow facility (below) of left eye, with changes produced by drinking water, during the 10 years preceding the development of field loss.

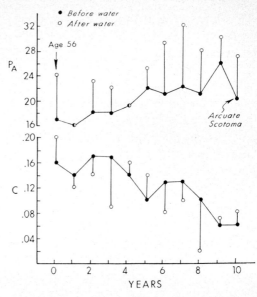

FIG. 4. Patient 2. Intraocular pressure (above) and outflow facility (below) of left eye, with changes produced by drinking water, during the 10 years preceding the development of field loss.

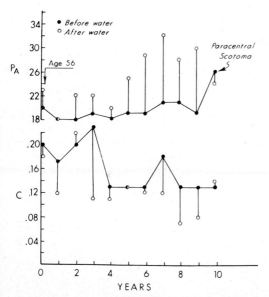

FIG. 3. Patient 2. Intraocular pressure (above) and outflow facility (below) of right eye, with changes produced by drinking water during the 10 years preceding the development of field loss.

period of the study. Intraocular pressure and outflow facility are plotted, along with the changes in these parameters following water-provocative testing.

## DISCUSSION

The present study confirms the high prevalence of abnormalities of aqueous dynamics in close relatives of patients with primary open-angle glaucoma. Thus, about 10 to 12% of these patients have an intraocular pressure $\geq 22$ mm Hg, and about 30% have a $P_0/C$ ratio greater than 100 after water. The cumulative percentages (i.e., present on one or more examinations) are much higher.

Three patients developed glaucoma during the 10-year period of study: an incidence of about 5%. All were over 40 years of age, ranging from 53 to 74 years at the time of diagnosis. Of the 62 patients followed up for 10 years, 35 were $\geq 40$ years of age at their first examination. The incidence among those relatives over 40 years of age, therefore, is

9%. Added to the 10% prevalence of glaucoma in relatives over 40 years when first examined (1), the incidence of glaucoma approaches 20% in close relatives over 40 years of age. This is less than the 40 to 50% incidence predicted by dominant inheritance, but begins to approach the 25 to 30% incidence predicted by the recessive inheritance of a gene with relatively high frequency in the population.

*Intraocular pressures.* Ocular hypertension has long been associated with open-angle glaucoma and loss of visual field. Leydhecker (4) reported that field defects developed in 52% of eyes with intraocular pressures < 20 mm Hg within seven years. However, most other studies (5, 6) indicate a much lower incidence of visual damage associated with elevated intraocular pressure. The present study agrees more closely with the latter findings. Of eyes followed up for five years, 18 had baseline intraocular pressures $\geq$ 22 mm Hg (Schiøtz), while 13 had applanation pressures at this level. Only one of these eyes developed field loss during the five-year follow-up period. In the group followed for 10 years, there were 16 eyes with Schiøtz pressures $\geq$ 22 mm Hg and 11 with applanation pressures at this level at the time of their initial evaluation. Three of these eyes developed field loss: an incidence of 27%. However, three eyes which developed field loss had initial intraocular pressures below 22 mm Hg. Thus, an ocular hypertension of $\leq$ 22 mm Hg (applanation) in a patient with normal visual fields may indicate a likelihood of about one in four of field loss within 10 years. This criterion, however, will identify only about half of the eyes in which damage is likely to develop during this period. These conclusions apply only to eyes with pressures between 22 and 30 mm Hg, since patients who had intraocular pressures $\geq$ 30 mm Hg were referred for treatment at their first examination.

*$P_0/C$ ratio.* A $P_0/C$ ratio $\gtreqless$ 100 after the patient has drunk water is a characteristic finding in eyes with glaucomatous damage. At the time of their baseline examination, four of the six eyes which suffered field loss, i.e., at least one eye of each of the three patients in whom damage developed, had $P_0/C$ ratios > 100. There were, however, 25 other eyes that did not develop visual damage within 10 years but demonstrated this finding at the time of their first examination. Thus, the index $P_0/C$ >100 appears to be a poor predictor of veentual field loss.

*Development of field loss.* The four eyes of the two patients who could be followed up for 10 years preceding field loss hardly constitute a large enough survey from which to draw definite conclusions. Nevertheless, the alterations in their aqueous dynamics during this time are remarkably similar. In contrast to the rest of the series, which showed little change in pressure or outflow facility, the eyes developing field loss underwent a progressive impairment in outflow facility, followed by the progressive elevation of intraocular pressure after outflow facility reached very low levels. Even when outflow facility was relatively good, the drinking of water resulted in a marked reduction in outflow. As outflow facility began to decrease, intraocular pressure was still only slightly elevated, but water provocation produced a marked rise in pressure. With further impairment in outflow, unprovoked pressures began to rise progressively, eventually reaching sufficiently high levels to cause optic nerve damage.

Thus, progressive changes with time, rather than a specific level of abnormality in pressure or outflow, may provide the most significant evidence of impending field loss. These observations, if confirmed by more extensive studies, may be of importance in the detection and diagnosis of glaucoma.

### SUMMARY AND CONCLUSIONS

A 10-year evaluation of close relatives of

patients with primary open-angle glaucoma is presented. The incidence of glaucoma, including those cases present at the first examination and those developing during the study, is about 19% in relatives 40 years of age or older at the time of their first evaluation.

The prevalence of abnormalities in aqueous dynamics is much higher in relatives of glaucoma cases than in the general population, but changes only slightly over 10 years. Ocular hypertension ($P_A \geq 22$ mm Hg with normal visual fields) at baseline evaluation appears to be a poor indicator of later visual damage. About three-quarters of such eyes retain normal fields 10 years later. Furthermore, only about half of the eyes in which damage developed are identified by pressures at this level on first examination. A $P_0/C$ ratio $\geq 100$ after drinking water identifies most patients who eventually develop field loss, but also characterizes many eyes that do not do so; and is, therefore, not an accurate predictor of damage.

Eyes followed up for 10 years, with eventual field loss, demonstrate a progressive decrease in outflow facility, followed by a period of marked increase in intraocular pressure after the subject has drunk water. With a further decrease in outflow, unprovoked pressures begin to rise rather rapidly and eventually reach a level where visual damage occurs.

Supported by Grants EY-00336 and EY-00004, National Eye Institute, National Institutes of Health, Bethesda, Md.

## REFERENCES

1. BECKER B, KOLKER AE and ROTH FD. Glaucoma family study. *Am J Ophthalmol* **50**: 557, 1960.
2. KOLKER AE and MOSES RA. Glaucoma family study: One year follow-up. *South Med J* **54**: 1115, 1961.
3. BECKER B. Intraocular pressure response to topical corticosteroids. *Invest Ophthalmol* **4**: 198, 1965.
4. LEYDHECKER W. Die Zuverlässigkeit der Diagnose des glaucoma simplex im Frühstadium. *Doc Ophthalmol* **20**: 214, 1966.
5. LINNÉR E and STROMBERG U. Ocular hypertension, in: Leydhecker W (Ed), "Glaucoma: Tutzing Symposium." Basel, S Karger, 1967.
6. ARMALY M. Ocular pressure and visual fields. *Arch Ophthalmol* **81**: 25, 1969.

angle-closure glaucoma because ocular tensions and optic disks are normal at the time of examination (7).

Acute attacks need intensive management in properly equipped hospitals. Attacks that have been brought under control can easily relapse, and angles that have opened can not only close again, but are then likely to remain closed despite further intensive treatment. If patients were to report quickly, most angles would reopen with miotics alone, but there are few such favorable cases. For emergency treatment I favor heavy doses of acetazolamide: 500 mg i.v. accompanied by 500 mg orally, followed by 500 mg orally at 8-hr intervals.

The aim of the intensive acetazolamide therapy is to depress ciliary body secretion rapidly so that, with the assistance of some fluid escape from the posterior chamber via uveoscleral pathways, the pressure in the posterior chamber becomes less than in the anterior chamber. For a short time the pupil block acts in the reverse direction, so as to diminish the convexity of the iris sufficiently to open the angle. In this way, angles frequently open even when pupils remain considerably dilated and resistant to miotics.

Osmotic therapy is very valuable, and the type most suited to routine use in any particular hospital must be determined. I am not convinced that the sudden drop in pressure by osmosis is as efficient at opening angles as the lowering of pressure by acetazolamide. I am investigating a parallel series, but there are so many other factors involved that a controlled trial in sufficient numbers is proving very difficult.

*Fixed pupils.* When patients report late with acutely high intraocular pressures, the pupil dilates from ischemic paresis and even necrosis of the iris constrictor muscle. The mechanism has been described by Tyner and Scheie (7), and more recently by Charles and Hamasaki (8).

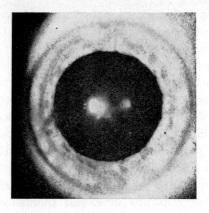

FIG. 1.  Pupil widely dilated after 10% phenylephrinee eydrops.

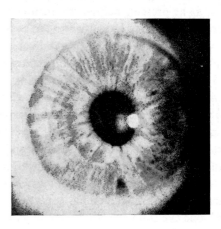

FIG. 2.  Phenylephrine pupil dilatation reversed by 0.5 % thymoxamine eyedrops. No other miotics were used.

This form of pupil dilatation is similar to that caused by the tropine alkaloids in that the sphincter becomes paretic, while the dilator, in suffering much less necrosis, continues to act and the iris folds into the angle (9). This intensifies the angle closure produced by the iris convexity from the pupil block. The pupil becomes virtually fixed and does not constrict with miotics.

*Thymoxamine.* This new and interesting substance is being tested to see if it will produce iris muscle dilator paresis. It acts as a sympathetic α-inhibitor (10) and can be administered in the form of eye drops. The optimum strength is under investigation but 0.5% is effective. It dramatically reverses wide mydriasis produced by 10% phenylephrine eyedrops (11) (Fig. 1 and 2) and also causes miosis in normal eyes.

In primary angle closure glaucoma, a combination of thymoxamine and miotics may activate the paretic sphincter sufficiently to produce pupil constriction and draw the iris away from the occluded angles, but the miosis produced is likely to be incomplete owing to iris atrophy and partial sphincter destruction.

The routine use of thymoxamine following diagnostic pupil dilatation by phenylephrine should be a valuable safeguard against iatrogenic acute angle closure. This form of angle closure is very dangerous because pupils are usually very widely dilated and unresponsive to miotics. The iris ischemia produced by the high intraocular pressure is aggravated by the vasoconstriction due to phenylephrine.

## SUMMARY

Primary angle-closure glaucoma remains a very destructive disease for eyes and vision. The most significant advance in prevention was the recognition of the efficacy of prophylactic peripheral iridectomy on the fellow eye.

At present, the possibility of preventing most attacks of acute glaucoma in the first eye appears remote. The prevention of benign intermittent attacks developing into destructive acute angle closure glaucoma depends upon better education, not only of the general public, but also of medical practitioners in general and ophthalmologists in particular.

For acute angle-closure glaucoma, much less eye damage could result from quicker presentation, more accurate diagnosis and more determined treatment. Patients need admission to hospital for intensive acetazolamide therapy, osmotic treatment, miotics and careful supervision as preludes to surgery.

Special investigations were conducted in the Glaucoma Unit of the Hospital with the help of Dr. Magda Horvat and the cooperation of my hospital colleagues.

Supported by the J. Bruce Hamilton Fellowship of the Ophthalmic Research Institute of Australia and Research Project No. 13 of The Royal Victoria Eye and Ear Hospital, Melbourne.

## REFERENCES

1. GORDON BL. The problem of glaucoma. *Arch Ophthalmol* **19**: 515, 1938.
2. PERKINS ES. Laser iridotomy. *Br Med J* **2**: 580, 1970.
3. LOWE RF. Primary angle closure glaucoma: a review of provocative tests. *Br J Ophthalmol* **51**: 727, 1967.
4. LOWE RF. The natural history and principles of treatment of primary angle closure glaucoma. *Am J Ophthalmol* **61**: 642, 1966.
5. LOWE RF. Acute angle closure glaucoma. The second eye. *Br J Ophthalmol* **46**: 641, 1962.
6. LOWE RF. Primary creeping angle closure glaucoma. *Br J Ophthalmol* **48**: 544, 1964.
7. LOWE RF. Acute glaucoma. Missed diagnosis. *Med J Aust* **2**: 782, 1963.
8. TYNER GS and SCHEIE HG. Mechanism of the miotic resistant pupil with increased intraocular pressure. *Arch Ophthalmol* **50**: 572, 1953.
9. CHARLES CT and HAMASAKI DI. The effect of intraocular pressure on the pupil size. *Arch Ophthalmol* **83**: 729, 1970.
10. LOWE RF. Angle closure, pupil dilatation and pupil block. *Br J Ophthalmol* **50**: 385, 1966.
11. BIRMINGHAM AT and SZOLCSÁNYI J. Competitive blockade of adrenergic α-receptors and histamine receptors by thymoxamine. *J Pharm Pharmacol* **17**: 449, 1965.
12. MAPSTONE R. Safe mydriasis. *Br J Ophthalmol* **54**: 690, 1970.

of age. This had not been the rule before, and as a result many definite cases of glaucoma were discovered by ophthalmologists working in private practice. This again is the answer to the question of how blindness from glaucoma can be prevented. The ideal would be that every patient over the age of 40 should obtain his reading glasses from an eye specialist, and that tonometry be performed routinely.

If the oculist sees his patient only in the afternoon, he will miss a still greater number of cases of early glaucoma. However, I feel that under-referrals might be preferable to over-referrals, because if too many cases are classified as suspicious and it is found out later that glaucoma is in fact absent, confidence in eye specialists is lost and the whole mass screening is discredited. However, this is a very personal decision and I imagine that other ophthalmologists would prefer a high referral rate so that no patient with early glaucoma is overlooked. My own attitude to this question has changed in the course of the years from one of favoring a high referral rate to a more lenient attitude, after I found so many mild cases which should not have been classified as possible glaucomas. Of course, every patient with a progressive field loss who has been overlooked by someone else and is discovered by one of us will tend to change our attitude towards a more strict one in order to detect the maximum number of cases.

Perhaps nothing should be done about glaucoma detection and the patient should be left to decide for himself whether to see an ophthalmologist or not. We might conclude this if we consider the difficulties involved in mass screening, in selection of methods and in the definition of what glaucoma is or at what stage it begins, and if we consider the large number of mild glaucomas which develop slowly and are relatively harmless.

Nevertheless, I think that a decision to do nothing about early detection is wrong. There are recent statistics about the frequency of definite glaucoma which confirm this. Thus statistical analysis of 106,605 patients of various eye specialists in Germany showed that 12.1 % of them had glaucoma. When the results of one week of the ophthalmological practice of 116 eye specialists were pooled, it was found that among 6,374 patients who came for a first examination declaring that they just wanted glasses, 3 % had glaucoma. These percentages do not refer to mass screenings of the total population, but to people looking for ophthalmological advice. They are sufficiently high to remove any doubts of the need for mass screening.

CONCLUSIONS

To avoid blindness from glaucoma, the following steps seem appropriate.

1) In countries where the percentage of ophthalmologists is very high, the best way to prevent blindness from glaucoma and the best means of early detection of the disease is to persuade the public to consult an eye specialist, and not an optometrist, for glasses. Ocular tensions should be checked at each visit. There is no doubt that some early cases will be missed, for example if the patient happens to have a normal tension on some particular visit or when the clinic hours of the eye specialist fall at the time of day when relatively low tensions are prevalent. But I think that this is the wisest method, if the eye specialist himself can make the diagnosis and then treat the patient accordingly.

2) In countries with a small number of ophthalmologists per unit of population, the public should be informed about glaucoma and the need to have their eye tensions checked. There should be centers where tonometry can be obtained free of charge and where further examinations of suspicious cases can be carried out. Such institutions exist, for example, in many eastern countries, including Russia.

3) The use of mobile units carrying out mass screening of sections of the population seems to me less advisable. They would need to repeat the same population study every few years in order to find new cases of glaucoma and also to screen those who have, in the meantime, reached the age of 40. X-ray mass screening is mandatory in West Germany. However, this is not considered as a social measure to protect the individual, but rather as a check on the spreading of an infectious disease. Glaucoma detection is more comparable to the early diagnosis of cancer in females or to diabetes prevention. Such examinations are left to the individual's decision. The help which the state can give is to make people aware of glaucoma, to explain its symptoms and consequences and to offer a free examination.

4) All these efforts will be of no avail if ophthalmologists working in private practice are not constantly trained to treat glaucoma properly. Some doctors of the older generation still believe that pressures of 25 mm Hg are normal, and they will probably not offer adequate treatment to their glaucoma patients. The effect of drugs is not checked often enough, or too soon, after administration of mitotics. The visual field is checked by nonstandardized, nonreproducible methods and not often enough. The damage due to glaucoma is estimated from inspection of the optic disk instead of by careful studies of the visual field. These are perhaps the most frequent mistakes.

### REFERENCES

1. LEYDHECKER W. "Glaukom. Ein Handbuch." Berlin, Springer-Verlag, 1960, p 666.
2. LEYDHECKER W. Zur Verbreitung des Glaucoma simplex in der scheinbar gesunden, augenärztlich nicht behandelten Bevölkerung. *Doc Ophthalmol* **13**: 359, 1959.
3. LEYDHECKER W. Die soziale Bedeutung und Häufigkeit des Glaukoms. *Klin Monatsbl Augenheilkd* **135**: 188, 859, 1959.
4. LEYDHECKER W. The technique and organization of mass screening for glaucoma. *Am J Ophthalmol* **51**: 248, 1961.
5. LEYDHECKER W. Die Zuverlässigkeit der Frühdiagnose des Glaucoma simplex nach 7 Jahren retrospektiv beurteilt. *Ber Dtsch Ophthalmol Ges* **67**: 230, 1965.
6. LEYDHECKER W. Die Zuverlässigkeit der Diagnose des Glaucoma simplex im Frühstadium. *Doc Ophthalmol* **20**: 214, 1966.

We believe that our i.v. provocative test provides a more reliable method for detecting cases of suspected open-angle glaucoma than the commonly used water-drinking test. One reason for this may be that in the i.v. administration of fluid in amounts proportional to the body weight of the individual, the ocular response is obtained under standardized and hence, comparable physiological conditions. Therefore the observed changes in intraocular pressure reflect only the hydrodynamic condition of the individual eye. More precise information on this aspect requires, in addition, values of other parameters such as facility of outflow (C) and outflow (F) which can be obtained by means of tonography. When tonography is performed the scleral rigidity and its viscoelastic behavior should be particularly taken into consideration since such behavior during the stress of our i.v. provocative test has not been established. Naturally, in a screening program for chronic simple glaucoma in a community, problems such as these arise only for those cases where there is still some doubt about the diagnosis of glaucoma. Nevertheless, this does not minimize the potential value of the water infusion test as an aid in the diagnosis of chronic simple glaucoma.

# THE GLAUCOMATOUS OPTIC DISK

J. FRANÇOIS

Ophthalmological Clinic, University of Ghent, Ghent, Belgium

One should be very cautious when interpreting an ophthalmoscopic picture. Indeed, it must supplement, but it can seldom replace a comprehensive study of all the clinical information. This is particularly true with regard to the so-called "glaucomatous" disk.

NORMAL OPTIC DISK AND PHYSIOLOGICAL CUP

*Anatomical data.* The optic nerve begins beyond the lamina cribrosa, where the axons take their myelin sheath.

When the scleral opening is narrow, the axons are pressed together and the optic disk is flat. When the opening is larger, the axons are more spread out and leave a depression in the center, the bottom of which is constituted by the lamina cribrosa (physiological excavation).

The central vessels of the retina, which pass through the papillary depression, penetrate without anastomosing with the vascular system of the head of the optic nerve (Fig. 1). This system is important and largely anastomosed with the vessels of the choroid, the arteries of the Zinn-Haller circle and the vessels of the periphery as of the axial system of the optic nerve. Indeed, at the level of the lamina cribrosa, we find the vascular circle of Zinn-Haller generally incomplete, and formed by the short posterior ciliary arteries. The peripheral vascularization of the optic nerve depends on the pial vessels, while the central vascularization depends on the central artery of the optic nerve or in any case on an axial vascular system, which anastomoses with the vessels of the Zinn-Haller circle. These vessels are also joined by recurrent branches from the choroid. The optic disk, the circumpapillary retina, the lamina cribrosa and the anterior part of the optic nerve are supplied by an arterial anastomotic network, which does not supply the retina itself.

*Ophthalmoscopic data.* The optic disk has a diameter of $1.6224 \pm 0.0153$ mm (1). It is rose-colored, sometimes reddish. Its borders are distinct and its surface plane. The retinal vessels emerge from its central portion.

Generally a so-called physiological excavation exists. It has been recorded in 77% of the cases (2), in 73% of 5,000 normal subjects (3) and in 80% of 3,370 normal subjects (4). In 34% (4) the excavation was deep enough to make the lamina cribrosa visible. In 10% the excavation was large and deep.

The physiological depression is partial and central. There is a smooth slope from the border of the depression to the center. The vessels are never bent either at the level of the depression or at the approach of the scleral ring. If the depression is whitish, the periphery of the disk is always pink.

According to Goldmann (1) who studied 20 cases, the depth of the physiological excavation (distance between the surface of the

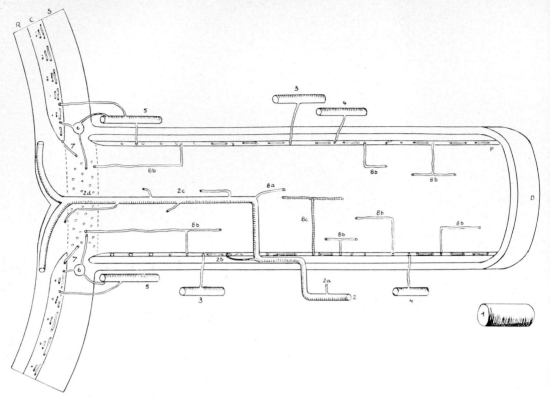

FIG. 1.  Survey of the vascularization of the orbital optic nerve. R = retina, C = choroid, S = sclera, P = leptomeningeal arterial plexus with its peripheral nerve supply, D = dural sheath. 1 = ophthalmic artery, main source of all the arterial branches, 2 = central retinal artery, 2a = extraneural branch, 2b = arachnoidal branch for the leptomeningeal plexus, 2c = intraneural branches or precocious retinal branches (inconstant, variable in size and small in number), 2d = absence of branches at the level of the lamina cribrosa, 3 = ciliary arteries (branches for the leptomeningeal plexus and the nerve), 4 = muscular arteries (branches for the leptomeningeal plexus and the nerve), 5 = posterior short ciliary arteries (branches for the leptomeningeal plexus, the choroid and the arterial circle of Zinn-Haller), 6 = arterial circle of Zinn-Haller, 7 = recurrent arterial twigs to the lamina cribrosa, 8 = peripheral and central optic nerve supply, 8a = occasional central branch from the central retinal artery, 8b = peripheral supply with an anterior or a posterior branch or both, 8c = one of these may reach the center of the nerve and, if important in size, realize a central optic nerve artery. Variations of 2c, 8a, 8c are frequent.

retina and the lamina cribrosa) is approximately $0.72 \pm 0.077$ mm in hyperopic or emmetropic eyes and 0.39 mm in myopic eyes. Its width is variable. Exceptionally it occupies more than 60% of the disk surface (5).

Some authors (4, 6, 7) thought that the physiological depression may increase with age. Others, on the contrary, believed that it disappeared during senescence (8). It is at present thought that the physiological excava-tion does not change during life (2, 9, 10).

Some authors also believed that a senile excavation of the disk could exist. But Goldmann (1) has shown that it actually was a pseudo-excavation, because of the increased transparency of the papillary tissue. On slit-lamp examination one receives the impression of an excavation, as the scleral edge casts a shadow on the lamina cribrosa. However, when the course of the nervous fibers are

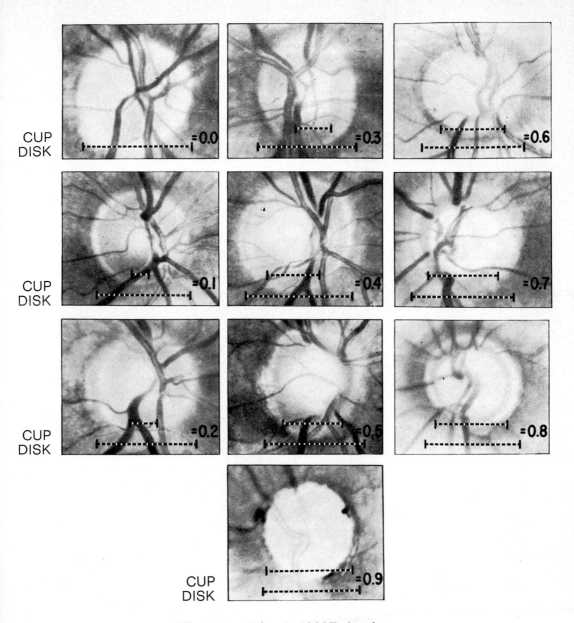

Fig. 2. Cup : disk ratio of M.F. Armaly.

traced on the temporal side and if they slope smoothly down to the central depression, the disk can be considered physiological.

Finally, the physiological excavation is never accompanied by perimetric defects.

Measurements with the aid of a graticule give an exact idea of the relative size of the physiological (or glaucomatous) excavation in relation to the disk diameter (2, 11, 12). But it is Armaly (13) in particular who has shown the importance of the cup:disk ratio and suggested a very convenient photographic procedure (Fig. 2). These ratios, which may be 0.5, 0.7 etc., are not distributed according to a Gaussian curve in normal subjects. In 45% of the cases, the physiological excavation occupies less than 1/10 of the disk diameter and in 67% of the cases less than 3/10. Moreover, in 92% of the cases, the ratio is exactly the same in both eyes.

So there exist "cup:disk" ratios of 0.3, which are pathological; and others, of course more exceptional, of 0.8 or even 0.9, which are not.

Consequently it is not right to say that each cup reaching two-thirds of the optic disk is suspect, since the physiological depression is generally less than one-half of the disk diameter. Among 4,231 patients between 14 and 75 years of age, Hollows and Graham (14) found 102 subjects with big cups (2.2%); 54% of these had no glaucoma, 27% had positive glaucoma, and 19% had intraocular hypertension without functional defects ($P_0 \geq 21$ mm Hg).

On the other hand, as neither age nor sex has any influence on this ratio, it is probably congenital, and genetically determined. According to Armaly (13) the heredity should be polygenic (plurifactorial): multiple genes with additive expression.

### GLAUCOMATOUS CUP OF THE OPTIC DISK

The optic nerve is the greatest victim of glaucoma. Its alterations can be observed on the one hand by ophthalmoscopic examination, and on the other hand by the evaluation of the visual field. Therefore, the correlation between the papillary aspect and its eventual perimetric manifestation is one of the most important problems in glaucoma.

To realize perfectly the alterations of the disk, the pupil has to be dilated. However, before doing so, it is necessary to know the opening of the angle of the anterior chamber.

If the angle is large, there is no danger of producing a mydriasis. If the angle is narrow, dilatation of the pupil must be avoided. If it is nevertheless necessary, the mydriasis should

be limited to a minimum. Atropine must never be used: only neosynephrine together with glycerol. At the end of the examination a strong miotic must be instilled.

Examination of the optic disk should be made: 1) with the ophthalmoscope to examine the scleral border, the emergence of the vessels, the color of the disk and the appearance of the lamina cribrosa, and also to search for the presence of a cup, of capillaries and of a circumpapillary halo; 2) with the slit lamp. The stereoscopic view and the light slit permit a precise evaluation of the level differences and the depth of an eventual cup. 3) Photography is important, because it allows one to note the changes which occur over the years. Moreover it provides a document, on which the cup:disk ratio can be measured. However, it gives no information about the depth of the excavation, which can only be appreciated by stereophotography. Photography may sometimes be misleading, because the disk color depends on the film, the exposure time and the absorption of light by more or less transparent media.

Contrary to what was expected, it seems that fluoroangiography has not made any valuable contribution to our understanding of glaucoma.

*Characteristics of the glaucomatous disk.* The glaucomatous cup of the optic disk has many characteristics: 1) The scleral border of the disk is clearly visible. Its sharp internal rim seems to hang over the bottom of the excavation. 2) The excavation is total and involves the whole of the area. 3) One has to modify the focusing of the ophthalmoscope by several diopters in order to see the lamina cribrosa, which constitutes the bottom of the excavation. As we know, one diopter corresponds to 0.3 mm and sometimes we find excavations of 1.6 to 2 mm (level difference of five or six diopters). 4) The emergence of the central vessels is displaced towards the nasal side. Furthermore, these vessels are partially hidden at the lateral side of the deep excavation. 5) The disk becomes white and atrophic. 6) Around the disk, there may be a halo, due to the circumpapillary atrophy of the choroid. This atrophy is secondary to the ischemia and the sclerosis of the vessels of the Zinn-Haller circle. 7) The capillaries of the disk have disappeared. 8) A spontaneous pulse of the central retinal artery, or one produced by slight finger pressure on the globe, proves that the intraocular pressure is more or less equal to the diastolic arterial pressure. 9) It is not unusual to find newly formed anastomoses, wound at the level of the nasal part of the optic disk. 10) In myopic eyes only a slight depression, but not a real excavation, will be seen.

Between this characteristic glaucomatous cup and the physiological excavation, there are obviously a great number of intermediary conditions. The glaucomatous cup may, indeed, begin with a deepening of the physiological excavation (1). On the other hand, ocular hypertension has to exist for a long time before the alterations and the excavation of the disk appear. Leydhecker (15) thinks that 10 years are necessary when the hypertension is moderate.

It is not so much the grade of the excavation which is important, but rather the change in the cup:disk ratio; for every increase of the diameter of the cup is pathologic, even if the ophthalmoscopic appearance is still that of a classical physiological excavation. This change of the depression can only be appreciated by serial photography.

Moreover, a difference between the cup:disk ratios of both eyes, especially if it is above 0.2, has much more pathologic significance than the relative size of the excavation itself.

A central depression which becomes pathologic does not always increase uniformly in all axes. Generally the excavation increases first at the inferior temporal side, where it

soon reaches the scleral rim. A grayish pit without vessels is formed, which corresponds closely to the Bjerrum arciform scotoma in the superior visual field.

More rarely, the excavation increases at the superior temporal side, where it does not reach the scleral border. In this case a bend of the vessels is usually seen.

Often the glaucomatous cup affects both temporal segments, and has a kidney-like aspect, the vascular hilum being represented by the emergence of the central vessels. The temporal rim is then very steep.

More rarely, the cup occupies the whole of the disk to form a plate. This aspect is seen especially in myopic eyes.

Initially the distance between the level of the retina and that of the lamina cribrosa is the same in the glaucomatous cup as in the normal disk. It is only later that the lamina cribrosa is pushed back.

The evolution of a glaucomatous cup after normalization of the pressure is generally stationary. We have never seen it disappear. Its apparent disappearance in exceptional cases may be due to proliferation of glial tissue (16–18). Amsler and Rumpf (19), and Werner and McDougald (20) have observed the disappearance of the excavation after an antiglaucomatous operation.

The aspect of the disk can vary according to the clinical type of glaucoma. In congenital glaucoma, very deep disk excavations without perimetric defects may be seen. Furthermore a decrease in the depth and width of the excavation may be observed after a successful goniotomy (18).

In closed-angle glaucoma the disk does not have time to excavate if the pressure increases very quickly. The nervous fibers are destroyed before their supporting tissue disappears. Therefore, the disk becomes white. The atrophy of the optic nerve with its more total and more anarchic visual field defects prevails over the cupping.

In open-angle glaucoma, excavation precedes atrophy. Moreover, there is often a great difference in the appearance of both disks. A progressive disappearance of the capillaries of the disk is also seen, especially in some sectors, which often allows us to predict the site of the perimetric defects.

*Differential diagnosis.* We have already discussed the physiological excavation.

Generally the colobomatous pit is easily recognized, although the glaucomatous excavation may sometimes have the same aspect. The coloboma of the optic nerve, which may be accompanied by visual field defects (21), is congenital and larger than the disk. It is surrounded by an irregular pigmentary ring and often accompanied by ocular or systemic anomalies.

Primary or secondary optic atrophy are characterized by very red perimetric defects, by normal ocular pressure and by normal outflow facility.

A disk excavation due to intracranial compression of the optic nerve has been mentioned in cases of tumor or calcified carotid (15). But, in this case the excavation of the disk may be due to arteriosclerosis of the vessels of the optic nerve.

Pallor of the disk with excavation may be seen in pseudopapillitis vascularis, but the disease starts with signs of optic nevritis or papillitis.

*Correlations between the glaucomatous cup and the visual field.* Some facts are now well established.

1) Perimetric defects, sometimes very discrete, may exist in the absence of any excavation of the disk (22), and even when the disk seems to be completely normal (23–25). According to Shutt et al. (10) visual field defects are found in 34% of glaucomas without excavation of the disk. These facts prove that it is always necessary to determine the visual field of a glaucomatous patient. 2) A glaucomatous cupping may exist and increase in the absence of visual field defects (18, 26). Shutt et al. (10) found no perimetric defects in 12% of glaucomas with disk excavation. These findings are explained by the fact that the excavation is produced at the expense of the astroglial cells or fibers, that is to say the supporting cells (27). This factor also accounts for a possible decrease in the excavation after normalization of the pressure (27). 3) When there are visual field defects, the cup:disk ratio is generally greater (28, 29).

4) Examination of the disk allows us to predict the seat of the perimetric defects in 72% of the cases (30), but in 28% of the cases there is no correlation. If the vascular condition is examined in the two groups, it is found to be abnormal in 20% of the cases in the first group, and in 50% of the cases in the second. When there are glaucomatous disk changes together with obvious narrowing of the retinal arteries, examination of the disk does not permit us exactly to predict the defects of the visual field. 5) When the disk is pale or atrophied with or without excavation, there are always visual field defects (22).

*Genesis of the glaucomatous cupping.* The pathological changes of the disk observed in glaucoma depend, in the first place, on pre-existing anatomic conditions. When glaucoma enlarges the normal depression of the disk, the pathological aspect will be different in emmetropic or myopic eyes. In myopia a deep glaucomatous excavation is impossible, since the distance between the surface of the retina and the lamina cribrosa is only 0.39 mm.

On the other hand, we must take into account the very rich capillary vascularization of the disk, which has a large number of anastomoses with vessels outside the eyeball.

When the intraocular pressure increases, the blood of the disk is driven out towards other territories which are not influenced by the ocular pressure.

Therefore, it is likely that the destruction of the visual fibers, or of their supporting tissue, by glaucoma is not due directly to the compression of axons on the border of the scleral canal, but to an insufficiency of vascularization (ischemia). This view also explains why in "glaucoma without pressure," the same ophthalmoscopic, perimetric and anatomic alterations are seen as in glaucoma with hypertension, since the mechanism is the same (vascular insufficiency). Moreover, it explains why the decrease of systemic arterial hypertension may heighten the functional defects of a glaucoma, till then well equilibrated (24).

In summary, vascular changes in the head of the optic nerve may give the same anatomical and clinical signs, but may depend on three different mechanisms: ocular hypertension, hypotension of the ophthalmic artery and local capillary disease, which also explains glaucoma without pressure.

Regardless of whether the glaucomatous cupping is due to an insufficient blood supply to the disk, it is produced, at least initially, at the expense of the supporting glial tissue to the nervous fibers, since important excavations may exist without visual field defects (31). Afterwards, the fibers of the optic nerve also disappear, but for a long time the distance between the level of the retina and the lamina cribrosa remains the same as in normal subjects, viz. 0.66 mm (1).

The pressing back of the vessels towards the nasal side is more like a sinking of the vessels and is also due to the disappearance of the supporting tissue (1).

A direct effect of the ocular pressure, compressing the nervous fibers on the resistant rim of the scleral ring, does not explain glaucoma without pressure, and consequently not glaucoma with hypertension. Furthermore, there is not a single argument in favor of a primary disease of the nervous tissue.

#### GLAUCOMA WITHOUT PRESSURE

There are cases where hypertension is intermittent (32), where it is only nocturnal (33), where the provocative tests are positive (32), where the scleral rigidity is decreased, especially as seen in myopic eyes (32) and where the tonography is abnormal. All these cases are not glaucomas without pressure, but are true glaucomas. Moreover, it is always essential to make a diurnal pressure curve for at least three days. An eye, the pressure of which has always been low, for example 11 mm Hg, has a glaucoma from the moment that the tension increases, say, to 19 mm Hg (34).

Perkins (35) and Winstanley (36) examined 58 patients (103 eyes), presumed to be affected by glaucoma without pressure. The diagnosis could be maintained with the aid of tonography, provocative tests, etc., for only four eyes.

#### SIGNIFICANCE OF THE CUPPING OF THE DISK

1) Eyes having a normal disk, may support moderate ocular hypertension for a number of years without deterioration of the visual field. 2) Eyes which already have a restricted pathologic cupping of the disk tolerate ocular hypertension better than those with total excavation. 3) When glaucoma is very advanced, the disk deeply excavated and the visual field narrowed, the condition can only remain stationary when the ocular pressure is reduced below the statistically normal limits (31, 37, 38). Even then optic atrophy may continue to develop and cause blindness. 4) In any case, the appearance of the disk must be the guide for adequate treatment in glaucoma, because the pressure level does not have the same importance, whether or not the disk is normal (37). When the cupping of the disk becomes wider during treatment, it is absolutely necessary to decrease the pressure level obtained medically. For an identical tonometric reading, the force acting on the papillary surface, stretched out by the excavation, is much higher than when the surface is flat (39). On the other hand, the stretch of the capillaries

and the nervous fibers in the excavated sectors of the disk increases the surface of each element and so, indirectly, subjects it to a higher effect of the pressure.

In other words, the first effect of an excavation is to increase the surface of the disk, which is transformed into a "hemisphere." For an ocular pressure of 30 mm Hg, the disk supports a force of 0.7 g when the surface is flat, and of 1.4 g when it is excavated. Identical reasoning applies to the stretched capillaries and nervous fibers.

Furthermore, when the disk has a more fragile sector, viz the temporal segment, the pressure, which is theoretically transmitted equally in all directions, will nevertheless exert a much higher pressure on the fragile sector, the surface of which is enlarged. The nasal segment offers a better resistance, probably because of the protective role of the central retinal vessels, as long as they are surrounded by their connective sheath.

## REFERENCES

1. GOLDMANN H. La papille, in: Busacca A, Goldmann H and Schiff-Wertheimer S (Eds), "Biomicroscopie du corps vitré et du fond d'oeil." Paris, Masson et Cie, 1957, p 339.
2. HOLLOWS FC and McGUINESS R. The size of the optic cup. *Trans Ophthalmol Soc NZ* **19**: 33, 1967.
3. FORD N and SARWAR M. Features of clinically normal optic disk. *Br J Ophthalmol* **47**: 50, 1963.
4. WITUSIK W. Types of physiological excavation of the optic nerve head. *Ophthalmologica* **152**: 57, 1966.
5. PICKARD R. The alteration in size of the normal optic disk cup. *Br J Ophthalmol* **32**: 355, 1948.
6. PROCKSCH M. Ueber die Altersveränderung der physiologischen Exkavation. *Klin Monatsbl Augenheilkd* **122**: 168, 1953.
7. COLENBRANDER MC. Measurement of the excavation. *Ophthalmologica* **139**: 491, 1960.
8. PICKARD R. The clinical course of cavernous atrophy and its relation to the normal enlargement of the optic disc cup. *Trans Ophthalmol UK* **55**: 599, 1935.
9. SYNDACKER D. The normal optic disk. Ophthalmoscopic and photographic studies. *Am J Ophthalmol* **58**: 958, 1964.
10. SHUTT HKR, BOYD TAS and SALTER AB. The relationship of visual fields, optic disk appearance and age in nonglaucomatous and glaucomatous eyes. *Can J Ophthalmol* **2**: 83, 1967.
11. PARR JC. Clinical estimation of optic disk cupping, with description of a graticule. *NZ Med J* (Suppl) **16**: 93, 1966.
12. PARR JC. Clinical estimation of optic disk cupping. *Trans Ophthalmol Soc NZ* **18**: 93, 1966.
13. ARMALY MF. Genetic determination of cup/disk ratio of the optic nerve. *Arch Ophthalmol* **78**: 35, 1967.
14. HOLLOWS FC and GRAHAM PA. Intraocular pressure, glaucoma and glaucoma suspects in a defined population. *Br J Ophthalmol* **50**: 570, 1966.
15. LEYDHECKER W. Glaukom. "Ein Handbuch." Berlin, Springer Verlag, 1960.
16. ELSCHNIG A. Ueber Glaukom. *Albrecht von Graefes Arch Ophthalmol* **120**: 94, 1928.
17. SALZMANN M. Die präpapilläre Bindegewebswucherung bei Glaukom und ihr Verhältnis zur Retinitis proliferans. *Albrecht von Graefes Arch Ophthalmol* **140**: 629, 1939.
18. SHAFFER RN. New concepts in infantile glaucoma. *Can J Ophthalmol* **2**: 243, 1967.
19. AMSLER M and RUMPF J. Schwankungen der glaukomatösen Exkavation. *Klin Monatsbl Augenheilkd* **97**: 688, 1936.
20. WERNER LE and MacDOUGALD TJ. Low tension glaucoma. Its diagnosis and treatment. *Trans Ophthalmol Soc UK* **71**: 439, 1951.
21. EISUM EF. Crater-like hole in the optic disk. *Acta Ophthalmol (Kbh)* **35**: 200, 1957.
22. TRAQUAIR HM. "An introduction to clinical perimetry." London, H Kimpton, 1948.
23. NORDMANN J, LOBSTEIN A, GERHARD J and BENCK P. Le test à la cortisone dans le glaucome simple à champ visuel normal. *Ophthalmologica* **150**: 46, 1965.
24. FRANÇOIS J and NEETENS A. Increased intraocular pressure and optic nerve atrophy. The Hague, Ed Junk, 1966.
25. LAVERGNE G and JOACHIM M. Déficits périmétriques et altérations papillaires dans le glaucome à angle ouvert débutant. *Bull Soc Belge Ophthalmol* **146**: 364, 1967.
26. CHANDLER P and GRANT M. "Lectures on glaucoma." Philadelphia, Lea and Febiger, 1965, p 327.
27. SHAFFER RN. The role of the astroglial cells in glaucomatous disk cupping. *Doc Ophthalmol* **26**: 516, 1969.
28. ARMALY MF. Cup/disk ratio in early open-angle glaucoma. *Doc Ophthalmol* **26**: 526, 1969.
29. ARMALY MF. The correlation between appearance of the optic cup and visual function. *Trans Am Acad Ophthalmol Otolaryngol* **73**: 898, 1969.
30. AULHORN E and HARMS H. Papillenveränderung und Gesichtsfeldstörung beim Glaukom. *Ophthalmologica* **139**: 279, 1960.
31. ETIENNE R. "Les glaucomes." Marseilles, Ed Diffusion Générale de Librairie, 1969.
32. NORDMANN J and GERHARD JP. Au sujet du glaucome sans hypertension. *Bull Soc Ophthalmol Fr* **57**: 443, 1957.
33. MATTEUCCI P. Considerazioni sul glaucoma senza ipertensione. *Atti 37 Congr Soc Ottal Ital* **10**: 168, 1948.
34. FRIEDENWALD JS. Symposium: Primary glaucoma. I. Terminology, pathology and physio-

logical mechanisms. *Trans Am Acad Ophthalmol Otolaryngol* **53**: 169, 1949.

35. PERKINS ES. Discussion on low-tension glaucoma. *Proc R Soc Med* **52**: 429, 1959.

36. WINSTANLEY J. Discussion on low-tension glaucoma. *Proc R Soc Med* **52**: 433, 1959.

37. CHANDLER P. Long term results in glaucoma therapy. *Am J Ophthalmol* **49**: 221, 1960.

38. LEE PF. Importance of status of visual field and optic disc in management of open-angle glaucoma. *Am J Ophthalmol* **53**: 435, 1962.

39. VILLASECA A. The impact of intraocular pressure on the glaucomatous disc. A theoretical study based on hydrostatic principles. *Arch Ophthalmol* **67**: 769, 1962.

# PRELIMINARY OBSERVATIONS ON THE APPEARANCE OF THE OPTIC DISK IN GLAUCOMA

RALPH E. KIRSCH and DOUGLAS R. ANDERSON

Departments of Ophthalmology, University of Miami School of Medicine and
Mount Sinai Hospital, Miami, Florida, USA

In pursuing our goal, the prevention of blindness, and in seeking out the glaucomatous patient in need of therapy, whether in developed or developing nations, the most important diagnostic considerations are the appearance of the optic disk, the state of the visual fields and tonometry.

Tonometry is valuable and necessary, but Linnér and Leydhecker have described the difficulties which it may cause. Visual field testing is subjective, and subjective data are often open to criticism. Field testing is frequently complicated by many variables with which we are all familiar. The worsening of cataracts can mislead us; furthermore, field testing, which is time-consuming, can only be carried out by a trained and skilled examiner.

On the other hand, examination of the disk is an objective examination and when pursued with diligence may prove to be, if a clear view is obtainable, the single most dependable sign in the diagnosis of glaucoma.

The broadest goal of the present investigation was to attempt to determine if it is possible to take a single look at a disk and to differentiate by that single look between a normal disk and a glaucomatous disk. In this study the disks have been examined by all possible clinical and photographic techniques.

We studied two groups of patients, one with known normal (nonglaucomatous) eyes having normal applanation tension, fields and tonography and the second group of known glaucomatous eyes with definitely elevated applanation tension, glaucomatous field defects and impaired outflow facilities. Thus we eliminated from consideration any borderline cases in which the eye was not clearly normal or clearly glaucomatous. We studied 70 eyes in the normal group and 80 in the glaucomatous group.

In normal eyes, Elschnig (1) gave his classic typing of the physiologic cup, namely, funnel-form excavation, cylindric-form excavation, dish-form excavation, excavation with gradually sloping lateral wall and atypical excavation.

In studying our normal eyes we were able to divide the disks into two groups, those with flat surfaces and those with physiologic cups. The latter group could be divided into: 1) round cup, 2) horizontally-oval cup and 3) atypical cup.

Elschnig (1) has stated that a disk is glaucomatous only if its cup extends to the margin and if the wall of the cup is steep there. The majority of modern clinicians still agree with this statement.

We found that the disks in glaucomatous eyes fell into three groups. The first and most obvious group included disks with a huge cup which was generally round, extended to the disk margin and left no surface tissue remaining; there was extensive undermining of the cup, walls, general nasal displacement of the vessels, and a sickly, dusky gray color of the base of the cup.

The second group showed an incomplete cup not extending to the margin everywhere. These had a generally vertically-oval cup with disk surface depression, that is, surface depression extending to the margin, usually inferiorly. This is probably what Chandler and Grant (2) described as saucerization and probably what others have described as enlargement of the cup extending to the margin. Chandler and Grant believe that the physiologic cup first enlarges, usually downward and temporally, reaching the inferior temporal margin. They add that in some eyes the cup enlarges only upward or may enlarge both up and down. This group includes disks which are certainly clearly definable as glaucomatous, and it was in this group that we first became aware of the tendency for the early glaucomatous cup to be vertically-oval.

This realization, then, led us to our definition of the third and earliest group of glaucomatous disks, those in which the only abnormal finding was a vertically-oval cup. This cup need not extend to the disk margin at all, may be surrounded by apparently healthy tissue and the disk surface may be normal or only subtly depressed. This sign, the vertically-oval cup, we now believe constitutes an early and important diagnostic criterion of the glaucomatous disk.

The glaucomatous disk may thus be identified if it has: 1) a vertically-oval cup, 2) a vertically-oval cup with disk surface depression or 3) a complete glaucomatous cup.

These changes all have in common a single pathologic anatomic mechanism, namely, disk tissue loss. This tissue loss may occur at the cup rim, on the disk surface and in the wall of the cup. Our concept of the development of this tissue loss is that it is a dynamic process which occurs in all three locations simultaneously, though first seen clinically at the cup rim where it produces the vertically-oval cup.

We have made an observation concerning tissue loss in the cup wall and its relationship to so-called undermining (ampulliform excavation). Our study indicates that if there is undermining with healthy surface tissue remaining and forming a round boundary for the cup, the undermining is almost surely physiological, whereas if there is no surface tissue remaining or that which does remain outlines a vertically oval cup, the undermining represents glaucoma.

Since hearing the first presentation of our data in Los Angeles in May 1971, Becker (personal communication) reviewed the disk data in his own large series of open-angle glaucoma cases in St. Louis and confirmed statistically what we found clinically concerning the vertically-oval cup.

The concept of the vertically oval cup in early glaucoma is clinically useful. When a new patient has a large but incomplete cup of the disk which is round or horizontally oval the likelihood of glaucoma immediately decreases. On the other hand a small but vertically oval cup is considered to indicate glaucoma until proved otherwise.

The possibility that this vertical cupping of the disk could serve usefully as an adjunct in glaucoma screening in both developed and developing nations should be borne in mind. For now, let each of us examine every optic disk under the most ideal conditions available to us, and with meticulous care, in an attempt to decide if it is normal or glaucomatous and to look particularly for the early sign of the vertically-oval cup. This is one more way in which we shall contribute to the prevention of blindness from glaucoma.

## REFERENCES

1. Elschnig A. "Encyclopaedie der Augenheilkunde." Leipzig, ECW Vogel, 1904, p 292 (translated by EVL Brown, Chicago, American Medical Association).

2. Chandler PA and Grant WM. "Lectures on glaucoma." Philadelphia, Lea and Febiger, 1965, p 14.

# THE DIAGNOSIS AND ADRENERGIC THERAPY OF OPEN-ANGLE GLAUCOMA

ROBERT W. HART and MAURICE E. LANGHAM

Applied Physics Laboratory, Johns Hopkins University, Silver Spring, Maryland and Johns Hopkins Hospital, The Wilmer Institute, W. K. Kellogg Foundation Laboratories, Baltimore, Maryland, USA

The general problem posed by glaucoma diagnosis and therapy is illustrated in Fig. 1. Each "characteristic point" represents the intraocular pressure ($P_0$) and the tonographic coefficient of outflow facility ($C_T$) of either a normal eye or an untreated eye which has been diagnosed as glaucomatous (primary, open-angle). Glaucomatous eyes may be dif-

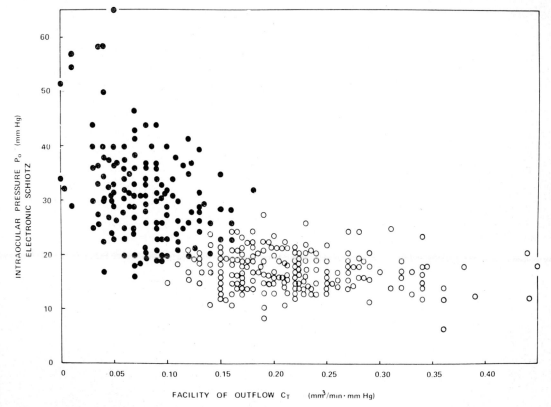

FIG. 1. Intraocular pressures and coefficients of tonographic outflow facility of normal (open circles) and glaucomatous eyes (closed circles). Taken from ref. 13.

ferentiated from normal eyes by the tendency of their $P_0$ and $C_T$ values to lie outside the domain defined for normal eyes. *Pari passu*, with the development of glaucoma the $P_0$ and $C_T$ values of the individual patient describe a mean path, or trajectory, that moves upwards and to the left on the $P_0$-$C_T$ diagram. Recognition of such a trajectory provides a basis for early diagnosis of the glaucomatous process. The inhibition of this trajectory is tantamount to preventive treatment of glaucoma; the reversal of the glaucoma trajectory implies successful medical therapy.

Differentiation between glaucomatous and normal eyes is better accomplished in terms of both parameters $P_0$ and $C_T$ rather than in terms of either one alone (1). In this respect it is important to recognize that $P_0$ and $C_T$ reflect quite different features of aqueous humor dynamics, because $P_0$ is a steady state property while $C_T$ is a nonsteady state property. $P_0$ is the equilibrium pressure at which the rates of inflow and outflow of aqueous humor are equal in the individual eye. On the other hand, $C_T$ is a coefficient derived from the rate of return of the intraocular pressure to equilibrium after $P_0$ has been increased by the weight of the tonometer resting on the cornea. $C_T$ is expressed as the average excess rate of loss of aqueous humor per unit of increased pressure and has the dimensions of $mm^3/min \cdot mm\ Hg$. Eyes with either a pressure exceeding 25 mm Hg or a tonographic coefficient less than $\sim 0.15$ should be considered as suspect for glaucoma (Fig. 1). However, when $P_0$ exceeds 25 mm Hg and at the same time $C_T$ is less than 0.15 the likelihood of glaucoma is much increased. Thus the measurement of both the transient response $C_T$ and the steady state parameter $P_0$ provides a more discriminating tool in the diagnosis and management of open-angle glaucoma than the measurement of either parameter alone.

Clinical use has been made of the empiri-cal coefficient $P_0/C_T$. Thus, in the above example, values of $P_0/C_T$ exceeding 166 would be considered glaucoma-suspect. The clinical importance of $P_0/C_T$ (or alternative relationships between the steady state value $P_0$ and the transient pressure response of the eye) in the diagnosis and prognosis of open-angle glaucoma cannot be overemphasized. However, the separation of normal and glaucomatous eyes in Fig. 1 is based on the traditional criteria of reduced visual field and characteristic pathological changes at the optic disk. An abnormal $P_0/C_T$ is generally not recognized until structural and functional changes have been established. Consequently, at the time the diagnosis is made, significant changes in $P_0$ and $C_T$ of the individual eyes will already have occurred. It is the trend of the time course of the $P_0$-$C_T$ trajectory that facilitates recognition of the glaucoma process before visual impairment and abnormal disk structure sets in. On this basis we must conclude that a $P_0$-$C_T$ trajectory giving rise to a diagnosis of glaucoma precedes visual loss. Consequently, if we could define the trajectories for individual eyes, we would have a powerful method for the early diagnosis of glaucoma. This possibility is here illustrated by describing the time course of $P_0$ and $C_T$ values associated with the development of open-angle glaucoma in an individual subject.

The patient, a woman aged 44 years, was first seen in 1967 during a glaucoma-screening program of glaucoma-prone families. Her mother, aged 75 years, had established open-angle glaucoma for at least 15 years, and had suffered severe visual loss in spite of medical treatment and surgical intervention. At the time of the first examination of the daughter the visual fields and optic disks were normal, the anterior chambers were deep and the angles open (grade III to IV) with no pigment deposition on the trabecular meshworks. The intraocular pressure measured by both the Goldmann applanation and the Schiøtz elec-

TABLE 1. *l-epinephrine data for human eyes[a]*

| Source of data | Dose and time | Number of eyes | Before treatment[b] | | | After treatment[b] | | | |
|---|---|---|---|---|---|---|---|---|---|
| | | | $\langle P_0 \rangle$ | $\langle C_T \rangle$ | $\langle \lambda \rangle$[c] | $\langle P'_0 \rangle$ | $\langle C_T \rangle$ | $\langle \lambda \rangle$[c] | $\langle \lambda - \lambda' \rangle$ |
| Becker et al. (16) | Daily for three months | 37 (glaucomatous) | 21.9 | 0.145 | | 17.1 | 0.20 | 12.5 | + 0.3 |
| | Six months | 27 (glaucomatous) | | | 12.8 | 17.2 | 0.22 | 13.0 | – 0.2 |
| Kitazawa[d] (15) | Twice daily for seven days  0.06 M | 40 (glaucomatous) | 22.4 ± 0.99 | 0.16 ± 0.011 | 13.3 | 21 ± 0.95 | 0.19 ± 0.013 | 13.6 | – 0.3 |
| | 0.12 M | | 23.9 ± 1.25 | 0.14 ± 0.006 | 13.3 | 18.7 ± 0.93 | 0.21 ± 0.015 | 13.3 | 0 |
| | 0.25 M | | 23.8 ± 0.95 | 0.13 ± 0.007 | 13.0 | 17.8 ± 0.88 | 0.21 ± 0.022 | 13.0 | 0 |
| | 0.5 M | | 24.2 ± 0.46 | 0.15 ± 0.006 | 13.6 | 18.6 ± 0.96 | 0.26 ± 0.025 | 14.4 | – 0.8 |
| Richards and Drance (9) | One application 6 to 8 hr post dose | 9 (glaucomatous) | 22.4 | 0.09 | 11.6 | 14.9 | 0.20 | 11.6 | 0 |
| Prijot (10) | One application 24 hr post dose | 25 (normal) | Data as reported for individual eyes | | 14.0 ± 1.2 | Data as reported for individual eyes | | 13.7 ± 2.4 | + 0.3 |
| Langham et al. (3) Langham (2) | 0.25 M one application 6 hr post dose | 6 (normal) | 14.6 ± 0.9 | 0.28 ± 0.04 | 13.1 | 11.4 ± 1.1 | 0.48 ± 0.06 | 14.8 | – 1.7 |
| Langham et al. (3) | 24 hr post dose | 6 (normal) | | | | 12.0 ± 1.2 | 0.37 ± 0.06 | 13.3 | – 0.2 |

[a] Range $P_0 > 9$ mm Hg, $C_T \leq \frac{1}{2}$ mm³/min·mm Hg.

[b] $\langle \rangle$ denotes average value for the number of eyes indicated ± SD where available, $P_0$ in mm Hg, $C_T$ in mm³/min·mm Hg, $\lambda$ in (mm Hg)$^{\frac{1}{2}}$.

[c] $P_T$ calculated from the 1957 Friedenwald tonometer calibration equations.

[d] For these data the "before treatment" values are given instead of the values for the control (i.e. untreated eye).

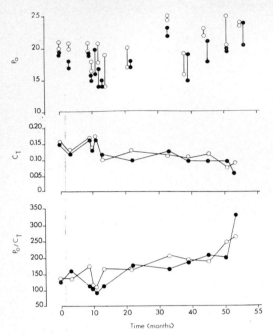

FIG. 2. Intraocular pressures and coefficients of tonographic outflow facility in a patient with developing clinically diagnosed open-angle glaucoma (see text). Intraocular pressures were measured by both Goldmann applanation and Schiøtz indentation tonometric procedures. The vertical bars relate the two pressure readings on the individual eye. The bottom graph gives the $P_0/C_T$ values, where $P_0$ is the Goldmann applanation pressure.

tronic indentation tonometer was approximately 20 mm Hg, and $C_T$ was 0.15 mm³/min·mm Hg in both eyes. Thus $P_0$ and $C_T$ and $P_0/C_T$ (133) were within the range of normal values. On the other hand, pressure cup studies made at this time on both eyes, using the experimental and analytical procedures described by Langham (2), indicated abnormally low pressure-regulatory capacity. A summary of further examinations from 1967 through 1971 is given in Fig. 2. $P_0$ showed significant variations typical of early glaucoma, whereas $C_T$ showed a significant steady drift to lower and more abnormal values over the same period. Values of the empirical coefficient $P_0/C_T$ reflected the long-term development of abnormality, again sug-

gestive of the glaucomatous process. However, no visual loss or pathological changes were seen within the optic disk until the 50th month, when only moderate cupping and minimal disturbance of retinal vessels were observed (Fig. 3). Visual fields measured by Goldmann perimetry were normal at the 36th month, but at the 50th month a superior arcuate defect in the left eye was found by the same procedure, and significant enlargement of the blind spot in both eyes was found at this time by the tangent screen technique. Depression of retinal function typical of glaucoma was confirmed by Harms static perimetry. In this patient the long-term trend of the tonographic data was obviously indicative of the glaucomatous process well before the development of significant visual loss.

The object of therapy of glaucoma in terms of the $P_0$-$C_T$ relationship is to displace the $P_0$-$C_T$ point representing the untreated pathological eye into the domain of normality. Different displacements will be desired, depending on the pressure and outflow coefficient of the untreated eye. Thus, for example, mere reduction of $P_0$ (without changing $C_T$) may suffice for an eye with elevated pressure but normal facility, whereas increases in $C_T$ will also be needed for eyes in which $P_0$ is elevated and $C_T$ is depressed. Ideally, it should be possible to anticipate drug effects in terms of trajectories on Fig. 1, since a particular family of trajectories characterizes a particular drug.

It is therefore important to determine the kinds of trajectory associated with the various adrenergic drugs, so that a medication can be selected which will lead to the desired changes of pressure and outflow facility. Recent theoretical and experimental studies (3–5) make it possible to achieve this goal.

In general, adrenergic drugs are categorized according to their influences on the two types of adrenergic receptors, and this provides a valuable organizational framework. Thus, drugs which primarily enhance *a*-receptor

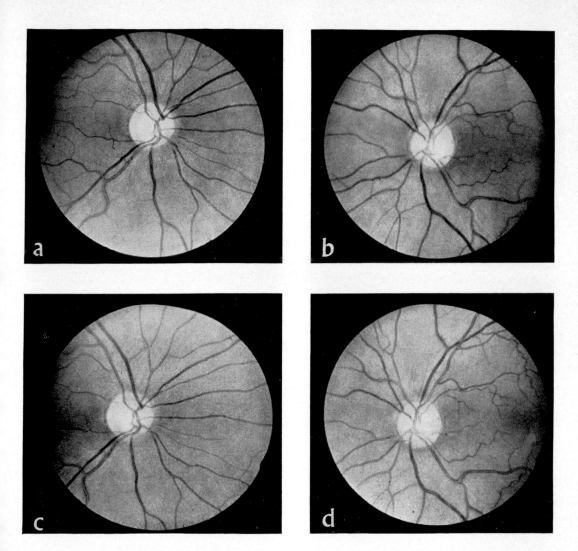

FIG. 3. Fundus photographs taken during development of clinically diagnosed open-angle glaucoma. These photographs relate to the same patient as described in Fig. 2. a and b) photographs of left and right eyes, respectively at the 23rd month after the initial examination; c and d) corresponding photographs taken at the 46th month when field loss in both eyes was first established.

action (e.g., the adrenergic transmitter nor-epinephrine, and the α-adrenergic potentiator protriptyline) lower the intraocular pressure and increase the facility of outflow (and dilate the pupil) in a characteristic way. The effects of these drugs can therefore be represented in Fig. 1 in terms of a characteristic family of curvilinear trajectories corresponding to decreasing $P_0$ and increasing $C_T$ (3).

Furthermore, drugs which primarily enhance β-receptor action (e.g., salbutmol, and relatively low concentrations of isoproterenol), when applied topically to the eye, induce decreased intraocular pressure without pupil dilatation. Moreover, the decreased pressure induced by these agents may be associated with little change in the tonographic outflow facility (3). The ability of salbutamol to decrease pressure without causing pupil dilatation in human eyes is analogous to the action of isoproterenol, but the properties of these two compounds differ in that isoproterenol causes tachycardia whereas salbutamol does not (6). The effects of drugs which lower $P_0$ but have little effect on $C_T$ can be represented on the $P_0$-$C_T$ diagram in terms of almost, if not exactly, vertical lines.

Epinephrine, the adrenergic agonist widely used in glaucoma, has both α- and β-agonistic activity and causes decreased intraocular pressure, with a variable degree of both pupil dilatation and increase of $C_T$. Initial induction of decreased intraocular pressure by epinephrine in normal and glaucomatous eyes has been reported to occur without significant increase in $C_T$, whereas continued administration of this drug has been found to decrease $P_0$ and increase $C_0$ in both normal and glaucomatous eyes (7–9). Thus, the effect of epinephrine, with its combined α- and β-action, can be represented on the $P_0$-$C_T$ diagram in terms of trajectories intermediate between the α- and β-trajectories.

These positive effects of the adrenergic drugs contrast with the negative qualities of pilocarpine, the drug most often currently employed in the present treatment of glaucoma, which has little, if any, effect on $P_0$ and $C_T$ in normal eyes, in spite of a marked effect on pupil constriction and accommodation (10).

From the theoretical investigations of Hart (4, 5) it has been possible to develop equations of the $P_0$-$C_T$ trajectories which agree with a large body of published data. The underlying mechanism is regarded as vasomotor, and the adrenergic responses may be thought of as being primarily vasoconstrictor (α) and vasodilator (β), which is in keeping with their known physiological effects. The relationship of these vasomotor actions to the determination and regulation of intraocular pressure follows from the basic concept that the rate of aqueous humor is dependent on and proportionate to the rate of blood flow to the ciliary processes, and that the outflow resistance of the living eye is dependent on the extent to which blood fills the intrascleral plexus (where both aqueous humor and blood drain from the eye). For the present purpose, it is sufficient to present the equations of the trajectories and briefly to explain the component parameters. Attention is focused primarily on the action of epinephrine because it has been used extensively and considerable data are available.

Epinephrine (except in quantities so small that only β-action is elicted) is regarded as equally enhancing the responses of the α- and β-vasomotor mechanisms. This assumption leads theoretically to the family of trajectories defined by

$$\lambda = \frac{(1+\beta\, C_T)\,(P_T - P_O)}{\sqrt{P_T - P_V} - \sqrt{P_O - P_V}}$$

where $P_T$ is the average pressure during tonography, $P_V$ is the pressure in the episcleral veins (assumed for calculational purposes to be 7 mm Hg) and the constant β reflects the sensitivity of aqueous outflow resistance to blood flow. Various considerations have indicated that $\beta \simeq 3$ mm Hg/min·μl can be regarded as normal for the human eye.

The parameter λ is related to the relative ability of the drug to affect vasoconstriction vis-à-vis vasodilatation (as well as to other factors such as ocular rigidity, which we suppress). Thus, since epinephrine is here regarded as enhancing α- and β-receptors equally, λ should be found to be a constant (unaffected by the drug) and defines the particular trajectory describing the effect of epinephrine on the pressure and outflow facility. Application to the action of epinephrine on normal and glaucomatous eyes is summarized in Table 1. The results from the five separate studies include 86 patients with open-angle

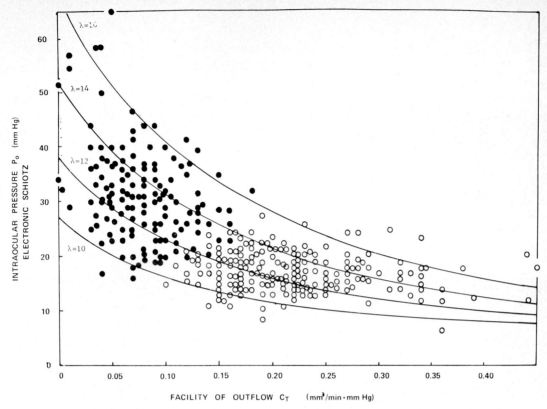

FIG. 4.   Theoretical $P_0$-$C_T$ trajectories for increasing values of λ. Ideally, the effect of a drug in an individual eye would be characterized by a trajectory relating pre- and post-treatment values of pressure and $C_T$. Experimental evidence suggests that drugs with comparable α- and β-agonist activity give rise to this family of trajectories.

glaucoma and 37 normal subjects. In both normal and glaucomatous eyes in all series of studies the application of epinephrine caused both a decrease in intraocular pressure and an increase in the tonographic coefficient of outflow facility $C_T$. The important finding is that λ did indeed remain essentially unchanged in all five studies.

The observation that the combined α-β-agonistic actions of epinephrine can be understood in terms of equal α- and β-responses has an important implication with respect to glaucoma therapy because it defines the trajectories for these drugs on the $P_0$-$C_T$ diagram, examples of which are shown in Fig. 4. Moreover, different eyes having a common sensitivity ratio should define a

common trajectory so that data from various sources can be organized accordingly. In Fig. 5 three trajectories are compared with the relevant data, the upper point of a pair denoting the average* ($P_0$, $C_T$) values before treatment and the lower point of the pair denoting the corresponding values at some time after treatment. Most of the data pertain to the middle (λ = 13.25) curve, with which we have associated all of the data for which the λ of the untreated eye is calculated to lie in the range 13 to 13.3. The lower curve (λ =

---

*   The data for individual eyes show considerable variability, no doubt arising partly from measurement error and random fluctuations, as well as from individual differences in β, $P_V$ and ocular rigidity.

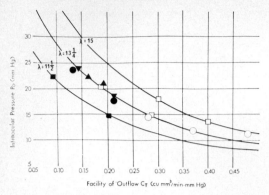

FIG. 5. Comparison of theoretical trajectories with the clinically observed effects of *l*-epinephrine on intraocular pressure and tonographic coefficient of outflow facility. Solid points represent glaucomatous eyes, open points represent normal eyes. The open squares (□) are taken from ref. 12 and the solid squares from refs. 11 and 14. The open and solid triangles (△ and ▲) and the solid circles (●) are taken from ref. 15 and the open circles (○) are taken from ref. 3.

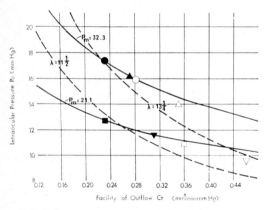

FIG. 6. Effects on groups of normal human eyes, different mean initial pressures, of *l*-norepinephrine alone (upper data group) and of *l*-norepinephrine potentiated with protriptyline (lower data group) as compared with calculated trajectories. The observed results fit the constant $P_m$ trajectories (as predicted by the theory), but do not fit the constant λ-trajectories which describe the effects of *l*-epinephrine (cf. Fig. 5). These data are taken from ref. 3. The solid points represent the mean $P_0$-$C_T$ values before treatment and the corresponding open points represent the $P_0$-$C_T$ values after treatment with norepinephrine.

11.5) is in good accord with data between 11.25 and 11.75, namely those of Richards

and Drance (11) (λ = 11.6), and the upper curve (λ = 15) is in good accord with the mean of Prijot's points (12) which fall between 15 and 15.3.

A similar analysis shows that certain drugs which primarily enhance α-receptor activity can be represented by a corresponding family of trajectories defined by

$$(P_0 - P_V)\left[\frac{(P_T - P_0)(1 + \beta\, C_T)}{\sqrt{P_0 - P_V}\,[\sqrt{P_T - P_V} - \sqrt{P_0 - P_V}]} - 1\right] = \text{constant } P_m$$

These are illustrated by Fig. 6, where they are compared with normal eye data for *l*-norepinephrine alone and in combination with protriptylene (3).

## CONCLUSION

The utilization of the $P_0$-$C_T$ trajectory concept not only provides a powerful means for the early diagnosis of glaucoma, before irreversible damage is detected, but also provides a logical approach to evaluation of the mechanisms through which drugs favorably influence ocular hypertension. Moreover, the close agreement between the theoretically derived trajectories and the observed effects of α- and β-adrenergic agonists in both glaucomatous and normal eyes lends strong support to the underlying concept of neurovascular control of intraocular pressure.

Supported by U.S. Public Health Service Research Grants EY-00476–06 and NS 07226–04, National Institutes of Health, Bethesda, Md.

## REFERENCES

1. BECKER B and SHAEFFER RN. "Diagnosis and therapy of the glaucomas." St Louis, CV Mosby, 1965.
2. LANGHAM ME. Manometric, pressure-cup and tonographic procedures in the evaluation of intraocular dynamics, in: Leydhecker W (Ed), "Twentieth international congress of ophthalmology, Munich, 1966. Glaucoma, Tutzing Symposium." Basel, S Karger, 1967.
3. LANGHAM ME, KITAZAWA Y and HART RW. Adrenergic responses in the human eye. *J Pharmacol Exp Ther* **179**: 47, 1971.

4. HART RW. Theory of nervous regulation of intraocular pressure. *Appl Phys Lab Tech Digest* **9**: 2, 1970.
5. HART RW. Theory of neural mediation of intraocular dynamics. *Bull Math Biophys* (in press).
6. CULLUM VA, FARMER JB, JACK D and LEVY GP. Salbutamol: a new selective β-adrenoceptive receptor stimulant. *Br J Pharmacol* **35**: 141, 1969.
7. BALLANTYNE EJ and GARNER LL. Improvement of the coefficient of outflow in glaucomatous eyes. *Arch Ophthalmol* **66**: 314, 1961.
8. WEEKERS R, DELMARCELLE Y and GUSTIN J. Treatment of ocular hypertension by adrenalin and diverse sympathomimetic amines. *Am J Ophthalmol* **68**: 216, 1969.
9. BECKER B and LEY AP. Epinephrine and acetazolamide in therapy of the chronic glaucomas. *Am J Ophthalmol* **45**: 639, 1958.
10. WILLETTS AS. Autonomic effector drugs and the normal eye. *Am J Ophthalmol* **68**: 216, 1969.
11. RICHARDS JSF and DRANCE SM. The effect of 2 percent epinephrine on aqueous dynamics in the human eye. *Can J Ophthalmol* **2**: 259, 1967.
12. PRIJOT E. Contribution à l'étude de la tonographie. *Doc Ophthalmol* **15**: 1, 1961.
13. GRANT WM. Clinical measurements of aqueous outflow. *Arch Ophthalmol* **46**: 113, 1951.
14. DRANCE SM, in: Paterson, Miller and Paterson (Eds), "Drug mechanisms in glaucoma." London, Churchill, 1966, p 60.
15. KITAZAWA Y. Dose response analysis of ocular hypotensive effects of epinephrine and norepinephrine. *Am J Ophthalmol* (in press).
16. BECKER B, PETIT T and GAY AJ. Topical epinephrine therapy of open-angle glaucoma. *Arch Ophthalmol* **66**: 219, 1961.

# DIAGNOSTIC AND THERAPEUTIC ASPECTS OF EARLY CHRONIC SIMPLE GLAUCOMA

ERIK LINNÉR

Department of Ophthalmology, University of Umeå, Umeå, Sweden

Glaucoma concerns every ophthalmologist. To the patient, his vision—and not his intraocular pressure—is the essential problem. My report will, however, deal with glaucomatous changes in the anterior part of the eye.

*Intraocular pressure.* Considerable effort has been made in trying to define normal intraocular pressure. While the results obtained using the Schiøtz tonometer and the applanation tonometer vary considerably, nevertheless good overall agreement is noted (1). Even if the accuracy of measuring intraocular pressure is satisfactory, there are still problems. For example, repeated measurements indicate successively lower values of intraocular pressure and it is not quite clear which value is the best one. In addition, the intraocular pressure varies throughout the course of the day. Can a single measurement be used? Which time of the day gives the most reliable pressure reading? The difference in intraocular pressure between the two eyes of the same individual can give some information of clinical value. A difference of more than 4 mm Hg occurs in only 3% of non-glaucomatous individuals (1).

The upper limit of normal intraocular pressure is of great clinical importance. It has been studied in a large number of individuals in order to define the borderline between normal and pathologically elevated intra-ocular pressure. The steady level of intra-ocular pressure is determined by a combination of three factors: formation of aqueous humor, resistance to aqueous outflow and episcleral venous pressure. Intraocular pressure is therefore the result of a complex system. It is not clear *a priori* which type of statistical distribution variations in intra-ocular pressure might follow.

Conventional statistical methods are the type most commonly used. These analyses are based on the assumption that intraocular pressure in healthy human eyes is distributed according to a normal Gaussian curve. The upper normal limit of intraocular pressure has been chosen as three times the standard deviation above the mean value. However, there are considerable discrepancies among various studies (1).

It is now appreciated that the statistical variation of intraocular pressure is not symmetrical in a Gaussian manner, but shows a skew deviation with a large number of high-pressure readings (2). If we assume that intra-ocular pressure is normally distributed, then the large number of people having high intra-ocular pressure reflects the inclusion of early glaucoma cases belonging to a different statistical population.

Clinically it is not clear whether moderately elevated intraocular pressure is sufficient for making the diagnosis of early glaucoma. This question can be elucidated by following cases with moderate ocular hypertension over a long period of time. Such a longitudinal study has been carried out and some results of a ten-year follow-up are presented here. Previous results obtained after periods of $1\frac{3}{4}$ and 5 years have been reported (3, 4). The basic material of that study consisted of 152 subjects with moderate ocular hypertension, detected in a mass survey conducted by Dr. Strömberg. A total of 7,275 subjects over 40 years of age were examined using the Schiötz tonometer. In the group with ocular hypertension, the average intraocular pressure was five to six scale readings with 7.5 g weight (21.9 to 25.8 mm Hg) (5).

During this 10-year period the subjects, though kept under clinical observation, were not given any antiglaucomatous treatment unless it was indicated. In all, eight men and six women were started on glaucoma therapy, some of them by other ophthalmologists.

The group included in this report consists of 92 subjects who were with us for 10 years of observation. Their average age was 68 years, and they did not receive any treatment. The intraocular pressure had a tendency to decrease with time, the overall decrease being about 2 mm Hg. The facility of outflow showed the same tendency, the decrease being about 0.02 µl/min per mm Hg.

This simultaneous decrease in intraocular pressure and facility of outflow is compatible with a reduction in aqueous flow. The assumption is that there is no change in episcleral venous pressure or other outflow pathways. In this group of individuals with ocular hypertension, it was estimated that the rate of aqueous flow diminished from 3.2 µl/min to 2.3 µl/min during the 10-year period, i.e., to 72% of the initial value. The same tendency toward a reduction in aqueous flow in higher age groups was also found in normal subjects (6).

The relationship between the factors determining the steady level of intraocular pressure and its decrease in higher age groups is not clear. I do not think in fact that it is possible to define a clear borderline between the physiological changes in aqueous humor dynamics in older individuals and the pathological changes associated with early glaucoma. No tendency toward an increase in cupping of the optic disk was observed. Examination of the visual field using a tangent screen showed no progressive field changes.

The following conclusion can be drawn from this 10-year study: a moderately elevated intraocular pressure can be present for a least 10 years without any further elevation, and without any further clinical evidence of early chronic simple glaucoma. Such cases of ocular hypertension are worth considering when one is trying to define the borderline between normal and pathologically elevated intraocular pressure.

*Tonography.* This method has been widely used for 20 years and has given results of great interest. However, these are mostly statistical results obtained from groups of subjects. There are still many unsolved errors and uncertainties. Tonographic results are difficult to assess for the individual patient. I think a tonographic tracing as a single test is of limited value in an individual who might be a borderline case of early glaucoma.

*Capsular exfoliation.* Pseudoexfoliation, senile exfoliation, fibrillopathia epitheliocapsularis and fibrillopathy are different names for the same lesion. To the best of my knowledge, the first description of this lesion was published in 1917 by Lindberg in Finland (7) who found four positive cases out of 60 examined. The frequency has been a matter of discussion and a considerable variation between different countries has been reported. The results of a new investigation reported at this meeting (8) suggest that early detection of exfoliation is important from a clinical point of view. It is essential that a slit lamp examination be carried out in a dark room, and that the pupil be dilated. According to Aasved, the lesion could not be detected before dilatation in five out of 48 eyes (8).

The clinical course of eyes with exfoliation can be expected to be different from that of eyes without this lesion. If the patient shows exfoliation, but no other evidence of glaucoma, he ought to be considered as a glaucoma suspect and kept under careful observation. This is because he might develop a rapidly progressive glaucoma with high intraocular pressure, glaucomatous cupping of the optic disk and visual field defects within a rather short time.

*Therapeutic aspects.* Glaucoma treatment is a lifelong occupation for the patient, and considerable inconvenience cannot be avoided. A prerequisite for rational therapy is that we be able to detect very early cases of chronic simple glaucoma and to differentiate between these and nonglaucomatous cases. With our present knowledge we are not able to draw a clear borderline between the glaucomatous eye and the normal one. Consequently, it is not easy to give clear and simple recommendations as to when glaucoma treatment should be started. Careful clinical judgment is required for each case. Clinical observation over a long period of time may be necessary before a clear diagnosis can be made. Both the advantages and the disadvantages should be considered before lifelong therapy is started.

Supported by grants B68-14X-589-02, K70-14X-589-03A, B71-14X-589-04B from the Swedish Medical Research Council.

## REFERENCES

1. GLOSTER J. "Tonometry and tonography." London, J & A Churchill Ltd, 1966.
2. LEYDHECKER W. Zur Verbreitung des Glaucoma Simplex in der scheinbar gesunden, augenärztlich nicht behandelten Bevölkerung. *Doc Ophthalmol* **13**: 359, 1959.
3. LINNÉR E and STROMBERG U. The course of untreated ocular hypertension. *Acta Ophthalmol* **42**: 836, 1964.
4. LINNÉR E and STRÖMBERG U. Ocular hypertension. A five-year study of the total population in a Swedish town, Skövde. *Glaucoma Symp, Tutzing Castle 1966.* Basel, Karger, p 187, 1967.
5. STRÖMBERG U. Ocular hypertension. *Acta Ophthalmol [Suppl] (Kbh)* **69**: 1962.
6. LINNÉR E. The rate of aqueous flow in human eyes with and without senile cataract. *Arch Ophthalmol* **61**: 520, 1959.
7. LINDBERG JG. Kliniska undersökningar över depigmenteringen av pupillaranden och genomlysbarheten av iris vid fall av åldersstarr samt i normala ögon hos gamla personer. *Diss Helsingfors*, 1917.
8. AASVED H. The geographical distribution of fibrillopathia epitheliocapsularis, so-called senile exfoliation or pseudoexfoliation of the anterior lens capsule. *Acta Ophthalmol (Kbh)* **47**: 792, 1969.

# ASPECTS OF
# GLAUCOMA THERAPY IN A DEVELOPING COUNTRY (NIGERIA)

OYIN OLURIN

Department of Ophthalmology, University College Hospital, Ibadan, Nigeria

Primary glaucoma, excluding congenital glaucoma, is the second commonest cause of blindness in eye clinic patients in Ibadan. It accounts for 20.7% of 1,000 consecutive blind Nigerian patients seen at the University College Hospital in Ibadan (O. Olurin, in preparation). It is conceivable that glaucoma is no more prevalent in Nigeria than in other countries, but certain features of the disease as seen here make it stand out as an important cause of visual disability.

Glaucoma is more prevalent in Nigeria in the younger age groups than is generally found in other racial groups (1, 2). Of a group of 220 patients with primary glaucoma, 59 (26.8%) were under 21 years of age. Intraocular tensions tend to be more difficult to control in younger patients. Patients with glaucoma suffer severe loss of vision due to late presentation. The local peasant population is still largely illiterate, and it is possible that patients are unaware of, or careless about, the gradual loss of vision and field which is a feature of chronic glaucoma. Primary acute congestive glaucoma, which causes pain and so brings patients for early treatment in other countries, is seldom encountered in Nigerians, but chronic glaucoma with open angle or chronic angle closure is the form usually seen. In many patients, the disease has been present for two, three or more years before medical consultation. Even literate patients often present with blindness in one eye and marked loss of field in the better eye. It would appear that the disease progresses rather more rapidly in these patients than in other population groups. This observation is further emphasized by the evidence of rapid deterioration of visual field in defaulting patients and the experience of other workers treating Negro patients with glaucoma (1, 3, 4). Our criterion for blindness is a visual acuity of "count fingers" or less at three feet in the better eye, in conformity with previous studies (5). Even by these criteria, which do not take into account the loss of visual field, which is often gross, we found 203 (40.6%) of a random sample of 500 patients with primary glaucoma to be blind in both eyes, and a further 197 (39.4%) to be blind in one eye. With such advanced disease at presentation, only very few patients can be helped with any form of therapy.

Medical treatment is the therapy of choice, and this takes the form of miotics, pilocarpine 1 to 4%, with or without physostigmine 0.25%. A limited number of patients are treated with echothiopate iodide (PHOSPHOLINE IODIDE®) 0.012 to 0.05%. Patients with open-angle glaucoma are treated with 1% epinephrine

(1 % ADRENALINE®) with or without the addition of miotics. Many patients are found initially to respond well to miotics alone, with a fall in intraocular tensions and some improvement of symptoms. A few weeks later, 50 to 60 % of these patients require oral acetazolamide (DIAMOX®) in doses of 250 mg to 1 g daily as an adjunct. Control of ocular tension can still be difficult in about 20 % of patients even with full medical therapy. Such patients are often offered surgery.

Furthermore, surgery is also offered to patients who default repeatedly, to young patients (under 41 years of age), patients with chronic angle closure, and those who find drops intolerable. In this environment, many patients who still have good field and vision worthy of preservation refuse surgery. There is considerable evidence, including our own, that surgery for glaucoma in the Negro patient is fraught with disappointing results (1, 6–9). In 40 % of Nigerian patients who undergo surgery there is satisfactory control of ocular tension. In a further 30 %, it was found necessary to continue postoperatively with miotic drops and oral Diamox. In the remaining 30 %, surgery was of no avail. Certain factors appear to be responsible for the relatively poor surgical result. A racial characteristic due to heavy iris pigmentation, marked reaction of the negroid eye to trauma (9), and increased formation of scar tissue (9–11) are considered to be significant etiological factors. Possible means of minimizing these factors include the use of surgical antiglaucoma procedures which cause minimal trauma to the eye, and the early postoperative application of topical corticosteroids. Of the various filtering procedures in use, we found sclerodiathermy and iridectomy (10) to be most rewarding. Iris inclusion operations have been found to be unsatisfactory in Negro eyes (13). Lately, Ben-Sira and Ticho (14) described the complete excision of Tenon's capsule from the area of drainage, and have claimed good results. Of possible relevance is the fact that glaucoma filtering operations are less successful in younger patients who have thick Tenon's capsule. Nevertheless, other workers maintain that the presence of Tenon's capsule is essential for successful filtering operations (15). We have not been able to assess the efficacy of this modification in our patients. Gorin (16) has suggested the use of a thin conjunctival flap and avoidance of handling of Tenon's capsule during limbosclerectomy. We are employing this technique and are evaluating its efficacy.

Certain practical difficulties are encountered in treating patients with glaucoma in developing countries, including Nigeria. Hospital dispensaries are often overcrowded and patients are unable to purchase their drugs outside the hospital. Prepacked drops and tablets are dispensed to patients in eye clinics to ensure that these patients obtain their drugs in good time and in sufficient quantities. The default rate is remarkably high. This may be accounted for by the long distances traveled by patients to specialist units. Furthermore the patients are often in the lower economic strata and cannot afford repeated visits. In some parts of Nigeria, distances are so vast that follow-up is very difficult and medical treatment often fails (I. S. Bahr, personal communication). Illiterate patients fail to understand the nature of their disease even after adequate explanation, and default if they do not get the dramatic improvement which they expect, or think they have been permanently cured when symptoms improve with miosis and, sometimes, with spectacles. Facilities for ophthalmic consulation are also clearly inadequate in developing countries, including Nigeria, where there are only 24 ophthalmologists, two separate eye hospitals and a few other eye units attached to general hospitals in the bigger towns serving a population of over 50 million people. These and the few opticians are the only facilities available in the country.

Programs for the prevention of blindness in many developing countries are not operative. Effective measures in preventing blindness from glaucoma by early detection of cases are virtually nonexistent. A recent field survey done in this unit (O. Olurin, in preparation), offering eye examinations to adults at their place of work, and to patients attending hospital for conditions other than ocular problems, revealed that glaucoma can be detected early in unsuspecting adults. The problem of preventing blindness from glaucoma is enormous, and present facilities to cope with it are evidently inadequate. The population requires education on the importance of early medical consultation and on the provision of more facilities for ophthalmic consultation and treatment in well-staffed and equipped units. To be able to fulfil these obligations, many developing countries require expanded training programs for medical and paramedical ophthalmic personnel. Such measures would go a long way towards minimizing loss of vision from glaucoma.

## REFERENCES

1. McNair SS. Chronic simple glaucoma in the Negro. *Am J Ophthalmol* **34**: 70, 1951.
2. Neuman E and Zauberman H. Glaucoma survey in Liberia. *Am J Ophthalmol* **59**: 8, 1965.
3. Rouse HKJ. *Mississippi Doctor* June 1937.
4. Packer H, Deutsch AR, Lewis PM, Oglesby CD and Cheij AC. A study of the frequency and distribution of glaucoma. *JAMA* **171**: 1090, 1959.
5. Olurin O. Etiology of blindness in Nigerian children. *Am J Ophthalmol* **70**: 533, 1970.
6. Quere MA, Diallo J, Razafunjato R and Heitz R. Le problème du glaucome primaire chez l'African de race noire. Analyse critique de la litérature. *Doc Ophthalmol* **20**: 230, 1966.
7. Berson D, Zauberman H, Landau L and Blumenthal M. Filtering operations in Africans. *Am J Ophthalmol* **67**: 395, 1969.
8. Quere MA. Results of primary glaucoma surgery in Negroes. *Am J Ophthalmol* **70**: 150, 1970.
9. Welsh NH. Failure of filtration operations in the African. *Br J Ophthalmol* **54**: 594, 1970.
10. Blumenthal M. Corneal keratoplasty in Tanzania. *Am J Ophthalmol* **65**: 762, 1968.
11. Bourell P. Keloids in the African. *Med Trop (Mars)* **27** (Suppl): 1, 1967.
12. Scheie HG. Peripheral iridectomy with scleral cautery for glaucoma. *Arch Ophthalmol* **61**: 291, 1959.
13. Cassady JR. Results of iridencleisis in the Negro and white races. *Arch Ophthalmol* **62**: 239, 1959.
14. Ben-Sira I and Ticho U. Excision of Tenon's capsule in fistulizing operations on Africans. *Am J Ophthalmol* **68**: 336, 1969.
15. Sugar HS. Surgical treatment of chronic open angle glaucoma. *Am J Ophthalmol* **59**: 656, 1965.
16. Gorin G. Use of a thin conjunctival flap in limbosclerectomy. *Ann Ophthalmol* **3**: 258, 1971.

# ACUTE OPEN-ANGLE GLAUCOMA
# DUE TO LATENT IRIDOCYCLITIS

## GEORGE GORIN

Albert Einstein School of Medicine, Yeshiva University and Glaucoma Clinic, Manhattan Eye and Ear Hospital, New York, New York, USA

The pattern of intraocular pressure at the onset of acute iridocyclitis is unpredictable. Acute iridocyclitis may begin with ciliary pain, photophobia, periciliary flush and low tension. Slit-lamp examination reveals many keratic precipitates (KP), flare and cells in the aqueous. The low intraocular pressure may be due to suppression of aqueous formation, which is the response of the ciliary processes to a severe inflammatory insult. This is accompanied by pronounced vasodilation of the vessels of the ciliary processes with possibly increased permeability of the small capillaries, leading to formation of a scanty, albumin-laden aqueous.

The clinical response of the condition to corticosteroids, accompanied by a return of the subnormal tension to normal level, suggests that the transient hypotony is due to suppression of the capability of the ciliary processes to produce aqueous.

On the other hand, we have observed cases of clinically very mild iridocyclitis without any objective slit-lamp findings in the early stage, without KP, flare or ciliary flush. The chief complaint is either transient recurring blackouts of vision in older people or rainbow colors around light in younger people. Both types of symptom occur in one eye, which appears white, has very high tension and a wide angle. The above symptoms are due to compression of the central retinal artery in old people and to stretching of the cornea with subsequent edema in younger people.

These cases present a diagnostic and therapeutic problem when high tension persists and there is danger of permanent closure of the central retinal artery. In the two cases described the true nature of the condition was successfully determined with the aid of 0.125% echothiopate (PHOSPHOLINE®) iodide. Because there was no satisfactory response to several drugs used singly and in combination, a mild iridocyclitis was suspected, causing neither objective nor subjective symptoms, but exerting an irritative effect on the ciliary processes. In such a case high intraocular pressure develops as a result of overstimulation of the ciliary processes instead of the hypotony seen in severe aqueous-suppressing iridocyclitis. This would explain the absence of cyclitic symptoms and the high intraocular pressure.

In both cases several instillations of 0.125% echothiopate iodide was followed by the appearance of cyclitic pain, numerous fresh KP and 3+ flare, accompanied by a moderate reduction in tension. Once iridocyclitis was unmasked, treatment with acetazolamide (DIAMOX®), epinephrine and corticosteroid drops led to the gradual normalization of tension and clearing of cyclitic symptoms.

Case 1 was a 70-year-old woman who had recurrent blackouts of vision with a tension of 70 mm Hg in the right eye. Case 2 was a 50-year-old man who developed tearing in the right eye and saw colored rings around the light. Both patients were treated as chronic simple glaucoma cases by the referring physician without results. Symptoms in both were controlled after the iridocyclitis became manifest with the use of echothiopate iodide by routine treatment of secondary glaucoma due to iridocyclitis. In the first case filtering surgery was considered after the tension remained high for two weeks (between 60 and 70 mm Hg). Once tension became normalized there was no recurrence. In the second case (intraocular tension of 50 mm Hg) there were many recurrences, which could be controlled with acetazolamide, epinephrine and steroid drops. To prove the validity of the diagnosis, KP and flare were produced during the third attack by instillation of ecothiopate iodide.

### DIFFERENTIAL DIAGNOSIS

Before the appearance of KP and flare the following diagnostic possibilities were considered: 1) unilateral chronic simple glaucoma; 2) traumatic glaucoma; 3) glaucomatocyclitic crisis of Posner and Schlossman.

1) Chronic simple glaucoma could not be excluded with certainty, although it is rare for one eye to have chronic simple glaucoma of such severity while the other eye is entirely normal. As a matter of fact, both cases were treated unsuccessfully as chronic simple glaucoma. 2) Traumatic glaucoma was excluded because of lack of history of trauma and absence of angle recession on gonioscopic examination. 3) Differentiation of the well-established entity of glaucomatocyclitis crisis can be made on the following grounds:

It was never established that glaucomatocyclitic crisis has cyclitis as an underlying etiology. The only indication of a cyclitic origin is the finding of one or two KP without aqueous flare. This lack of cyclitic reaction is the distinctive characteristic which makes the Posner-Schlossman syndrome a separate entity whose etiology is still obscure, and not simply a secondary glaucoma due to iridocyclitis.

The two cases described above began with a unilateral high intraocular pressure in wide-angle eyes without the presence of even one KP or flare. In both cases ecothiopate iodide characteristically produced a full blown iridocyclitis with many KP, 3+ flare and cells in the aqueous. This reaction was not observed in typical cases of the Posner-Schlossman syndrome.

# PROLONGED RELEASE MEDICATION
# IN THE TREATMENT OF EYE DISEASE

SIDNEY LERMAN

Department of Ophthalmology (Experimental), McGill University, Montreal, Quebec, Canada

The present day medical therapy of ocular disease consists of the local application of drugs in the form of eye drops or ointment. Although ointments generally ensure a more prolonged contact of the specific drug with the eyeball in comparison with eye drops, there are still certain problems with this form of treatment. For example, in the medical therapy of glaucoma, it is well known that it is difficult if not impossible to obtain continuous 24-hr control of the disease by eye drops or ointment. Furthermore, the use of eye drops or ointment is a relatively wasteful procedure with respect to the amount of drug employed. There is also the relatively rare problem of certain individuals who display extreme sensitivity to cholinergic drops. In such cases it would be advantageous to have a form of therapy in which the minimum amount of drug is applied to the eye. Another problem is the fact that certain patients frequently forget to apply the medication as directed, resulting in poor control of the disease.

A new form of prolonged release therapy is currently under investigation. The drug to be delivered to the eye is incorporated into a very thin pledget which is capable of releasing the drug at a relatively constant rate over a specific time period. This device (known as the OCUSERT®, Fig. 1) is inserted into the inferior cul-de-sac and can be left there for varying periods of time; i.e., 24 hr or longer.

In order to test the hypothesis that prolonged release medication would require a much lower drug concentration and would be at least as effective in the therapy of glaucoma, a study was performed utilizing a simulated form of sustained release pilocarpine therapy.

## MATERIALS AND METHODS

Patients with well-documented open angle glaucoma, each acting as his own control, were the subjects of this study. Each patient had an initial complete glaucoma examination in which the pupillary size was measured, and applanation, Schiøtz tonometry, visual field studies and gonios-

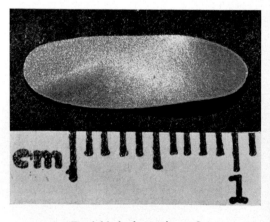

FIG. 1.   Erodable hydrocortisone Ocusert.

TABLE 1. *Results of a clinical trial with sustained release pilocarpine[a]*

| Pilocarpine dose | Pupil diameter (mm) | | | | Change in pupil diameter (mm) | | Tension (mm Hg) | | | | C, coefficient of facility of outflow | | Δ C | |
| --- | --- | --- | --- | --- | --- | --- | --- | --- | --- | --- | --- | --- | --- | --- |
| | Initial | | Final | | | | Initial | | Final | | | | | |
| | OS | OD | OS | OD | OS | OD | OS | OD | OS | OD | OS | OD | OS | OD |
| Instillations without Ocusert | | | | | | | | | | | | | | |
| 1 drop, 4% solution, both eyes at 9 AM and 1:30 PM | 1.50 | 1.25 | | | | | 17 | 15 | 15 | 15 | 0.14 | 0.11 | | |
| | | | 0.50 | 0.50 | 1.00 | 0.75 | 12 | 12 | 11 | 10 | 0.23 | 0.15 | 0.09 | 0.04 |
| Instillations with Ocusert (OD) | | | | | | | | | | | | | | |
| 1) OD, 40 µg/drop, 20 drops/hr for 5 hr[b] | 1.75 | 1.75 | | | | | 14 | 11 | 12 | 10 | 0.20 | 0.10 | | |
| OS, control[e] | | | 0.50 | 1.75 | 1.25 | 0.00 | 8 | 10 | 10 | 12 | 0.32 | 0.18 | 0.12 | 0.08 |
| 2) OD, 3.3 µg/drop, 20 drops/hr for 5 hr[c] | 2.00 | 2.00 | | | | | 15 | 14 | 13 | 13 | 0.13 | 0.13 | | |
| OS, control[e] | | | 1.00 | 1.50 | 1.00 | 0.50 | 14 | 15 | 15 | 15 | 0.22 | 0.13 | 0.09 | 0 |
| 3) OD, 0.6 µg/drop, 20 drops/hr for 5 hr[d] | 2.00 | 2.00 | | | | | 11 | 11 | 12 | 12 | 0.13 | 0.11 | | |
| OS, control[e] | | | 1.50 | 1.50 | 0.50 | 0.50 | 12 | 10 | 14 | 13 | 0.23 | 0.15 | 0.10 | 0.04 |

[a] Our patient was a 67-year-old woman who had received 4% pilocarpine drops four times a day in both eyes for 13 years. She was taken off all drugs for two weeks, and afterward received Diamox for one week prior to the clinical trial.
[b] Equivalent to 2 drops of 4% pilocarpine.
[c] Equivalent to 2 drops of 0.3% pilocarpine.
[d] Equivalent to 2 drops of 0.067% pilocarpine.
[e] Control, Isoptotears only.

copy were performed. In most cases the patient was then taken off all therapy and placed on acetazolamide (DIAMOX®) for one week in order to maintain control of his intraocular pressure. At the end of one week the patient was re-evaluated by applanation and Schiøtz tonometry and tonography. He was then given one drop of pilocarpine in one eye and a drop of 0.5% Isoptotears in the other. The drops were instilled at 9 AM and treatment was repeated at 1:30 PM. The pupillary response, the pressure response and outflow changes were recorded. The patient then returned at weekly intervals (while still under acetazolamide therapy if required) at which time one eye received a form of simulated prolonged release pilocarpine therapy while the other received the placebo consisting of Isoptotears. The simulated prolonged release pilocarpine therapy consisted of pilocarpine hydrochloride in 0.5% Isoptotears made up in varying concentrations and instilled into the eye at the rate of one drop every 3 min for a total of 100 drops over a period

of 5 hr. The total amount of pilocarpine hydrochloride that the patient received by this method was noted as the equivalent amount the patient would receive if he had been given one drop of a specific concentration of pilocarpine hydrochloride twice during the 5-hr period under investigation, as shown in the results. The pupillary response, applanation and Schiøtz tension readings at the beginning and end of the experimental period and the outflow measurements were also noted. Decreasing concentrations of simulated prolonged release pilocarpine were given to each patient as noted in the results. The applanation readings were done every 15 min in the control and experimental eye and tonography was performed at the beginning of the experimental period prior to the instillation of any drops and at the end of the 5-hr experimental period.

RESULTS

The results of these studies on typical patients

TABLE 2. *Results of a clinical trial with sustained release pilocarpine[a]*

| Pilocarpine dose | Pupil diameter (mm) | | | | Change in pupil diameter (mm) | | Tension (mm Hg) | | | | C, coefficient of facility of outflow | | ΔC | |
| | Initial | | Final | | | | Initial | | Final | | | | | |
| | OS | OD | OS | OD | OS | OD | OS | OD | OS | OD | OS | OD | OS | OD |
|---|---|---|---|---|---|---|---|---|---|---|---|---|---|---|
| Instillations without Ocusert 1 drop, 4% solution, both eyes at 9:20 AM and 12:20 PM | 2.50 | 2.50 | | | | | 12 | 12 | 12 | 12 | 0.11 | 0.13 | | |
| | | | 0.75 | 1.00 | 1.75 | 1.50 | 6 | 8 | 10 | 9 | 0.13 | 0.20 | 0.02 | 0.07 |
| Instillations with Ocusert (OD) 1) OS, 40 µg/drop, 20 drops/hr for 5 hr[b] | 2.50 | 2.50 | | | | | 11 | 12 | 12 | 13 | 0.11 | 0.15 | | |
| OD, control[e] | | | 5.00 | 2.00 | 0.50 | dilated | 8 | 7 | 12 | 10 | 0.13 | 0.26 | 0.02 | 0.11 |
| 2) OS, 3.3 µg/drop, 20 drops/hr for 5 hr[c] | 3.50 | 3.50 | | | | | 10 | 11 | 11 | 10 | 0.12 | 0.12 | | |
| OD, control[e] | | | 4.50 | 4.00 | dilated | | 9 | 9 | 13 | 9 | 0.13 | 0.19 | 0 | 0.07 |
| 3) OS, 0.67 µg/drop, 20 drops/hr for 5 hr[d] | 3.00 | 3.00 | | | | | 9 | 10 | 12 | 12 | 0.20 | 0.14 | | |
| OD, control[e] | | | 5.50 | 5.00 | dilated | | 9 | 8 | 13 | 8 | 0.19 | 0.17 | 0 | 0.03 |

[a] Our patient was an 85-year-old man with a history of open angle glaucoma since June 1967; he received 4% pilocarpine drops four times a day in both eyes and had normal visual fields.

[b,d,e] See Table 1 for explanation.

[c] Equivalent to 2 drops of 0.1% pilocarpine.

are shown in Tables 1 and 2. The changes in intraocular pressure, seen both by applanation and Schiøtz readings, while more marked in the eye receiving the pilocarpine hydrochloride, were also significant in the eyes receiving the placebo (Isoptotears). This was probably due to the multiple instillation of drops in either eye. However, the facility of outflow changes were significantly different in the eyes receiving the varying concentrations of sustained release pilocarpine therapy in contrast with the eyes receiving the placebo therapy.

## DISCUSSION

The results of this study indicate that an apparent minimum effective dose for pilocarpine therapy in the form of simulated sustained release medication (100 drops over a 5-hr period) ranges between 10 and 30 µg/hr. This would be equivalent to a 24-hr dose of 240 to 720 µg. This compares with a total dose of 1,500 µg/day for a patient who is receiving 1% pilocarpine three times a day, to 6,000 µg in a patient receiving 4% pilocarpine three times a day. The total amount of pilocarpine hydrochloride given to the patient by conventional means is thus greater by a factor ranging between 10 and 25, than if the simulated prolonged release medication is used. Moreover, if some form of prolonged release medication could be developed in the treatment of glaucoma, the total amount required for the individual patient would be significantly less than 1 mg for 24 hr and for the average patient would range between 0.25 and 0.5 mg over a 24-hr period. Preliminary studies with a 24-hr sustained release pilocarpine Ocusert indicate that this device can control the intraocular pressure. Furthermore, this form of therapy, in contrast to eye drops, permits a continuous effect on intraocular pressure, with a total dose of pilocarpine over a 24-hr time period of 240 to 480 µg.

Relevant to the findings reported above, we have also performed studies on rabbits utilizing an erodable hydrocortisone Ocusert in the treatment of experimental phlyctenular keratitis. The Ocusert was an oval pledget measuring $5 \times 14$ mm and consisted of a matrix containing 10% hydrocortisone acetate. The entire Ocusert would be completely dissolved in 24 hr, hence the name "erodable Ocusert." The Ocuserts were soaked in saline overnight to eliminate the initial spike of steroid release which results from hydration. Thereafter, 20 µg of hydrocortisone was released per hour for a maximum of 24 hr. The Ocuserts were inserted into the inferior cul-de-sac of the rabbit eye once a day. This was compared with the usual forms of medication consisting of hydrocortisone acetate 2.5% in the form of an ointment and of prednisolone (PREDNEFERIN®) in the form of eye drops. The effects of these various forms of medication were examined in rabbit eyes in which an experimental form of phlyctenular keratitis was induced (1). The animals were observed daily and photographed on the third and sixth days of the experiment and on the 11th day prior to being killed. The eyes were also examined with the slit lamp during the course of the experiment. As soon as the animals were killed the eyes were removed and fixed in 10% formalin, sectioned and stained with hematoxylin and eosin. These studies indicated that the hydrocortisone Ocusert is a useful therapeutic agent in treating experimental

phlyctenular keratitis. Once again, the total dose of hydrocortisone applied to the eye over 24 hr by means of Ocusert therapy is significantly less than the amount of drug the eye would receive using conventional eye drops or ointment.

The results of the foregoing studies indicate that the Ocusert is an effective method of treating certain eye conditions. The advantages derived from utilizing this form of therapy are as follows:

1) A specific drug can be delivered to the eyeball at a relatively constant rate over a 24-hr period. 2) The total concentration of the drug applied to the eye by means of the Ocusert is much lower than with the present conventional forms of therapy. This would be advantageous in treating patients with a high degree of sensitivity to cholinergic drugs. The use of steroid Ocusert therapy, with its significantly lower total dose of steroid employed, might possibly be of help in those patients where prolonged steroid therapy leads to steroid glaucoma. 3) Aside from the continuous control of glaucoma and the much lower drug concentration required using the Ocusert, a further advantage of the 24-hr Ocusert, and particularly of Ocuserts designed for longer periods (up to a week), is in ensuring therapy in the unreliable patient who applies his medication in a more or less haphazard fashion.

Supported by funds from the ALZA Corporation manufacturer of Ocusert, Palo Alto, California and by a National Health Grant.

REFERENCE

1. DAVIS PL, WATSON JI and SAPP GA. Experimental phlyctenular keratitis. Can J Ophthalmol 5: 284, 1970.

earlier than if the disk is completely normal.

Finally, the answer to the question whether nurses should do tonometry: I would say, yes, they can learn it just as well as doctors.

With regard to screening, you have in some way to follow the population to know if they are later on to develop glaucoma. It is very important to know if it is a slowly progressing condition or if the progress is rather rapid, and this leads to the matter of economy. How often can you carry out screenings? I think this is a complicated problem.

DR. G. GORIN (*USA*): With regard to Dr. Olurin's comments, I analyzed 55 limbal sclerectomies performed in Manhattan Eye and Ear Hospital on 55 eyes, belonging to 38 black patients and 17 white patients. I modified the operation as follows: feeling that the main factor in the failure of filtering operations both in white and in black people is the presence of the Tenon's capsule. I didn't excise the latter. Instead, I made a very thin conjunctival flap without touching the Tenon's capsule. In other words, I aimed at forming a filtering bed not between the complex of conjuctiva, Tenon's capsule and sclera, but between the conjuctiva and Tenon's capsule. In addition, we made the scleral punch as anterior as possible, and away from the ciliary body. Our results before we started this program between 1967 and 1968 used to be 50% success. Now of these 55 eyes, 88% had excellent filtrations and for several years they continue to have very low tensions. The results continue to be similar in colored and white patients.

Dr. Sears and I would like to ask Dr. Kirsch two questions. Your observations about the vertically oval disk were very interesting, but all the patients concerned had glaucoma along with field defects, and I am therefore wondering about two things. First, do you think that this concept of yours about the glaucoma disk could be used as a parameter that would have predictive value for the development of glaucoma? Second, why would you be surprised to find this vertically oval cup, since probably this is the arcuate area?

DR. BLUMENTHAL: I would like to ask Prof. François if he thinks the supply to the optic nerve comes from the choroid or from the Zinn zonule.

DR. J. E. WOLFF (*South Africa*): I would like to ask Prof. François if he uses the ophthalmodynamometer to assess the prognosis of glaucoma clinically; I would also like to ask Dr. Kirsch if in his examination of the optic disk he dilates the pupils and prepares them to get a stereo picture of the fundus.

DR. LEYDHECKER: I would like to say that the pictures which Dr. Kirsch has shown of excavated disks in normal eyes with no glaucoma made me again rather doubtful about the possibility of early diagnosis of glaucoma from looking at the disk. There is another point which has been brought to my attention: What shall we do if a patient has a certain degree of ocular hypertension? Shall we treat him, and when shall we treat him? I feel that if the tension is between 20 and 24 mm Hg the patient may have glaucoma and damage to the optic nerve will follow. Such a patient, even with normal fields, should receive miotics.

DR. J. FRANÇOIS (*Belgium*): One should be very cautious when interpreting an ophthalmoscopic picture. What is important is not so much the appearance of the disk, but the change in appearance that you see during the year. Now, to Dr. Blumenthal, the vascularization of the optic disk is supplied by the circle of Zinn, and also by vessels coming from the choroid and from the vascular system of the optic nerve. In a case of glaucoma these vessels are compressed and ischemia develops. The vessels of the choroid also suffer; this is proved ophthalmoscopically by the fact that very often you have a halo around the disk which is due to alterations in choroidal vessels. Now, to Dr. Wolff, I do not think that a dynamometer is useful in glaucoma. Of course, we know that a slight pressure on the eyeball can give you a pulse of the artery but the dynamometer does not teach us more in glaucoma than in other cases, as it records only the pressure of the ophthalmic artery.

DR. R. E. KIRSCH (*USA*): To Dr. Sears' questions about the predictive value of the vertically oval cup, the answer is that all of the eyes that we have reported in this study already had a field defect, so that we really have no evidence bearing upon this point. However, our hope is, in the future, to get earlier glaucomatous cellular changes and gather some data on this matter. His next question: Why were we surprised concerning the vertically oval cup, since it is in the Bjerrum area? We were not surprised; it is just a clinical observation which was previously described as superior or inferior temporal enlargement of the cup, and we are just calling attention to the simple, easily observable clinical sign. To Dr. Wolff: we dilate the pupils for stereophotography. I think the safest answer would be the least amount of drug that would produce the maximum dilation.

tion around the tear will result in a false sense of security. Excessive reaction may well induce a secondary tear along its margin. The combined use of peripheral cryotherapy or surface diathermy with photocoagulation will achieve a satisfactory result.

Multiple areas of atrophic degenerative change in the equatorial or postequatorial areas are accessible to light coagulation but the extensive use of this or any other method in the temporal half of the retina must be assessed in relation to the risk of visual damage by macular pucker, an uncommon but serious complication (Fig. 1). In the instance illustrated it followed retinal detachment surgery involving a long radial retinal break but it can appear after light coagulation to a simple, flat tear.

If a single retinal tear is of any great dimension and certainly if there is evidence of eversion of the retinal edges, consideration should be given to the use of local plombage since this will ensure choroidoretinal apposition at the margin of the tear, will achieve a small volume reduction, will relax vitreous traction and will minimize the risk of failure of the initial treatment.

When equatorial or preequatorial degenerative changes are too extensive in relation to the circumference of the globe to enable them to be adequately treated by local intervention a technique of circumferential treatment must be adopted. This can be carried out by means of cryotherapy or light coagulation and in either instance not more than one half of the circumference of the globe should be treated at one time. Our usual technique is to treat the half of the globe including the major degenerative changes and to allow a period for consolidation of about a month before undertaking the remainder of the treatment. The presence of retinal degenerative changes is especially important in the fellow eye when a retinal detachment has occurred in the first eye and more particularly when surgi-

cal intervention has been unsuccessful.

More complicated problems do arise and I should like to introduce the possibility of prophylactic surgery more radical in nature than may seem at first sight to be indicated. If a surgical intervention or a number of interventions have been undertaken on the first eye and have been unsuccessful, this is a warning that similar treatment undertaken on the fellow eye, should the need arise, may meet with equal disappointment. In such circumstances we have undertaken an encircling procedure with a silicone rubber band to produce a gentle indentation, and with cryotherapy in areas of particular retinal weakness, in the hope that the circumferential nature of the procedure and the volume reduction achieved will minimize the chances of a more severe condition developing. Vitreous degeneration, vitreous retraction and the development of further retinal lesions in the equatorial zone all predispose to the development of a retinal detachment, even in an eye that has had limited prophylactic treatment. An example

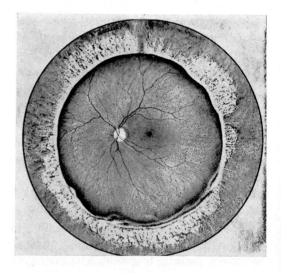

FIG. 2. Treatment with circling buckle for equatorial degeneration because of loss of fellow eye due to retinal detachment following photocoagulation without buckle.

of this procedure is given by a case in which the first eye developed massive vitreous retraction following photocoagulation, scleral resection and an encircling procedure done consecutively. The patient presented for further advice about treatment to the already affected eye and this was considered to be impossible. He had equatorial weakness in the fellow eye including three small retinal lesions. A prophylactic encirclement was decided upon. The result is illustrated in Fig. 2 and the patient retains a corrected visual acuity of 6/5 with a reasonably full visual field well over three years after treatment. The indications are infrequent in relation to the amount of retinal surgery carried on at our unit but the results in 15 procedures have led to only one disappointment and this followed over-enthusiastic surgery in which the indentation was more radical than had been intended.

In the case of giant retinal tears our discouraging experience has made us wonder whether in spite of the absence of any evident indications for treatment in the fellow eye it may not be justified by the poor prognosis. Two cases will serve to illustrate this point. In the first case a patient attended for treatment with a giant retinal tear in the right eye (Fig. 3). Anatomical replacement of the retina was possible but because of the extent of the treatment restoration of the central vision was incomplete. Seven years later the patient reported symptoms in his healthy fellow eye which had been kept under careful observation. There was a giant retinal tear in the equatorial zone in the temporal half of this eye and surgical treatment failed with the ultimate complication of massive vitreous retraction (Fig. 4).

In the second case a nasally placed giant retinal tear was successfully treated by means of a large meridional plomb together with encirclement (Fig. 5). Observation of the fellow eye revealed, some two years later, an early retinal detachment in the upper nasal

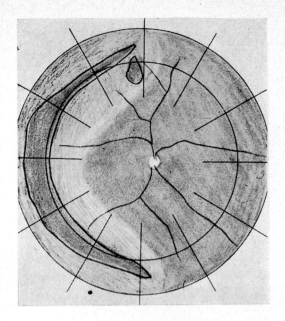

FIG. 3. Right eye. Giant retinal tear; anatomical replacement following operation but without complete restoration of central vision.

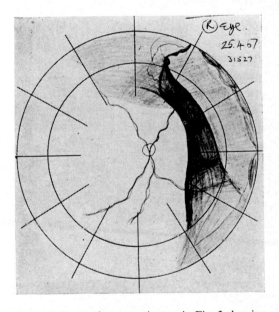

FIG. 4. Left eye of same patient as in Fig. 3 showing a giant retinal tear that appeared seven years later. Surgical treatment was unsuccessful.

quadrant with an associated peripheral tear or dialysis (Fig. 6). These two cases, not unusual in character among those with a giant

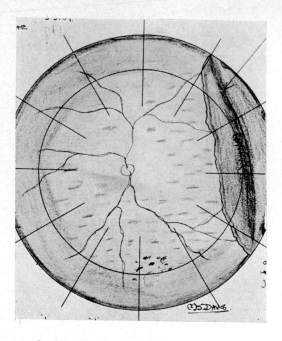

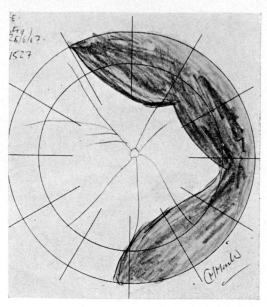

FIG. 5.  Nasally placed giant retinal tear in right eye successfully treated by means of a large meridional plomb together with encirclement.

FIG. 6.  Same patient as in Fig 5, showing an early detachment two years later in the upper nasal quadrant.

retinal tear, make one wonder whether a prophylactic encircling procedure would have been helpful in the management of the fellow eye.

I should like to thank my colleagues in the Retina Unit at the High Holborn branch of Moorfields for their help and Dr. Peter Hansell and his staff in the Department of Audio-Visual Communication at the Institute of Ophthalmology in London for the illustrations.

## REFERENCES

1. CUENDET JF.   Mod Probl Ophthalmol (Basel) 3: 46, 1965.
2. WAGNER H.   Ein bisher unbekanntes Erbleiden des Auges (Degeneratio hyaloideo-retinalis hereditaria), beobachtet im Kanton Zürich. Klin Monatsbl Augenheilk 100: 840, 1938.
3. BLACH RK.   The hereditary hyalo-retinopathies. Br J Ophthalmol 53: 136, 1969.
4. SPIRA C.  in: McPherson A (Ed), "New and controversial aspects of retinal detachment." New York, Harper & Row, 1968.

# PREVENTIVE TREATMENT OF THE PREHOLE STAGE OF RETINAL DETACHMENT

LORIMER FISON

Moorfields Eye Hospital, London, England

When discussing any type of treatment, it is necessary to mention the method of examination since recognition of the detailed clinical features is entirely dependent on specialized examination. The three basic methods of fundus examination are all used: binocular indirect ophthalmoscopy with a fully dilated pupil provides the basis from which a drawing of each fundus is made, scleral indentation supplying more information about the far periphery of the retina and its probable attachments to the vitreous; direct ophthalmoscopy with its greater magnification permits particular features already observed to be examined in detail; and finally examination by the slit lamp microscope with the three-mirror genioscope is used to study fundus features stereoscopically again, but at a far greater magnification. The fine structures of the retina can be resolved, thus further refining the completeness of the fundus diagram.

Subsequent detailed observation of the vitreous, including its fluidity, direction of motion during ocular movements, and strands and attachments all contribute basic knowledge for the estimation of the physical state of the retina. Unfortunately a method of studying the physiological state of the peripheral retina is not yet available since fluorescein angiography is at present applicable only to the more central areas of the retina.

In the future, when a method of assessing the state of the peripheral retinal blood supply has been developed, we will be better able to decide which areas require prophylactic strengthening.

The eyes at risk of developing a retinal detachment include those whose fellow eyes have had a detachment of the retina, because the condition is often bilateral, and those eyes which are myopic or aphakic. Blunt injury may increase the probability. There may be no symptoms preceding the detachment.

Lattice degeneration is probably the most common clinical appearance in the prehole stage. It may be minimal in extent or it may cover a large area of the peripheral retina. Frequently, patches of lattice do not demonstrate definite holes, but may show pits of partial thickness from ruptured degenerate cysts.

U-shaped tears occurring in the absence of lattice degeneration present an especially difficult problem in clinical observation. Only occasionally is there an evident prehole raising of the retina without actual tear formation. At times there is appreciable disturbance in the vitreous at one particular spot, which may indicate the presence of an early vitreoretinal traction. It is sometimes possible to trace vitreous bands to the retina, at the area where a retinal hemorrhage can be seen, thus giving a clue to the site of pathology.

Juvenile giant tear formation has a strong bilateral tendency but it is most unusual to find any abnormal vitreous or retinal signs in the opposite eye at the time the detachment occurs in the first eye. The time interval before appearance of the detachment in the second eye may vary from one month to two years. Giant tear may be a giant dialysis of the retina, or a giant U-tear formation in the retina when the only prehole sign in the opposite eye would be vitreous traction.

Indications for preventive treatment include: 1) lattice degeneration in both eyes with evident vitreous traction; 2) lattice degeneration in the second eye; 3) raised retina from vitreous traction or a patch of retinal hemorrhage in the second eye of a patient with detachment from U-tear formation in the first eye; 4) raised retina from vitreous traction in a postoperative eye with a U-tear elsewhere in the fundus; 5) the opposite eye of a giant dialysis—particularly in a juvenile; 6) the site of removal of an intraocular foreign body by the posterior route; 7) the opposite eye when cataract extraction is planned, there having been a retinal detachment in the first aphakic eye; 8) retinoschisis which presents a specially difficult problem for prophylaxis.

Retinoschisis may be considered a prehole condition since it may change its eventual nature to a frank retinal detachment. Most cases of retinoschisis change slowly so that any progress may best be observed by serial drawing, photographs and charted fields. If the central area is not damaged and there are no apparent holes, the retinoschisis is left alone. If, however, drawings and fields show progressive change, there is a strong indication for preventive treatment.

Preventive treatment consists simply in applying a light damaging injury to the retina and its pigment layer and to the choroid over the area of degenerate retina or hole, in order to weld these three layers into one firm scar. The general intention is to place such a reaction over a patch or broad area, taking in a small margin of apparently normal retina and thereby achieving a firm secure edge. Multiple, small, separated scars are to be avoided since scar tissue traction between adjacent patches may well develop with subsequent secondary retinal hold formation.

Cryosurgery lends itself to peripheral lesions, to eyes with unclear media and to structures inaccessible to a photocoagulator. Photocoagulation is specially suitable for lesions behind the equator of the eye and in accessible areas short of the far periphery where extreme accuracy is essential.

The green argon laser is likely to find a more prominent place in the future. Its color spectrum is better absorbed by the hemoglobin of the blood thus making it more applicable than the original red ruby laser. Coagulation with the green argon laser should produce the adhesive reaction even if the pigment layer of the retina is deficient.

# THE NATURAL HISTORY OF
# THE RETINOPATHIES OF RETINAL DETACHMENT
# AND PREVENTIVE TREATMENT

NORMAN E. BYER

Department of Ophthalmology, University of California School of Medicine, Los Angeles, California, USA

The retinal break is the final common pathway in the retinopathies which lead to retinal detachment. Approximately 50% of the breaks resulting in detachment are caused by vitreous traction which is not associated with visible preexisting retinopathy (excluding, therefore, lattice degeneration). About 30% are caused by lattice degeneration (of this group about 70% are tractional and 30% are nontractional). The remaining 20% are nontractional, non-"lattice" breaks including dialyses.

Isolated retinal breaks, lattice degeneration and senile retinoschisis are the most common types of retinopathy associated with retinal detachment. They are also the three retinopathies for which prophylactic treatment is most frequently recommended.

*Isolated retinal breaks* (those not associated with lattice degeneration or retinoschisis). The most useful manner in which such breaks may be further subdivided is to differentiate them into symptomatic and asymptomatic groups. This division is of prognostic value in regard to the risk of retinal detachment. a) Symptomatic retinal breaks: Pischel (1) showed that no more than 30% of eyes with symptomatic breaks lead to retinal detachment. Such breaks produce symptoms because they are caused by vitreoretinal traction or produce some degree of hemorrhage at the time of their occurrence. Because of such traction, these breaks are either horseshoe tears or breaks with free opercula. The increased likelihood of hemorrhage is based upon the fact that they tend to be comparatively larger in size than asymptomatic breaks. b) Asymptomatic retinal breaks: These are very common lesions being found in 5.8% of a large clinical series and some reports state a higher prevalence. These breaks tend to be very small but occasionally may be larger than one disk in diameter. Of these breaks, 76% are round holes without operculum and this type tends to occur in the decades prior to age 30. The 10% which are of the horseshoe type tend to appear after the age of 40. The quadrant of predominance for asymptomatic breaks is the inferior temporal. Asymptomatic retinal breaks are more common than retinal detachment by a ratio of 83:1. The risk of a patient with such a break of developing a retinal detachment from this cause is, therefore, no more than 1 to 2%.

*Lattice degeneration.* This peripheral vitreoretinal degeneration has been shown by a number of studies (both clinical and histological) to be present in about 8% of the population. This high prevalence rate occurs prior to the age of 20. It is important to remember that, on the basis of both clinical and histologic surveys, the white lines for which the disease has been named are present in only 20% of the cases. In 29% of patients, one or more retinal breaks are found in association with these lesions. These are almost always of the small round, atrophic, non-operculated variety. Lattice degeneration tends to be located in the vicinity of the 12:00 and 6:00 meridians preferentially. It is also significantly associated with myopia. Lattice degeneration is more common than retinal detachment by a ratio of 110:1. However a number of independent studies have shown that only about 30% of patients with retinal detachment also have lattice degeneration. Therefore the real risk of developing a retinal detachment from preexisting lattice degeneration is no more than 0.5%. When retinal detachment does occur from this disease, it occurs in one of two ways. In about 70% of such cases a tractional tear of the horseshoe type develops suddenly, usually with symptoms, along the posterior edge or the ends of a lattice degenerative lesion. In about 30% of the cases the detachment develops slowly and often asymptomatically as the result of the small atrophic round holes mentioned earlier.

*Senile retinoschisis.* This peripheral intra-retinal degenerative lesion has been found to be present in 3.7% of the general population over the age of 10 and in 7% of those older than 40. It is bilateral in 82% of cases and the maximal involvement tends to be in the inferior temporal quadrant. It is significantly associated with hyperopia. It usually begins in the fourth decade but may begin in the third decade. A small number of the cases, about 8%, show breaks in one of the layers, almost always the posterior. On rare occasions, breaks may be seen in both layers of the split retina and in some of these cases this can lead to retinal detachment. The only other danger to vision from senile retinoschisis is

fortunately also rare and results from the slow progression of the splitting process until it approaches the posterior pole. Because of its subtle clinical appearance, the presence of retinoschisis is usually overlooked and the diagnosis missed. Senile retinoschisis is more common than retinal detachment by a ratio of about 50:1. However, since not more than 5% of retinal detachments originate from this disease the actual risk of having a detached retina from previous retinoschisis is approximately 0.1% or less.

PROGRESSION OF RETINOPATHIES

The only accurate way of assessing the long-term significance of these lesions is to observe the natural behavior of individual lesions over a long period of time, in the absence of any form of prophylactic therapy. Such follow-up studies are being carried out by the author and data on their present status are shown in Table 1. In each of the two cases of subclinical retinal detachment indicated in Table 1, the subretinal collection of fluid adjacent to the lattice lesion measured approximately four disk diameters in diameter and resulted from small round holes. These patients are still being observed without treatment. None of the 17 cases with new round holes are being treated. It is evident from these studies that the changes which have been observed are generally of minor importance. It is particularly important that no retinal detachments have yet been seen in this study of 281 patients with retinopathies observed for from three to eight years.

INDICATIONS FOR PROPHYLACTIC
TREATMENT

Any list of indications for treatment is somewhat arbitrary depending upon the point of view of the author. The accumulation of direct and indirect evidence as reviewed in this paper tends to substantiate the view that the three retinopathies discussed rarely lead to

398

TABLE 1. *Progression of retinopathies*

| Lesion type | Changes observed | No. of patients |
|---|---|---|
| Asymptomatic retinal breaks (85 patients, observed for from three to eight years) | Retinal detachment (general or local) | 0 |
| | Enlargement | 0 |
| | Pigmentation | 1 |
| | New breaks in other areas | 8 |
| Lattice degeneration (146 patients, observed for from three to eight years) | Clinical retinal detachment | 0 |
| | Subclinical retinal detachment | 2 (very small) |
| | New horseshoe tear | 1[a] |
| | New round hole | 17 |
| | New white lines | 21 |
| | New lesion | 11 |
| Senile retinoschisis (50 patients, observed for from three to seven years) | Retinal detachment | 0 |
| | Posterior extension[b] | 3 |
| | Lateral extension[b] | 11 |
| | New holes | 3 |
| | New areas involved | 8 |

[a] This was an exception to the group because the observation period was only one year. This lesion was promptly treated.
[b] In both posterior or lateral extension, the amount of extension was clinically estimated as slight.

retinal detachment. For this reason, I consider the following conservative indications to be a reasonable guide to prophylactic treatment in most cases:

*a) Asymptomatic retinal breaks*: 1) prior to cataract surgery, or if aphakic; 2) if breaks are large enough or posterior enough so that they might be difficult to close if the retina detached; 3) any horseshoe tear larger than $\frac{1}{2}$ disk diameter; 4) history of detachment of the first eye, and one of the following: a family history of detachment, multiple breaks in the second eye, or if surgery on the first eye was unsuccessful.

*b) Lattice degeneration*: 1) with adjacent horseshoe tear; 2) prior to cataract surgery or if aphakic; 3) history of detachment in first eye and one of the following: a family history of detachment, the lattice had a similar appearance and location as that which caused detachment in the first eye, or if surgery on the first eye was unsuccessful.

*c) Senile retinoschisis*: 1) with definite retinal breaks in both layers; 2) with marked posterior extension near the posterior pole with evidence of increasing enlargement toward the macula.

With regard to prophylactic treatment in cases of lattice degeneration, it is accepted by many that the presence of lattice degeneration per se is not a sufficient reason for treatment, but lattice degeneration associated with round atrophic holes is more dangerous and should be treated. It is true that such round holes do occasionally lead to retinal detachment. The comparative risk in the two groups can be analyzed approximately as follows. Statistically not more than 0.5% of cases of lattice degeneration lead to retinal detachment. As stated earlier, when retinal detachment results from lattice degeneration, around 70% of the cases are caused by traction tears at the borders of the lattice lesions, and around 30% are caused by atrophic round holes within the lesions. Thus detachments due to traction tears account for 0.35% and those caused by round holes account for 0.15%. We may probably assume that the risk of a traction type detachment is spread equally over the total group of patients who have lattice, since histologically all lattice lesions are characterized by abnormal attachments of vitreous to the edges of the lesions. In patients with lattice degeneration without atrophic round holes, we may estimate the risk to be 0.35%*. However the risk of retinal detachment from the round holes of lattice is spread only over those patients who have such holes, namely about 30% of the total patients who have lattice degeneration. This risk is therefore about 0.50%**. However this group of patients (those with lattice plus round holes) also share the risk of retinal detachment from tractional tears. Therefore their total risk is the combination of these two, about 0.85%***. In conclusion it may be stated that lattice with round holes appears to have a higher risk of leading to detachment, but that in either case (with or without such holes) the risk is still less than 1%. In addition it must be pointed out that detachments due to the small round holes of lattice have a better prognosis than those due to traction tears.

Prophylactic treatment therefore is probably not any more necessary when atrophic round holes are present in cases of lattice degeneration than when they are absent.

In summary, prophylactic treatment is of foremost importance in cases of symptomatic retinal breaks, and secondarily in some cases of the three forms of retinopathy discussed, and in a few other rather rare instances. With the passing of more time and with the above noted lesions under continued observation, a more complete and satisfactory picture of their natural history will be expected to emerge.

---

\* .35/100.
\*\* .15/30.
\*\*\* .35 + .50.

REFERENCE

1. PISCHEL DK. The risk of untreated retinal holes. *Mod Probl Ophthalmol* **4**: 128, 1966.

# A NATIONAL STUDY ON THE PREVENTION OF RETINAL DETACHMENT

I. C. MICHAELSON and R. STEIN (Coordinators)

Departments of Ophthalmology, Hadassah University Hospital and Hebrew University–Hadassah Medical School, Jerusalem, Chaim Sheba Medical Center, Tel-Hashomer and Tel Aviv University Medical School, Israel

The development of an idiopathic retinal detachment is preceded by a series of pathological events, which usually occur over a number of years. The predetachment phase and the retinal detachment together are referred to as the retinopathy of retinal detachment. The events are consecutive and finally lead to detachment of the retina from the pigment epithelium in a certain number of cases. There is only incomplete knowledge, however, regarding the following: 1) prevalence of retinal hole formation; 2) circumstances that may be associated with retinal holes leading to retinal detachment; 3) discovery of cases potentially in need of preventive treatment; 4) effectiveness of treatment in preventing retinal detachment developing from retinal holes; 5) incidence and prevalence of idiopathic retinal detachment.

Hitherto, efforts to gain more information about these questions have been attempted by individual ophthalmologists or by individual departments. The prevalence of retinal detachment has been investigated in the Canton of Zurich on the basis of 196 detachments that occurred between 1949 and 1955 (1).

The National Study on the Prevention of Retinal Detachment has been conducted in all the 15 hospital eye departments in Israel since 1962. Each month, each department transmits the following information to the central secretariat:

1) A list of all cases of idiopathic detachment admitted that month which includes a) general ocular information—whether the affected eye is myopic or aphakic and whether an idiopathic retinal detachment has previously affected the other eye, and b) information regarding shape, size and situation of the retinal hole.

2) A list of all cases of retinal hole treated preventively which includes the type of information detailed in (a) and (b) above.

3) Investigation sheets with regard to patients suspected by the examiner of suffering from the retinopathy of retinal detachment without retinal detachment. These are generally completed with respect to "fellow" eyes, i.e. the unaffected eye of one whose other eye has suffered from idiopathic retinal detachment; myopic and aphakic eyes and eyes showing the fundal appearance of detachment retinopathy found by chance or because of certain symptoms. The investigation sheets, which are completed for cases the examiner chooses, are sent to the central secretariat. After the information contained in them has been filed, they are returned to each department where they remain until, in the course of succeeding months or years,

further information is added. In this way, an attempt is made to determine the natural history of the predetachment phase in as many cases as possible. To date, over 608 such eyes have been followed up over a period of one to four years.

*Hole prevalence studies.* Several of the departments (in the Rothschild Hospital, Haifa, and Hadassah University Hospital and Shaare Zedek Hospital, Jerusalem) have studied the prevalence of retinal holes in certain groups of nondetached eyes: fellow eyes, myopic eyes and nonmyopic eyes.

Perhaps the most interesting results of the National Study have been with regard to our knowledge of the natural history of the retinopathy. This chiefly concerns the determination of the kind of hole in a flat retina which is worthwhile closing preventively because it is more likely to lead to a detachment. To ascertain this knowledge, two types of prevalence were compared: prevalence of flat retina with holes, arranged according to hole-types (size, shape, situation) and to eye-type (myopic, nonmyopic, fellow eye); and prevalence of detached retina with holes, arranged according to similar hole type and eye type. As a result, it has been possible to assemble detachment/hole ratio tables, the purpose of which is to formulate the degree of advisability of hole closure. These tables, being a comparison of two prevalences do not, however, take into account the age of the retinal hole. Dr. Neumann will bring forward evidence suggesting the significance of this point (2).

Analysis of the accumulating data in this study have already been reported (3–7 and S. Merin et al., in preparation). Dr. Stein will, in this session, discuss the effect of preventive therapy (8) and Dr. Neumann, the natural history of detachment retinopathy (2).

*The suitability of Israel for this project.* Israel is thought to be a suitable country for this kind of research because: a) It is large enough to give significant statistical results.

The project deals with the Jewish population of 1,886,000 who were present in the country on 1 January 1960. Subsequent immigrants were not included in this cohort, which was augmented for later years by the 2% natural increase. This cohort amounted to 2,341,047 in 1971. b) It is small enough to permit the close cooperation necessary between the various eye departments if all cases of retinal detachment are reported. There are 15 hospital eye departments in Israel. It would not be possible to obtain exact figures on the incidence of retinal detachment and the effect on this incidence of a known number of prophylactic treatments if patients go to different ophthalmologists for diagnosis, preventive treatment and perhaps a subsequent detachment, and if these ophthalmologists were not in a position to pool their findings. c) The nation-wide study has made ophthalmologists "retinal detachment prevention minded," and retinal clinics have been set up wherein "cases at risk," in particular, are examined and followed up (i.e. fellow eyes, myopic-aphakic eyes and patients with complaints suggestive of detachment retinopathy).

Supported by the U.S. Department of Health, Education, and Welfare, Public Health Service, Bureau of State Services, Grant No. CD-IS-10.

### REFERENCES

1. BOHRINGER HR. Statistisches zu Häufigkeit und Risiko der Netzhautablösung. *Ophthalmologica* **131**: 331, 1956.
2. NEUMANN E, HYAMS S, BARKAI S, FEILIER V, IVRY M, JEDWAB E, KRAKOWSKI D, MAYTHAR B, SCHARF J and ZINGER L. The natural history of retinal holes with special reference to the development of retinal detachment and the time factor involved. *Isr J Med Sci* **8**: 1424, 1972.
3. MICHAELSON IC and STEIN R (Coordinators). National scheme in the prevention of retinal detachment. *Int Congr Ophthalmol, New Delhi, 1962.*
4. MICHAELSON IC and STEIN R (Coordinators). A national cooperative study in the prevention of retinal detachment. A preliminary report. *Mod Probl Ophthalmol* **4**: 135, 1966.
5. MERIN S, FEILER V, HYAMS S, IVRY M, KRAKOWSKI D, LANDAU L, MAYTHAR B, MICHAELSON IC, SCHARF J, SCHUL A and SER I. The

fate of the fellow eye in retinal detachment. *Am J Ophthalmol* **71**: 477, 1971.

6. AV-SHALOM A, BERSON D, GOMBOS GM, LANDAU L, MICHAELSON IC and ZAUBERMAN H. The vitreo-retinopathy associated with retinal detachment among Africans. *Am J Ophthalmol* **64**: 387, 1967.

7. HYAMS SW, FRIEDMAN Z and NEUMANN E. The peripheral retina in myopia with particular reference to retinal breaks. *Br J Ophthalmol* (in press).

8. STEIN R. The effect of treatment in the prevention of retinal detachment. *Isr J Med Sci* **8**: 1429, 1972.

# THE NATURAL HISTORY OF RETINAL HOLES WITH SPECIAL REFERENCE TO THE DEVELOPMENT OF RETINAL DETACHMENT AND THE TIME FACTOR INVOLVED

E. NEUMANN, S. HYAMS, S. BARKAI, V. FEILER, M. IVRY,
E. JEDWAB, D. KRAKOWSKI, B. MAYTHAR, J. SCHARF and L. ZINGER

Eye Departments, Rothschild Municipal–Government Hospital, Haifa, Government Hospital, Poriah, Chaim Sheba Medical Center, Tel-Hashomer, Hadassah University Hospital, Jerusalem, Shaare Zedek Hospital, Jerusalem, Assaf Harofe Government Hospital, Zerifin, Rambam Government Hospital, Haifa and Donolo Government Hospital, Jaffa, Israel

The following report is based on information gathered from all of the eye departments in Israel, as part of the Israel National Study on the Prevention of Retinal Detachment which began in 1962 (1–3), and which has already been referred to by Prof. Michaelson.

The main purpose of this study is to assess the possibility of preventing retinal detachment. Basic to the problem of selection of cases for preventive treatment is a knowledge of the prevalence of retinal holes and retinal detachments in the general population and in certain groups of eyes prone to retinal detachment. In addition, it is essential to be able to distinguish those holes which will eventually lead to retinal detachment from those which will not.

The prevalence of retinal holes in eyes examined *post mortem* and in the general population is between 5 and 10% (4–6). In Israel, prevalence studies have been carried out on various groups of eyes such as myopic eyes, fellow eyes* and aphakic eyes (7–10).

Table 1 shows the prevalence of retinal holes in the general population in Israel and in three groups of eyes within the population, myopes, nonmyopes and fellow eyes. This

---

\* A "fellow eye" is the undetached eye of a patient who has had a retinal detachment in one eye.

TABLE 1.  *Prevalence of retinal holes and retinal detachment in Israel*

|  | Myopia | Nonmyopia | Fellow eyes | Total |
|---|---|---|---|---|
| No. of eyes under study | 600,000 | 3,400,000 | 7,000 | approx. 4,000,000 |
| Prevalence of detachments |  |  |  |  |
|   No. of eyes | 5,500 | 1,500 | 700 | 7,000 |
|   Ratio | 1:109 | 1:2266 | 1:10 | 1:570 |
| Prevalence of eyes with holes (no. of eyes) | 74,000 | 327,800 | 1,330 | 360,000 |
| Detachment/hole ratio | 1:13.5 | 1:218 | 1:1.9 | 1:51.4 |

TABLE 2.   *Prevalence of various types of retinal hole*

| Type of hole | Nonmyopic eyes (%) | Myopic eyes (%) | Fellow eyes (%) | General population (%) |
|---|---|---|---|---|
| Peripheral horseshoe holes | — | 1.7 | 1.8 | 0.3 |
| Peripheral round holes | 5.5 | 3.7 | 10.0 | 5.2 |
| Other horseshoe holes | — | 2.3 | 2.2 | 0.5 |
| Other round holes | 2.2 | 4.7 | 5.0 | 3.0 |

TABLE 3.   *Detachment/hole ratio in myopic eyes*

| Type of hole | Prevalence of eyes with holes | Prevalence of eyes with detachment | Detachment/hole ratio |
|---|---|---|---|
| Peripheral horseshoe holes | 10,200 | 280 | 1/36 |
| Peripheral round holes | 22,200 | 560 | 1/40 |
| Other horseshoe holes | 13,800 | 2,950 | 1/4.7 |
| Other round holes | 28,200 | 1,700 | 1/17 |

study involves the Jewish population of Israel on 1 January 1960, totaling 1,882,600 people and their descendants; immigrants since that date are excluded. The group studied is estimated to have numbered 2,250,035 people in 1969. The figure of 2,000,000, involving about 4,000,000 eyes, is taken as a rough estimate for our purpose. Based on an annual incidence of 240 primary retinal detachments and knowing the ages of patients with retinal detachments and their average life expectancy, we estimate that in our population sample there are about 7,000 eyes which have or have had a retinal detachment. The prevalence of retinal detachment is therefore 7,000/4,000,000, that is 1:570. The prevalence of retinal holes in Israel is about 9%, so that the number of eyes with retinal holes in the general population is about 360,000. The detachment/hole ratio is therefore 1/51. Thus, about 2% of retinal holes in Israel develop retinal detachment.

The next three columns of Table 1 show the figures for myopia, nonmyopia and fellow eyes. The prevalence of retinal detachment in myopia is 1:109, in nonmyopia is 1:2,266 and in fellow eyes, 1:10. The ratio between the number of eyes with retinal detachment and the number of eyes with retinal holes is 1:13 in myopia, 1:218 in nonmyopia and 1:1.9 in fellow eyes. These are overall ratios which do not take into account the type of retinal break, a factor of considerable importance in the selection of cases for preventive treatment. It would be impossible to treat the 74,000 myopic eyes with holes in Israel, or for that matter the approximately 7,000,000 such eyes in the USA.

Table 2 shows the prevalence of various types of retinal hole in the same groups of eyes as appear in Table 1. The type of break most frequently found is a peripheral round hole in a fellow eye (10%). On the other hand, a peripheral horseshoe break is found in only 0.3% of the total population of eyes.

Table 3 shows detachment hole ratios for various types of holes in myopic eyes. Based on a prevalence of 1.7% the number of myopic eyes with peripheral horseshoe holes in the group under review is 10,200. The number of myopic eyes with detachment due to this type of hole in this group was 280. Therefore, for every myopic eye with a detachment caused by a peripheral horseshoe hole, there

**405**

TABLE 4. *Detachment/hole ratio in nonmyopic eyes*

| Type of hole | Prevalence of eyes with holes | Prevalence of eyes with detachments | Detachment/hole ratio |
|---|---|---|---|
| Peripheral round holes | 187,000 | 135 | 1:1385 |
| Other round holes | 74,000 | 330 | 1:224 |

TABLE 5. *Detachment/hole ratio in fellow eyes*

| Type of hole | Eyes with holes | Eyes with detachments | Detachment/hole ratio |
|---|---|---|---|
| Peripheral horseshoe holes | 126 | 16 | 1:8 |
| Peripheral round holes | 700 | 16 | 1:44 |
| Other horseshoe holes | 154 | 96 | 1:1.6 |
| Other round holes | 350 | 32 | 1:11 |

TABLE 6. *Detachment/hole ratio in all groups of eyes studied*

| Type of hole | Myopic | Nonmyopic | Fellow eyes | All eyes |
|---|---|---|---|---|
| Peripheral horseshoe holes | 1:36 | ? | 1:8 | 1:29 |
| Peripheral round holes | 1:40 | 1:1385 | 1:44 | 1:270 |
| Other horseshoe holes | 1:4.7 | ? | 1:1.6 | 1:4.6 |
| Other round holes | 1:17 | 1:224 | 1:11 | 1:66 |

are 35 eyes with this type of break but without a detachment. Similarly, the detachment/hole ratio for peripheral round holes is 1:40, for equatorial horseshoe holes 1:4.7 and for equatorial round holes 1:17.

In order to avoid an impossible statistical situation in eyes with multiple holes, with and without detachment, only the most dangerous looking break in each eye was considered. For this purpose horseshoe breaks were considered more dangerous than round breaks and equatorial breaks more dangerous than those in the periphery.

Table 4 shows the detachment/hole ratio in nonmyopic eyes. The detachment/hole ratio with regard to peripheral round holes is 1:1,385 and with regard to equatorial round holes 1:224. The number of horseshoe holes in eyes without detachment is far too small to be of statistical significance in the size of sample we have so far been able to explore.

Table 5 shows the detachment/hole ratios for various types of holes in "fellow eyes." The detachment/hole ratio is highest for equatorial horseshoe holes, 1:1.6, and lowest for peripheral round holes, 1:44.

Table 6 summarizes the detachment/hole ratios for various types of hole in the four groups of eyes under study. It is clear that preventive treatment is a practical proposition in any type of eye with an equatorial horseshoe hole (see third line in the Table) and in fellow eyes with any type of hole except a peripheral round one.

These tables are intended to give an indication of the danger of various types of retinal holes in certain groups of eyes with regard to development of retinal detachment. They do not take into account other parameters such as the quadrant which is affected, or the age and sex of the patient, because the number of cases available so far is not large enough to be of statistical significance. Other important factors such as the state of the vitreous and family history of detachment are more difficult to classify, but should be taken into account for each individual case.

The tables are based upon studies of the prevalence of long-standing, mostly asymptomatic retinal breaks and they can be used in the selection of cases for preventive treatment only on the assumption that most detachments are caused by old breaks. If old breaks do cause detachments a detachment/hole ratio of 1/10, for example, means that one out of every ten eyes with a certain type of hole will eventually develop a detachment. On the other hand, if only fresh breaks, i.e., breaks less than two to three weeks old, cause detachments, a detachment/hole ratio of 1/10 means that for every ten eyes with this type of hole, one eye developed a detachment soon after the hole was formed and the other nine eyes will not develop detachment unless a new hole forms.

The truth probably lies somewhere between these two possibilities, but to date there is no proof that old breaks play a significant role in the etiology of retinal detachment, and such proof will have to be supplied if preventive treatment is to continue on present-day lines.

The literature on the fate of untreated retinal holes in sparse and often fails to make a clear distinction between fresh and old breaks. The only large series is that of Byer (5) which was published in 1967. Smaller series were reported by Gonin (11) and by Vogt (12) in 1934, by Knapp (13) and by Gramstrom (14) in 1943 and by Colyear and Pischel (15) in 1956. These reports contain only two fully documented cases in which an old retinal break led to the formation of a retinal detachment, and in one of these cases trauma was a precipitating factor. In all other cases, including those reported by Colyear and Pischel (15), a detachment occurred either

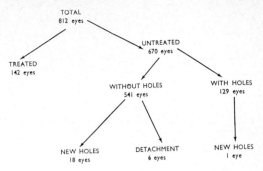

FIG. 1. Results of a one- to four-year follow-up study on prevention of retinal detachment.

within two weeks of the formation of a fresh retinal break, or not at all. The longest follow-up was eight years.

The Israel National Study on the Prevention of Retinal Detachment includes a follow-up of the retinopathy of retinal detachment. The retinal hole/detachment tables described by Michaelson (3) are in effect an epidemiological study of detachment retinopathy achieved by the comparison of two prevalences. It is a horizontal study. The study to be discussed here is a follow-up of 812 eyes and is a complementary vertical study. These eyes have been examined at least once a year over a follow-up period of one to four years (Fig. 1). One hundred and forty-two eyes with retinal holes were treated. The 670 untreated eyes included 129 eyes with retinal holes and 541 eyes without holes: these 670 eyes consisted of 377 fellow eyes, 97 myopic eyes (49 of them aphakic) and 196 eyes examined because the patient complained of muscae or flashes. During the follow-up period, six eyes developed retinal detachment, but in none of them had a hole been present when the eye was examined six weeks to one year before the detachment occurred. In 19 additional eyes a fresh hole appeared, unaccompanied by a detachment. It is clear that all six detachments occurred from relatively fresh holes, but it is not possible to draw conclusions concerning the fate of untreated re tinal holes because many of the more d angerous-looking holes were treated (the gro up of 142 eyes).

At the Rothschild Hospital it has been our p olicy not to treat retinal holes unless there is some extraneous factor such as glaucoma, s ubluxation of the lens, myopia-aphakia with vi treous loss or the insistence of the patient o n being treated. So far we have under study 108 eyes with untreated breaks during a follow-up period of one to six years (average 37 months). About half of these cases are "high risk" eyes such as fellow eyes, aphakic eyes and eyes with recent vitreous detachment. The other half were asymptomatic myopic eyes. These 108 eyes contained 153 holes, two-thirds of them equatorial (in position), one-third horseshoes (in shape) and one-third larger than one-quarter of the disk diameter (in size).

Three detachments have occurred so far, two of them in eyes with a fresh retinal break accompanied by a vitreous hemorrhage, while the patient was still in bed in hospital. In the third case a giant horseshoe hole occupying an entire quadrant in a myopic eye caused a detachment six weeks after its incidental discovery. Excluding the traumatic detachment mentioned earlier, this represents the second recorded case in which an old break was seen to cause a detachment.

In view of the paucity of recorded evidence that old breaks cause detachments, one must at least consider the possibility that the majority of detachments occur only a short time after the formation of a retinal hole and that the "freshness" of a retinal hole may be the decisive factor in determining the need for preventive treatment. The scale of present-day prophylactic treatment, with its occasional failures and complications, emphasizes the need for more information regarding the role of old, as opposed to fresh, retinal holes in the etiology of retinal detachment. If we can provide statistical evidence

that the incidence of retinal detachment in Israel has been reduced by prophylaxis, the extent of this reduction may be an indication of the importance of old breaks as a cause of retinal detachment.

## REFERENCES

1. MICHAELSON IC, STEIN R, FELSENTHAL W, HAUER I, IVRY M, KALLNER G, KURZ O, SACHS R and SINAI E. A national cooperative study in the prevention of retinal detachment—a preliminary report. Ophthalmologica 2: 1356, 1962.
2. MICHAELSON IC, STEIN R, FELSENTHAL W, HAUER I, IVRY M, KALLNER G, KURZ O, SACHS R and SINAI E. A national cooperative study in the prevention of retinal detachment—a preliminary report. Mod Probl Ophthalmol (Basel) 4: 135, 1966.
3. MICHAELSON IC, STEIN R, BARKAI S, BERSON D, FELSENTHAL W, HAUER I, IVRY M, KALLNER G, KURZ O, LIEBLING S, NEUMANN E, SACHS W and SPEYER H. A national cooperative study in the prevention of retinal detachment. Ann Ophthalmol 1: 49, 1969.
4. RUTNIN U and SCHEPENS C. Fundus appearance in normal eyes. IV. Retinal breaks and other findings. Am J Ophthalmol 64: 1063, 1967.
5. BYER NE. Clinical study of retinal breaks. Trans Am Acad Ophthalmol Otolaryngol 71: 461, 1967.
6. FOOS RY and RAYMOND AA. Retinal tears and lesser lesions of the peripheral retina in autopsy eyes. Am J Ophthalmol 64: 643, 1967.
7. OKUN E. Gross and microscopic pathology in autopsy eyes. III. Retinal breaks without detachment. Am J Ophthalmol 17: 369, 1961.
8. HYAMS S and NEUMANN E. Peripheral retina in myopia with particular reference to retinal breaks. Br J Ophthalmol 53: 300, 1969.
9. MERIN S, FEILER V, HYAMS S, IVRY M, KRAKOWSKI D, LANDAU L, MAYTHAR B, MICHAELSON IC, SCHARF J, SCHUL A and SER I. The fate of the fellow eye in retinal detachment. Am J Ophthalmol 71: 477, 1971.
10. FRIEDMAN Z, NEUMANN E and HYAMS S. The vitreous and peripheral retina in aphakia. A study of 200 nonmyopic, aphakic eyes. Br J Ophthalmol (in press).
11. GONIN J. Cited in ref. 15.
12. VOGT A. Freischwebender Lochdeckel der Netzhaut, eine Form von Glaskörperprüfung. Mit Beobachtungen über latente foramina retinae. Klin Monastbl Augenheilkd 92: 577, 1934.
13. KNAPP A. Peripheral retinal holes without detachment. Arch Ophthalmol 30: 585, 1943.
14. GRAMSTROM KO. Retinal hole observed 15 months before detachment of the retina. Acta Ophthalmol (Kbh) 21: 204, 1943–1944.
15. COLYEAR BH and PISCHEL DK. Clinical tears in the retina without detachment. Am J Ophthalmol 41: 773, 1956.

# THE EFFECT OF TREATMENT IN THE PREVENTION OF RETINAL DETACHMENT

R. STEIN, V. FELLER–OFRY and A. ROMANO

Department of Ophthalmology, Chaim Sheba Medical Center, Tel-Hashomer, Israel

Despite the progress made during the last decade in the surgical treatment of retinal detachment, few would claim today that surgery is preferable to prevention. The first prerequisite for effective prevention of retinal detachment is the ability to recognize those situations which will probably lead to retinal detachment, and those in which such an event is unlikely. This recognition depends chiefly on the nature of prehole degeneration, the appearances and situation of the hole and the state of the vitreous. In order to help solve this problem, all the eye departments in Israel initiated a scheme in 1960 known as "A National Cooperative Study in the Prevention of Retinal Detachment." This study has three main sections: a) the assessment of the incidence of retinal detachment; b) the natural history of the retinopathy of retinal detachment, essentially a recognition of holes which lead to retinal detachment; and c) an assessment of the effect of artificial closure of retinal holes on the incidence of retinal detachment. Points a and b have been discussed by Dr. Michaelson et al. and Dr. Neumann et al., respectively. We here refer to point c: the effect of preventive treatment.

*Decision to treat.* Despite the information regarding the advisability of retinal hole closure which may be found in the detachment/hole ratio tables (1), and which is mentioned in Dr. Neumann's lecture, the temperament of the ophthalmologist still remains an important factor. A cautious ophthalmologist may leave an equatorial horseshoe tear untreated if he can be certain that a) there is no vitreous traction of the flap and b) the edges of the tears are adherent to the pigment epithelium. In such a case, he would have to limit the daily activity of the patient and keep him under close observation.

More difficult is the decision as to whether to treat an eye with a lesion low in the danger scale, such as an equatorial round hole, in a fellow or myopic eye. Our policy is to close such holes if they are one-quarter of a disk diameter or more in size, if the operculum is still adherent and pulled by the vitreous and if, as a consequence of this, the patient complains of flashes. This is especially serious if the condition is found in a fellow eye, or in the eye of a patient with a family history of retinal detachment. Some ophthalmologists may decide not to treat a peripheral hole if it is not operculated, or even an equatorial hole if it is covered with solid vitreous which can act as a tampon. We usually choose to treat these two types because they are potentially dangerous. Experience has shown that they may remain quiescent for months or even years, but then suddenly they become detached if fluid vitreous enters the subretinal

TABLE 1. *Annual incidence of retinal detachments and number of eyes treated preventively*

| Year | Rate per 100,000 population | No. of eyes treated preventively |
|------|------|------|
| 1962 | 9.4 | 158 |
| 1963 | 9.0 | 210 |
| 1964 | 8.1 | 187 |
| 1965 | 8.6 | 127 |
| 1966 | 8.7 | 180 |
| 1967 | 8.2 | 182 |
| 1968 | 10.8 | 180 |
| 1969 | 9.5 | 181 |
| 1970 | 9.2 | 156 |
| 1971 | 9.3 | 117 |

space. A dense pigment scar around such holes may be a manifestation of a spontaneous cure and a safeguard, thus making treatment unnecessary.

*The effect of preventive treatment.* The annual incidence of idiopathic cases of retinal detachment in Israel between the years 1962 and 1971 is shown in Table 1. The results take into account an annual population increase of 2%. The population which was 1,920,252 in 1962 rose to 2,341,047 in 1971. The annual number of preventively treated cases in the same period is also indicated.

In 1967, the method of collecting data from each of the departments in the country was radically changed. This probably accounts for the difference in incidence during the three-year periods 1964–66 and 1969–71: 8.1, 8.6 and 8.7, as compared with 9.5, 9.2 and 9.3. The higher incidence in 1962–63 as compared with 1964–66 is probably due to the fact that the effect of the treatments had not yet been felt. The unexpectedly high figure for 1968 results from the fact that cases were not reported in 1967 because of the shortcomings of the organization, but were reported in 1968. During that period a total of 1,678 preventive treatments (average, 168) were carried out. Since 1970, the number of preventively treated cases per year has fallen considerably. In a treated population the annual incidence of idiopathic retinal detachment is apparently about 9.3/100,000. Unfortunately, there are no comparable figures available in Israel or elsewhere for an untreated population.

REFERENCE

1. MICHAELSON IC and STEIN R. A study in the prevention of retinal detachment. *Ann Ophthalmol* 1969.

# RETINOSCHISIS AS PREHOLE STAGE
# IN THE RETINOPATHY OF RETINAL DETACHMENT

O. KURZ and J. REIF

Ophthalmological Department, Beilinson Medical Center and
Tel Aviv University Medical School, Petah Tikva, Israel

Retinoschisis is a splitting of the sensory retina which, in the acquired adult form, cleaves in the plexiform layer, and in the congenital form, in the nerve fiber layer (1). Clinical and pathological experience have led to the distinction of a number of clinical entities, as shown in Table 1.

The symptomatic form of retinoschisis constitutes one form of the prehole stage of detachment retinopathy. Cystoid degeneration of the retina and vitreous pull cause separation of the retinal layer. In the following stage a break may occur in the external, the internal or both retinal lamellae. The hole in the external layer appears as a round, reddish area, with a sharp grayish-white margin (Fig. 1). Internal to this area are the vessels of the inner retinal layer. Eventually, a break in the inner layer with or without operculum completes the perforation of the retina. While an isolated rupture in the internal layer need not cause a detachment, an isolated rupture in the external retinal lamella may lead to retinal separation. The surgical closure of such a lamellar break is therefore imperative. After reattachment of the retina, the outlines of the previous lamellar break may still be distinguished by circumscribed pigmentation (Fig. 2).

In the relationship between idiopathic reti-noschisis (2, 3) and retinal detachment, the following possibilities are encountered (Table 2).

TABLE 1. *Retinoschisis*

| | |
|---|---|
| Primary | Symptomatic (evolutionary in development of retinal detachment) |
| | Idiopathic Infantile (hereditary, juvenile) Juvenile acquired (presenile) Senile (2, 3) |
| Secondary | In old retinal detachment Over choroidal tumors In other conditions (Coats' disease, etc.) |

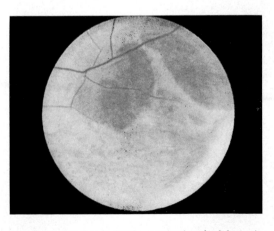

FIG. 1. Large break in the external retinal layer in a 63-year-old female with retinoschisis and retinal detachment.

411

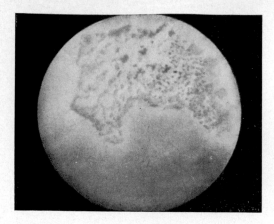

FIG. 2.   Same eye after reattachment.

a) Detachment by soulèvement, that is by elevation of the retina which surrounds the cyst, often leading to retinal disinsertion in the lower temporal periphery (4). b) Detachment by hole formation in the adjacent degenerated retina. c) Detachment by perforation of the cyst wall. d) The incidental appearance of a rhegmatogenous detachment due to hole formation in other parts of the fundus not involved in the existing retinoschisis. Here the causal relationship is a general tendency of the eye to undergo degenerative changes.

We have tried to clarify this relationship in 23 patients with presenile and 10 with senile retinoschisis. Table 2 shows the causal relationship between the detachment and retinoschisis, consecutive or nonconsecutive, which we observed in 14 of the 23 presenile patients. Table 3 describes the sex, age and refraction of the 33 patients of retinoschisis under study. The majority of eyes showed typical demarcation lines. All eyes showing a progression of the detachment, especially such as to endanger the macula, were operated upon. Two cases of rhegmatogenous detachment were independent of the existing retinoschisis (nonconsecutive).

In the senile group there was only one case of retinal detachment adjacent to the cyst.

The frequently used classification of congenital hereditary retinoschisis in children and of acquired senile retinoschisis in adults, does not seem to be satisfactory. Additional types

TABLE 2.   *Relationship of retinoschisis to retinal detachment*

| | No. of cases with consecutive detachment | | No. of cases with nonconsecutive detachment, "independent" detachment due to breaks in other parts of the retina |
| | By "soulèvement" (elevation of adjacent retina and disinsertion) | By other types of hole formation | |
|---|---|---|---|
| Presenile | 8 | 3 | 2 |
| Senile | 1 | 1 | — |

TABLE 3.   *Idiopathic retinoschisis*

| Age | | Age groups | | | | | Refraction | | | |
| M | F | 20 to 29 | 30 to 39 | 40 to 49 | 50 to 60 | 61+ | M | E | H | Bilateral |
|---|---|---|---|---|---|---|---|---|---|---|
| Presenile (23 cases) | | | | | | | | | | |
| 13 | 10 | 10 | 7 | 6 | — | — | 16 | 4 | 3 | 7 |
| Senile (10 cases) | | | | | | | | | | |
| 8 | 2 | — | — | — | 8 | 2 | 3 | 4 | 3 | 3 |

of juvenile and presenile forms of the disease have been identified (5). We believe that the distinction between infantile, presenile and senile forms of retinoschisis conforms more closely to the clinical picture. In the presenile group, which approximately covers the age range of 20 to 40 years, the typical location is the temporal lower quadrant, and the consecutive detachment is often limited by demarcation lines.

In the senile group retinoschisis usually begins temporally and spreads slowly along the periphery toward the macula. This type is encountered mainly after the age of 50.

## REFERENCES

1. ZIMMERMAN LE and NEUMANN G. The pathology of retinoschisis, in: McPherson A (Ed), "New and controversial aspects of retinal detachment." New York, Harper, Hoeber Medical Division, 1968, p 400.
2. SHEA M, SCHEPENS CL and VON PIRQUET SR. Retinoschisis. I. Senile type. *Arch Ophthalmol* **63**: 1, 1960.
3. BYER NE. Clinical study of senile retinoschisis. *Arch Ophthalmol* **79**: 36, 1968.
4. WEVE H. The relation between the layer, isolated cysts and retinal detachment. *Arch Augenheilkd* **109**: 49, 1935.
5. OKUN E and CIBIS PA. Retinoschisis. Classification, diagnosis and management, in: McPherson A (Ed), "New and controversial aspects of retinal detachment." New York, Harper, Hoeber Medical Division, 1968, p 424.

# PREVENTION OF RETINAL DETACHMENT
# IN HIGH MYOPIC APHAKIC EYES

GIORA TREISTER

Chaim Sheba Medical Center, Tel-Hashomer, Israel

It is generally recognized that aphakia considerably increases the probability of retinal detachment and that the higher the myopia, the greater is the tendency to develop a detachment. The risk is greatest when both of these predisposing factors, i.e., high myopia and aphakia, are present. Preventive treatment is therefore of special significance in this specific group of eyes. The present report deals with the incidence and clinical features of retinal breaks and detachments in high myopic aphakic eyes, and describes the efficacy of preventive treatment.

## MATERIALS AND METHODS

This series included 374 eyes with a myopia of –8.0 D or greater, or an aphakic refraction of +6.0 D or less. In 164 of these eyes a pro-phylactic barrage was performed at least three months prior to the extraction of the lens, and in the remaining 210 eyes the lens was extracted without any preceding preventive treatment. The aphakic refraction and the calculated preoperative refraction of both groups are shown in Table 1. The indications for preventive treatment are given in Table 2.

The prophylactic treatment consisted of creating a new ora serrata by diascleral diathermy coagulations that were set in two to three rows in a hatchlike pattern at the central border of all retinal degenerations, including the degeneration itself. In eyes in which the lens opacity prevented ophthalmoscopic control, the barrage was performed blindly at the level of the vortex veins, which approximately corresponds to the central border of

TABLE 1. *Refraction of the prophylactically treated and untreated eyes*

| Aphakic refraction (D) | +6.0 | +5.0 | +4.0 | +3.0 | +2.0 | +1.0 | +0.0 | –1.0 | –2.0 | –3.0 | –4.0 or more |
|---|---|---|---|---|---|---|---|---|---|---|---|
| Preaphakic refraction (D)[a] | –8.5 | –10.0 | –11.5 | –13.0 | –15.0 | –16.5 | –18.0 | –20.0 | –21.5 | –23.0 | –25.0 or more |
| Prophylactically treated eyes | 6 | 10 | 10 | 31 | 24 | 20 | 19 | 17 | 10 | 9 | 8 |
| Prophylactically untreated eyes | 45 | 38 | 40 | 35 | 28 | 16 | 4 | 2 | 1 | 1 | — |

[a] Preaphakic refraction was calculated from the aphakic correction using the formula: Preaphakic correction = (aphakic correction – 11.25) / 0.62. In the case of astigmatism, half of this value was added to the spherical refraction.

**414**

TABLE 2. *Indications for prophylactic treatment*

| Clinical indications | No. of eyes |
|---|---|
| Lattice degeneration with or without microholes and erosions associated with vitreoretinal adhesions, vitreous detachment and traction or both | 20 |
| Snail track degeneration with above-defined vitreous pathology | 25 |
| Cobble stones nearly all around, peripheral pigmentation, sclerotic areas of thin retina, and vitreous pathology as above | 38 |
| One of the above changes, even though less extensive and intensive, occurring in the fellow eye, a detachment or a complicated cataract probably in consequence of a detachment | 62 |
| Fundus not visible because of progressed cataract but vitreoretinal pathology of the above-defined types in the other eye | 19 |

the equatorial zone. In young high myopes, lamellar scleral resections or imbrications were performed in preference to simple application of diathermy.

At least three months later, and in many cases only after years (i.e., when the cataract had progressed sufficiently), the lens was extracted intracapsularly by the tumbling method. If α-chymotrypsin was used, it was injected under the iris and along its lower half at a concentration of 1:5,000 using 0.4 to 0.6 cm³ of solution. Two min later the anterior chamber was irrigated with saline. A round pupil extraction was carried out in all cases, and mannitol was used to reduce the intraocular pressure. The incision was closed with five to eight corneoscleral sutures.

The selection of cases for preventive treatment depended on the pathology of the fundus and not on the degree of myopia. Though the existence of a serious situation was assessed by the same criteria as those employed for eyes not awaiting a lens extraction, the indications of danger were more liberal in this group. Strong indications were: extensive lattice degenerations in the equatorial zone

with or without microholes; retinal erosions associated with traction of a detached vitreous; snail tracks occupying large areas, particularly if found in young high myopes awaiting clear lens extraction; extensive cobblestone degeneration with sclerotic thinned retinal areas and vitreoretinal adhesions. If surgery was to be performed on the fellow eye of one with a retinal detachment, even less pronounced fundus pathology would be regarded as an indication of the need for preventive treatment. Fifteen patients with 28 eyes had a clear lens extraction for the correction of high myopia. The follow-up-period in the presented sample varied from 2 to 10 years. The patients' hospital sheets, outpatient clinical records, repeated check-ups and checks at the National Central Registry of Retinal Detachment in Jerusalem, were used to evaluate the results.

RESULTS AND COMMENTS

Table 3 illustrates the effect of preventive barrage on the incidence of retinal detachment. Of 210 eyes not preventively treated, 17 (8.1%) developed retinal detachment, compared to only four (2.5%) of the 164 prophylactically treated eyes. In the four cases which developed retinal detachment, in spite of preventive treatment, two were due to macular holes and two to nasal equatorial tears in the lower quadrant in areas that had

TABLE 3. *Incidence of retinal detachment in prophylactically treated and untreated high myopic aphakic eyes*

| | No. of eyes | No. of detachments |
|---|---|---|
| Prophylactically treated eyes | 164 | 4 (2.5%) |
| Prophylactically untreated eyes | 210 | 17 (8.1%) |
| After exclusion of six eyes with retinal detachment due to a macular hole | | |
| Prophylactically treated eyes | 162 | 2 (1.2%) |
| Prophylactically untreated eyes | 206 | 13 (6.3%) |

TABLE 4. *Time lapse between lens extraction and retinal detachment*

| | Months | | | |
|---|---|---|---|---|
| | 1 to 6 | 7 to 12 | 13 to 36 | 37 to 60 |
| No. of eyes | 7 | 4 | 7 | 3 |

not been prophylactically treated. Since a retinal detachment caused by a macular hole could not have been prevented by peripheral barrage, these cases were not included in the statistical evaluation of the effect of preventive treatment. The corrected results are shown in the lower part of Table 3.

The rate of retinal detachment of 8.1% (or 6.3%, corrected) in the nonprophylactically treated group is probably an underestimation of the actual incidence in aphakic high myopic eyes since this group was strongly influenced by the selective exclusion of the more seriously affected eyes that were subjected to preventive treatment. On the other hand, the 2.5% rate (or 1.2%, corrected) found in the prophylactically treated eyes may be an underestimation of the efficacy of the treatment since this group comprised eyes that were regarded as particularly seriously affected.

Of 164 patients with prophylactic treatments, only one developed a detachment due to an excessive administration of diathermy. No other complication of the preventive barrage was observed.

About 30% of the detachments occurred within the first six months and about 50%

within the first year after lens extraction. There was no relationship between the time interval and the development of complications, either during the lens extraction or in the postoperative period (Table 4).

The incidence of retinal detachment in eyes treated with α-chymotrypsin for the lens extraction was more than twice as high as in those where the enzyme was not used (Table 5). This rather unexpected finding led us to examine the possibility that other operative complications such as vitreous loss could have been responsible for the higher incidence of retinal detachment associated with the use of α-chymotrypsin. However, it was found that chymotrypsin had been employed in only one eye out of three with a detachment following vitreous loss. Statistical calculations also excluded the possibility that the average age of the patients with detachments after lens extraction using chymotrypsin was different from that in which chymotrypsin was not used.

Table 6 shows the influence of vitreous loss and of free vitreous in the anterior chamber on the incidence of retinal detachment. The former was found in 8% of the high myopic eyes and the latter in 9%. Both anterior vitreous loss and free vitreous in the anterior chamber were found more frequently (14 and 28%, respectively) in eyes that developed retinal detachment than in those which did not (8 and 7%, respectively). Ten percent of the eyes that had suffered vitreous loss, and 17% of the eyes with free vitreous in the

TABLE 5. *Effect of α-chymotrypsin in lens extraction on the incidence of retinal detachment in high myopic aphakic eyes*

| Method of extraction | No. of eyes | Retinal detachments | | Total | |
|---|---|---|---|---|---|
| | | Prophylactically treated | Untreated | No. | % |
| With chymotrypsin | 262 | 4 | 14 | 18 | 6.9 |
| Without chymotrypsin | 112 | | 3 | 3 | 2.7 |

TABLE 6.  *State of the anterior vitreous membrane in detached and undetached high myopic aphakic eyes*

| Condition of eye | No. of eyes | Intact vitreous membrane | | Vitreous in the anterior chamber | | After vitreous loss | |
|---|---|---|---|---|---|---|---|
| | | No. | % | No. | % | No. | % |
| Undetached | 353 | 298 | 85 | 29 | 8.0 | 26 | 7.0 |
| Detached | 21 | 12 | 58 | 6 | 28 | 3 | 14 |

TABLE 7. *Circumferential and radial distribution of retinal breaks in 21 retinal detachments in high myopic aphakic eyes*

| Location of breaks | Holes | Tears | Total No. | % |
|---|---|---|---|---|
| Circumferential | | | | |
| Temporal, upper | 3 | 1 | 4 | 15 } 22 |
| Temporal, lower | 1 | 1 | 2 | 7 |
| Nasal, upper | 9 | 5 | 14 | 50 } 78 |
| Nasal, lower | 5 | 3 | 8 | 28 |
| Radial | | | | |
| Peripheral | 5 | 1 | 6 | 17 |
| Equatorial | 13 | 9 | 22 | 66 |
| Central | | 6 | 6 | 17 |

anterior chamber, developed retinal detachment, while only 4% of the eyes with an intact vitreous membrane became detached.

Seventy-eight percent of the retinal breaks found in the detached aphakic high myopic eyes were located in the nasal hemiretina; 50% of them were in the upper, and 28% in the lower nasal quadrant. Sixty-four percent of the retinal breaks were in the equatorial zone and 18% near the ora serrata. The ratio of round holes to horseshoe tears was about 2:1 (Table 7). The high incidence of central holes was conspicuous: they were present in nearly 30% of the detached high myopic aphakic eyes, which constituted 18% of all breaks in our study.

### DISCUSSION

Our results give clear evidence of the efficacy of prophylactic treatment in the prevention of retinal detachment. Assuming an incidence of retinal detachment of 10 to 12% in high myopic aphakic eyes, there should have been 35 to 42 detachments in our sample of 347 eyes. In fact, after exclusion of six detachments due to macular holes, only 15 detachments were observed. This means that from 20 (5.7%) to 27 (6.4%) cases of retinal detachment had been prevented. We are aware of the fact that this result was achieved at the expense of preventive barrage carried out in 164 eyes, of which 135 to 142 would probably never have developed retinal detachment and were therefore needlessly treated. This discrepancy between investment and gain reflects the dilemma of every ophthalmologist wishing to try preventive methods, if he has to decide whether to treat a retinal lesion or not. We are also aware of an alternative to preventive barrage prior to lens extraction; namely extraction of the lens without being concerned about any pathologies present (with the exception of a tear) and reevaluation of the situation after the lens extraction. Nevertheless, the inherent uncertainties of the evaluation will not have changed.

Though the equatorial barrage was done in our series with diathermy, since a suitable cryo-unit was not available at the time, there is no doubt that cryopexy would have been just as effective. We do not like photocoagulation for an all-around barrage since it is apt to overheat the vitreous which—especially in young people—is sensitive to heat. Photocoagulation was used only for circumscribed areas that may have been overlooked during diathermy treatment.

Our data do not indicate that vitreous loss at the time of extraction is more dangerous than the presence of free vitreous in the anterior chamber.

The fact that the incidence of retinal detachment was 2.5 times greater in eyes in which chymotrypsin was used at the time of the lens extraction, was unexpected. In an investigation on nonmyopic aphakic eyes, in which 918 eyes were operated on for cataract with the use of chymotrypsin, 11 (1.2%) later developed detachments (L. Berar, unpublished data). However, during the same period of 302 extractions performed without the use of the enzyme, detachment occurred in only two (0.66%) cases. Chymotrypsin may possibly induce an inflammatory reaction in the peripheral retina, which is the counterpart of the pars planitis shown by Schepens to play a major role in the development of retinal detachment in aphakic eyes.

Thirteen eyes of the nonprophylactically treated group escaped the detection of danger signs before retinal detachment occurred.

Further investigation showed that in three eyes the detachment had developed within the first six weeks, at a time when a thorough examination of the fundus had not yet been possible. Three patients were discharged after the extraction without having been instructed to return for an examination. In the seven remaining cases the seriousness of the ophthalmoscopic findings was misjudged.

In four eyes the fundus was not visible prior to the extraction; and in seven, the tear leading to detachment was at the edge of a circumscribed lattice degeneration. Although the tear was noticed before the extraction in four of these eyes, it was not treated. In the remaining three, the hole was overlooked. In two eyes multiple holes occurring in an area of snail tracks were the cause of the detachment; and in three others, the tear developed in an atrophic retinal area that otherwise appeared innocuous. It seems that human psychological factors on the part of both the doctor and the patient, as well as our inability to distinguish between dangerous and harmless lesions in all cases, determine an irreducible number of detachments that are not preventable.

# VISUAL RESULTS AFTER TREATMENT OF RHEGMATOGENOUS RETINAL DETACHMENT

J. CHARAMIS and G. THEODOSSIADIS

Athens University Eye Clinic, Athens, Greece

Due to sophisticated innovations that have become available during the last few years, anatomical restoration of the retina is achieved in a higher proportion of cases today than at the time of Gonin's first successful treatment of rhegmatogenous retinal detachment. Nevertheless, functional restoration of the retina, the main purpose of the operation, has no kept pace with these developments. The many factors influencing postoperative visual acuity include: 1) macular detachment and its duration; 2) existence of vitreoretinal adhesion in the posterior pole; 3) the number of retinal tears and especially their distribution; 4) macular puckering syndrome; 5) primary optic atrophy immediately following retinal detachment surgery (1); and 6) gradual occlusion of the central retinal artery (1). In addition to the above known factors, there are other unknown ones which may influence postoperative visual acuity.

The present study discusses the functional results, the changes in refraction and the reasons for functional failure in 198 cases of retinal detachment successfully operated on from 1968 to 1970 at the Athens University Eye Hospital. We defined successfully treated patients as those who have a complete anatomical reattachment of the retina for one year or more, and have achieved a visual acuity of at least 20/200 or 6/60.

*Functional results.* Table 1 shows both the anatomical and functional results in all the cases undergoing surgery. One hundred and forty-four out of 198 patients with retinal detachment had a detachment that included the macula.

The degree of postoperative improvement in visual acuity following surgery for retinal detachment varies greatly with the patient's age (Table 2). Those who were under 40 years of age responded less favorably following the operation than older patients, confirming the findings of Jay (2) and Hudson (3).

The most important factor influencing the functional results following the operation is the length of time elapsing between macular involvement and surgery. Results are less favorable in cases where the macula had been detached for more than a month. In contrast, there are no significant variations in visual

TABLE 1. *Anatomical and functional results of 230 retinal detachment operations*

| Period of study | vi/1968 to vi/1970 | |
|---|---|---|
| Total no. examined patients with retinal detachment | 246 | |
| Not operated | 16 | |
| Operated | 230 | |
| Anatomical success | 198 | 86% |
| Functional success (visual acuity after operation > 0.1) | 180 | 78% |

TABLE 2. *Percent improved and mean improvement of visual acuity after retinal detachment surgery*

| No. of patients | Macular involvement | Age (years) | Time elapsed until operation (days) | Mean visual acuity improvement | % improved |
|---|---|---|---|---|---|
| 13 | + | < 40 | d ≤ 15 | + 0.26 | |
| 12 | + | < 40 | 15 < d ≤ 30 | + 0.23 | |
| 17 | + | < 40 | 30 < d | + 0.24 | 88.2 |
| 26 | + | ≥ 40 | d ≤ 15 | + 0.33 | |
| 34 | + | ≥ 40 | 15 < d ≤ 30 | + 0.42 | |
| 42 | + | ≥ 40 | 30 < d | + 0.15 | |
| 10 | − | < 40 | d ≤ 30 | + 0.06 | |
| 5 | − | < 40 | 30 < d | 0 | 42.6 |
| 24 | − | ≥ 40 | d ≤ 30 | − 0.02 | |
| 15 | − | ≥ 40 | 30 < d | + 0.04 | |
| TOTAL 198 | | | | | |

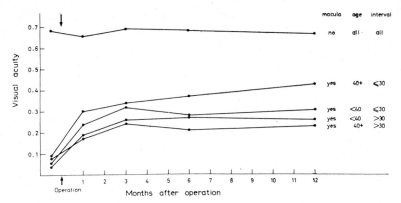

FIG. 1. Mean visual acuity before and after operation in groups of patients with retinal detachment.

acuity after the operation among patients whose macula had been detached for 15 to 30 days (3). Fifty-four of 198 patients had no macular detachment, and in this group the functional results were influenced neither by the patient's age nor by the duration of detachment.

Fig. 1 shows the mean development of post-operative visual acuity in the various groups compared to their mean preoperative visual acuity. Significant improvement in cases of macular detachment occurs mainly during the first month after the operation. Nevertheless, improvement may continue beyond the first month, although to a lesser extent.

In cases where the macula is not detached there are no clear time trends. A month after the operation there was a decrease of visual acuity which, however, was restored three months after the operation.

The percent of cases with involvement of the macula who showed improvement are shown in Table 3. No change or deterioration occurred during various successive time intervals. By the end of the first postoperative month, more than 115 of the patients had significantly improved visual acuity which, in a number of cases, continued to improve beyond the first month. However, 30 patients showed improvement even a year after the

TABLE 3. *Changes of visual acuity in a group of patients with retinal detachment and macular involvement during successive intervals of time in 144 patients (%)*

| Changes | Before and after operation | First to third month | Third to sixth month | Sixth to twelfth month | After twelve months |
|---|---|---|---|---|---|
| Improvement | 82.2 | 45.7 | 22.0 | 14.5 | 21.3 |
| No change | 16.9 | 53.4 | 72.9 | 82.9 | 76.6 |
| Deterioration | 0.9 | 0.9 | 5.1 | 2.6 | 2.1 |

TABLE 4. *Refractive changes in patients originally hypermetropic or emmetropic and myopic*

| Preoperative condition | Before operation | After operation | | |
|---|---|---|---|---|
| | | After one month | After six months | After one year |
| Hypermetropia and emmetropia (72 patients) | + 2.88 | + 3.81 | + 3.47 | + 3.20 |
| Myopia (48 patients) | − 5.49 | − 3.57 | − 4.00 | − 4.59 |

operation. Of these 30 patients, 18 were younger than 30 years of age. This observation is very important for it helps considerably in prognosis.

Our patients received surgical treatment according to their specific needs. Our surgical procedures of choice were: a) buckling with scleral infolding, b) Custodis-Lincoff method, c) Paufique method and d) encircling procedure. In patients with limited retinal detachment, there was no difference in postoperative visual acuity with any of these procedures. The same cannot be said, however, for cases where tears were found in different quadrants of the eye.

*Postoperative refractive changes.* The refractive changes occurred mainly in patients who had been operated on by a scleral infolding, with or without a simultaneous encircling procedure. The study was limited to those patients whose refraction was known preoperatively or had been measured by retinoscopy (macula not detached). Using the scleral infolding procedure is known occasionally to produce changes in both the spherical and the cylindrical corrections.

Patients with refractive changes who had hypermetropia or emmetropia, or were myopic before the operation are listed in Table 4. Both an increase of hypermetropia and a decrease of myopia were observed after the operation. However, these variations are rather temporary because the refractive ability does not approach the preoperative level until one year after the operation (Fig. 2). The above changes are more obvious among myopic patients, suggesting that the myopic eye undergoes a greater expansion than the hypermetropic or the emmetropic one.

Table 5 shows variations in refractive changes of the cylinder. These data suggest that cylinder correction changes are more prominent than sphere changes in patients treated with the scleral infolding procedure. The cylinder in those cases is rather prominent and does not change with time (4–6). Cases successfully operated on by either the Custodis-Lincoff or the Paufique procedure developed a temporary astigmatism which decreased or disappeared completely in about six months.

*Reasons for functional failure.* Eighty-six

**421**

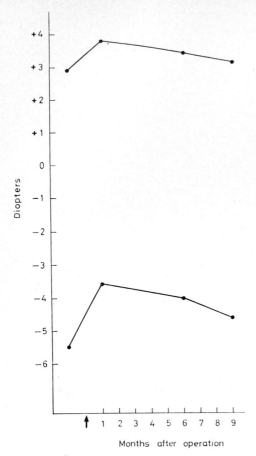

FIG. 2. Refractive changes in patients originally a) hypermetropic or emmetropic and b) myopic.

TABLE 5. *Mean values of absolute changes of cylinder in 120 patients with retinal detachment in successive intervals of time. Mean values of absolute changes (diopters)*

| Before and after operation | Up to six months after operation | Six to nine months after operation |
| --- | --- | --- |
| 2.04 | 0.63 | 0.33 |

percent of all the patients operated on for retinal detachment, achieved anatomical success whereas only 78% achieved functional improvement. This discrepancy of 8% may be due to the following factors: a) creation of folds of the macula (eight cases); b) existence of a vitreoretinal adhesion in the macular area (two cases); c) high intraocular pressure during and immediately after the operation, which influences the circulation in the central retinal artery especially in older patients (two cases); d) persistent postoperative inflammation (one case); e) destruction of the pigment epithelium in the area of the macula (three cases). The decrease of visual acuity in cases of long-standing detachments in the posterior pole can be attributed to the destruction of the pigment epithelium. This lesion is easily observed using fluorescein angiography.

### REFERENCES

1. SCHEPENS C. Postoperative visual loss (discussion), in: McPherson A (Ed), "New and controversial aspects of retinal detachment." New York, Harper, 1968, p 494.
2. JAY B. The functional cure of retinal detachments. *Trans Ophthalmol Soc UK* **85**: 101, 1965.
3. HUDSON JR. Functional results of retinal detachment surgery, in: McPherson A (Ed), "New and controversial aspects of retinal detachment." New York, Hoeber, 1969.
4. GIVNER I and KARLIN D. Alterations in refraction and their clinical significance. *Eye Ear Nose Throat Mon* **37**: 676, 1958.
5. ROSENTHAL ML. Discussion on Pischel DK. A method of scleral resection for retinal detachment, in: Schepens CL (Ed), "Importance of the vitreous body in retina surgery with special emphasis on reoperations." St Louis, CV Mosby, 1960, p 165.
6. CURTIN BJ and SHARER DM. Aniseikonia following retinal detachment. *Am J Ophthalmol* **47**: 468, 1959.

# THE SURGICAL TREATMENT OF
# RETINAL DETACHMENTS WITHOUT DRAINAGE OF
# SUBRETINAL FLUID

## M. WALLACE FRIEDMAN

Department of Ophthalmology, Mount Zion Hospital, San Francisco, California, USA

There seems to be little doubt that drainage of subretinal fluid is one phase of retinal detachment surgery during which the retinal surgeon is most likely to run into trouble. Of the multiplicity of methods available, no one method is completely satisfactory. Perforation of the eye for release of subretinal fluid is a troublesome procedure, for which no technique is absolutely safe (1, 2).

The complications of the drainage of subretinal fluid are many, varied and well known. They may be listed as follows: 1) Drainage of subretinal fluid may certainly give rise to intraocular hemorrhage (3). The bleeding may be subretinal, retinal or intravitreal (4). The bleeding site can be either traumatized choroidal vessels or an injured sclerotic retinal vessel (5). The vortex veins are particularly dangerous sites and prone to bleeding (4).

2) A most serious complication is retinal incarceration. This can be precipitated in three ways: a) by sudden release of subretinal fluid; b) by tearing the choroid with a needle electrode when the escape of subretinal fluid stops (no new opening should ever be made in the choroid without making sure, by ophthalmoscopy, that there is still subretinal fluid to be evacuated); and c) by choroidal rupture occurring in an area where the sclera is either very weak or absent (6).

3) Fluid may be drained from the wrong side of the retina. While fluid is released the break might be open and fluid from the vitreous cavity may continue to escape through the break and out of the eye via the choroidal perforation (7).

4) After perforation, some fluid may be drawn back into the eye by negative pressure (from a pool of subretinal fluid, saline and blood from episcleral vessels). This could induce a subretinal hemorrhage and the danger of intraocular infection (8).

5) If, at the time of perforation, a choroidal hemorrhage occurs, blood may accumulate at the posterior pole, with resultant macular degeneration (8).

6) Both retina and choroid may become incarcerated in the scleral incision if subretinal fluid is drained too quickly or if the incision is closed too late (4). An incarceration, with or without a new hole in the retina made at the time of drainage, may lead to redetachment (3).

7) Another potential complication is a proliferation of connective tissue that probably begins in the episclera and extends into the vitreous cavity through the perforation made for drainage. In such cases, the retina may finally become firmly reattached to the site of the perforation (9).

8) Production of iatrogenic holes in the retina (5), commonly by Walker-type pins, is a complication frequently seen as a cause of surgical failure.

It was my impression, when going over my own operated retinal detachment cases, that the most frequent cause of failure was a complication encountered during the act of draining subretinal fluid. This started me looking in other directions for alternative procedures which would reduce the danger of fluid drainage.

In 1965 I started to use, in indicated cases, the external buckle technique of Custodis (10). This operation was again reported at the Second Conference of the Retina Foundation (11), and has since been modified many times, particularly by Lincoff, McLean and Naro (12, 13).

To Lincoff, the most intriguing aspect of the Custodis operation was that it did not call for drainage of subretinal fluid. Dr. Lincoff's modification was made possible by the development of suture material with spatula needles, so that long intrascleral mattress sutures could be placed, and by the availability of Dow-Corning silicone sponges for explants. Finally, cryotherapy was substituted for diathermy.

in the customary manner with continuous ophthalmoscopic control using the binocular indirect ophthalmoscope. Tenotomy is rarely done. Limbal conjunctival incision is used.

After accurate localization of the circumferential and radial extremes of the breaks, the broad mattress sutures are placed. The number and directions of the sutures vary with the direction (radial or circumferential) of the area to be buckled and the length of the area. Cryotherapy is used to surround all retinal breaks under direct observation.

The sponge explant is placed under the mattress sutures and the position is checked by ophthalmoscopy. If the position is correct, the sutures are tied. If the sponge needs to be moved, the sutures are replaced. Drainage of subretinal fluid is not required if the buckle is in proper position beneath the hole.

The advantages of not draining are considerable. A detachment operation bears no more trauma than a strabismus procedure. Eliminating perforation of the choroid eliminates in turn the risk of hemorrhage, intraocular infection and prolapse of retina and vitreous. Without decompression, one rarely encounters choroidal detachment, and the uveitic response appears to be less.

### TECHNIQUE

The technique which I currently use for operation without drainage is essentially that of Lincoff. The exposure and localization is done

### INDICATIONS

In Table 1, the situations where subretinal fluid should be drained are compared with those for which release of fluid is not indi-

TABLE 1. *Comparison of situations requiring drainage with those for which drainage is not indicated*

| Drainage required | Drainage not indicated |
|---|---|
| Longstanding detachment | Detachment of recent origin |
| Posterior break | Breaks at equator or anterior |
| Large break | Breaks less than 1 hr on clock |
| Multiple breaks in different quadrants | Breaks in one quadrant or single break |
| Evidence of vitreous band and preretinal organization | No vitreous traction |
| Inferior breaks | Horizontal or superior breaks |
| Aphakic | Phakic |
| Recent or threatened detachment of macula | Macula not detached |

TABLE 2. *Complications of release of subretinal fluid in retinal detachment surgery (no. of cases)*

| Nature of complication | With drainage | Without drainage |
|---|---|---|
| Reattachments | 57 | 79 |
| Reattachments after additional photocoagulation | 15 | 12 |
| Reattachments after repositioning buckle | 12 | 4 |
| Reattachments after later drainage | 4 | 2 |
| Failures | 12 | 3 |
| TOTAL | 100 | 100 |

TABLE 3. *Results of retinal detachment surgery (no. of cases)*

| Range of visual acuity achieved | With drainage | Without drainage |
|---|---|---|
| 20/20 to 20/30 | 31 | 33 |
| 20/40 to 20/50 | 20 | 39 |
| 20/60 to 20/70 | 13 | 15 |
| 20/80 or worse | 36 | 13 |
| TOTAL | 100 | 100 |

TABLE 4. *Complications arising after retinal detachment surgery; comparison of 100 cases in which subretinal fluid was drained with 100 cases without drainage*

| Nature of complication | Drainage | Non-drainage |
|---|---|---|
| Severe muscle imbalance | 6 | 4 |
| Granuloma in operative site | 3 | 4 |
| Exposed explant material | 3 | 2 |
| Intraocular hemorrhage | 4 | 0 |
| Intraocular infection | 2 | 0 |
| Retinal incarceration (unintentional) | 2 | 0 |
| Vitreous loss | 2 | 0 |
| Iatrogenic holes | 3 | 0 |
| Preretinal organization (MUR) | 6 | 0 |

cated. The "drainage list" was originally compiled by Edward and Norton (14).

## ADVANTAGES

The complications of release of subretinal fluid are shown in Table 2. A major advantage of this procedure is that these complications can be avoided. In addition, I have found the following advantages: 1) Surgical time is shortened, thereby reducing the anesthesia risk and postoperative morbidity. 2) The procedure is technically easier, making it easier for an inexperienced assistant, such as a new resident, to be of value. 3) Reoperations are easier. Since there has been minimal tissue manipulation and destruction, the revision of a scleral buckling procedure can be done safely.

## RESULTS

In order to give added meaning to the material presented above, a comparison has been made between the last 100 cases with drainage and the last 100 cases without drainage. The results are shown in Tables 3 and 4.

## REFERENCES

1. PISCHEL DK. In: Schepens CL and Regen CDJ (Eds), "Controversial aspects of the management of retinal detachment." Boston, Little, Brown and Co, 1965, p 250.
2. SCHWARTZ A. Drainage of subretinal fluid. *Am J Ophthalmol* **47**: 98, 1959.
3. FRANCOIS J. Complications in retinal detachment surgery, a panel discussion, in: McPherson A (Ed), "New and controversial aspects of retinal detachment." New York, Hoeber, 1969, p 487.
4. KLOTI R. Complications in retinal detachment surgery, a panel discussion, in: McPherson A (Ed), "New and controversial aspects of retinal detachment." New York, Hoeber, 1969, p 486.
5. BIETTI GB. Complications in retinal detachment surgery, a panel discussion, in: McPherson A (Ed), "New and controversial aspects of retinal detachment." New York, Hoeber, 1969, p 483.
6. MALBRAN ES. In: Schepens CL and Regen CDJ (Eds), "Controversial aspects of the management of retinal detachment." Boston, Little, Brown and Co, 1965, p 249.
7. SCHEPENS CL. Present status of scleral buckling operation, in: McPherson A (Ed), "New and controversial aspects of retinal detachment." New York, Hoeber, 1969.
8. SHEA M. Complications common to all surgical procedures, in: Schepens CL and Regen CDJ (Eds), "Controversial aspects of the management of retinal detachment." New York, Little, Brown and Co, 1965, p 217.
9. HUDSON JR. Complications in retinal detachment surgery, a panel discussion, in: McPherson A (Ed), "New and controversial aspects of retinal detachment." New York, Hoeber, 1969, p 486.

**425**

10. CUSTODIS E. Bedeutet die Plombenaufnähung auf die Sklera einen Fortschritt in der operativen Behandlung der Netzhautablösung. *Ber Dtsch Ophthalmol Ges* **58**: 102, 1953.

11. CUSTODIS E. Scleral buckling without excision and polybiol implant, in: Schepens CL (Ed), "Importance of the vitreous body in retinal surgery with special emphasis on reoperation." St. Louis, CV Mosby, 1969, p 175.

12. LINCOFF H, McLEAN KM and NARO H. Cryo-surgical treatment of retinal detachment. *Trans Am Acad Ophthalmol Otolaryngol* **68**: 412, 1964.

13. LINCOFF H. Full thickness scleral buckling with silicone-sponge implant, in: McPherson A (Ed), "New and controversial aspects of retinal detachment." New York, Hoeber, 1969, p 293.

14. EDWARD WD and NORTON MD. Complications in retina and retinal surgery, in: "Symposium on retina and retinal surgery." St Louis, CV Mosby, 1969, p 222.

# RETINAL DETACHMENT ASSOCIATED WITH PROLIFERATIVE RETINOPATHIES (SICKLE CELL DISEASE, RETROLENTAL FIBROPLASIA AND DIABETES MELLITUS)

MORTON F. GOLDBERG

Department of Ophthalmology, University of Illinois Eye and Ear Infirmary, Chicago, Illinois, USA

This communication reviews the pathogenesis and treatment of retinal detachment associated with three types of proliferative retinopathy: sickle cell diseases, retrolental fibroplasia and diabetes mellitus. These diseases have much in common: an underlying retinal ischemia, development of retinal neovascularization, temporal predilection in the eye, spontaneous vitreous hemorrhage, marked vitreous degeneration and traction, hole formation in the retina and retinal detachment. Of these three diseases, the prognosis for retinal reattachment and restoration of useful vision appears to be best in retrolental fibroplasia, presumably because the active disease process is no longer operational at the time of detachment or at the time of surgery.

## SICKLE CELL DISEASES

*Pathogenesis of retinal detachment in PSR* (1–3). The somewhat fortuitous combination of several factors has made the study of proliferative sickle retinopathy (PSR) relatively straightforward and has thereby provided a useful, easily understood model of proliferative retinopathy leading to retinal detachment. Many features of this model can be applied to other proliferative retinopathies, such as retrolental fibroplasia and diabetes

mellitus, which take their origin similarly from an underlying retinal ischemia. Other somewhat similar diseases also seem to be based on underlying retinal ischemia, and include certain forms of carotid artery insufficiency (4, 5), pulseless disease (6), radiation retinitis (7) and retinal sarcoidosis (8).

The availability of stereoscopic indirect ophthalmoscopy, scleral indentation and photographic fluorescein angiography has permitted more detailed analysis of PSR than has been possible in the past. In addition, patients with these sickling disorders develop initial (as well as end-stage) retinal abnormalities during the second, third and fourth decades of life. Thus, unlike the situation that ordinarily prevails in retrolental fibroplasia, both the ophthalmoscopic and photographic techniques have been available for use in most circumstances. Using these, it has been possible to separate PSR from the incorrectly inclusive entity of Eales's disease.

Of the variety of inherited diseases characterized by intravascular sickling, two—sickle cell hemoglobin C (SC) disease and sickle cell thalassemia (S thal)—are especially affected with PSR (3, 9). The sequence of events in PSR in these diseases begins with arteriolar and capillary occlusions (Fig. 1) particular-

427

## PROLIFERATIVE SICKLE RETINOPATHY

I ARTERIOLAR OCCLUSIONS

II A–V ANASTOMOSES

III NEOVASCULAR PROLIFERATIONS

IV VITREOUS HEMORRHAGE

V RETINAL DETACHMENT

FIG. 1. Stages of proliferative sickle retinopathy

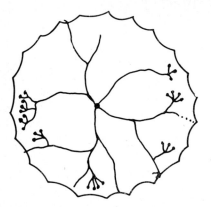

FIG. 2. Schematic diagram of PSR in Stage III. Neo-vascular proliferations arise at equator at site of pre-existing arteriolar occlusions.

ly in the temporal periphery of the retina (between the equator and the ora serrata) (1). The precise factors responsible for this vaso-occlusion (Stage I) are not known, but they are presumably related to the presence of sickled, rigid erythrocytes which either direct-ly or indirectly result in vascular shutdown. These cells may possibly act as microemboli, or they may increase the viscosity of the blood so that thrombosis is induced. In terms of ultimate pathogenetic consequences this stage of retinal ischemia is apparently similar to that observed in early diabetic retinopathy and in early retrolental fibroplasia (RLF).

Secondly, arteriolar-venular anastomoses (Stage II) arise at the sites of previous vaso-occlusions. As in the case of diabetic retinop-athy, these shunt vessels appear to be en-largements of preexisting capillaries rather than true neovascular growths. Evidence in favor of this interpretation is provided by trypsin digestion studies of whole mounted retinas; and by fluorescein angiography, in which profuse leakage of dye through the vessel wall, a valuable sign of true neovascu-larization, is absent.

Subsequently, true neovascularization (Stage III) occurs at the sites of preexisting Stage I and II lesions (Fig. 2). Early neovascular growths are frequently fan-shaped and are often supplied by only one major feeding arteriole and one major draining venule. In time, additional feeding and draining vessels appear. The retinal quadrants of predilection for development of Stage III lesions are superotemporal > inferotemporal > supero-nasal > inferonasal. This pattern is precisely that which is observed in proliferative dia-betic retinopathy (PDR) (10), and is similar to that observed in RLF (11). As is frequent-ly, or perhaps always, the case in the early neovascularization of PDR and RLF, the newly formed blood vessels of PSR grow into or towards a zone of retinal ischemia, as demonstrated by fluorescein angiography (1, 11, 12). During this early phase the blood vessels remain flat on the surface of the retina, but ultimately appear to be pulled forward into the vitreous chamber, perhaps by con-traction and collapse of the overlying ad-herent vitreous.

Spontaneous regression of these new vessels has not been observed. If this observation is confirmed by study of additional cases of PSR with prolonged follow-up, it will represent a significant point of departure from the not uncommon spontaneous regressions of neo-vascular tissue that are observed in PDR (13) and RLF (14).

At varying, unpredictable intervals, the neo-vascular patches give rise to vitreous hemor-rhage (Stage IV). The hemorrhages may be

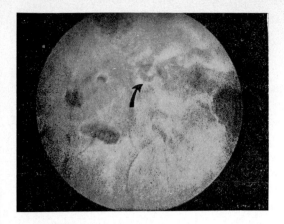

FIG. 3. Horseshoe tear (arrow) in retina with PSR. Vitreous band is attached to flap of tear. Retina is still flat. Note surrounding black chorioretinal scars (so-called "black sunbursts").

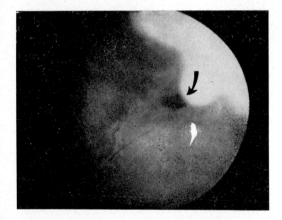

FIG. 4. Detached retina in PSR. Note tear (arrow) adjacent to white vitreous sheet of fibrous tissue.

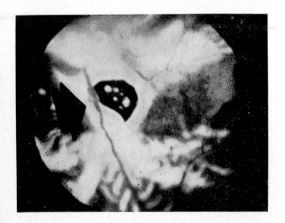

FIG. 5. Detached retina in PSR. Arrow points to tear in retina.

miniscule, in which case no symptoms occur (2). The small volume of blood is converted into gray-white fibrous tissue overlying, and frequently obscuring, the newly formed blood channels. Fluorescein angiography is the best technique for demonstrating these vessels.

Progressive neovascularization of the retina occurs either because of further vascular growth in the individual patch with subsequent additional hemorrhages or because of the circumferential formation of new vascular patches in the equatorial plane of the globe. Massive vitreous hemorrhage may then occur obscuring all details of the fundus, and may or may not reabsorb.

As a result of progressive vitreous degeneration with band and membrane formation, small to moderate sized retinal holes and tears develop (Fig. 3). These are frequently observed subjacent or adjacent to the neovascular and fibrous proliferations, where they are often obscured by the overlying opaque or translucent vitreous (15). Obscuring of retinal breaks by vitreous sheets or membranes is also commonly observed in RLF and in diabetes (Fig. 4).

Since neovascular tissue, regardless of etiology, constantly transudes large volumes of fluid into the vitreous, as demonstrated by fluorescein angiography, it is possible that this tissue contributes directly to the vitreous degeneration. Rhegmatogenous retinal detachment (Stage V) then develops initially around the retinal breaks but ultimately involves the entire retina (Fig. 5).

*Therapy of retinal detachment in PSR* (15). When buckling an eye which has a propensity for intravascular sickling, several considerations beyond those ordinarily employed in the surgical reattachment of a retina must be borne in mind.

a) In PSR, holes and tears are often obscured by opaque or translucent membranes in the vitreous. Careful scleral indentation, performed in conjunction with the binocular

**429**

indirect ophthalmoscope and the 3-mirror fundus contact lens, is invaluable in demonstrating these breaks in the retina. In RLF similar obscuring of retinal tears by opacities in the vitreous has been reported by Farris and Brockhurst (16). Successful reattachment of the retina obviously requires closure of all breaks. As a matter of surgical thoroughness, therefore, such membranes and all neovascular and fibrous proliferations should be treated with cryotherapy and, whenever possible, should be included on the buckled area, even when retinal breaks are not identified in the immediate vicinity of the membranes and proliferations.

b) The vitreous membranes in PSR often exert profound traction on the retina, and may actually take the form of circumferential bands with a purse-string configuration. In most cases, nullification of this traction requires a broad, high buckle and an encircling band. Because of complications to be discussed below the encircling band should not be excessively tightened. The buckle itself should not interfere with the vortex veins.

c) The ocular tissues in PSR are ischemic even prior to the onset of retinal detachment. With the exception of drainage of subretinal fluid, most surgical maneuvers employed in the scleral buckling operations contribute to further ischemia during the operative and immediate postoperative periods. A variety of responsible mechanisms prevail, including the reduction of vascular perfusion by raised intraocular pressure. Consequently, measures designed to improve delivery of blood and oxygen to the tissues of the eye are indicated.

In a series of 10 eyes with retinal detachments caused by PSR, Ryan and Goldberg (15) noted six with ischemic signs following scleral buckling. This rate of postoperative ischemia compared unfavorably with the 3% incidence of postoperative ischemia noted in 100 buckled eyes having normal hemoglobin. Complications of the induced ischemia in the

eyes with sickle hemoglobin included phthisis or prephthisis in four instances. Only two of these eyes had 20/25 vision or better after operation. In this series two eyes underwent prolonged and extensive but successful buckling procedures after the patients were prepared for surgery by treatment with partial exchange blood transfusion and a variety of other prophylactic measures. Ordinarily, in patients with SC disease essentially none of the total hemoglobin is normal; and in patients with S thal only 5 to 40% of the total hemoglobin is normal (3). Because of the dangers associated with the sickling which is commonly observed during parturition and during general surgical procedures, therapeutic elevation of normal hemoglobin to 60% of the total or greater has been recommended (15). Although risks of serum hepatitis and septicemia are incurred by partial exchange blood transfusion, this technique, possibly in combination with other prophylactic measures, currently appears capable of eliminating postoperative ischemia and necrosis in the eye as well as elsewhere in the body.

Since anterior necrosis can cause visual disability that negates the effect of an otherwise anatomically successful buckling procedure, several prophylactic measures are currently recommended prior to buckling an eye with PSR. Because the number of eyes operated upon has been small, it has been impossible to assess the relative efficacies of these procedures. In addition to partial exchange blood transfusion they include: local, retrobulbar anesthesia (without added sympathomimetics), stellate ganglion block, pupillary dilation with parasympatholytics only, lowered intraocular pressure (through the use of osmotic agents and carbonic anhydrase inhibition), supplemental oxygenation via a nasal catheter, avoidance of rectus muscle traction or detachment, preservation of the integrity of the long posterior ciliary vessels and the vortex veins, minimization of tightness of the encircling band and performance of subretinal fluid drainage whenever possible (15).

Available data are limited, but do not indicate that a scleral exoplant has advantages (or disadvantages) over a scleral implant. Because diathermy occludes vessels, shrinks sclera and raises intraocular pressure, it is less preferred for inducing the chorioretinal adhesion in detachments caused by PSR than is cryotherapy.

### RETROLENTAL FIBROPLASIA

*Pathogenesis of retinal detachment in RLF.*
Retinal ischemia is the hallmark of the early phases of RLF (11) just as it is in PSR (1, 2) and PDR (17). In the case of RLF ischemia is produced by a vaso-occlusive effect of excessive oxygenation on the immature retinal vasculature (18) (Fig. 6). Since the temporal vasculature is the most immature in the newborn premature infant the major effects of hyperoxia begin temporally. This anatomic predilection for the temporal portions of the retina is similar to that observed in PDR (10) and PSR (1) but for obviously different reasons.

The precise reasons why oxygen induces vaso-obliteration of immature retinal capillaries are unknown but may include a direct cytocidal effect on the immature capillary endothelium (19), pressure on the capillary caused by swollen surrounding retinal tissue (20) and possibly other factors.

Following return to normal environmental oxygen levels, the premature infant's peripheral ischemic retina becomes relatively hypoxic since it no longer obtains sufficient oxygen from surrounding tissues, including the choroid. Tortuosity of the retinal vasculature is seen (Stage I) (21). Budding of the capillary endothelium occurs and an advancing wave-front of neovascular tissue grows towards the ischemic retina which lies between the equator and the ora serrata (Fig.

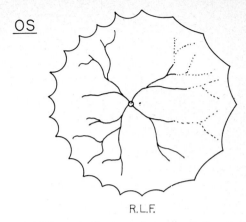

FIG. 6. Schematic diagram of retrolental fibroplasia in acute stage of oxygen toxicity. Dotted lines indicate occluded arterioles in retinal periphery.

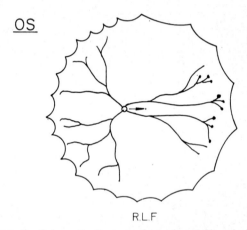

FIG. 7. Schematic diagram of retrolental fibroplasia during stage of retinal neovascularization. New vessels arise at sites of previous arteriolar occlusions. Arrow indicates temporal dragging of macula.

7). Again, the parallelism between RLF and PSR is apparent. However, in the case of RLF a considerable number (up to 60%) of eyes show spontaneous regression of the neovascular tissue (14), unlike the ordinarily progressive situation prevailing in PSR. When the neovascularization in RLF is progressive, however, local hemorrhage and fibrous proliferations occur (Stage II) (21, 22).

This acute, active phase of RLF may often be observed between the third and tenth weeks of life (14, 19) and may last for three to six months (23). If progression continues rapidly, early retinal detachment may occur and may, if localized, cause retinal folds or may involve the entire retina (Stages III, IV, V) (21). Proliferated fibrous and neovascular tissue and contracted vitreous can cause a complete retrolental membrane having no potential for restoration of vision (so-called Stage V of RLF active phase (21).

Alternatively, in cases with milder involvement the retina may remain quiescent for some years leaving only mild residual signs in the retinal periphery or causing only permanent retinal artery tortuosity (24).

At one time, it was felt that the condition of the eyes became quiescent after the age of six years (19) and that retinal holes only rarely led to late rhegmatogenous retinal detachment (25). Recently, it has become apparent that progressive vitreous and retinal changes may sometimes develop long after the onset of the quiescent phase and may result in retinal detachment during the second and third decades of life (11, 16, 23, 26, 27). Tasman and Annesley, for example, reported eight retinal detachments in five patients with RLF between the ages of 9 and 19 (26). Faris and Brockhurst subsequently reported 55 retinal detachments in 37 patients (16). Two-thirds of their patients were between the ages of 6 and 15, two were less than six years of age and 10 were over 16 years of age. Tasman (11) found cicatricial RLF in 0.9% of a group of 995 randomly selected patients between the ages of 9 and 22 years. Of 46 randomly selected expremature patients 20% had evidence of cicatricial RLF. In another series of 69 patients with known cicatricial RLF 16, or 23%, had retinal detachment.

In these series multiple retinal breaks were responsible for the detachments, and were usually located in the temporal periphery, near the equator. Tasman found them most commonly in the superotemporal quadrant (11). They were almost always round or horseshoe-shaped. Dialyses were rarely observed (16). In the series of Faris and Brockhurst (16) breaks were not found in 18 of 55 eyes with retinal detachments, presumably because of obscuring by overlying vitreous membranes similar to those in PSR (15). Residual areas of retinal neovascularization, similar to PSR, were also frequently observed in the temporal periphery.

*Therapy of retinal detachment in RLF.* Despite the obscuring of many retinal breaks and the presence of vitreous membranes and traction phenomena, the available data suggest that routine scleral buckling procedures are successful in reattaching such retinas in approximately 90% of cases (11, 16). Surgical complications attributable to RLF could not be identified in the reported series even though high myopia characterizes the cicatricial phase of RLF. Of 15 eyes subjected to buckling operations by Tasman, 12 (80%) had 20/50 or better vision and only two (13%) had 20/200 or less (11). In the series of Faris and Brockhurst, 25 of 45 eyes (55.5%) had postoperative improvement in central vision (16). There was no postoperative visual improvement in 13 eyes (28.8%) and three eyes (6.6%) deteriorated (visual data were not available for the remaining eyes) (16). The prognosis for this type of detachment is considerably better than that for the detachment of PSR (15) despite the many similarities between the two diseases. It is possible that the improved prognosis for RLF reflects normal vascularization of nonretinal ocular tissues in patients who are young and otherwise healthy. In addition, their active ocular disease is for the most part a thing of the past by the time retinal detachment occurs. Conversely, retinal detachment in PSR occurs in a milieu in which the nonretinal ocular tissues are constantly abnormally perfused, and in which the retinal disease is continually evolving, presumably because of the chronic assault of sickled erythrocytes.

As in the case of the retinal detachment of PSR (15), Faris and Brockhurst (16) often found it necessary to make their scleral underminings wider and longer than usual in order to buckle adequately the areas of vitreoretinal adhesions.

Since chronic changes in the retinas of ex-premature babies occur years (and decades) after the acute phase of RLF, affected individuals should be considered at risk for the rest of their lives. Periodic peripheral fundus examinations are obviously indicated.

### DIABETES MELLITUS

*Pathogenesis of retinal detachment in PDR.* Dobree (13) has described how proliferative lesions in the diabetic retina begin as a collection of fine, naked vessels (Stage I), progress through a stage of vascular proliferation with connective tissue formation (Stage II) and terminate in a stage of regression of the vascular systems with contracture of the connective tissue components (Fig. 8). It is of interest that neovascular proliferations of Stage II frequently grow into or towards a zone of retinal ischemia as demonstrated by fluorescein angiography (17). In this respect, as in others, PDR resembles PSR and RLF.

The following observations were made by Dobree in a further study on 112 eyes with PDR: Vitreous retraction was present in 78.8%, retinovitreal bands in 29.3%, thickening of the posterior vitreous face in 14.3%, retinal detachment in 10.6%, retinoschisis in 6.3%, and flat holes in 2.7% (28). The important role of contracting vitreous in the production of retinal breaks and retinal detachments was also stressed by Davis (29), Tolentino et al. (30), and Madsen (31). In their view, the presence of neovascular tissue in the vitreous chamber and the occurrence of retinal detachment were caused not so much by an active anterior growth of the neovascular tissue as by a more passive effect of contracting vitreous, which had become adherent to the neovascular tissue and retina (28–31). Retinoschisis and retinal holes also appear to develop as the result of vitreous traction (Fig. 9).

In a detailed classification of the advanced fibrotic stages of PDR, McMeel (32) described two common types, "fibrovascular proliferative tissue" and "avascular proliferative tissue," and an infrequent iatrogenic type which arose at the borders of photocoagulation scars. The "fibrovascular" variety of

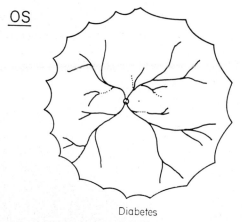

FIG. 8. Schematic diagram of early stage of diabetic retinopathy. Dotted lines indicate occluded arterioles in posterior pole.

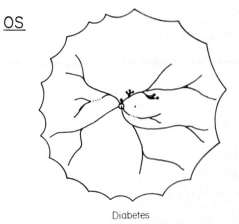

FIG. 9. Schematic diagram of proliferative diabetic retinopathy. Neovascular tissue arises at sites of previously occluded arterioles.

fibrotic tissue was most frequently observed and was found in association with abnormal new vessels on the surface of the retina or disk, or with those vessels which extended into the vitreous chamber. The "avascular" variety was further divided into three types: a) a direct extension from the fibrovascular variety; b) vitreous membranes unassociated with fibrovascular tissue (vitreoretinal bridges); and c) preretinal membranes, also known as preretinal organization or thickening of the posterior hyaloid face (32). Traction on the retina was observed with all forms of fibrotic proliferations except with the thickened posterior hyaloid face and with the iatrogenic type (32).

McMeel (32) carefully distinguished between traction detachments in PDR, which were not caused by retinal breaks, and detachments, which were, in fact, directly caused by retinal breaks. Of 653 diabetic eyes with classifiable fibrotic proliferations, 284 (43%) also had detachments of the traction variety. These detachments had a more progressive course when caused by proliferations of the fibrovascular type rather than when caused by those of the avascular type (32). McMeel observed that 284 of 381 (75%) diabetic eyes with retinal detachment were nonrhegmatogenous (traction variety), and approximately 20% were rhegmatogenous. The remainder were not classified.

Characteristics of the traction detachment in PDR included the following: a) The elevated retina was confined to the posterior fundus and infrequently extended more than two-thirds of the distance to the equator; b) the retina was taut and had a shiny surface; c) concentric demarcation lines were often seen, indicating that extension of the detachment was common; and d) there was no shifting of subretinal fluid or mobility of the retina (32). A spontaneous decrease in extent of the traction detachment occurred in 5% of 284 eyes (32).

In contrast, rhegmatogenous detachments in PDR had the following characteristics: a) the borders of the detachment usually extended to the ora serrata; b) the surface of the retina had a dull, greyish appearance; and c) the retina undulated due to retinal mobility and some shifting of subretinal fluid (32). In McMeel's series, localization of retinal holes was complicated by several of the following factors, which were commonly observed in the diabetic population: a) poor dilation of the pupil; b) lens opacities; c) increased vitreous turbidity; d) vitreous hemorrhage; e) similarity in appearance between holes and small, round intraretinal hemorrhages; f) retinal breaks were often obscured by overlying proliferative tissue (similar to the situation prevailing in PSR and RLF) or lay within deep crevices between sharp retinal folds; and g) the retinal breaks were invariably small (32).

McMeel also noted that retinal holes occurred infrequently in the elevated retina once a traction detachment had occurred. Surprisingly, the area of the detachment remained unchanged after hole formation (32). Despite the retinal break, the detachment continued to resemble that of the traction variety in all other respects. Six such cases were followed by McMeel for six months to eight years without formation of rhegmatogenous characteristics (32). Madsen also noted that localized traction detachments sometimes remained unchanged for several years (31). Assessment of surgical results must take such data into consideration.

*Therapy of retinal detachment in PDR.* Okun and his colleagues operated on retinal detachments in PDR with or without holes when the macula detached or appeared imminently endangered (33–35). Surgery was delayed as long as the detachment remained localized and reassessment was performed every three to four months (35). McMeel and Schepens also used the presence of concentric demarcation lines and, where documented, progression of the detachment, as indications for surgery (36). Contraindications to surgery included: a) extensive preretinal fibrosis obscuring the fundus; b) vitreous blood obscuring the fundus; and c) chronic detachment with dense preretinal membrane formation (35).

Surgical results vary from author to author. Dobree reported 12 total retinal detachments in PDR of which only one, of undefined type, underwent surgery successfully (28). The single successful case redetached one year after an encircling operation.

Pannarale (37) reported anatomical success in seven of eight eyes, six of which had visual improvement, after encircling procedures. Scott (38) advocated the use of encircling bands at the ora serrata, with or without scleral resection.

Okun and colleagues (33–35) utilized a variety of surgical techniques with follow-ups ranging from six months to 12 years. Encircling operations with scleral resection were performed on 38 eyes and 63% obtained useful vision, which was defined as the ability to move about in familiar surroundings. Encircling operations, without scleral resection but with plombage, were performed on 14 eyes; 75% obtained useful vision. Episcleral encircling bands alone were inserted in 25 eyes, just anterior to the equator; 75% obtained useful vision. Scleral resection alone was performed in three eyes and all obtained useful vision. Visual results with and without the presence of retinal breaks and with and without drainage of subretinal fluid appeared to be similar (35).

McMeel (32) reported surgical results on eyes with the rhegmatogenous variety of retinal detachment in PDR. When the breaks were found at the equator, a scleral undermining was performed with implantation of silicone and placement of an encircling silicone band. For posterior holes, a thick silicone implant was used in order to indent the choroid maximally. There was a follow-up of six months to four years. Nine of the eleven retinas were reattached. Data on visual acuity were not reported. Late complications included: a) traction detachments in areas outside the scleral buckle (three eyes); b) anterior segment ischemia (one eye), a complication which has been reported in 60% of eyes with SC hemoglobin after buckling operations, but in only 3% of eyes with normal hemoglobin (15); c) cataract (one eye); and d) infection (one eye).

McMeel and Schepens (36) also reported on scleral resection alone for traction detachments in PDR. A 3-mm-wide scleral resection of almost full thickness was created for 180 to 270 degrees around the globe at its equator, usually on the temporal side. No attempt was made to place the resected area at the site of the traction detachment itself. Ultrasound studies performed in four eyes showed either a shortening of the anteroposterior diameter of 1 mm (in two eyes) or no change (in two eyes). Of eight eyes treated in this fashion, 87% (seven eyes) maintained or improved their vision postoperatively (36).

A certain percentage of diabetic retinal detachments may remain unchanged in extent for a prolonged period of time, and some may actually spontaneously decrease in extent (31, 32, 36). Because anatomic success rates in large series have not been available, because results vary from author to author and because control observations on visual acuities in untreated eyes with traction detachment have not been reported, a final assessment of the operative results for diabetic retinal detachment is not possible at this time.

## CONCLUSIONS

Retinal detachments are common late complications of the proliferative retinopathies that characterize sickle cell diseases, retrolental fibroplasia and diabetes mellitus. Vitreous traction, with or without retinal hole formation, is frequently, if not always, responsible for detachment of the retina.

Surgical therapy of such retinal detachments is particularly difficult in sickle cell diseases and in diabetes mellitus. Extensive series of studies with detailed and controlled data concerning ultimate visual acuity and anatomic reattachment of the retina are not yet available. Final conclusions regarding the indications for, and the efficacy of, various surgical procedures must therefore be held in abeyance.

## REFERENCES

1. GOLDBERG MF. Classification and pathogenesis of proliferative sickle retinopathy. *Am J Ophthalmol* **71**: 649, 1971.
2. GOLDBERG MF. Natural history of untreated proliferative sickle retinopathy. *Arch Ophthalmol* **85**: 428, 1971.
3. GOLDBERG MF, CHARACHE C and ACACIO I. Ophthalmologic manifestations of sickle cell thalassemia. *Arch Intern Med* **128**: 33, 1971.
4. KNOX DL. Ischemic ocular inflammation. *Am J Ophthalmol* **60**: 995, 1965.
5. KNOX DL. Ocular aspects of cervical vascular disease. *Surv Ophthalmol* **13**: 245, 1969.
6. SKIKANO S and SHIMIZU K. "Atlas of fluorescence fundus angiography." Philadelphia, WB Saunders, 1968, p 58.
7. HAYREH SS. Post-radiation retinopathy. A fluorescence fundus angiographic study. *Brit J Ophthalmol* **54**: 705, 1970.
8. ALGUERE P. Fluorescein studies of retinal vasculitis in sarcoidosis. Report of a case. *Acta Ophthalmol (Kbh)* **48**: 1129, 1970.
9. WELCH RB and GOLDBERG MF. Sickle-cell hemoglobin and its relation to fundus abnormality. *Arch Ophthalmol* **75**: 353, 1966.
10. TAYLOR E and DOBREE JH. Proliferative diabetic retinopathy, site and size of initial lesions. *Br J Ophthalmol* **54**: 11, 1970.
11. TASMAN W. Vitreoretinal changes in cicatricial retrolental fibroplasia. *Trans Am Ophthalmol Soc* **68**: 548, 1970.
12. BALODIMOS MC, REES SB, AIELLO LM, BRADLEY RF and MARBLE A. Fluorescein photography in proliferative diabetic retinopathy treated by pituitary ablation, in: Goldberg MF and Fine SL (Eds), "Symposium on the treatment of diabetic retinopathy." Public Health Service Publication no 1890, Washington, DC, Superintendent of Documents, 1969, chap 16.
13. DOBREE JH. Proliferative diabetic retinopathy. Evolution of the retinal lesions. *Br J Ophthalmol* **48**: 637, 1964.
14. COHEN J, ALFANO JE, BOSHES LD and PALMGREN C. Clinical evaluation of school-age children with retrolental fibroplasia. *Am J Ophthalmol* **57**: 41, 1964.
15. RYAN SJ and GOLDBERG MF. Anterior segment ischemia following scleral buckling in sickle cell hemoglobinopathy. *Am J Ophthalmol* **72**: 35, 1971.
16. FARIS BM and BROCKHURST RJ. Retrolental fibroplasia in the cicatricial stage. The complication of rhegmatogenous retinal detachment. *Arch Ophthalmol* **82**: 60, 1969.
17. GOLDBERG MF. Natural history of diabetic retinopathy. *Isr J Med Sci* **8**: 1311, 1972.
18. PATZ A. The continuing role of the ophthalmologist in the premature nursery. *Arch Ophthalmol* **85**: 129, 1971.
19. DUKE-ELDER S and DOBREE JH. "Diseases of the retina." London, Henry Kimpton, 1967.
20. ASHTON N, GRAYMORE C and PEDLER C. Studies on developing retinal vessels. *Br J Ophthalmol* **41**: 449, 1957.
21. Joint Committee for the Study of Retrolental Fibroplasia. A classification of retrolental fibroplasia. *Am J Ophthalmol* **36**: 1333, 1953.
22. ZACHARIAS L, CHISHOLM JF JR and CHAPMAN R. Visual and ocular damage in retrolental fibroplasia. *Am J Ophthalmol* **53**: 337, 1962.
23. FARIS B, TOLENTINO FI, FREEMAN HM, BROCKHURST RJ and SCHEPENS CL. Retrolental fibroplasia in the cicatricial stage. Fundus and vitreous findings. *Arch Ophthalmol* **85**: 661, 1971.
24. BAUM JD. Retinal artery tortuosity in ex-premature infants. *Arch Dis Child* **46**: 247, 1971.
25. REESE AB and STEPANIK J. Cicatricial stage of retrolental fibroplasia. *Am J Ophthalmol* **38**: 308, 1954.
26. TASMAN W and ANNESLEY W JR. Retinal detachment in the retinopathy of prematurity. *Arch Ophthalmol* **75**: 608, 1966.
27. TASMAN W. Retinal detachment in retrolental fibroplasia. *Mod Probl Ophthalmol (Basel)* **8**: 371, 1969.
28. DOBREE JH. Evolution of lesions in proliferative diabetic retinopathy: An 8 year photographic survey, in: Goldberg MF and Fine SL (Eds), "Symposium on the treatment of diabetic retinopathy." Public Health Service Publication no 1890, Washington, DC, Superintendent of Documents, 1969, chap 5.
29. DAVIS MD. Vitreous contraction in proliferative diabetic retinopathy. *Arch Ophthalmol* **74**: 741, 1965.
30. TOLENTINO FI, LEE PF and SCHEPENS CL. Biomicroscopic study of vitreous cavity in diabetic retinopathy. *Arch Ophthalmol* **75**: 238, 1966.
31. MADSEN PH. Ocular findings in 123 patients with proliferative diabetic retinopathy. III. Changes in the posterior segment of the eye. *Doc Ophthalmol* **29**: 351, 1971.
32. MCMEEL JW. Diabetic retinopathy: fibrotic proliferation and retinal detachment. *Trans Am Ophthalmol Soc* (in press).
33. OKUN E. Discussion on treatment techniques of photocoagulation, in: Goldberg MF and Fine SC (Eds), "Symposium on the treatment of diabetic retinopathy." Public Health Service Publication no 1890, Washington, DC, Superintendent of Documents, 1969, p 632.
34. OKUN E and FUNG W. Therapy of diabetic

retinal detachment, in: "Symposium on retina and retinal surgery." St Louis, CV Mosby Co, 1969, chap 21.

35. OKUN E.   Scleral buckling in diabetic retinal detachment, in: Okun E et al, "Current concepts in treatment of diabetic retinopathy—a stereoscopic presentation." St Louis, CV Mosby Co, 1971.

36. McMEEL JW and SCHEPENS CL.   Treatment of traction detachment of the retina by scleral resection. Presented at the Wilmer Residents Association Meeting, Baltimore, 1971 (in press).

37. PANNARALE MR.   Indications et resultats des traitements operatoires des decollements retiniennes des sujets diabetiques. *Mod Probl Ophthalmol* (*Basel*) **8**: 511, 1969.

38. SCOTT JD.   Surgery of advanced diabetic retinopathy. *Mod Probl Ophthalmol* (*Basel*) **8**: 505 1969.

binocular vision. Yet, with the exception of a few isolated case reports, no meaningful data are available to indicate the rate of spontaneous or therapeutically-induced recovery of vision in an amblyopic eye after loss of the sound eye, and to what extent this recovery really depends on previous attempts to improve vision in amblyopic eyes, at least temporarily, in childhood. Such information should be collected on a worldwide basis by one of the international ophthalmological organizations. Until such knowledge becomes available, we have the obligation to treat amblyopia until the best possible visual result is reached.

Supported in part by Research Grant EY-00274 from the National Eye Institute, Bethesda, Md.

## REFERENCES

1. BURIAN HM. Eyedness, handedness and refractive error in relation to strabismic amblyopia. *Wiss Z Karl-Marx-Universität Leipzig Math Naturw Reihe* **18**: 236, 1969.
2. HELVESTON EM and VON NOORDEN GK. Microtropia: a newly defined entity. *Arch Ophthalmol* **78**: 272, 1967.
3. VON NOORDEN GK and MAUMENEE AE. Clinical observations on stimulus deprivation amblyopia (amblyopia ex anopsia). *Am J Ophthalmol* **65**: 220, 1968.
4. RYAN SJ and VON NOORDEN GK. Further observations on the aspiration technique in cataract surgery. *Am J Ophthalmol* **71**: 626, 1971.
5. PICETTI B and FINE M. Keratoplasty in children. *Trans Pac Coast Otoophthalmol Soc* **46**: 153, 1965.
6. BROWN SI. Corneal transplantation in the anterior chamber cleavage syndrome. *Am J Ophthalmol* **70**: 942, 1970.
7. SACHSENWEGER R. Über die Ursachen der Schielamblyopie. *Klin Monatsbl Augenheilkd* **147**: 488, 1965.
8. GILES CL. Retinal hemorrhages in the newborn. *Am J Ophthalmol* **49**: 1005, 1960.
9. WEIDEN H. Über Netzhautblutungen bei Neugeborenen mit unterschiedlichem Geburtsablauf. *Klin Monatsbl Augenheikd* **156**: 363, 1970.
10. BONAMOUR G. Le prognostic éloigne des hémorrhagies rétiniennes du nouveau-né. *Bull Mem Soc Fr Ophtalmol* **62**: 227, 1949.
11. BANGERTER A. "Amblyopiebehandlung," 2nd edn. Basel, S Karger, 1955.
12. LANG J. Der kongenitale oder frühkindliche Strabismus. *Ophthalmologica* **154**: 201, 1967.
13. VON NOORDEN GK and BURIAN HM. Visual acuity in normal and amblyopic patients under reduced illumination. I. Behavior of visual acuity with and without neutral-density-filter. *Arch Ophthalmol* **61**: 533, 1959.
14. AWAYA S and VON NOORDEN GK. Visual acuity of amblyopic eyes under monocular and binocular conditions: further observations. *Trans 2nd Int Orthopt Cong, Amsterdam, 1971* (in press).
15. GREGERSEN E and RINDZIUNSKI E. "Conventional" occlusion in the treatment of squint amblyopia. *Acta Ophthalmol* **43**: 462, 1965.
16. FLETCHER MC, SILVERMAN SJ, BOYD J and CALLAWAY M. Biostatistical studies: comparison of the management of suppression amblyopia by conventional patching, intensive hospital pleoptics, and intermittent office pleoptics. *Am Orthopt J* **19**: 40, 1969.
17. ALLEN HF. Incidence of amblyopia (editorial). *Arch Ophthalmol* **77**: 1, 1967.

# SCREENING FOR AMBLYOPIA

## SCREENING FOR AMBLYOPIA IN CHILDREN UNDER THREE YEARS OF AGE IN ISRAEL

I. NAWRATZKI, M. OLIVER and E. NEUMANN

Department of Ophthalmology, Hadassah University Hospital, Jerusalem and Department of Ophthalmology, Rothschild Municipal–Government Hospital, Haifa, Israel

During the past few years, screening of young children has been introduced in many parts of Israel. This report summarizes the results of screening of children under the age of three in Jerusalem, Beersheba and Haifa.

### MATERIALS AND METHODS

The screening was performed in all three cities in the Mother and Child Care Clinics which are part of a national institution providing periodic examinations of children from birth to kindergarten. In Jerusalem and Beersheba the examinations were performed by an orthoptist, and in Haifa by an ophthalmologist and an orthoptist. Children in whom amblyopia, strabismus or any other eye disease was suspected were referred to the outpatient eye clinics of the different hospitals where they were further examined by an ophthalmologist, an orthoptist and an optometrist.

The screened population included 13,028 children, of whom 4,718 were from Jerusalem, 1,910 from Beersheba and 6,400 from Haifa. The attendance rate of the children at the Mother and Child Care Clinics was highest in Beersheba (about 90%), somewhat less in Haifa (80%) and lowest in Jerusalem (60%).

Identical methods were used in all three cities. Comprehensive case histories were taken and the Hirschberg test and cover test for near vision were routinely used. Criteria for amblyopia were: 1) a unilateral tropia, confirmed by the cover test and 2) an obvious difference in the behavior of the child when one eye was covered compared to that when the other eye was covered. Treatment consisted of occlusion or mydriatics in the good eye, or a combination of both.

### RESULTS

The prevalence of amblyopia, as defined above, was 0.53 % and no significant difference was found among the three cities (Table 1). When comparing the results of treatment of amblyopic children, marked differences in

TABLE 1. *Prevalence of amblyopia in 13,028 children*

|  | No. of cases | Prevalence (%) | Esotropia | Exotropia |
|---|---|---|---|---|
| Jerusalem | 23 | 0.5 | 21 | 2 |
| Beersheba | 11 | 0.5 | 10 | 1 |
| Haifa | 40 | 0.6 | 31 + (5[a]) | 4 |
| TOTAL | 74 | 0.53 | 67 | 7 |

[a] With hypertropia or hypotropia.

TABLE 2.  *Results of treatment of amblyopia with unilateral tropia*

| | Total | Alternation | Good visual acuity, no alternation | Improved treatment continued | No cooperation[b] | Satisfactory results No. | % |
|---|---|---|---|---|---|---|---|
| Jerusalem | 23 | 4 (1[a]) | 2 | 4 | 13 | 10 | 44 |
| Beersheba | 11 | 5 (5[a]) | 2 | 0 | 0 | 7 | 63 |
| Haifa | 40 | 25 | | 1 | 14 | 26 | 65 |
| TOTAL | 74 | 34 (6[a]) | 4 | 5 | 27 | 43 | 58 |

[a]  Good visual acuity.
[b]  Nonattendance, under treatment or treated elsewhere.

cooperation, and hence in the rate of success, were found (Table 2). Cooperation was highest in Haifa and lowest in Jerusalem. Of all the children treated 34 showed alternation. In 10 of the children who cooperated in visual acuity tests, equal vision was achieved in both eyes; four of them did not alternate. Under the heading of improvement, there are five children still under treatment, but who already show some alternation. Of the 74 children with amblyopia, 58% benefited from the treatment.

The incidence of strabismus without amblyopia, as well as of other eye diseases in need of treatment or observation is shown in Table 3. There were 170 such cases, that is, a prevalence of 1.3%.

TABLE 3.  *Eye diseases other than amblyopia in 13,028 children*

| | |
|---|---|
| Esotropia | 74 |
| Exotropia | 63 |
| High myopia | 11 |
| Congenital cataract | 4 |
| Retinitis pigmentosa | 4 |
| Subluxated lens | 3 |
| Microcornea | 3 |
| Chorioretinitis (including Coats' disease) | 2 |
| Congenital glaucoma | 1 |
| Aniridia | 1 |
| Dysautonomia | 1 |
| Retinoblastoma | 1 |
| Tay Sachs | 1 |
| Unilateral exophthalmus | 1 |
| TOTAL | (1.3%)170 |

## DISCUSSION

It was difficult to diagnose amblyopia in children under three years of age because there was a lack of cooperation in visual acuity tests and because the cover test is not reliable (1). Despite the fact that unilateral tropia may exist without amblyopia, the diagnosis was based on unilateral tropia because the cover test was the only one which could be performed in all children. Therefore, only cases of amblyopia associated with tropia were detected, and orthophoric cases may have been overlooked, especially those with anisometropia in whom near vision is unimpaired. A new test described by Rose (2) may improve the early diagnosis in these cases, but it was introduced only recently, and was not used in this screening program.

The rate of prevalence of amblyopia of 0.5% in children under three years of age in a control group in the Beersheba children rose to 0.9% a year later and had risen to 1.8% by the time the children reached five years of age. This discrepancy was due mainly to a high incidence of orthophoria in the five-year-old children. These variations in prevalence are similar to those observed in children in the United States (0.3 to 1.9%) (5) and are in part due to the differences in the methods used.

It may be assumed that in cases with unilateral tropia, amblyopia is of the more severe type. The prevalence of 0.56% in our series is in keeping with the 0.45% of children with vision under 6/18 reported by Gansner (3) who screened 11,000 children between the ages of four and six.

The difference in results of treatment reflects the varying degrees of cooperation. In Jerusalem, where cooperation was lowest, other medical services are available, and some of the children may have been treated elsewhere. In Beersheba there is only one hospital to which all children were referred. The presence of an ophthalmologist at the time of the screening in Haifa may have convinced the parents of the importance of following the treatment advised. The good results (58% of the 74 children treated) agreed with other results of treatment reported later.

The importance of amblyopia (5) as one of the most obvious examples of preventable blindness is generally accepted, and the desirability of its early detection is well known (4, 6, 7). In a child under three years, no treatment is necessary other than occlusion or mydriatics to the good eye. This treatment is inexpensive and more easily imposed than in older children. The eccentric fixation is not yet firmly established at this early age, and recurrence of amblyopia has been found less frequently in cases treated early (8). Nevertheless, until our methods of diagnosis are improved, it will continue to be desirable to reexamine five-year-old children in kindergarten.

In view of these findings, it is important to consider the financial aspect of this type of screening program in Israel. Each year 70,000 children are born and if 20 are screened in 1 hr, then 3,500 working hours (i.e. two or three full-time employees) per year would be required to screen every child. The screening could be carried out by an orthoptist working with a nurse and a secretary. Taking into account that about 8% of the children are referred to the outpatient clinic for further examinations, each of which requires about half an hour's work by an orthoptist, a refractionist and an ophthalmologist, these 5,600 cases would require 2,700 working hours. One full-time and one part-time doctor would be needed for this. The total cost for all the personnel required to screen our population of children would be IL 60,000 to 70,000 for a year or IL 1 for each child examined! About 2%, or 1,400 children, would have a pathological finding that should be treated or at least observed. From these, we could anticipate that at least 350 children would have amblyopia and 175 or more of them would benefit from treatment.

A person who has amblyopia with a visual acuity less than 6/60 in one eye and subsequently loses his good eye in an accident, is entitled to compensation of 80% of his salary for the rest of his life. Even if his vision improves later, very expensive reeducation is often necessary and he is limited in his choice of profession.

We feel that IL 70,000 is not too extravagant a sum to spend to save at least 175 children from this disease. This cost may be still further reduced in the future because the screening may ultimately be carried out by the nurses already working in the Mother and Child Care Clinic. In this way every child could be tested with very little extra effort. However, this can only be done when the specialized team has acquired enough experience to teach nurses who have not previously been trained in ophthalmological work.

In areas where screening for amblyopia is taking place, there is increased awareness in the population. During the past year many children, apart from those who had been screened, were referred to us by doctors, nurses or parents. We also have the impression that the attendance rate at the Mother and Child Care Clinic is higher this year than last, perhaps because of our screening program.

## REFERENCES

1. OLIVER M and NAWRATZKI I. Screening of pre-school children for ocular anomalies, Parts I, II. *Br J Ophthalmol* (in press).
2. ROSE L. New method of detecting amblyopia. *J Pediatr Ophthalmol* (in press).
3. GANSNER I. Zur Haüfigkeit der Schielamblyopie. *Ophthalmologica* **155**: 234, 1968.
4. NAWRATZKI I and OLIVER M. Screening for amblyopia in children under 3 years of age.

*1st Congr Int Strabismus Assoc, Acapulco, Mexico, March 1970*, p 167.
5. DUNLAP E. Introduction. Symposium on current aspects of amblyopia. *Am Orthopt J* **21**: 5, 1971.
6. MME. SARINGUET-BADOCHE. Quinze années de plé-optique. Résultats à longue écheance. *Bull Soc Ophthalmol Fr* **70**: 495, 1970.
7. WILSON G. The practical management of suppression amblyopia. *Am Orthopt J* **21**: 21, 1971.
8. FRANÇOIS J, cited in ref 6.

# OBSERVATIONS ON THE PREVALENCE OF AMBLYOPIA IN AFRICAN CHILDREN

## Y. YASSUR, S. YASSUR, S. ZAIFRANI, U. SACHS and I. BEN-SIRA

Department of Ophthalmology, Hadassah University Hospital, Jerusalem, Israel

A survey for the detection of amblyopia was performed in Rwanda on 1,550 African pupils from 10 to 18 years of age. Eighteen (1.2%) were unilaterally amblyopic (visual acuity of 6/12 or less). Of the 18 amblyopic eyes, 11 (61%) had myopia or myopic astigmatism. This corresponds to the high rate of myopia found among the refractive errors in Rwanda. Four (23%) eyes were hypermetropic and three (16%) were emmetropic.

Of the 18 amblyopic eyes, eight (44%) were exotropic, five (28%) esotropic and five (28%) did not deviate. All the exotropic eyes were myopic or emmetropic. It seems possible that the high rate of exotropia can be attributed partly to the high rate of myopia and myopic astigmatism, partly to the age of the pupils examined and partly to the fact that none of the children had previously been treated. However, it is likely that there are still other factors that could not be clearly identified in the present study.

Larger scale screening for the early detection of amblyopia among Africans is recommended because the prevalence of amblyopia is not negligible and its early therapy is worthwhile. By such screenings one can also detect cases of organic defective vision which could be treated surgically. In practical terms, however, such screening programs are still very difficult because there are many other problems in the country such as the organization of national health services, the mental attitude and cooperation of parents (a very important factor in treatment) and a general lack of eye clinics and medical staff.

# SCREENING FOR AMBLYOPIA

S. DELTHIL and J. SOURDILLE*

Ministry of Health, Paris, France

We recently produced a film that emphasizes the difficulties of examining visual acuity in young children. It was filmed both in a kindergarten, using a group of children aged three to six years, and in an ophthalmologic laboratory. The measurement of vision at this age, as in adults, depends on the successful measurement of various visual functions. The use of subjective methods that require difficult responses from children leave a great margin of uncertainty. On the other hand, some objective methods are not completely reliable, while others produce strong reactions of fear in many children. Our study was therefore begun in the normal environment of the kindergarten so that the most precise responses could be obtained.

*Distance visual activity.* Only strictly accurate visual charts permit a precise evaluation of visual acuity. Directional charts such as those of Snellen or Sjögren may give some false responses. The letters we have selected are very precise if two conditions are fulfilled: 1) each letter should be presented separately and 2) the response should be by analogy, that is, the child has to designate a similar letter that is placed before him. This eliminates errors of both expression and reflection. In the three year-old age group, these games result in an accurate measurement of visual acuity and in those children whose vision is normal, we obtained a response of 6/6. Our film shows the principal precautions that should be taken during the test.

*Near visual acuity.* This is very difficult to assess, even if Rodenstock's R5 instrument is used.

*Color vision* is both interesting and easy to study with pseudoisochromatic tables if the method of analogy is used.

*Visual fields.* Most of the reliable instruments now in use are too complex to be used for children. However, tachytoscopic methods with simpler instruments give good results. Mesotropic vision can also be evaluated in this way.

*Objective methods.* These are probably the most reliable type presently available. Electroretinography is extremely precise, but because it must be done under anesthesia, it is reserved only for the more severe types of defect. Optokinetic nystagmus offers great promise for the future. This method requires an electro-oculographic record and a nystagmo-exciter which retain the attention of the children.

## CONCLUSION

Although diagnosis of visual defects is still difficult in young children, good results have been obtained by performing the tests in the kindergarten and by using more accurate instruments. Thus, younger age groups can be examined, treatment can be undertaken sooner and children with serious visual handicaps can be directed to special schools at an early age.

* Address for reprints: 46 rue de Naples, Paris VIIIème, France.

# TREATMENT OF AMBLYOPIA

## AMBLYOPIA THERAPY IN AN UNDERDEVELOPED AREA

### ALBERT M. POTTS

Eye Research Laboratories, University of Chicago, Chicago, Illinois, USA

The available tools for the treatment of amblyopia are few and unsophisticated. They consist of correction of refractive errors, removal of physical obstruction to light passage (congenital cataract, ptosis) and the judicious use of patching. It is not proposed to deal with pleoptics in this discussion.

The two prerequisites for the effective use of these tools are early referral and enough social organization around the child to insure continued use of therapeutic measures. Both are largely dependent upon social factors. The level of parents' education and the availability of early pediatric consultation determine early referral. Parents' understanding and daily parental availability determine the continued use of glasses and patching.

In recent years we have studied amblyopia therapy in two classes of population with widely divergent backgrounds and mores. The University of Chicago Clinics are private clinics, and are utilized by middle class patients of the four-state metropolitan area (Illinois, Indiana, Wisconsin and Michigan). Fees are equal to or higher than those charged by private physicians in the area. Four years ago the University established a pilot-project pediatric clinic in a neighboring area characterized by low income, crowded housing and high crime rate. The clinic serves only residents of the area, and no fees are charged. The ophthalmology section of this clinic as well as that of the University Clinic is staffed by University Hospital personnel, so that methods and approach are the same in both. It is thus a fair assumption that the chief differences between the two clinic populations are social ones.

We have therefore reviewed the records of 25 consecutive amblyopia patients from the University Clinic (Group A), and a similar series of 25 consecutive patients from the neighborhood clinic (Group B). We have paid particular attention to the age at which first treatment was sought (from us or elsewhere) and the length of follow-up for each child. Results are shown in Tables 1 and 2.

It is clear that although Group B sought help at a later time than Group A, the difference between overall means is less impressive than if one expresses this figure as percent seeking help at under five years of age. If one takes five years as a boundary beyond which success diminishes rapidly, Group A has 76% seeking help before five years whereas in Group B the number is 40%.

An equally impressive figure concerns persistence with therapy. Of Group A 20% were lost to follow-up after a mean time of 1.1 years. In Group B 68% were lost to follow-up after a mean time of 0.7 years.

The implication of these figures is that, of

TABLE 1. *Amblyopia therapy in a group of middle-income patients*

| Patient no. | Age at first treatment | Length of treatment (years) | Lost to follow-up after x years |
|---|---|---|---|
| 1 | 17.0 | 1.0 | — |
| 2 | 4.5 | 12.5+ | — |
| 3 | 2.5 | 10.5 | — |
| 4 | 3.8 | 7.25 | — |
| 5 | 6.0 | 2.0– | 1.0 |
| 6 | 5.0 | 5.5 | — |
| 7 | 6.0 | 1.0 | — |
| 8 | 1.0 | 2.2 | — |
| 9 | 2.5 | 1.8 | 1.8 |
| 10 | 3.0 | 5.0 | — |
| 11 | 1.5 | 3.6 | — |
| 12 | 1.0 | 3.2 | — |
| 13 | 1.5 | 1.6 | — |
| 14 | 1.8 | 2.5 | — |
| 15 | 3.0 | 1.2 | — |
| 16 | 4.5 | 1.5 | 1.5 |
| 17 | 6.0 | 2.3 | — |
| 18 | 0.8 | | — |
| 19 | 2.0 | 0.25 | — |
| 20 | 3.0 | 3.0 | — |
| 21 | 4.0 | 1.0 | 1.0 |
| 22 | 5.0 | 1.0 | — |
| 23 | 2.9 | 0.75 | — |
| 24 | 2.3 | 0.2 | 0.2 |
| 25 | 2.0 | 0.3 | — |

TABLE 2. *Amblyopia therapy in a group of low-income patients*

| Patient no. | Age at first treatment | Length of treatment (years) | Lost to follow-up after x years |
|---|---|---|---|
| 1 | 5.0 | 0.5 | 0.5 |
| 2 | 6.0 | 0.8 | 0.8 |
| 3 | 2.0 | 0.9 | 0.9 |
| 4 | 7.0 | 0.1 | 0.1 |
| 5 | 5.0 | 1.3 | 1.3 |
| 6 | 14.0 | 0 (1 visit) | 0 |
| 7 | 0.9 | 0.8 | 0.8 |
| 8 | 1.8 | 1.5 | — |
| 9 | 5.0 | 2.0 | — |
| 10 | 6.0 | 1.5 | — |
| 11 | 5.0 | 0.3 | 0.3 |
| 12 | 1.1 | 1.5 | 1.5 |
| 13 | 2.0 | 0.3 | 0.3 |
| 14 | 2.0 | 0.9 | — |
| 15 | 11.0 | 0.2 | 0.2 |
| 16 | 5.0 | 1.2 | — |
| 17 | 3.0 | 0.1 | 0.1 |
| 18 | 3.0 | 1.3 | 1.3 |
| 19 | 3.0 | 2.0 | — |
| 20 | 13.0 | 0.8 | 0.8 |
| 21 | 5.0 | 3.0 | — |
| 22 | 7.0 | 2.0 | 2.0 |
| 23 | 5.0 | 0.6 | 0.6 |
| 24 | 4.0 | 4.5 | — |
| 25 | 5.0 | 0.1 | 0.1 |

Group A, 61 % are available for the time required for therapy and at an age that promises success. In Group B this figure is reduced to 13%.

The conclusion seems inevitable that social factors conspire sharply to reduce the effectiveness of amblyopia therapy even under reasonably ideal circumstances. In the social environment of our underdeveloped area, represented by Group B, only one patient in eight is likely to present early enough and to persist long enough to allow treatment to proceed. Furthermore, even the best and most prompt treatment is not effective in 100% of cases. Amblyopia therapy is therefore disastrously wasteful in our Group B.

The author wishes to acknowledge the technical assistance of Miss Stephanie M. Melkin and Mrs. Edith G. Goldman.

Supported in part by Public Health Service Research Grant EY-00416 from the National Eye Institute, Bethesda, Maryland.

## TREATMENT OF AMBLYOPIA

### I. NAWRATZKI

Department of Ophthalmology, Hadassah University Hospital, Jerusalem, Israel

The present methods of treatment of amblyopia are of two types. The first excludes the use of the good eye so that the amblyopic eye must be made to look and fix. The second deals with reversion of eccentric fixation.

The first method employs occlusion, full or part time, filters and mydriatics to the good eye. Miotics administered to the amblyopic eye, especially in cases of high hypermetropia or astigmatism, may replace glasses. The blurring of the good eye by mydriatics can be enhanced by strong concave or convex lenses, while a reading correction in front of the amblyopic eye may encourage its use for near vision (1).

The second group includes the use of strong prisms in front of the amblyopic eye and pleoptics. In the inverse prism method, introduced by Pigassou and Garypuy (2), the good eye is occluded and in the amblyopic eye, the image of the fixed object is shifted in the direction of the eccentric fixation. The separation of the line of vision from the real object, together with a constant divergence, seems to restore the proper fixation pattern, and consequently good vision. Because the moving of fixation towards the macula occurs gradually, the power of the prisms should change accordingly (3).

Pleoptics aim mainly at stimulating the macula by after-images, flashing of symbols and Haidinger brushes. Occlusion of the amblyopic eye between treatments and dazzling of the paramacular areas of eccentric fixation at the time of treatment serve to discard the abnormal fixation pattern.

The practicability of the methods described depends on the age of the patient and the degree of amblyopia.

Under the age of three, mydriatics and occlusion by patching the good eye, are the methods of choice, adding if necessary miotics to the amblyopic eye. From the age of three on, when glasses are more easily accepted, various filters or high power lenses in front of the good eye together with atropine may be added. If eccentric fixation persists, the inverse prism method is adequate for the young, while pleoptics are suitable only for children over six years of age.

Blurring of the good eye by other means than patching or occluders is useful as long as the visual acuity in the amblyopic eye is better than the blurred vision of the good eye. Otherwise the child will continue to use the dominant eye. The limit for filters and mydriatics is 6/21. If high-plus lenses for near vision are added to the amblyopic eye, then even an eye with 6/60 vision may take up fixation.

The prism therapy used for eccentric fixation is rather difficult for the patient with visual acuity under 6/60, while pleoptics are suitable even at 3/60.

During the last 10 years, most of these methods have been used in the treatment of amblyopia at the Eye Department of the Hadassah University Hospital, and 217 of the cases treated can now be assessed. In this paper we report only the results of our treatment relating to visual acuity.

### METHODS

Visual acuity was tested with Snellen, number or illiterate E charts. 6/9 was considered good visual acuity since most children do not read 6/6 on these charts; 6/12 is satisfactory, although 10 cases with 6/12 were apparently treated for other reasons.

Three age groups were considered. In the first, treatment was started before the age of three, in the second, between three and six years and in the third, after six years of age.

Methods of treatment were occlusion of the good eye including filters, mydriatics, pleoptics preceded by occlusion of the amblyopic eye and inverse prisms. In combined treatment, inverse prisms always followed unsuccessful pleoptics or occlusion.

### RESULTS

The results relating to visual acuity are given in Table 1. Thirty-one percent achieved good visual acuity (6/9); another 17%, satisfactory visual acuity (6/12); and in 49 cases, vision remained unchanged. In 15 other cases improvement occurred though visual acuity still remained low.

TABLE 1. *Visual acuity in 217 cases before and after treatment*

| Before treatment | After treatment | | | | |
|---|---|---|---|---|---|
| | 6/9 | 6/12 | 6/18 to 24 | 6/30 to 60 | < 6/60 |
| 6/12 | 9 | *1* | 0 | 0 | 0 |
| 6/18 to 24 | 25 | 15 | *14* | 0 | 0 |
| 6/30 to 60 | 18 | 13 | 27 | *40* | 0 |
| < 6/60 | 3 | 1 | 5 | 11 | *4* |
| Unknown | 12 | 7 | 8 | 2 | 2 |
| TOTAL | 67 (31%) | 37 (17%) | 54 (25%) | 53 (24%) | 6 (3%) |

Numbers in italics indicate the number of cases with no change in visual acuity.

TABLE 2. *Final visual acuity after treatment*

| Age at onset of treatment (years) | 6/9 | | 6/12 | | 6/18 to 24 | | 6/30 to 60 | | < 6/60 | | Total no. |
|---|---|---|---|---|---|---|---|---|---|---|---|
| | No. | % | No. | % | No. | % | No. | % | No. | % | |
| < 3 | 22 | 42 | 13 | 24 | 10 | 19 | 6 | 11 | 2 | 4 | 53 |
| 3 to 6 | 28 | 40 | 10 | 14 | 16 | 25 | 14 | 20 | 1 | 1 | 69 |
| > 6 | 16 | 18 | 12 | 14 | 24 | 28 | 31 | 37 | 3 | 3 | 86 |
| Unknown | 1 | | 2 | | 4 | | 2 | | — | | 9 |
| TOTAL | | | | | | | | | | | 217 |

TABLE 3. *Duration of treatment*

| Age at onset of treatment (years) | < 6 months | 6 to 12 months | > 12 months |
|---|---|---|---|
| < 3 | 4 | 10 | 45 |
| 3 to 6 | 11 | 16 | 47 |
| > 6 | 21 | 28 | 46 |
| TOTAL | 36 | 43 | 138 |

TABLE 4. *Alternation after treatment*

| Age at onset of treatment (years) | Yes | No |
|---|---|---|
| 0 to 2 | 12 | 14 |
| 2 to 3 | 12 | 17 |
| 3 to 4 | 9 | 17 |
| 4 to 6 | 4 | 37 |
| > 6 | 2 | 65 |
| TOTAL | 39 | 150 |

Table 2 summarizes the results of treatment according to the age at which it was begun. In the youngest age group, 66% of the children achieved satisfactory results. This figure fell to 54% in those who started treatment at three to six years of age; and to 32% in those who started treatment when they were over six years old.

There was no difference in the length of treatment in the three age groups (Table 3). However, the large number of patients who were treated for a short period in the older group may be misleading since patients who subsequently discontinued the treatment have been included.

The data presented in Table 4 suggest that alternation is not a good criterion of success, even in the youngest age group. The number of cases with good visual acuity without alternation is quite high; moreover the older the child is, the less he alternates.

**457**

TABLE 5.    *Results of different types of treatment in 217 cases of amblyopia*

| Visual acuity | Occlusion including mydriatics | Pleoptics | Inverse prism | Combined | Unknown | Total |
|---|---|---|---|---|---|---|
| 6/9 | 60 | 1 | 1 | 4 | 1 | 67 |
| 6/12 | 28 | 4 | 1 | 4 | 0 | 37 |
| 6/18 to 24 | 28 | 5 | 4 | 12 | 5 | 54 |
| 6/30 to 60 | 11 | 14 | 9 | 19 | 0 | 53 |
| < 6/60 | 2 | 0 | 1 | 3 | 0 | 6 |
| TOTAL | 129 | 24 | 16 | 42 | 6 | 217 |

TABLE 6.    *Comparison of results using different methods of treatment*

| Visual acuity | Occlusion mydriasis | | Pleoptics and inverse prisms | | Unknown | Total |
|---|---|---|---|---|---|---|
| | No. | % | No. | % | | |
| 6/9 to 12 | 88 | 41 | 15 | 7 | 1 | 104 |
| 6/18 to 24 | 28 | 13 | 21 | 10 | 5 | 54 |
| 6/30 and less | 13 | 6 | 46 | 21 | — | 59 |
| TOTAL | 129 | | 82 | | 6 | 217 |

Treatment by pleoptics alone was successful in 5 of 24 cases; by inverse prism alone in 2 of 16 cases; and by a combination of both in 8 of 42 cases (Table 5).

Forty-one percent of the cases improved with occlusion alone, while another 7% benefited from pleoptics and inverse prisms (Table 6).

### DISCUSSION

The improvement of vision to 6/9 to 6/12 in 48% of 217 cases treated is in keeping with the results obtained by other authors. Fletcher (4) states that roughly 50% of preschool- and schoolchildren have a good prognosis— the former slightly better. Limpaecher (5) and François (6) were more successful. Their criteria of success were similar to ours: 5/10 or 20/30, if there is more than one or two lines difference between the two eyes.

It is generally found that results are better when treatment is started early (4, 7) although there are findings to the contrary (5, 8). It does seem, however, that there is relatively little difference between groups beginning treatment before three years of age and those starting between three and six years. This is especially true when the follow-up is for more than six months, as Fletcher (4) and Gregerson and Rundziunski (9) have pointed out.

In all age groups the duration of treatment was generally more than 12 months. This is contrary to the report of Zelawska-Rybusowa (10) who found that the necessary length of treatment in very small children was several months, whereas in the older children it was 1 to 1½ years. This may be due to a difference in cooperation. In our series there was an average interruption in treatment of three to six months for each child, the treatment having been stopped for various reasons.

As in reports by others (7, 11–13) occlusion therapy was the most useful treatment; and 41% of 217 children benefited from it. Inverse prism therapy, as advised by Pigassou, is a method nearly as simple as conventional occlusion, and with the introduction of the press-on-prisms the cost of changing the prism has been reduced and the cosmetic problem resolved. Nevertheless, when used as the only treatment, it was not superior to pleoptics. A combination of both seemed more promising. In our series of 83 patients who received additional treatment after unsuccessful occlusion, 15 patients (18%) achieved good visual acuity. The low rate of success with inverse prisms contradicts an early report (3). This is probably due to the fact that this series includes cases in which treatment had been discontinued, mainly for cosmetic reasons, since press-on-prisms were not yet available.

Reports on methods of treatment and their results are controversial, as recently pointed out by Wilson (7). Each method has its value, but it depends greatly on those who give and those who receive treatment. Occlusion therapy still seems to be the most useful method, and it can be applied easily. The results in preschool children are similar in both age groups, under three and between three and six years. Still it is preferable to begin this treatment as early as possible because it is much easier to induce a small child to accept it, and it does not disturb him psychologically. All the other more sophisticated methods may be considered for a later stage, if occlusion therapy has failed or amblyopia is discovered at an advanced stage. If eccentric fixation is well established, inverse prisms therapy is advisable as the most simple method, but additional pleoptics may be required.

## REFERENCES

1. BERRONDO P. Brève revue des méthodes pour mettre en bascule les yeux des enfants strabiques convergents. *Bull Soc Ophtalmol Fr* **68**: 250, 1968.
2. PIGASSOU R and GARYPUY J. Treatment of eccentric fixation. *J Pediatr Ophthalmol* **4**: 35, 1967.
3. NAWRATZKI I and OLIVER M. Eccentric fixation managed with inverse prism. *Am J Ophthalmol* **71**: 549, 1971.
4. FLETCHER MC, SILVERMANN SJ, BOYD J and CALLAWAY M. Biostatistical studies, comparison on the management of suppression amblyopia by conventional patching, intensive hospital pleoptics and intermittent office pleoptics. *Am Orthopt J* **19**: 46, 1967.
5. LIMPAECHER E. Amblyopia therapy, methods and results. *Am Orthopt J* **19**: 97, 1969.
6. FRANÇOIS J, GOES F and JAMES M. Statistical results in the treatment of strabismic amblyopia. *Bull Soc Belge Ophtalmol* **151**: 351, 1969.
7. WILSON G. The practical management of suppression amblyopia. *Am Orthopt J* **21**: 21, 1971.
8. NAWRATZKI I and OLIVER M. Screening for amblyopia in children under 3 years of age. *Ist Cong Int Strabismus Assoc, Acapulco, March 1970*, p 167.
9. GREGERSON E and RUNDZIUNSKI E. Conventional occlusion in the treatment of squint amblyopia. *Acta Ophthalmol (Kbh)* **43**: 462, 1965.
10. ZELAWSKA-RYBUSOWA H. Über die Behandlung der Amblyopie mit exzentrischer Fixation beim einseitigen Begleitschielen bei Kindern, Jugendlichen und Erwachsenen. *Klin Monatsbl Augenheilkd* **4**: 486.
11. GOULD A, FISHKOFF D and GALIN M. Active stimulation, a method of treatment of amblyopia in the older patient. *Am Orthopt J* **20**: 39, 1970.
12. VERLEE D and IACOBUCCI I. Pleoptics versus occlusion of the sound eye. *Am J Ophthalmol* **63**: 244, 1967.
13. VON NOORDEN G. Occlusion therapy in amblyopia with eccentric fixation. *Arch Ophthalmol* **73**: 776, 1965.

# CLASSIFICATION AND TREATMENT OF AMBLYOPIA IN NIGERIA

## I. RÉTHY

Lagos University Teaching Hospital, Lagos, Nigeria

In describing treatment of amblyopia in Lagos, we need a precise definition of the syndrome in etiologic terms. We must exclude those organic visual defects resulting from intoxications and from protein and vitamin deficiencies which abound in Africa and may involve definite and final loss of light sensitivity. Organic loss of vision has nothing in common with the etiology of functional amblyopia.

We define amblyopia as diminished visual acuity without a decrease in light perception. In the "Recommendations for the standardization of terminology" (1), functional amblyopia was considered as a special case in a group of amblyopias. Here the term amblyopia refers to the functional type only, namely perceptual deficit of a functional type that is consequently alterable. Functional impairment of visual acuity can be divided into two main groups: 1) active inhibition; 2) passive inability due to "nonuse," according to Burian (2) (Fig. 1).

The active type of amblyopia was classified on the basis of its location, namely retinal or central inhibition. The differentiation was made possible by use of a new instrument, the "Contrastoscope." It compares the central light sensitivity under photopic conditions by decreasing the diameter of 10 light spots until the threshold of normal light perception is reached. The light and contrast of the light spots against the background are kept constant. Patients with retinal inhibition exhibit diminished light sensitivity. The degree of the loss of light sensitivity is related to the eccentricity of the fixation. Patients with central fixation and passive or active reduction of form vision exhibit completely normal light sensitivity (Fig. 2).

The Contrastoscope can be used as an indicator of the effectiveness of treatment by inverse occlusion. Covering the deviated eye alleviated and diminished the active inhibition exerted on the retina, and the number of light spots seen on the Contrastoscope

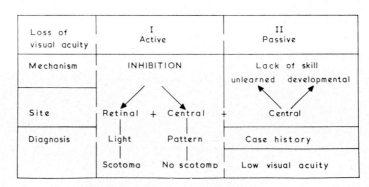

FIG. 1. Classification of functional amblyopia on the basis of the pathophysiology.

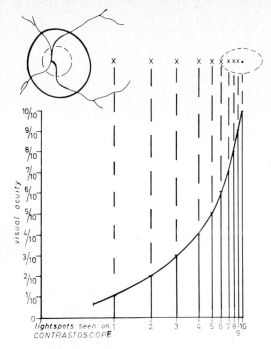

FIG. 2. Relation of the maximal visual acuity occurring in active retinal inhibition to the light spots seen on the screen of the Contrastoscope.

increased after the occlusion treatment.

Complete disappearance of the inhibition, the scotoma, coincided with the ability to see the last and smallest light spot on the Contrastoscope. This was the indication for the beginning of gradual active use of the formerly inhibited amblyopic eye. Simple exercises with ball and with drawing for gradually increasing periods were applied to overcome the passive part of the amblyopia. The exercises were combined with direct occlusion of the fixating eye, gradually increasing until it could be fully employed.

In Lagos, the active type of inhibition is infrequent in comparison with its prevalence in temperate climates; and its cause, esotropia, is also rare in this region. The 40 cases of esotropia included 13 unilateral cases, eight of which showed an eccentric fixation. The small number of cases treated does not permit a statistical evaluation.

Bilateral uncertain fixation is a new feature detected only during the last two years. Most of these 21 patients had symmetrical but very poor visual acuity. Their main complaint was difficulty in reading. Visual acuity was approximately 6/36 in 18 males and three females from 10 to 36 years of age. No refractive error was detectable in atropine cycloplegia. Single letters were rarely seen better. Slow reading of the visual chart was invariably present, the slowness being most conspicuous during the Wirt test, which showed varied and diminished stereoacuity. Fixation reflex was uncertain: the foveola did not follow the Visuscope star. The fixation shift was usually in the same direction in both eyes, so as to preserve the parallel position of the eyes. There were no signs of squint; however, convergence ability was extremely poor in some cases. On redrawing simple figures, the trace was shifted either horizontally or vertically at the level of a four-year-old child. The Worth test sometimes revealed alternating suppression.

REFERENCES

1. LINKSZ A. "Report on terminology. Working Group I of International Strabismus Symposium 1966." Basel, S Karger, 1968, p 267.
2. BURIAN HM. Pathophysiologic basis of amblyopia and its treatment. *Am J Ophthalmol* **67**: 1, 1969.
3. RÉTHY I. Lichtwahrnehmungsänderung durch die Okklusionstherapie exzentrisch fixierender Schielaugen. *Klin Monatsbl Augenheilkd* 1967, p 568.

# STIMULUS DEPRIVATION AMBLYOPIA

## KENNETH WYBAR*

Hospital for Sick Children, Great Ormond St., London, England

In an international discussion on amblyopia it would be an omission to fail to stress the important step forward in an understanding of the sensory anomalies of squint by the use of the term amblyopia ex anopsia which was featured in the German literature in the 19th century and subsequently in the English literature in the present century. It is, of course, a curious mixture of Greek and Latin which has a somewhat contradictory literal meaning (vision which is dull, or has the edge taken off it, without loss of eyesight). By convention it has come to mean the defective vision which results from disuse of the eye. It is natural that the term was received enthusiastically at a time when squint was ceasing to be regarded simply as a cosmetic deformity which was "corrected" in adolescence by a tenotomy of one or other of the horizontal rectus muscles. It must be appreciated, however, that the recognition of amblyopia in squint originated much earlier when in the 18th century G. L. Leclerc, Comte de Buffon, the French naturalist, sought to explain the development of squint as an attempt to escape from the difficulties arising from the reception of different impressions of the same object (1). This view was not wholly correct, because it tended to regard amblyopia as the cause and not the result of the squint. It was, at least, a distinct advance from the view predominantly held at that time that a squint was essentially a muscular deformity.

The term amblyopia ex anopsia came to be applied indiscriminately to all forms of amblyopia but it is now recognized that there are three main forms: the suppression amblyopia of an active inhibitional nature which occurs in squint (strabismic amblyopia), the suppression amblyopia of a more passive inhibitional nature which occurs when there is a marked difference in the refractive errors of the two eyes (anisometropic amblyopia) and the amblyopia which follows true disuse of one eye (stimulation deprivation amblyopia) (2). It is obvious that the term amblyopia ex anopsia can be retained legitimately only in the last of these three forms of amblyopia, so that it is synonymous with stimulation deprivation amblyopia. The present contribution is limited to this form of amblyopia.

The experimental studies of Hubel and Wiesel (3–6), in which newborn kittens were deprived of all forms of visual stimulation to one or both eyes during the first few months of life, shed considerable light on the mechanism of stimulus deprivation amblyopia in man. Such a conclusion, of course, is reached only by an analogy, and it is often unwise to apply the results of animal work to the clinical sphere. In this instance, however, it appears

---

* Author's address: Welbeck House, 62 Welbeck St., London, England.

to be a reasonable application. This is further supported by the findings of Von Noorden (7) in which young monkeys, which, unlike kittens, have a similar visual mechanism to that of man, show a form of stimulus deprivation amblyopia which is essentially the same as that found in kittens. Hubel and Wiesel (3, 4) found that newborn kittens thus deprived of visual stimuli showed evidence of a profound degree of amblyopia with degenerative changes in the lateral geniculate body and with functional changes in the visual cortical receptor fields. On the other hand, in the adult cat, a similar degree of visual deprivation produced no such changes. With the present state of knowledge, it is not certain to what extent anomalies in the lateral geniculate body are relevant to an understanding of the amblyopic process of man, but the cortical changes are of great interest. In the normal kitten about 80% of the cells of the visual cortex are driven by both eyes but after a period of visual deprivation only a small number of the cells are so driven. Indeed, most of the visual cells which remain responsive to the deprived eye act in an abnormal way, so that there is a lack of precise receptive-field orientation and a pronounced decline in responsiveness after repeated stimulations.

In the clinical sphere there are several conditions which foster the production of a stimulus deprivation amblyopia in early life, such as dense congenital cataract, extensive corneal opacification resulting from an inflammatory change or more commonly from part of the anterior chamber cleavage syndrome, and ptosis. Ptosis must be sufficient to completely cover the eye, so that it is usually associated with some other abnormality such as a marked hemangioma of the upper lid, since a straightforward congenital ptosis, as a general rule, permits the retention of vision in downward gaze.

When a congenital cataract is complete, insufficient light enters the eye to permit accurate foveal fixation, so that there is a failure of development of fixation in association with the development of an intense stimulus deprivation amblyopia, and usually also of an ocular type of nystagmus. Unfortunately, once these changes are established, technically successful cataract surgery is seldom followed by a satisfactory visual result, even when it is followed by the fitting of a contact lens (particularly when the cataract is of a uniocular nature so that ordinary spectacle lenses are unable to combat the anisometropia which is inevitable in uniocular aphakia), and by the application of intensive occlusion therapy. These clinical findings, in conjunction with the results of experimental occlusion in kittens and young monkeys, therefore infer that there is a critical period in the visual development (including the development of foveal fixation) which is limited to the early weeks of life. This determines success or failure, and it is thus essential to carry out effective treatment at a sufficiently early stage. This emphasizes the necessity of embarking upon surgical treatment of the cataract as soon as possible. The commonly stated difficulty in operating early because of the small size of the eye with a consequently shallow anterior chamber (particularly when there is some degree of microphthalmos) should be disregarded, because this may be overcome by a carefully planned surgical method.

It is essential, however, in advocating such a policy to take due regard of the hazards which may be experienced in its application to a cataract which is part of the rubella syndrome. It is well recognized that a rubella cataract is liable to carry a worse prognosis than an uncomplicated congenital cataract. A recent survey showed an incidence of postoperative complications of 45% in rubella cases (8) as compared with a figure of 5% in nonrubella cases (9). The principal cause of this poor prognosis is a severe and persistent postoperative uveitis, which often assumes the form of an endophthalmitis with a particularly intense anterior uveitis leading to the formation of extensive posterior synechiae, with the attendant risk of a pupil-block glaucoma; to the formation of peripheral anterior synechiae; and in many cases to what appears on superficial examination to be a thick persistent posterior capsule but which is in reality an inflammatory retrolental membrane. The exact cause of this prolonged inflammation is not known with certainty. Dudgeon (10) showed that there is evidence of virus activity within the lens until well into the second year of life. It is therefore reasonable to assume that the endophthalmitis follows a liberation of the infective agent from the lens reservoir into other regions of the eye. It might, therefore, be advisable to postpone cataract surgery in rubella cases until the age of at least 18 months, when the virus is less likely to be active. However, such a policy determines the acceptance of an intractable stimulus deprivation amblyopia, which is a disastrous occurrence when it affects both eyes.

It seems reasonable, therefore, to suggest operating early in a uniocular cataract and on one eye in a bilateral cataract, even when of the rubella type. The second eye in the bilateral cases should be subjected to early surgical treatment only when the first eye has made a satisfactory response (11). It is natural that the concern over stimulus deprivation amblyopia, on the one hand and severe endophthalmitis, on the other hand, in rubella cataract has relegated the technique of the operation to an unimportant role (provided it is carried out adequately), but this is almost certainly an unjustified assumption. It would, of course, be ideal to remove the lens completely by the intracapsular method [and this is a feasible proposition with the availability of chymotrypsin (ZONULYSIN®) and cryosurgery], but this is considered an unwarranted procedure in early childhood because of the liability of vitreous displacement (or loss) even

with faultless technique with, inevitably, short-term and long-term complications. Hence a technique must be adopted which removes as much as possible of the lens material without any disruption of the posterior capsule of the lens and without the delay of several days which is sometimes advocated between opening the anterior lens capsule and removing the lens material, despite the fact that it is technically easier to remove the lens material after such an interval.

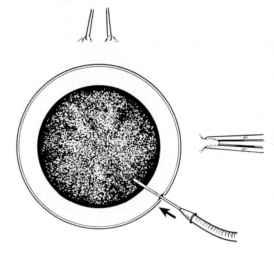

FIG. 1. Aspiration of congenital cataract (stage 1). Insertion of needle attached to reservoir of saline into anterior chamber.

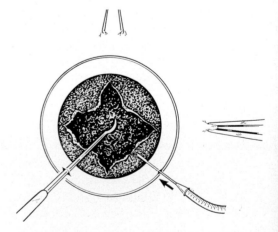

FIG. 2. Aspiration of congenital cataract (stage 2). Opening of anterior lens capsule with discission needle.

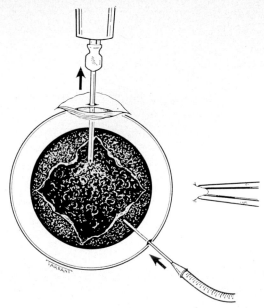

FIG. 3. Aspiration of congenital cataract (stage 3). Aspiration of lens material with Scheie needle.

The following technique offers a satisfactory method of approaching the problem: 1) A needle attached to a reservoir of saline is inserted into the anterior chamber by a limbal approach. The rate of entry of saline into the anterior chamber is readily controlled throughout the operation (Fig. 1). 2) A discission needle is inserted into the anterior chamber by a limbal approach, and the anterior capsule of the lens is opened widely by a cruciate incision so that some of the lens material is brought forward into the anterior chamber (Fig. 2). 3) A Scheie aspiration needle is inserted into the anterior chamber by an *ab externo* approach after the reflection of a conjunctival flap, at 12 o'clock, and the material within the capsule and within the anterior chamber is removed by repeated aspirations while the normal depth of the anterior chamber is maintained by the entry of saline at a controlled rate from the reservoir (Fig. 3).

The treatment of the stimulus deprivation amblyopia following an opacification of the cornea in early life is almost invariably un-

rewarding, because of the difficulty in carrying out a keratoplasty at a sufficiently early stage, quite apart from the fact that in many cases the corneal opacification is only part of the abnormality of the eye. The early establishment of stimulus deprivation amblyopia in corneal opacification is illustrated by a child who sustained an injury to the right eye at birth during a high forceps delivery. The cornea of the right eye was found to be more or less completely opaque when the eyelids opened about three days after birth following a subsidence of edema and hemorrhage. This opacification gradually resolved within a few weeks, and some months later it was limited to two faint deep crescentic linear scars in the nasal part of the cornea and to one more dense deep crescentic linear scar in the temporal part which were the result of localized ruptures of Descemet's membrane. On the temporal side the rupture had been particularly extensive, with the result that the free end of Descemet's membrane was detached and floated within the aqueous of the anterior chamber, with the formation of a triangular-shaped recess between the detached membrane and the overlying corneal stroma. Despite the complete clarity of the rest of the cornea including the whole of the central part there was a marked degree of amblyopia and the unaided vision of 1/60 and N36 improved only to 2/60 and N24 with the correction of a high degree of hypermetropic astigmatism ($+6.00$, $95°$) in the absence of any obvious eccentric fixation. The amblyopia was not essentially of the strabismic type, since there was only a small degree of right exotropia, which was almost certainly secondary to the amblyopia.

The recognition of the likely development of stimulus deprivation amblyopia in early life in a ptosis which is sufficient to cover the eye completely is important, because quite frequently such a case does not come into the province of the ophthalmic surgeon at a suf-

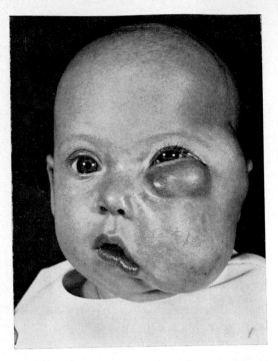

FIG. 4. Hemangioma of the left lower eyelid and cheek at age of three months.

ficiently early stage, particularly when it is complicated by a condition such as a hemangioma of the upper (or lower) eyelid. As a general rule a hemangioma of the eyelid responds best to masterly inactivity because of the spontaneous resolution which almost invariably occurs (Fig. 4–6). When, however, there is a risk of amblyopia, early treatment should be carried out to ensure some degree of opening of the palpebral fissure and this may be achieved by irradiation. A further point of importance in the management of a hemangioma of the eyelid is the likelihood of a sudden increase in the extent of the hemangioma some weeks or even months after birth as the result of a hemorrhage. In such a case, a lesion which is not sufficient to close the eyelids at birth may do so after an interval.

In conclusion, it should be recognized that a form of stimulus deprivation amblyopia may occur when the ocular abnormality is not sufficient to cause a complete "deprivation of

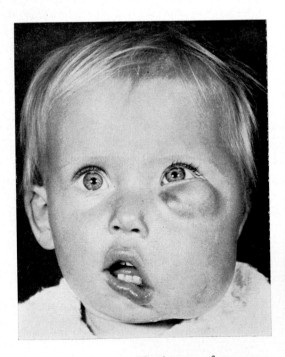

FIG. 5. Case shown in Fig. 4 at age of one year.

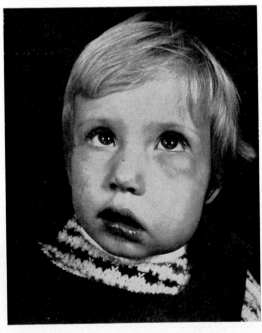

FIG. 6. Case shown in Fig. 4 and 5 at age of three years.

visual stimuli" although it is sufficient to detract from the quality of the retinal image. This is evident particularly in a partial unilateral cataract of congenital origin which frequently carries a poor visual prognosis, akin to that which occurs in a complete cataract, and which is in contrast to the satisfactory result usually obtained in partial bilateral cataracts of congenital origin, even when the surgical treatment is delayed for several years. It is reasonable to assume that the main cause of this distinction between the unilateral and bilateral cases is the failure of the development of adequate fixation in the affected eye in the unilateral cases because of any absence of a significant visual reward from its use. It is possible that some degree of amblyopia of disuse may occur, apart from any failure in the fixation mechanism, simply because of the poverty of the retinal image. In this way it is akin to the amblyopia which occurs in anisometropia and which is essentially the result of passive suppression, in contrast to the active suppression in strabismic amblyopia.

### REFERENCES

1. DE BUFFON GL. Sur la cause du strabismé ou les yeux louches. *Bull Mem Acad Sci* Suppl III, 1743.
2. VON NOORDEN GK and WYBAR KC. Stimulus deprivation amblyopia. *Am J Ophthalmol* **65**: 220, 1968.
3. HUBEL DH and WIESEL TN. Receptive fields of cells in striate cortex of very young, visually inexperienced kittens. *J Neurophysiol* **26**: 994, 1963.
4. HUBEL DH and WIESEL TN. Binocular-interaction in striate cortex of kittens reared with artificial squint. *J Neurophysiol* **28**: 1041, 1965.
5. WIESEL TN and HUBEL DH. Effects of visual deprivation on morphology and physiology of cells in the cat's lateral geniculate body. *J Neurophysiol* **26**: 978, 1963.
6. WIESEL TN and HUBEL DH. Comparison of the effects of unilateral and bilateral eye closure on cortical unit responses in kittens. *J Neurophysiol* **28**: 1029, 1965.
7. VON NOORDEN GK. Current concepts in amblyopia. *First Congr Int Strabismological Assoc, Acapulco, 1970.* London, Henry Kimpton, 1971, p 197.
8. SCHEIE HG, SCHAFFER DB, PLOTKIN SA and KERTESZ ED. Congenital rubella cataracts. Surgical results and virus recovery from intraocular tissue. *Arch Ophthalmol* **77**: 440, 1967.
9. SCHEIE HG, RUBENSTEIN RA and KENT RB. Aspiration of congenital or soft cataract; further experience. *Am J Ophthalmol* **63**: 3, 1967.
10. DUDGEON JA. Congenital cataract: Virological aspects. *Proc R Soc Med* **62**: 693, 1969.
11. HARCOURT RB and WYBAR KC. Congenital cataract: Surgical aspects. *Proc R Soc Med* **62**: 689, 1969.

# PREVENTION OF AMBLYOPIA
## CAUSED BY INCOMPLETE CONGENITAL CATARACT

S. MERIN and J. S. CRAWFORD

Department of Ophthalmology, Hadassah University Hospital, Jerusalem, Israel and Hospital for Sick Children
Toronto, Ontario, Canada

An eye with a complete (or total) congenital cataract may have poor visual acuity even after successful surgery, because of combined strabismic and deprivation amblyopia. It is less well known that an eye with an incomplete (or partial) congenital cataract may be similarly affected.

We recently (1) assessed the influence of the various properties of the incomplete congenital cataract, such as type, size and density, on visual acuity. Our purpose was to predict the visual acuity of the eye with an incomplete congenital cataract at the earliest possible age, and so to distinguish between those eyes which have a good visual prognosis and should be left alone, and those which should be operated on to prevent amblyopia.

We examined 57 patients who were old enough to allow their visual acuity to be measured.

A patient was said to have an incomplete congenital cataract if the cataract had been present since birth or early infancy, and the fundus could be visualized through the clear periphery of the lens. The type of cataract was determined with the help of the slit lamp, and its size with the slit lamp measuring device, by adjusting the length of the slit to the vertical diameter of the cataract. The density of the cataract was determined by a series of filters which were consecutively introduced

between the ophthalmoscope and the examined eye, until the combined density of the cataract and the filter did not allow the fundus to be visualized.

The 57 patients were assigned to two groups: those with unilateral and those with bilateral cataracts.

Twenty of the 23 patients with unilateral incomplete cataract had poor visual acuity. Most could see only hand movements or could just count fingers. The three patients with relatively good visual acuity had small anterior or posterior polar cataracts, the largest of which was 1.5 mm in diameter.

Table 1 shows that the visual acuity in most patients with unilateral incomplete cataract is poor, showing a similar pattern of visual acuity to that found in cases of unilateral complete congenital cataract.

In cases of bilateral, congenital, incomplete cataract, the morphologic type of the cata-

TABLE 1. *Visual acuity in the affected eye of 23 patients with unilateral incomplete congenital cataract*

| No. of patients | Visual acuity |
|---|---|
| 9 | Hand movements |
| 8 | Counting fingers |
| 1 | 6/120 |
| 2 | 6/60 |
| 3 | 6/24 to 6/9 |

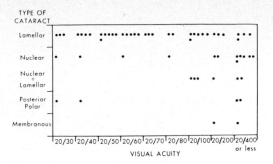

FIG. 1.    Correlation of the morphologic type of incomplete congenital cataract with visual acuity.

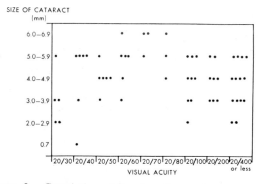

FIG. 2.    Correlation of the size of incomplete congenital cataract with visual acuity.

ract was not related to the resulting visual acuity. For instance, a patient with a lamellar cataract could have any visual acuity between 20/30 and 20/400 (Fig. 1).

The visual acuity unexpectedly bore no relationship to the size of the incomplete cataract. A patient with a 5.5 mm cataract might have almost any visual acuity. Poor visual acuity was found in eyes with large cataracts, and in others with cataracts as small as 2.0 mm (Fig. 2). That visual acuity is unrelated to the size of the cataract can also be proved by comparing the two eyes. In a patient with bilateral lamellar cataracts, the right cataract was 4.3 mm and the left 5.1 mm in diameter. However, the visual acuity was only 6/60 in the right eye, but 6/18 in the left (Fig. 3). Of 17 patients with cataracts of unequal size, seven had better visual acuity in the eye with the larger cataract, seven others in the eye with the smaller cataract, and in three the visual acuity was equal in both eyes.

The one factor clearly related to the visual outcome was the density of the cataract, that

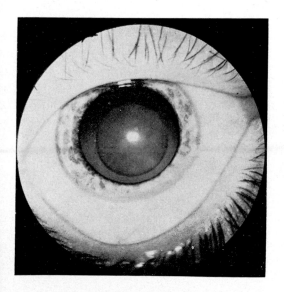
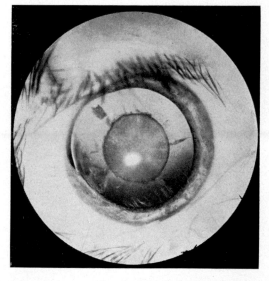

FIG. 3.    Bilateral lamellar cataracts in a patient who had an optical iridectomy in the right eye at the age of six months. The size of the cataract was 4.3 mm in the right and 5.1 mm in the left eye. The visual acuity was 6/60 in the right and 6/18 in the left eye.

469

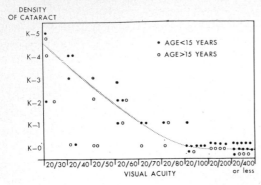

FIG. 4. Correlation of the density of the center of the cataract with visual acuity. The K-number indicates cataracts of different density, K-O being the most dense (when the fundus could not be seen through the lens even without a filter) and K-5 being the least dense cataract. The difference of 1 K-number is about 0.15 NDF. The patients were divided into two age groups.

is, the visual acuity was inversely related to the density of the cataract (Fig. 4). In 18 patients the visual acuity was unequal in the two eyes, and in each case the eye with the denser cataract, as measured by our filters, had the poorer visual acuity. A typical example is shown in Fig. 5.

We found that when the difference in density of the two cataracts was greater than 0.3 neutral density filter (NDF) (2K-filter numbers, see Fig. 4), strabismus with strabismic amblyopia always developed in the eye with the denser cataract even though the absolute density of the more severely affected lens might not be great.

Some of our patients had had an optical iridectomy, which seemed to have little effect on the visual acuity. Even if we assume that the worst cases from the group were chosen for this operation, only a limited number of eyes had good visual acuity as a result. This poor outcome was unrelated to the age at which the operation was performed (Fig. 6). Four patients with bilateral cataracts had optical iridectomy in one eye only, and in all four, the resultant visual acuity was less in the operated eye. Generally, the visual acuity depended on the density of the cataract, and was unrelated to whether an optical iridec-

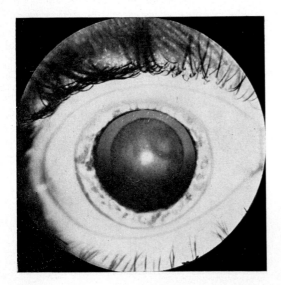 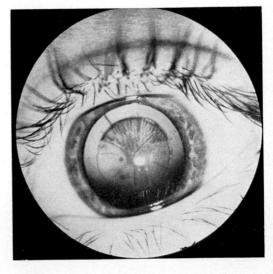

FIG. 5. Bilateral lamellar cataracts of different density. The cataract density was K-3 in the right and K-O in the left eye. The visual acuity was 6/15 in the right and 6/30 in the left eye. The eye with the denser cataract always had the poorer visual acuity.

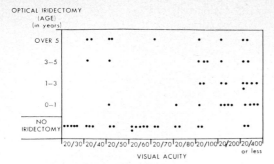

FIG. 6. Effect of optical iridectomy on visual acuity. Twenty-eight of the 37 eyes which had iridectomy have poor visual acuity, an effect not dependent on age at operation. The poorer visual acuity in operated cases is probably due to the fact that the poorer eye was operated on.

tomy was performed or not. Perhaps four or five cases benefited from the iridectomy (Fig. 6).

In summary, this study showed that: 1) The prognosis for the patient with unilateral incomplete cataract is generally as poor as the prognosis for the patient with unilateral complete congenital cataract. If not treated, both will develop monocular strabismus and combined strabismic and deprivation amblyopia. To prevent this, we should possibly follow von Noorden's advice for unilateral complete congenital cataracts, which is to operate very early in life (2). 2) The prognosis for the patient with bilateral incomplete cataract depends mainly on one factor, the density of the cataract. We believe that cataract extraction is indicated when the incomplete cataract is so dense that the fundus cannot be seen through it. Optical iridectomy cannot replace the cataract extraction and, by itself, does not improve the prognosis. 3) When the difference in density of the cataract between the two eyes is more than 2-K filters, or about 0.3 NDF, the eye with the denser cataract will behave like an eye with unilateral incomplete congenital cataract, and develop deep strabismic amblyopia.

## REFERENCES

1. MERIN S and CRAWFORD JS. Assessment of incomplete congenital cataract. *Can J Ophthalmol* (in press).
2. VON NOORDEN GK, RYAN SJ and MAUMENEE AE. Management of congenital cataracts. *Trans Am Acad Ophthalmol Otolaryngol* **74**: 352, 1970.

# SIGNIFICANCE OF NYSTAGMUS IN SUSPECTED BLINDNESS IN INFANCY

KENNETH WYBAR

Hospital for Sick Children, Great Ormond St., London, England

Possible blindness in infancy imposes a great responsibility on the ophthalmic surgeon because of the need to reach a conclusion at an early stage. The term "blindness" is used in a special sense, and is related essentially to the educational potential of the infant. Thus, a blind infant is regarded as one who is going to be dependent on a form of education which does not demand the use of sight. It follows that "blindness" is very variable: from true blindness (no perception of light) to blindness in the presence of quite reasonable peripheral visual function, permitting a considerable degree of independence in certain activities, although not sufficient for educational purposes.

We are here concerned with the role of nystagmus in the complex assessment of cases of suspected blindness in early life. The diagnostic significance of the congenital nystagmus which is present in many such cases and that of the nystagmus induced by visual stimuli (optokinetic nystagmus) are both considered.

Nystagmus which is present in early life is usually referred to as congenital nystagmus. Two distinct forms are distinguished by the rhythm (jerky or pendular) of the series of involuntary movements of the eyes, which constitute the disease.

Congenital jerky nystagmus is characterized by the appearance of a slow component in one direction and a fast component in the other. By convention the nystagmus is defined according to the direction of its fast component although, in fact, this is the recovery movement, and the slow component is the true one. The abnormal ocular oscillations are present to some extent within a few days of birth, but are readily overlooked so that their recognition may be delayed for several weeks or even months, until they become more obvious. It is usual for the nystagmus to continue in a marked form for a few years, but eventually it becomes less evident so that by early adult life it may be relatively slight. Even then there is a tendency at times for the nystagmus to assume its original prominent form, particularly in conditions of stress. A congenital jerky nystagmus is present in all positions of gaze (horizontal and vertical) but the direction of the nystagmus is almost invariably horizontal. A characteristic feature is that in one or more positions of gaze, there is a reduction in the nystagmus (the so-called "neutral zone") so that an attempt is made to utilize this point when looking at an object straight ahead by the adoption of a compensatory head posture with a transference of the "neutral zone" to a straight ahead position (Fig. 1). The mechanism concerned in the production of a congenital jerky nystagmus

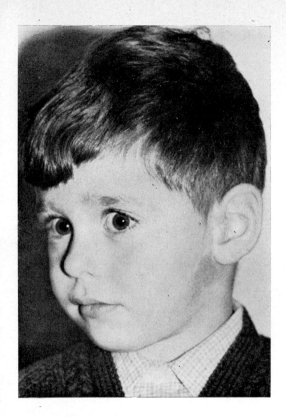

FIG. 1. Compensatory head posture in a child with congenital idiopathic nystagmus.

is not established, hence the frequent use of the attribute "idiopathic." It is, however, reasonable to regard the causative lesion as lying in the complex nervous mechanisms in the brain stem which are concerned in the centering and in the "steady fixation" of the eyes. Thus the nystagmus may be regarded as the result of an exaggeration of the fine persistent movements of the eyes (slow motion random drifts, rapid impulsive saccades which correct the position of the foveal image after the random drifts, and fine tremors) which occur during "steady" fixation, and which are essential to the maintenance of the perception of the retinal image.

A determination of the true nature of this form of nystagmus is of great importance because its development in early childhood quite frequently creates the impression of a gross impairment of vision. In fact, the long-term prognosis is surprisingly good, with a reasonable level of distant vision, particularly in the presence of an effective "neutral zone" and with a good level of reading vision, provided that the child is allowed to hold the print sufficiently near the eyes. In this instance, there is an almost invariable reduction in the nystagmus which occurs in a position of extreme convergence quite apart from the magnification which is provided in such a position of disjunctive gaze.

Congenital pendular nystagmus is characterized by the occurrence of rhythmic horizontal pendular oscillations which are equal in speed in both directions so that there is no distinction of slow and fast components. This is maintained when the eyes are looking forward, upward or downward and also to some extent on looking laterally. However, beyond a certain position of lateral gaze, the pendular oscillations tend to become replaced by jerky ones in which the fast component is in the direction of the lateral gaze (1). Despite the congenital nature of the nystagmus it is seldom evident in the early weeks of life because its apparent onset coincides with the usual time of the establishment of the fixation reflex. The determination of this form of nystagmus is of great importance because its development in early childhood signifies the presence of some underlying visual defect of a fairly severe form. It is unfortunate that congenital pendular nystagmus is sometimes included in the "idiopathic" category when there is no evidence of any obvious lesion of the eyes or the afferent visual pathways in infancy to account for it. This, of course, is in contrast to the congenital jerky nystagmus when the prefix "idiopathic" is legitimate, because it seldom proves to be of a progressive nature.

There are several conditions which cause visual impairment (or even blindness) in infancy and yet which elude detection. These

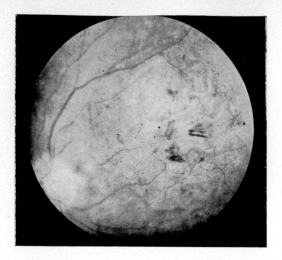

FIG. 2. Macular dystrophy as part of tapetoretinal degeneration.

include tapetoretinal degeneration, congenital cone dysfunction and ocular albinism.

Tapetoretinal degeneration is readily diagnosed on ophthalmoscopic examination when it shows the typical features of a retinitis pigmentosa. However, in the congenital form of the condition (Leber's amaurosis or retinal aplasia) there is frequently little or no abnormality of the fundi in the early stages, despite gross visual impairment or even blindness. In such cases the determination of the electroretinogram (ERG) is of critical importance in establishing the diagnosis because a diminution or extinction of the ERG response reflects the retinal dysfunction. The ERG only provides information about the outer retinal layers (retinal receptors and bipolar cells), and it represents to some extent a mass response. Thus, it may be normal unless more than half of the retina is defective. Special techniques are necessary in applying this electrodiagnostic method to young children (2). Tapetoretinal degeneration in early childhood may be present as a pigmentary disturbance of the macular area which suggests a macular dystrophy (Fig. 2). The more widespread involvement of the retina may become apparent only some years later in such a case, unless recourse is made to the ERG at an early stage.

Congenital cone dysfunction leads to gross disturbance of central vision in early childhood, although peripheral vision is spared because of the unimpaired function of the retinal rods. This is a difficult condition to diagnose because of the absence of any ophthalmoscopic abnormality. The ERG is also normal. However, the abnormal function of the retina is determined by a low ERG fusion frequency in response to a flickering light source.

Albinism is a readily recognized condition when it is of a generalized nature. There is almost invariably well-marked pendular nystagmus because the defective pigmentation of the eye as a whole causes a marked scattering of light rays within the eye so that the development of steady fixation fails. The diagnosis, however, is readily overlooked when albinism is partial and confined to the eye (ocular albinism), particularly as the characteristic light pigmentation of the fundus is quite frequently a normal feature in early childhood. It is therefore essential to examine the region of the root of the iris by retroillumination in order to detect the characteristic translucency of ocular albinism.

Optokinetic nystagmus may be regarded as a form of ocular movement activated by the visual cortex. In addition the adjacent areas also play an important role because a loss of function of the angular gyrus abolishes the optokinetic response. The brain stem "centers," particularly the reticular formation, are involved in quantitative integration of the optokinetic afferents. A relatively small lesion in the brain stem may thus be sufficient to abolish the ipsilateral optokinetic response. The presence of an optokinetic response is evidence of some form of visual function. It may, however, be attained even in the presence of a fairly gross retinal lesion. This is at variance

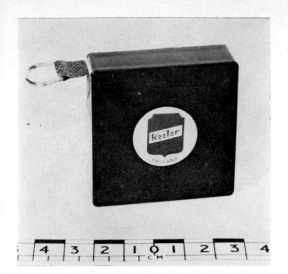

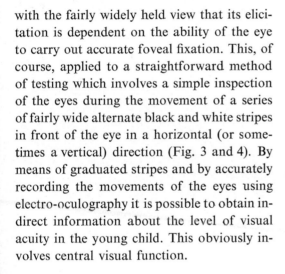

FIG. 3. Simple appliance for activating optokinetic nystagmus.

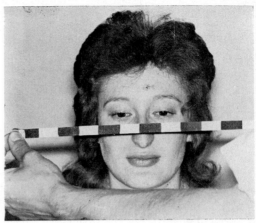

FIG. 4. Elicitation of optokinetic nystagmus.

with the fairly widely held view that its elicitation is dependent on the ability of the eye to carry out accurate foveal fixation. This, of course, applied to a straightforward method of testing which involves a simple inspection of the eyes during the movement of a series of fairly wide alternate black and white stripes in front of the eye in a horizontal (or sometimes a vertical) direction (Fig. 3 and 4). By means of graduated stripes and by accurately recording the movements of the eyes using electro-oculography it is possible to obtain indirect information about the level of visual acuity in the young child. This obviously involves central visual function.

An optokinetic response is not obtained consistently in the normal infant (certainly under the age of three months). It is essential for the visual stimulus to be of a type which excites recognition and for the subject to show a sufficient degree of attentiveness. The absence of an optokinetic response in early infancy on random testing should therefore be regarded with caution.

REFERENCES

1. HARCOURT RB.   Hereditary nystagmus in early childhood. *J Med Genetics* **7**: 253, 1970.
2. WYBAR KC and HARCOURT RB.   Role of electroretinography in investigation of impaired visual function in children. *Arch Dis Child* **43**: 658, 1968.

# EXPERIMENTAL AMBLYOPIA

## GUNTER K. VON NOORDEN

Wilmer Institute of Ophthalmology, Johns Hopkins University Medical School and Hospital,
Baltimore, Maryland, USA

Clinical, psychophysical and electrophysiologic data that have become available during the past 15 years have greatly enhanced our understanding of functional amblyopia and have shown it to be a complex disturbance of sensory and motor visual functions (1). Stimulus deprivation amblyopia has been studied less extensively than other conditions in the clinical laboratory because it is less frequently encountered in clinical practice. In addition, in spite of intensive study in the clinical laboratory, the basic seat and mechanism of amblyopia in human beings have remained virtually unknown.

Before discussing some of the more recent advances of basic research in this field and before defining the problems involved, we should clarify whether the various forms of amblyopia are caused by different cortical or subcortical mechanisms, or are merely

TABLE 1.  *Eliciting mechanisms in various forms of amblyopia*

| Type | Cause | Reversibility | Onset |
|---|---|---|---|
| Strabismic a. | Abnormal cortical interaction from different forms | Yes | Birth to 5 years |
| Anisometropic a. | 1. Abnormal cortical interaction from images of different optical quality<br>2. Form vision deprivation of the more ametropic eye with anisohypermetropia | Yes | Birth to 5 years |
| *Amblyopia ex anopsia*<br>Unilateral | 1. Abnormal cortical interaction from normal input through sound eye and "white noise" from deprived eye<br>2. Arrest of visual development or deterioration of innate visual functions | Partially | Birth to 5 years (?) |
| Bilateral | 1. Normal cortical interaction<br>2. Arrest of visual development or deterioration of innate visual functions | No | ? |
| Ametropia a. | 1. Normal cortical interaction<br>2. Mild form of visual deprivation | Yes | ? |

expressions of the same kinds of defect with different degrees of severity and reversibility.

Table 1 summarizes the causes for each condition and shows that one must differentiate between the effects of abnormal cortical interaction caused by differences in input from the two eyes and the effects of total lack of (or abnormally decreased) stimulation of one or both eyes. It is not known at this time to what degree these factors interact and, perhaps, augment the severity of one or the other clinical condition. However, such information is of vital importance to improve our understanding of amblyopia, and, it is hoped, eventually also our therapeutic methods.

## NEUROPHYSIOLOGIC STUDIES

Recently, developments in the basic sciences have made it possible to analyze excitatory and inhibitory neuronal activity in the cortical and subcortical centers of lower animals by means of intracellular recordings from microelectrodes inserted into the visual cortex or the lateral geniculate nucleus. With the advent of the electron microscope, it has also become possible to analyze the normal and abnormal ultrastructure of the central nervous system. Such research has already ascertained the neuron basis for binocular depth discrimination and retinal correspondence in the cat and monkey (2–4), has supplied evidence of a severe cortical functional anomaly in experimentally produced exotropia in cats (5), and is likely within the next decade to produce additional important information about other forms of experimentally produced strabismus in animals.

Basic research related to amblyopia has, in the past, been concerned mainly with the effects of various types of deprivation on the visual system. Only the changes produced by unilateral lid closure are here discussed, since this experimental condition is most likely to be comparable to similar clinical situations in man. Such experiments have been performed for more than 100 years (6) and have included neurophysiologic, physiologic, behavioral and biochemical studies.

Of special interest are the classical experiments of Wiesel and Hubel (7–11). After closing one eye by lid sutures in visually immature kittens during the first three months of life, these authors demonstrated profound functional changes in the visual cortex. Only a few cortical cells from the deprived eye could be activated and the majority responded only to stimulus from the normal eye. In the normal cat about 80% of the cortical cells from which recordings can be obtained are activated by either eye. These profound effects due to uniocular deprivation of vision were irreversible in kittens, and could not be produced in adult animals.

However, these findings cannot be transferred uncritically to explain the seat and mechanism of amblyopia ex anopsia in humans, since there are morphological and functional differences in the organization of the visual system in different vertebrate species. The monkey is a more appropriate model for visual comparison with man. Similar unpublished studies in our laboratories were performed by Dr. F. Baker on Rhesus monkeys. Amblyopia ex anopsia was produced by tarsorrhaphy after birth indicating that the neurophysiological defect described by Wiesel and Hubel (7–11) in cats not only occurs in primates as well, but may, in fact, be more severe. Of 40 cells in the striate cortex from which recordings were obtained through stimulation of the nondeprived eye, not a single unit responded to moving patterns in front of the deprived eye.

## MORPHOLOGIC STUDIES

In view of the severity of these defects of cortical function, one would expect to find their morphological equivalent by histological studies of the tissues involved. Indeed, with the light microscope, Wiesel and Hubel (7) and

**477**

Kupfer and Palmer (12) observed a marked decrease in the size of cells in all layers of the lateral geniculate body that received input from the deprived eye. However, no cortical morphologic changes were observed with the light microscope.

It is reasonable to assume that synapses, as the prime sites of neuron activity in the visual cortex, would be most likely to show morphological alterations in amblyopia. We recently completed a preliminary electron microscopic study of synaptic density and morphology in the visual cortex of a monkey with behaviorally proved amblyopia ex anopsia; and compared our observations with data obtained from comparable tissue of a normal monkey (13). Density and morphology of synapses were identical in comparable sections from cortical area 17 and 18 of both specimens. Thus, we were unable to identify the morphologic substrate for the severe functional cortical anomalies demonstrated by neurophysiological methods in animals deprived of form vision during visual immaturity, nor could we confirm anomalies of the cortical morphology described in such animals by other authors (14–18).

Current electron microscopic investigations in our laboratory are concerned with a more comprehensive study of the visual cortex, the lateral geniculate body and the retina of unilaterally visually deprived monkeys, in an effort to find the morphological substrate for disturbed function in this condition.

### BEHAVIORAL STUDIES

In a behavioral study of visually deprived monkeys we have performed unilateral lid closure in 10 Rhesus monkeys at various ages, in order to define the critical time at which interference with normal form vision stimulation no longer causes amblyopia (19). The animals were behaviorally trained by using the nondeprived eye to respond to Landolt rings of different sizes until visual acuity could

478

be determined. The previously closed eye was then opened, tarsorrhaphy was performed on the sound eye, and testing of the amblyopic eye was resumed. Severe forms of amblyopia can be produced in the monkey if lid closure is performed between birth and six weeks of age. Partial recovery occurred with lid closure between eight weeks and three months, while complete recovery occurred if the lid closure was performed at one year or older. Thus, the age of highest susceptibility to form vision deprivation in Rhesus monkeys is between birth and six weeks. Further behavioral study of this condition in monkeys should provide us with data that may be helpful in the evaluation of clinical situations in human beings by defining the exact age interval during which the primate's visual system is most sensitive to form vision deprivation.

### EXPERIMENTAL STRABISMUS

Whereas information regarding the basic mechanisms in form vision deprivation amblyopia is thus rapidly accumulating, the application of modern research techniques to the problem of strabismic amblyopia has in the past not been possible, since a suitable nonhuman model was lacking. The need arose to produce strabismic amblyopia in a species whose visual system is sufficiently similar to that of human beings to permit possible application of experimental data to clinical situations in man. We were able to produce strabismic amblyopia in two animals who were experimentally made esotropic during the first week of life (20). Amblyopia did not occur in a third monkey with an onset of artificially produced esotropia at age 17 months. Likewise, amblyopia could not be produced in two exotropic monkeys, one with an experimental onset of exotropia at age six days, and the other at age six months. The exotropic animals had developed an alternating fixation pattern. Thus, in these experiments, it appears that the time of onset of esotropia and the type of strabismus (esotropia or exotropia) are significant factors in determining whether amblyopia develops. This behavior is strikingly similar to that observed in the human strabismic patient in whom a direct relation exists between the occurrence of amblyopia, the age of onset of esotropia and the presence of a unilateral or an alternating fixation pattern. With these experiments a useful model has become available for further laboratory investigation. Further exploration of experimental amblyopia by modern neurophysiologic methods and by electron microscopy in monkeys may be of fundamental importance in improving our understanding of the site and mechanisms of similar disturbances in human beings.

Supported in part by Research Grant EY-00274 from the National Eye Institute, Bethesda, Maryland.

## REFERENCES

1. VON NOORDEN GK. Current concepts of amblyopia (Bielschowsky Lecture). *First Cong Int Strabismological Assoc.* London, Henry Kimpton, 1971, p 197.
2. BARLOW HB, BLAKEMORE C and PETTIGREW JD. The neural mechanism of binocular depth discrimination. *J Physiol* **193**: 327, 1967.
3. NIKARA T, BISHOP PO and PETTIGREW JD. Analysis of retinal correspondence by studying receptive fields of binocular single units in cat striate cortex. *Exp Brain Res* **6**: 353, 1968.
4. HUBEL DH and WIESEL TN. Stereoscopic vision in macaque monkey: cells sensitive to binocular depth in area 18 of the macaque monkey cortex. *Nature (Lond)* **225**: 41, 1970.
5. HUBEL DH and WIESEL TN. Binocular interaction in striate cortex of kittens reared with artificial squint. *J Neurophysiol* **28**: 1041, 1965.
6. GUDDEN B. Experimentaluntersuchungen über das peripherische und centrale Nervensystem. *Arch Psychiatr Nervenkr* **2**: 693, 1870.
7. WIESEL TN and HUBEL DH. Effects of visual deprivation on morphology and physiology of cells in the cat's lateral geniculate body. *J Neurophysiol* **26**: 978, 1963.
8. WIESEL TN and HUBEL DH. Single-cell responses in striate cortex of kittens deprived of vision in one eye. *J Neurophysiol* **26**: 1003, 1963.
9. WIESEL TN and HUBEL DH. Comparison of the effects of unilateral and bilateral eye closure on cortical unit responses in kittens. *J Neurophysiol* **28**: 1029, 1965.
10. WIESEL TN and HUBEL DH. Extent of recovery from the effects of visual deprivation in kittens. *J Neurophysiol* **28**: 1060, 1965.
11. HUBEL DH and WIESEL TN. The period of susceptibility to the physiological effects of unilateral eye closure in kittens. *J Physiol (Lond)* **206**: 419, 1970.
12. KUPFER C and PALMER P. Lateral geniculate nucleus: histological and cytochemical changes following afferent denervation and visual deprivation. *Exp Neurol* **9**: 400, 1964.
13. VON NOORDEN GK and DOWLING JE. Electronmicroscopic findings in the visual cortex of a form vision deprived monkey (preliminary report). *National Meeting of the Association for Research in Vision and Ophthalmology, Sarasota, Fla, 1971* (in press).
14. GLOBUS A and SCHEIBEL AB The effect of visual deprivation on cortical neurons: A Golgi study. *Exp Neurol* **19**: 331, 1967.
15. VALVERDE F. Apical dendritic spines of the visual cortex and light deprivation in the mouse. *Exp Brain Res* **3**: 337, 1967.
16. CRAGG BG. The effects of vision and dark-rearing on the size and density of synapses in the lateral geniculate nucleus measured by electronmicroscopy. *Brain Res* **13**: 53, 1969.
17. FIFKOVA E. The effect of unilateral deprivation on visual centers in rats. *J Comp Neurol* **140**: 431, 1970.
18. FIFKOVA E. Changes of axosomatic synapses in the visual cortex of monocularly deprived rats. *J Neurobiol* **2**: 61, 1970.
19. VON NOORDEN GK, DOWLING JE and FERGUSON DC. Experimental amblyopia in monkeys. I. Behavioral studies of stimulus deprivation amblyopia. *Arch Ophthalmol* **84**: 206, 1970.
20. VON NOORDEN GK and DOWLING JE. Experimental amblyopia in monkeys. II. Behavioral studies in strabismic amblyopia. *Arch Ophthalmol* **84**: 215, 1970.

# DISCUSSION

*Question from the floor*: How do you diagnose amblyopia in a child who may just need glasses?

DR. I. NAWRATZKI (*Israel*): After a complete eye examination and prescription of glasses if necessary, we check the cover test again after the child has worn the spectacles for a certain time. If he again shows a difference in behavior when covering the "good" eye, amblyopia is diagnosed.

*Question from the floor*: Is it necessary or desirable while patching a better eye in treating amblyopia, to give the eye a rest and leave both eyes open one day a week?

DR. NAWRATZKI: When treating a strabismic amblyopic eye by patching the better eye, we occlude the amblyopic eye at certain intervals but do not leave both eyes open at any time.

DR. A. E. SLOANE (*USA*): This is the method I follow when I want to permit the other eye to be used.

DR. G. K. VON NOORDEN (*USA*): I agree with both participants, and would like to add that this is not only desirable but utterly necessary if you include children up to the age of four-and-a-half. We have seen several instances where a fixating eye has been made permanently amblyopic by being occluded for too long without the fixation and vision being checked in between.

*Question from the floor*: Is patching for a few hours a day sufficient?

Dr. NAWRATZKI: This may be sufficient in the very small child under six months of age. In the older child, part time occlusion is indicated only in cases without strabismus.

DR. SLOANE: This, of course, has to be tailored to each individual case. In strabismus, certainly,

a couple of hours a day is quite worthless. In situations where there is no strabismus involved, where the visual acuity is at a fair level and where there is an attempt at binocularity, one can succeed with shorter periods. But the short periods are not nearly as helpful.

DR. NAWRATZKI: It is difficult to give a definite answer without taking into account other factors such as ametropia, etc.

DR. VON NOORDEN: If a 13-year-old child came to your office with an amblyopia which had never been treated before, would you treat it by occlusion or would you consider this child too old for improvement?

DR. NAWRATZKI: With a small-angle strabismus and eccentric fixation, I would still treat him by occlusion of the good eye; if necessary, and if he agrees, with an inverse prism in front of the amblyopic eye.

DR. VON NOORDEN: I have yet to see a child agree to any type of occlusion.

DR. SLOANE: Since our predictability of who can be helped and who cannot be helped is still not well defined, I never write off anybody as being in a hopeless situation without giving him a good trial. I vividly recall one youngster who, I thought, had strabismus and who, I felt, would never make any headway with occlusion. Some time later, he had an arrow shot into his good eye and his vision returned to 20/20. I am sure that if I had insisted, his vision could have been brought up before.

DR. VON NOORDEN: I certainly think that we should try therapy in children up to the age of 13 or 14 if they have never been treated before, even though I think everyone in the field will agree that the chances for success are extremely limited. But we have occasionally seen children over the age of ten improve two or three lines with occlusion treatment. I think, actually, that probably everyone, even an adult, would improve after prolonged occlusion, but it becomes a matter of inconvenience and social acceptance. These teenagers are very self-conscious and will just not put up with patching.

*Question from the floor*: Would you elaborate on the differentiation between functional and organic amblyopia?

DR. VON NOORDEN: We use two tests. The dark-filter test, which was originally used by Amman in Switzerland and reintroduced by Burian and myself for clinical ophthalmology, is of some value in differentiating between functional and organic components in a mild case of amblyopia. We use neutral density filter test No. 96 from Kodak with No. 2 and No. 0.5 neutral density filters mounted together between two pieces of glass. We hold them over the amblyopic eye for one minute. We then retest vision, and when this is drastically reduced, organic amblyopia is indicated. The other test is the binocular visual acuity test where we measure the visual acuity of the amblyopic eye while the healthy eye is open. This can be done with the haploscope described by Aulhorn, which I am sure not many of you have. There are only about three or four in existence. But you can use any type of polaroid image separation technique to test visual acuity monocularly while the other eye is open; we have usually found that in functional amblyopia, there is a considerable reduction in visual acuity of the amblyopic eye when the sound eye receives stimuli. This is not present in organic amblyopia.

*Question from the floor*: What is the true significance of hypermetropia in strabismus of early onset?

DR. NAWRATZKI: In our screening, we found a large percentage of high hypermetropia in amblyopic children, which may be statistically significant.

DR. VON NOORDEN: I suppose the questioner wants to know how often hypermetropia is of etiological significance in strabismus of very early onset, presumably between birth and six months of age. It is said that true accommodating strabismus characteristically occurs between the ages of two and three years. We have occasionally seen patients with congenital strabismus who had a significant hypermetropic refractive error and who, after correction, were orthophoric. These cases are rare but they do exist. However, hypermetropia usually does not play an important role in the etiology of congenital or early infantile squint.

DR. E. NEUMANN (*Israel*): The most significant factor in the etiology of strabismus in the 104 children fully investigated by us was hypermetropia. High hypermetropia was present in 18.4% and moderate hypermetropia in 30.7% of the 65 esotropias. This compares to 0.7% high hypermetropias and 5.8% moderate hypermetropias found among 600 eyes of newborn infants in the Haifa area (S. Zonis and B. Miller, personal communication).

Since it was recently found that most infants are born with a spastic accommodation which gradually resolves during the first six months of life (HAYNES H, WHITE BL and HELD R. *Science* **148**: 528, 1965), it seems logical to assume that accommodation does play an important role in the etiology of squint, even when congenital.

DR. SLOANE: When a child presents with strabismus and it is necessary to perform a complete cycloplegic refraction, I would have the mother put the drops into the fixing eye for several days. Assuming that I gave the appointment for two months hence, the mother would use the drops in the fixing eye, alone, for up to two days before the examination and then use it in both eyes. If during this period the atropine in one eye was sufficient to cause a fixation shift, I would know that the amblyopia would probably not be very deep, but if the strabismus did not alternate and go over into the nonatropinized eye, it would give me an idea of what was happening.

*Question from the floor*: What background luminence is used in the contrastoscope and what effect does the given change in background luminence have on your threshold findings?

DR. I. RÉTHY (*Nigeria*): The background illumination must strongly contrast with the light spots. We didn't measure the exact background illumination. Examination was done in a half darkened room and the light spots originated from a 200 w light. The contrast was so great that it did not matter if the room was completely dark, semidarkened or almost light.

To hold a child's attention to the light, we

begin with the larger lights and, to make sure the child is interested and responding to the test, we begin with the lights very close to the child and gradually move them back to 5 m from him. This test may also be important for the course of treatment. If the light sensitivity was first low, and the child then begins to see more light spots, it can be deduced that his prognosis is improving. This examination also directly indicates when to change from inverse to conventional occlusion. Sometimes inverse occlusion produces extreme changes in the light sense and in the behavior of the eccentrically fixating eye. Fixation may not become central immediately, and the child must learn to fixate. If amblyopia began very early and the child has never had the experience of fixating, he may relapse if the occlusion is changed abruptly from inverse to conventional, and then the amblyopic eye must again be occluded.

*Question from the floor*: Would you operate on a 10-year-old child with 20 degree convergence without glasses but fully corrected with glasses?

DR. VON NOORDEN: I certainly would not consider operating on such a child. He should be treated with glasses and not by surgery.

MR. K. WYBAR (*U.K.*): One would want to know what the measurement was for near distance and one would certainly want to know the refractive error. Now, one would assume that if this child s virtually orthophoric but wearing glasses for near distances, then the child must be considerably hypermetropic. If it remains with a 20 degree convergent squint without glasses, its binocular function cannot be perfect, and I would therefore agree not to operate because the child would probably develop a secondary divergence.

DR. RÉTHY: In my opinion, squint is a form of behavior and I would try to teach the child not to use his accommodation. Even if I find no refractive error after the use of atropine, there may be a high hypermetropic error not paralyzed by atropine and, with an overcorrection, the child may slowly learn to disaccommodate.

DR. NAWRATZKI: I want to ask Dr. Rethy if he does not get an adverse reaction. We often find that overcorrecting a hypermetropic patient or atropinizing him might cause the child to try to overcome the blurring by accommodation and more convergence.

DR. RÉTHY: The hypercorrection must be very, very carefully done and the child must be given a reward, otherwise the optical blur is a stimulus to accommodate.

*Question from the floor*: You are an ophthalmologist without orthoptic facilities in an understaffed country. How do you manage in the case of squint in a two-year-old child without any anomaly of the media, with special reference to the indication and timing of surgery?

MR. WYBAR: I would rely personally to a tremendous extent on the cover test. You can diagnose manifest and latent squints, and the degree of recovery will give you information about the fusional reserve and so on. You can assess how much your operation has done and also the angle of the squint.

DR. VON NOORDEN: Provided, of course, that the child is nonamblyopic, I would agree that you do not need an orthoptist to arrive at your sort of indication. All you need is a box full of prisms and your own hands to perform the prism cover test to measure the angle.

DR. E. AUERBACH (*Israel*): This is not really a question but a point I want to put forward. I am not astonished that there was practically no difference in the density of striate synapsis after monocular deprivation. This is the view expressed by Bishop, who found that practically all striate neutrons had a bilateral input. We confirmed this in our laboratory.

DR. VON NOORDEN: Yes, I would essentially agree with this theory, and the reason we did this study was mainly to use the electron microscope and look at the cortex. There have been many papers published in the past five years reporting more or less severe anomalies of the cortical spines, crippling of cortical spines, absence of cortical neurons and decrease of density of the cortical synapsis. I am referring mainly to the work of Globus and others.

*Question from the floor*: Would Dr. Wybar not agree that the electroretinogram (ERG) is meaningful only with visual evoked responses (VER)?

MR. WYBAR: I was talking about the tapetoretinal degeneration, i.e., the degeneration of the outer half of the retina. If it is sufficiently advanced, then it will show in the ERG test. You will have either an absence or a diminution of response. In the assessment of children with suspected blindness, the ERG should be combined with the VER, because you may be dealing with a condition in which you may have a normal ERG. For example, you may have optic atrophy and a perfectly normal ERG, but you will have diminished or lost cortical responses.

*Question from the floor*: Up to what age does Mr. Wybar advocate the aspiration technique for congenital cataracts featured in his film?

MR. WYBAR: I don't really think that there is any upper age limit for this, as long as you do not want to do it by the intracapsular method.

DR. VON NOORDEN: I think that the operation should be done as early as possible. We have now operated on several children at the age of two weeks, and operated on the other eye at the age of four weeks. By age six weeks they were wearing contact lenses. This can be done and I think it should be done in the presence of a complete cataract as early as you see this patient. As to the management of the rubella cataract, Mr. Wybar cited the figures of Scheie, according to which 45% develop severe intraocular complications. There are other figures published, including those from our Institute, which clearly contradict this experience. We have operated on a similarly large series of biologically proven rubella cataracts, and in our series we had only 5% intraocular complications. This was also reported by Boniuk. Therefore, in my opinion there is no reason to delay surgery even in the presence of rubella cataract.

*Question from the floor*: At what interval would you operate on the second eye in the case of a bilateral congenital cataract?

MR. WYBAR: If you have operated on one eye and the other one also needs an operation, you can do it shortly afterwards. I think you get your endophthalmitis or uveitis in the rubella cataract in a week at the most, and within two to three days the eye will start to show that it is reacting unfavorably. I personally wait a few weeks but I think it perfectly safe to operate after a week.

*Question from the floor*: Would you operate on a child five years old with bilateral congenital cataract and visual acuity 6/24 in each eye?

MR. WYBAR: Near visual acuity would guide me entirely on whether to operate on this child. If a child has bilateral lamellar cataracts with vision of 6/24 it will almost certainly have N5; and if the child has N5, he has enough vision to be educated in the normal way. He may need a certain amount of help as far as blackboards are concerned, but I am sure that a child is much better off with his vision without operation than relying on aphakic correction even with the use of contact lenses. If, on the other hand, the near visual acuity is not good because of the cataract, that would be an indication to operate. In order to get a satisfactory result, you would have to operate on both eyes.

DR. VON NOORDEN: I think it is not only the level of near vision but the way the child handles himself in school that is important. In the case of a partial congenital cataract, we should inquire carefully of the parents how much this child is excluded from normal activities with his peers in school, and we would base the time of surgery on that. There are many children with 6/30 who do very well at school until the age of eight or nine and suddenly find themselves unable to do certain things. This is then the time to operate. In a partial congenital cataract we don't have to fear amblyopia except, of course, when it exceeds a certain density. I would rather have the parents come and ask me to operate than push surgery on such a child. This is in contrast to complete congenital cataracts which, of course, should be operated upon immediately.

CORNI
CORN

S

Department of C

The maintenance o
tion resides in the e
serves both as a ph
fluid influx and as a
ling induced by ou
pump is involved in
mediated electrolyt
therefore of interest
changes occur in t
dothelial pump is a
swells. This questio
in previous studies
electrolyte concentr
whole layers of cor
bated in a changing
humor of an enuc
rabbit cornea, with
maintains normal tl
thelial surface is ba
fined medium (1).
preparation is an ex
ing the transendothe
lytes taking place d
The cornea obta
metabolism of gluco
plied from the aqueq
calculation of the
across the endotheli
bility coefficient for g
ular size, has show

# BASIC LABORATORY STUDIES

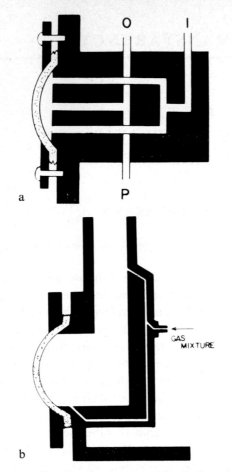

FIG. 1. Chambers for the corneal incubation. a) Perfusion chamber; I, inlet of perfusate; O, outlet of perfusate; P, connection to a manometer system. b) Bathing chamber. (Reproduced with permission from ref. 40).

*Incubation in a perfusion chamber.* After the cornea was clamped into a perfusion chamber (Fig. 1a), the specimen was placed in a moist chamber attached to a constant temperature water bath. The artificial anterior chamber behind the cornea was perfused with KEI medium (1) at a pH of 7.3 and an osmolarity of 303 mOsm/liter. Bicarbonate-Ringer's buffer was used for glucose transport studies. For experiments performed at body temperature, the cornea was maintained at 33 to 34 C. For low temperature experiments, the corneal temperature was maintained at 3 to 4 C.

*Incubation in a bathing chamber.* For glucose transport studies, the isolated cornea was held in a bathing chamber (Fig. 1b), and the whole specimen placed inside the moist chamber described above. The bathing medium, which consisted of 5 ml of bicarbonate-Ringer's solution containing glucose at a concentration of 6.7 mmoles/liter was circulated by bubbling through it a gas mixture consisting of 5% $CO_2$, 7% $O_2$ and 88% $N_2$. The pH of the medium was 7.3 and the osmolarity 296 mOsm/liter. The corneal temperature was maintained at 33 to 34 C.

*Removal of the epithelium and measurement of corneal thickness.* In some experiments the epithelium was removed prior to incubation. This was carried out by crushing the epithelium with rotating sandpaper and removing the cells with a scalpel. Corneal thickness was measured at various intervals during the incubation with a Maurice-Giardini pachometer (10).

*Measurement of corneal hydration.* After incubation, the cornea was removed from the chamber, with special precautions being taken to avoid evaporation or condensation of water. The epithelium and endothelium were scraped off and a stromal button was punched out with a trephine 9 mm in diameter. The button was placed in a small flask and tightly stoppered. Samples were weighed before and after desiccation *in vacuo* over $P_2O_5$ at 60 C for 24 hr. Hydration was expressed as the ratio of wet weight to dry weight.

*Electrolyte studies.* Measurement of electrolyte concentrations: After measuring the corneal hydration, an appropriate volume of extracting solution was pipetted into the flasks containing the dehydrated corneas. The extracting solution contained 0.1 N nitric acid, 10% glacial acetic acid and 250 ppm of lithium (Baird Atomic Inc., Cambridge, Mass.). The concentrations of sodium and potassium were determined in a Baird Atomic flame photometer, model KY 1, using an internal standard. Before each determination a recovery test was carried out using KEI medium. Chloride concentration was measured in a Buchler-Cotlove chloridometer (Buchler Instruments, Fort Lee, N.J.). For all three substances the extracting solution itself was used as a control for checking the zero concentration.

Measurement of evaporation from the cornea: During the perfusion of the cornea at body temperature (33 to 34 C), the anterior surface of the moist chamber was maintained at room temperature. Therefore, evaporation of water from the cornea and subsequent condensation on the inner surface of the moist chamber took place. This resulted in an increase in electrolyte concentration, the precise amount being estimated with Blue Dextran (Pharmacia, Uppsala) according to the method of Riley (11).

*Glucose transport studies.* Assay of radioactivity: The isotopes used for studies on transport across the endothelium were 3-O-methyl-$C^{14}$-glucose ($C^{14}$-MG) (specific activity, 10 mc/mmole) and $C^{14}$-L-glucose (specific activity 9.8 mc/mmole); both were obtained from the New England Nuclear Corp., Boston, Mass. The radioactivities of the bathing medium and of the perfusate were measured with a Tri-Carb liquid scintillation counter. After determining the corneal hydration, the tissue was extracted with distilled water under the same conditions as those described for electrolyte extraction. The isotope content of the extract was determined, and the data were calculated as counts/min per kg of tissue water.

Determination of endothelial permeability: After incubating the cornea in the perfusion chamber, the epithelium was removed and a small amount of isotope applied to the bare stromal surface. The efflux of isotope into the perfusate was measured and the endothelial permeability calculated according to the method of Mishima and Trenberth (12).

Uptake of isotopes: The cornea was incubated in a bathing chamber containing 10 μl of isotope solution (0.1 μc/μl). The volume of the bathing medium was 5 ml, giving a final isotope concentration of 0.02 mmole/liter. After an appropriate time interval, the isotope concentration in the corneal water was determined.

The bathing medium: The concentration of D-glucose in the standard bicarbonate-Ringer's basic medium was 6.7 mmoles/liter. Other glucose concentrations tested were 0, 3, 6, 9, 15 and 20 mmoles/liter. For concentrations lower than 6 mmoles/liter, glucose was replaced by sucrose. For higher concentrations, sodium chloride was replaced by glucose in order to maintain the normal osmolarity of the medium. In some experiments the glucose in the bathing medium was replaced by MG (Sigma Chemical Co., St. Louis, Mo.), as described in the text.

RESULTS AND DISCUSSION

*Electrolyte studies*

*Incubation at body temperature.* Corneas were incubated in a bathing chamber perfused with KEI medium at a rate of 20 μl/min. Four groups of experiments were performed. In Group A, corneas with intact epithelia were perfused for 3 to 5 hr and the electrolyte concentrations determined for the whole layers. In Group B, corneas were perfused for about 5 hr with epithelium intact; and in Group C, for 4 to 7 hr with the epithelium removed. In Group D, corneas devoid of epithelium were perfused for 6 hr in the presence of $10^{-5}$ M ouabain. The electrolyte concentrations in the whole cornea (Group A) and in

TABLE 1. *Perfusion of corneas with KEI medium at body temperature*

| | No. of experiments | Hydration | Sodium | Potassium | Chloride |
|---|---|---|---|---|---|
| A | 9 | 3.29 ± 0.15 | 165.1 ± 6.10 | 28.8 ± 2.58 | 99.6 ± 4.25 |
| | | | 543.2 | 94.7 | 327.7 |
| B | 11 | 3.49 ± 0.21 | 174.2 ± 1.72 | 19.2 ± 1.45 | 106.0 ± 1.75 |
| | | | 608.0 | 67.1 | 369.9 |
| C | 26 | 3.43 ± 0.24 | 183.8 ± 4.73 | 16.7 ± 1.38 | 110.6 ± 3.82 |
| | | | 630.4 | 57.3 | 379.4 |
| D | 8 | 5.04 ± 0.21 | 181.5 ± 6.78 | 9.4 ± 2.04 | 107.9 ± 6.07 |
| | | | 914.8 | 47.4 | 543.8 |

Values are averages and standard deviations. Upper line of each group is the electrolyte concentration in mEq per kg water and the lower is the electrolyte content in mEq per kg dry weight.

A: Whole cornea after 3 to 5 hr perfusion.
B: Corneal stroma after 5 hr perfusion with the epithelium.
C: Corneal stroma after 4 to 7 hr perfusion without the epithelium.
D: Corneal stroma after 6 hr of ouabain without the epithelium.

TABLE 2. *Perfusion of corneas with KEI medium, corrected for evaporation*

|   | Hydration | Sodium | Potassium | Chloride |
|---|---|---|---|---|
| A | 3.38 | 160.3 | 28.0 | 96.7 |
| B | 3.59 | 169.1 | 18.6 | 102.9 |
| C | 3.53 | 178.4 | 16.2 | 107.4 |
| D | 5.19 | 176.2 | 9.1 | 105.0 |

the corneal stroma (Groups B, C and D) are given in Table 1. In the first three groups, the corneal thickness remained normal during perfusion and the corneal hydration at the end of the experiment was within normal limits. In Group D, however, the increase in stromal hydration is significant; moreover, the stroma showed an increase in sodium and chloride with a concomitant loss of potassium.

The increase in electrolyte concentration in the cornea due to evaporation of water during perfusion was found to be 3.0 ± 1.1% in five separate determinations. These values were used in all calculations to correct for corneal hydration and electrolyte concentrations (Table 2).

*Incubation at low temperature.* In order to determine the passive ionic equilibrium between the corneal stroma and the medium, isolated corneas were perfused at a temperature of 3 to 4 C. These experiments were divided into five groups: in A and B, corneas with epithelium intact were perfused for 6 and 24 hr, respectively; in C and D, corneas devoid of epithelium were perfused for 24 and 48 hr, respectively; and in group E the epithelium was removed, the stromal surface covered with silicone oil and the preparation perfused for 24 hr. In Groups A and B (Table 3), the concentration of potassium in the stroma was nearly as high as that found when the tissue was incubated at body temperature (Table 1). This suggests that an electrolyte shift has occurred, induced by the low temperature incubation, the net result being a flow of potassium from the epithelial cells into the stroma. Therefore, incubation in the presence of the epithelium prevents the attainment of ionic equilibrium in the stroma, so that data from Groups A and B cannot be used for the estimation of equilibrium conditions. This view is further supported by the

TABLE 3. *Perfusion of corneas with KEI medium at low temperature*

|   | No. of experiments | Hydration | Sodium | Potassium | Chloride |
|---|---|---|---|---|---|
| A | 4 | 3.70 ± 0.12 | 180.2 ± 0.65<br>666.7 | 18.0 ± 1.00<br>66.6 | 108.3 ± 1.74<br>400.7 |
| B | 10 | 4.65 ± 0.57 | 179.5 ± 3.61<br>834.7 | 13.7 ± 0.76<br>63.7 | 106.7 ± 3.66<br>496.2 |
| C | 9 | 4.68 ± 0.24 | 182.0 ± 8.58<br>851.8 | 9.6 ± 1.10<br>45.0 | 107.4 ± 4.97<br>502.6 |
| D | 12 | 6.18 ± 0.46 | 173.8 ± 4.21<br>1,074.1 | 7.3 ± 0.84<br>45.1 | 108.3 ± 3.12<br>669.3 |
| E | 11 | 5.61 ± 1.88 | 169.5 ± 6.93<br>950.9 | 11.6 ± 3.23<br>65.1 | 105.4 ± 4.45<br>591.3 |

Values are averages and standard deviations. Upper line of each group is the electrolyte concentration in mEq per kg water and the lower line is the electrolyte content in mEq per kg dry weight.

A: 6 hr perfusion with the epithelium.
B: 24 hr perfusion with the epithelium.
C: 24 hr perfusion without the epithelium.
D: 48 hr perfusion without the epithelium.
E: 24 hr perfusion without the epithelium, the corneal surface immersed in silicone oil.

finding that the concentration of potassium was very low in tissues incubated without epithelium (Groups C, D and E). In all cases, the increase in hydration was accompanied by a loss of potassium and a rise in sodium and chloride.

*Equilibration of stromal sodium at low temperature.* Diffusional equilibrium of the corneal electrolyte was presumably reached in Groups C, D and E (Table 3), since no significant differences in the concentrations of the various electrolytes were found among the groups. The equilibrium condition for sodium was therefore analyzed by plotting its concentration as a function of the reciprocal of hydration (Fig. 2). The linear correlation was found to be significant. The regression equation for this relationship is

$$[Na]_d = 148.7 + 138.2 \frac{1}{H} \qquad (1)$$

where $[Na]_d$ is the concentration of sodium in the stroma in mEq/kg of tissue water and H is the hydration.

It will be recalled (Table 1) that when the corneal stroma swells in the presence of ouabain, the concentration of potassium is as low as that in stroma incubated at low temperature. It was therefore assumed that ionic equilibrium in the stroma had been reached, and the results of the ouabain experiments have therefore been included in Fig. 2, after correcting for evaporation. They have not, however, been included in the calculation of equation 1 since they did not significantly alter the results.

*Analysis of results.* The electrolytes in the corneal stroma are considered to reside in three compartments: a) within the keratocytes, b) bound to the stromal mucopolysaccharides and c) dissolved in the stromal fluid. By making certain assumptions, the present results may be used to analyze stromal swelling and the concomitant electrolyte changes in the stromal fluid when the latter

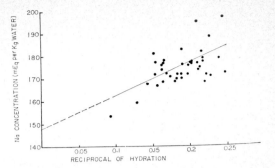

FIG. 2. Sodium concentration in the corneal stroma and tissue hydration at low temperature.

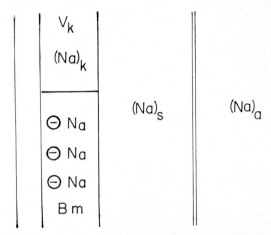

FIG. 3. A model of sodium distribution in the corneal stroma. For symbols see text. $[Na]_a$ is the sodium concentration in the bathing medium.

are at osmotic equilibrium with the aqueous humor.

The concentration of sodium in the corneal stroma (Fig. 3) may be expressed as

$$W[Na]_d = W \cdot V_k [Na]_k + W(1-V_k) [Na]_s + B \cdot m$$

where W is the weight of the stromal water, B is the content of bound sodium (in mEq/kg dry tissue), m is the weight of the dry tissue and $V_k$ is the volume occupied by the keratocytes. $[Na]_d$ is the concentration of sodium (in mEq/kg of water) found by direct measurement; $[Na]_s$ and $[Na]_k$ are the concentrations of sodium in the stromal fluid and in the keratocytes, respectively. Substitution of hydra-

**491**

tion (H) for W/m in equation 1 gives the following expression:

$$[Na]_d = [Na]_k \cdot V_k + (1-V_k) [Na]_s + B/H \quad (2)$$

In order to calculate changes in the concentration of sodium in the stromal fluid, $[Na]_s$, it is first necessary to derive values for bound sodium (B), the volume occupied by the keratocytes $(V)_k$ and the concentration of sodium in the keratocytes $[Na]_k$.

Bound sodium and sodium concentration in the stromal fluid at low temperature: When the corneas are incubated at low temperature and ionic equilibrium is reached in the stroma, any differences in sodium concentration between the keratocytes and the stromal fluid should disappear. This equilibrium condition can be expressed by transforming equation 2 into

$$[Na]_d = [Na]_s + B/H \quad (3)$$

A comparison of equations 1 and 3 leads to the conclusion that the concentration of bound sodium is about 138.2 mEq/kg dry wt, and is independent of tissue hydration. Otori (13) calculated the amount of bound sodium from the data of Mathews (14) and Anseth and Laurent (15), and obtained 35.7 mEq/kg of water at normal hydration. This value is in close agreement with the present one of 39.4 mEq/kg of water at normal hydration (3.5). The concentration in the stromal fluid is 148.7 mEq/kg of water, which is nearly equal to that of the bathing medium.

Volume and electrolyte concentration of keratocytes: In order to calculate these values, the assumption was made that the electrolyte concentration in the keratocytes is the same as that in the epithelium. Since the epithelium occupies 10% of the cornea, the latter concentration can be calculated from the data in Table 2 (Groups A and B). This gives the following values (mEq/kg in water): Na = 81 (90), K = 113 (102) and Cl = 41 (47), where the numbers in parentheses are those calculated from Otori's data (13). Direct measurement of the epithelium (13) gave values of Na = 57, K = 109 and Cl = 23 mEq/kg of

water after appropriate correction for evaporation. In consideration of these values, the range of concentration of electrolytes in the keratocytes was taken as Na = 57 to 90, K = 102 to 113 and Cl = 23 to 47 mEq/kg of water.

The volume occupied by the keratocytes $(V_k)$ may be calculated from the chloride concentration. If binding of chloride to mucopolysaccharides is neglected, the following equation applies:

$$[Cl]_d = [Cl]_k V_k + [Cl]_s (1-V_k) \quad (4)$$

The symbols have the same meanings as those used for calculating sodium in the equations above. Estimation of $[Cl]_s$ requires a Donnan ratio which is not precisely known. However, since chloride is considered to be evenly distributed and to have reached equilibrium during incubation at low temperature, $[Cl]_s$ may be obtained from the data in Table 3 (Groups C, D and E). Using the value of $[Cl]_k$ given above, the range of $V_k$ was found to be 3.7 to 5.2%, a value close to that estimated by Davson (4).

A similar calculation can be made using potassium concentrations. The amount of bound potassium is not known, but it was assumed to be present in similar proportion to sodium, namely about 1.5 mEq/kg of water at normal hydration. Using a stromal potassium concentration of 18.6 mEq/kg of water (Table 2, B) and assuming that the concentration in the stromal fluid is similar to that in the bathing fluid, one obtains a value of $V_k$ between 11 and 12.4%. Kaye (16), calculating the keratocyte volume from electron micrographs, arrived at a similar value.

The different values derived from sodium and potassium concentrations cannot be explained, but the range of $V_k$ should include all of these estimations. Therefore, a $V_k$ range of 3.7 to 12.5% was used for subsequent calculations. The data obtained on corneas incubated at body temperature without epithelium (Table 2, C) give a range of 2 to 10%

$1/V$ ($\times 10^{-6}$ mM/cm$^2$ per min)$^{-1}$

$-0.2$   $-0.1$

FIG. 6.   Linev
$V_{max} = 5.6$ n

TABLE 5.

| Tissue |
| --- |
| Lens |
| Red cell |
| Red cell |
| Small intestine |
| Small intestine |
| Heart muscle |
| Cornea |

neas, but sim
corneas devo

A Linweav
gives a straigl
$10^{-6}$ ($7.2 \times 10$
a $K_m$ of 8.0 (
parentheses ar
thelium. The
endothelium i
other tissues
ther support t
C$^{14}$-MG acros
mediated by c
present in othe

*Competition*
*glucose.* If the
the same carri
it should be p
petitive inhibiti
the medium (

for $V_k$. These slightly lower values may be due to damage caused to the keratocytes while the epithelium was being removed.

Sodium concentrations in the stromal fluid: Equation 2 may be used to calculate the possible range of sodium concentrations in the stromal fluid at body temperature. The data in Table 2 for Group B give values of 131 to 140 mEq/kg of water while those for Group C give 140 to 148 mEq/kg of water. Since the calculation uses a combination of the extreme limits of the range of keratocyte volumes, it is reasonable to assume that the actual stromal concentration is in fact within these limits.

The stromal concentration of sodium in a ouabain-treated cornea may be calculated by assuming that the $V_k$ is zero, due to cessation of the sodium pump in the keratocytes. A concentration of 149.4 mEq/kg of water is obtained, a value close to that of the bathing medium. In the swollen stroma incubated at low temperature, the concentration was 148.7 mEq/kg of water.

The above calculations suggest that when the normal thickness is maintained, the sodium concentration in the stromal fluid tends to be lower than that in the anterior chamber. Abolishing the endothelial pump either by incubation at low temperature or with ouabain leads to an increase in concentration reaching the level present in the aqueous humor. Since the Donnan ratio is not precisely known, it was neglected in this calculation. In any case, it would not have altered any of the conclusions reached on this point.

Consider for the moment a pump-leak system for sodium at the endothelium. The stroma has a swelling pressure (S) which tends to pull fluid across the endothelium into the stroma. This fluid flow may be expressed (17) as

$$J_v = L_p S - \sigma L_p RT\Delta C$$

where $J_v$ is the volume flow, $L_p$ is the hydraulic conductivity of the endothelium and $\sigma$ is the reflection coefficient for sodium (0.6). The concentration difference between the aqueous and the stromal fluid is $\Delta C$ and RT has the usual meaning. When the cornea maintains its normal thickness, $J_v$ should be zero. This may be expressed as

$$\Delta C_o = S_o/\sigma RT$$

where subscript o indicates steady state concentrations. For a normal swelling pressure ($S_o$) of 60 mm Hg (18, 19) and a reflection coefficient of 0.6 (17), one obtains $C_o = 5.3$ mEq/kg of water, the concentration in the aqueous being higher than that in the stroma. The maintenance of normal hydration thus requires an active pump to maintain the above concentration difference across the endothelium. Arrest or abolition of the pump allows sodium to flow into the stroma and the stromal concentration increases to the level present in the aqueous humor. The result is corneal swelling. The present analysis agrees with the model of a pump-leak system and strongly suggests that a sodium pump does indeed exist in the endothelium. Recent experiments (20) relating the ionic composition of the bathing medium to the degree of corneal swelling support this view.

### Transport of C$^{14}$-MG across the endothelium

*Permeability coefficients of C$^{14}$-MG and C$^{14}$-L-glucose.* Corneas were perfused at 33 to 34 C with bicarbonate-Ringer's buffer (glucose concentration, 6.7 mM) and the endothelial permeability to both radioactive substances was determined according to the method of Mishima and Trenberth (12). The coefficients obtained from eight separate experiments are given in Table 4, line one.

In another series of experiments, corneas were incubated in the bathing chamber and the uptake of C$^{14}$-MG was determined at various intervals up to 2 hr. These data provided an independent method for calculating

**493**

spectively, of the cornea and t, the time. Then the concentration of $C^{14}$-MG in the corneal stroma is given by $M_i = J_{total} \cdot A \cdot t/V$. Replacing $A/V$ by $1/Q$, where $Q$ is the stromal thickness, we obtain the following expression:

$$M_i/M_o = \left[\frac{V_{max}}{K_m + G + M_o} + K_d\right] \frac{t}{Q} \quad (6)$$

From the average ratio $M_i/M_o$ in Fig. 7 and equation 6, an average $K_d$ of $6.7 \pm 1.7 \times 10^{-6}$ cm/sec can be calculated for the diffusional permeability coefficient of the endothelium. The values used for the calculation were $V_{max} = 5.6 \times 10^{-6}$ mmole/cm² per min, $K_m = 8.0$ mM, $M_o = 0.02$ mM, $Q = 0.4$ to $0.08$ mm and $t = 20$ min. From the three curves shown in Fig. 7, $K_d$ values of 10, 8 and $6 \times 10^{-6}$ cm/sec, respectively, were calculated. The line for a $K_d$ value of six to eight fits the actual relationship reasonably well. The diffusional permeability coefficients thus calculated are in close agreement with that of L-glucose, a substance that is similar in molecular size to MG but is not transported by the carrier system (33, 34).

*Inhibition of $C^{14}$-MG uptake by ouabain and phlorizin.* The uptake of $C^{14}$-MG by the cornea was studied in the presence of ouabain ($10^{-5}$ M) using various concentrations of glucose in the medium. The uptake of $C^{14}$-MG was lower in the presence of glucose than in its absence (Fig. 8). Moreover, the average count ratio observed in these experiments agreed well with previous data calculated on the assumption of diffusional flux alone, using a $K_d$ of $8 \times 10^{-6}$ cm/sec. Since this value is close to that of the $K_d$ previously calculated, it was concluded that ouabain almost completely inhibited the carrier system.

The effect of phlorizin on the uptake of $C^{14}$-MG was similarly studied and the results are shown in Fig. 9. Maximum inhibition was found at a phlorizin concentration of $10^{-5}$ M, but even at concentrations as low as $10^{-7}$ M some inhibition was observed. When the up-

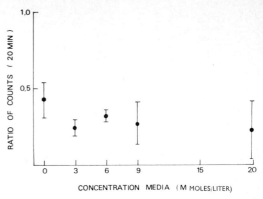

FIG. 8. Effect of ouabain on the uptake of $C^{14}$-MG across the endothelium. Ordinate: average and standard deviation of count ratios; abscissa: concentration of D-glucose in the bathing medium.

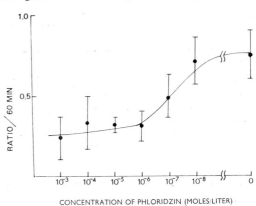

FIG. 9. Effect of phlorizin on the uptake of $C^{14}$-MG. Ordinate: average and standard deviation of count ratios after 60 min incubation; abscissa: concentration of phlorizin in moles/liter.

take was measured using various concentrations of glucose in the medium in the presence of both $10^{-3}$ and $10^{-5}$ M phlorizin, no effect of glucose was observed. This uptake can be accounted for by assuming diffusional flux alone, using a $K_d$ of 6 to $7 \times 10^{-6}$ cm/sec. These data indicate that the carrier transport system was completely inhibited by phlorizin.

## CONCLUSIONS

It has been established that nonmetabolizable MG is transported by the same carrier system as glucose (25–32). Both the saturation kinetics of the transport system and the competition between the two substances have been repeatedly shown in other tissues. Inhibition of this active transport by ouabain (35) and by phlorizin (36–38) has also been confirmed. All of these characteristics of MG transport have now been found in the corneal endothelium. The similarity of the apparent $K_m$ values between corneal endothelium and other tissues (25–29) indicates that the carrier systems are identical. Dependence of this transport on temperature, as shown by Hale and Maurice (9), strongly suggests that the transport requires active metabolic processes. The complete inhibition of transport by ouabain supports the view that this transport system is mediated through adenosine triphosphatase and is probably coupled to the sodium pump.

The diffusional permeability of the endothelium to glucose has not been determined, although it is assumed to be similar to that of other monosaccharides. The present value of $7 \times 10^{-6}$ cm/sec for MG agrees well with that expected from its molecular size. The similarity to the coefficient for L-glucose, which is transported by diffusion (33, 34), supports the validity of the above value. The apparent permeability coefficient at body temperature must be the sum of diffusional permeability and carrier-mediated permeability. From equation 5 the apparent permeability at a glucose concentration of 6.7 mM was calculated from the values of $V_{max}$ ($7 \times 10^{-6}$ mmole/cm$^2$ per min), $K_m$ (8 mM) and $K_d$ ($7 \times 10^{-6}$ cm/sec). The permeability coefficient of $15 \times 10^{-6}$ cm/sec calculated from these values is in good agreement with those found experimentally.

Nevertheless, the apparent permeability values obtained by Hale and Maurice (9) in efflux experiments is higher than the present value. The difference may be due, in part, to the higher temperature of the incubation medium in their experiments. The temperature effect in glucose transport indicates a $Q_{10}$ of about 2 (25). Therefore, the apparent permeability at 37 C would be higher by almost 40% than the present value.

Another factor to be considered is that of the experimental conditions used in the present investigation. In the uptake experiments, the isotope had not reached a steady state concentration in the cornea after only 20 min incubation. Therefore, the concentration in the whole stroma should have been lower than that in the posterior layer, which was in direct contact with the bathing medium. This uneven distribution in the stroma tends to minimize the apparent permeability values. It seems possible that in the efflux experiments, removal of the epithelium caused a reduction in glucose metabolism which could have led to an accumulation of glucose in the stroma; hence the efflux of MG may have been retarded by competitive inhibition with glucose. Riley (11) found the glucose uptake of rabbit cornea incubated at 37 C to be approximately 90 μg/cm$^2$ per hr. If the steady state concentration of glucose in the stroma is about half that in the bathing medium (39), the apparent permeability required by the endothelium to meet the metabolic needs of the tissue would be about $36 \times 10^{-6}$ cm/sec. This figure is about twice as high as the value found in the present study, a discrepancy which may be accounted for by the two factors discussed above, namely underestimation of the apparent permeability values and temperature differences.

The presence of facilitated transport of glucose across the endothelium has been clearly demonstrated in this investigation. The supply of glucose to the cornea from the aqueous humor can only be achieved through a metabolically active endothelium.

Figures and tables, not otherwise indicated, were reproduced from our papers in *Acta Soc Ophthalmol Jap* **75**: No 1 Suppl, 1971.

# REFERENCES

1. MISHIMA S and KUDO T. *In vitro* incubation of rabbit cornea. *Invest Ophthalmol* **6**: 329, 1967.
2. MAURICE DM. The cornea and sclera, in: Davson H (Ed), "The eye," 2nd edn. New York, Academic Press, 1969, p 489.
3. TRENBERTH SM and MISHIMA S. The effect of ouabain on the rabbit corneal endothelium. *Invest Ophthalmol* **7**: 44, 1968.
4. DAVSON H. The hydration of the cornea. *J Biochem* **59**: 24, 1955.
5. HARRIS JE and NORDQUIST LR. The hydration of the cornea. I. The transport of water from the cornea. *Am J Ophthalmol* **40**: 100, 1955.
6. HARRIS JE. The physiologic control of corneal hydration. *Am J Ophthalmol* **44**: 262, 1957.
7. LANGHAM ME and TAYLOR IS. Factors affecting the hydration of the cornea in the excised eye and the living animal. *Br J Ophthalmol* **40**: 321, 1956.
8. HARA T. Studies on the water and cation shift of the stored cornea. *Jap J Ophthalmol* **9**: 161, 1965.
9. HALE PN and MAURICE EM. Sugar transport across the corneal endothelium. *Exp Eye Res* **8**: 205, 1969.
10. MAURICE DM and GIARDINI AA. A simple optical apparatus for measuring the corneal thickness and the average thickness of the human cornea. *Br J Ophthalmol* **35**: 169, 1951.
11. RILEY MV. Glucose and oxygen utilization by the rabbit cornea. *Exp Eye Res* **8**: 193, 1969.
12. MISHIMA S and TRENBERTH SM. Permeability of the corneal endothelium to nonelectrolytes. *Invest Ophthalmol* **7**: 34, 1968.
13. OTORI T. Electrolyte content of the rabbit corneal stroma. *Exp Eye Res* **6**: 356, 1967.
14. MATHEWS MB. Structural factors in cation binding to anionic polysaccharides of connective tissue. *Arch Biochem Biophys* **104**: 394, 1964.
15. ANSETH A and LAURENT TC. Polysaccharides in normal and pathologic corneas. *Invest Ophthalmol* **1**: 195, 1962.
16. KAYE GI. Stereologic measurement of cell volume fraction of rabbit corneal stroma. *Arch Ophthalmol* **82**: 792, 1969.
17. MISHIMA S and HEDBYS BO. The permeability of the corneal epithelium and endothelium to water. *Exp Eye Res* **6**: 10, 1967.
18. HEDBYS BO and DOHLMAN CH. A new method for the determination of the swelling pressure of the corneal stroma *in vitro*. *Exp Eye Res* **2**: 122, 1963.
19. HEDBYS BO, MISHIMA S and MAURICE DM. The inhibition pressure of the corneal stroma. *Exp Eye Res* **2**: 99, 1963.
20. HODSON S. Evidence for a bicarbonate-dependent sodium pump in corneal endothelium. *Exp Eye Res* **11**: 20, 1971.
21. LONGSWORTH LG. Temperature dependence of diffusion in aqueous solution. *J Physiol (Lond)* **58**: 770, 1954.
22. MAURICE DM. The use of permeability studies in the investigation of submicroscopic structure, in: Smelser GK (Ed), "The structure of the eye." New York, Academic Press, 1961, p 381.
23. MISHIMA S and MAURICE DM. *In vivo* determination of the endothelial permeability to fluorescein. *Acta Soc Ophthalmol Jap* **75** (Suppl): 236, 1971.
24. LINEWEAVER H and BURK D. The determination of enzyme dissociation constants. *J Am Chem Soc* **56**: 658, 1954.
25. PATTERSON JW. A review of glucose transport in the lens. *Invest Ophthalmol* **4**: 667, 1965.
26. PARK CR, CROFFORD OB and KONO T. Mediated (nonactive) transport of glucose in mammalian cells and its regulation. *J Gen Physiol* **52**: 296, 1968.
27. FISHER RB and PARSONS DS. Glucose movements across the wall of the rat's small intestine. *J Physiol (Lond)* **119**: 210, 1953.
28. MORGAN HE, HENDERSON MF, REGAN DM and PARK CR. Regulation of glucose uptake in muscle. 1. The effects of insulin and anoxia on glucose transport and phosphorylation in the isolated perfused heart of normal rats. *J Biol Chem* **236**: 253, 1961.
29. RIKLIS E and QUASTEL JH. Effects of cations on sugar absorption by isolated surviving guinea pig intestine. *Can J Biochem Physiol* **36**: 347, 1958.
30. CRANE R. Intestinal absorption of sugars. *Physiol Rev* **40**: 789, 1960.
31. WILBRANDT W and ROSENBERG T. Concept of carrier transport and its corollaries in pharmacology. *Pharmacol Rev* **13**: 109, 1961.
32. STEIN WD. "The movement of molecules across cell membranes." New York, Academic Press, 1967.
33. CSÁKY TZ and FERNALD GW. Absorption of 3-methylglucose from the intestine of the frog, *Rana pipiens*. *Am J Physiol* **198**: 445, 1960.
34. LEFEVRE PG and MARSHALL JK. Conformational specificity in a biological sugar transport system. *Am J Physiol* **194**: 333, 1953.
35. CSÁKY TZ. Effect of cardioactive steroids on the active transport nonelectrolytes. *Biochem Biophys Acta* **74**: 160, 1963.
36. SMYTH DH and TAYLOR CB. The inhibition of glucose transport in the *in vitro* intestine by phlorizin. *J Physiol (Lond)* **130**: 11, 1966.
37. PARSONS BJ, SMYTH DH and TAYLOR CB. The action of phlorizin on the intestinal transfer of glucose and water *in vitro*. *J Physiol (Lond)* **144**: 387, 1958.
38. NEWEY H, PARSONS BJ and SMYTH DH. The site of action of phlorizin in inhibiting intestinal absorption of glucose. *J Physiol (Lond)* **148**: 83, 1958.
39. REIM M, LAX F, LICHTE H and TURSS RL. Steady state levels of glucose in the different layers of the cornea, aqueous humor, blood and tears *in vivo*. *Ophthalmologica* **154**: 39, 1967.
40. MISHIMA S. The function of the corneal endothelium in the regulation of corneal hydration, in: Langham ME (Ed), "The cornea, macromolecular organization of a connective tissue." Baltimore, Johns Hopkins Press, 1969, p 207.

# SYNTHETIC ACTIVITY OF CORNEAL ENDOTHELIUM

M. V. RILEY, S. A. HODSON and H. T. ORR

Institute of Biological Sciences, Oakland University, Rochester, Michigan, USA and Institute of Ophthalmology
London, England

The processes governing the control of corneal hydration lie in the endothelium, the single layer of cells that defines the posterior surface of the tissue and borders on the aqueous humor. Since the layer is permeable to water and salts, fluid is continually drawn into the corneal stroma by virtue of the prevailing imbibition pressure. Maintenance of a steady state of hydration, therefore, requires continuous "uphill" removal of water from the tissue. To date there is no clear indication of the specific mechanism which effects this, although the enzyme Na-K ATPase, which is frequently associated with active transport processes, has been identified in the endothelial cells (1). We studied the metabolism of the endothelial cells in an attempt to identify the nature of the synthetic processes previously investigated by autoradiographic methods (2) and to determine whether they might be related to the movement of ions or water across the cellular layer.

### METHODS

Cow eyes, obtained from a slaughter house, were transferred to the laboratory on ice. The corneas were removed by cutting around the limbus and then placed, epithelial side down, in a plastic egg-tray, thus forming cups which held the incubation medium. The tray was maintained at 37 C in a water bath and a 5% $CO_2$, 7% $O_2$, 88% $N_2$ gas mixture was passed over the corneas.

The incubation medium was that previously used in the study of corneal hydration in rabbits (3), but not including glutathione or adenosine. Glucose was present as indicated. One ml of the medium, brought to pH 7.5 by bubbling with the gas mixture, was pipetted into each "corneal cup."

Radioisotopes, ouabain or other inhibitors were added to this medium as described in the section on "Results." Preparations were incubated for 60 to 80 min.

After incubation the medium was drained off and the corneas were quickly rinsed in three changes of 0.15 M NaCl at 4 C. A cut was made with a razor blade at the periphery of the cornea, through Descemet's membrane and through approximately a quarter of the stromal thickness. Forceps were then used to grip a cut edge, pulling off the endothelium, Descemet's membrane and some stroma.

The material from 6 or 12 corneas was combined in 3 ml of 5% trichloroacetic acid and homogenized. The supernatant fluids were stored frozen.

G-25 Sephadex (Pharmacia Fine Chemicals Inc.) was packed in a 1.5 × 70 cm column after equilibration in either 0.01 M phosphate buffer or 0.01 M Tris buffer, each at pH 7.4.

Electrophoresis was carried out in phosphate or Tris buffers on cellulose acetate papers 12 × 2.5 cm. Polyvinylpyrrolidone was used to determine the extent of migration due to electroosmosis.

### RESULTS

Fig. 1 shows the pattern of radioactivity obtained on elution of the trichloroacetic acid

**499**

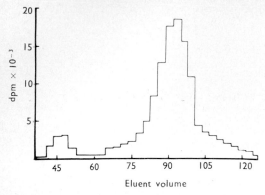

FIG. 1. Chromatography on Sephadex G-25-phosphate buffer of extract from corneal endothelium after incubation with $C^{14}$-glucose. Small, high molecular weight peak appears first, followed by the lower molecular weight compounds, mostly glucose.

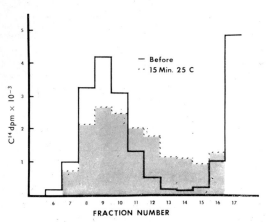

FIG. 2. Chromatography (Sephadex G-25-phosphate buffer) of extract from corneal endothelium before and after heating. Radioactivity is lost from the peak in fractions 7 to 11 and appears in the lower molecular weight range, fractions 12 to 15.

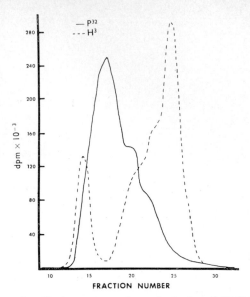

FIG. 3. Elution pattern from Sephadex G-25-Tris buffer of extract from corneas incubated in $H^3$-glucose and $P^{32}O_4$. Larger peaks of unmetabolized glucose and phosphate in later fractions not shown.

(TCA) extract on G-25 Sephadex in phosphate buffer. A single peak of activity appears shortly after the dead volume of the column, and is then followed by the much larger peak which represents small molecules, chiefly unmetabolized glucose.

The isolated fraction was found to be extremely labile. On rechromatography after very short periods of warming above 10 C, the elution pattern was distorted, indicating the presence of lower molecular weight fractions

and a breakdown of the initial compound. This is shown in Fig. 2.

The yield of radioactivity is increased, as might be expected, by preincubation of the corneas for 60 min in a glucose-free medium, thus depleting to a large extent the endogenous carbohydrate reserves (4). A further 5- to 10-fold increase in yield can be obtained by addition to the incubation medium of $2.10^{-5}$ M ouabain. The addition of actinomycin D or puromycin to both the preincubation and incubation media had no effect on the synthesis of the labeled compound.

Dual-isotope experiments were carried out to determine whether other metabolites were incorporated or could give rise to this same moiety. Sulfate was not incorporated and threonine and leucine showed negligible incorporation. Phosphate is incorporated in the TCA extract of corneal endothelium in more than one fraction. The use of Tris buffer in place of the phosphate buffer for elution of the G-25 Sephadex column yields partial resolution of three fractions resulting from incu-

**500**

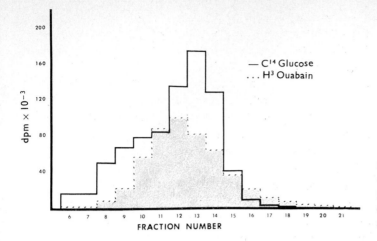

FIG. 4. High molecular weight range of elution pattern (Sephadex G-25-phosphate buffer) of extract from corneas incubated in C14-glucose and H3-ouabain.

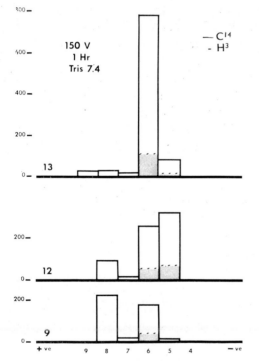

FIG. 5. Electrophoresis of fractions 9, 12 and 13 shown in Fig. 4. Origin at position 6.

bation with phosphate and also resolves the activity obtained from glucose into three fractions (Fig. 3). Whether all three of these glucose-derived fractions are heat-labile has not yet been determined.

When labeled ouabain is used in the incubation medium and the extract is run through the column with Tris, part of the ouabain is eluted in the same fraction as the glucose-labeled moiety (Fig. 4). Electrophoresis of these fractions yields the pattern shown in Fig. 5. The ouabain-containing fraction is less heavily charged than the other glucose-derived fractions that contain no ouabain.

To investigate the ion-binding capacity of the glucose-labeled fraction, a column of Biogel P-10 (Calbiochem) was equilibrated with $Na_2 ^{22}HPO_4$ (10 µM.) and an aliquot of the fraction was added and eluted with further $Na_2 ^{22}HPO_4$. The details of this method are to be published elsewhere, but the chief points are: 1) in the absence of any sodium-binding effect a steady flow of radioactivity exits from the column and 2) if sodium is

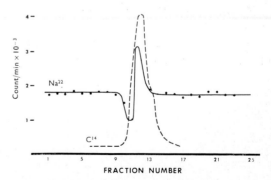

FIG. 6. Chromatography on Bio-Gel P-10 of C14-labeled fraction from corneal endothelium with continuous elution by $Na_2 ^{22}HPO_4$ (10 µM).

"bound" by the compound then a fluid low in sodium (Na$^{22}$) precedes it down the column, and when the complex exits the bound radio-activity registers as a volume of high counts. The results are shown in Fig. 6.

## DISCUSSION

Evidence for the synthesis of a macromolecule within the corneal endothelium was obtained in radioautographic experiments carried out by Hodson (2). Interest in this compound was stimulated by the unusual kinetics of synthesis and breakdown. It was found that over short periods of time synthetic activity was higher in the endothelium than in the stroma and epithelium, and that in cold-chase experiments the compounds in the endothelium showed rapid decay as compared with the constant levels that were maintained in the other layers.

It has been possible to isolate a TCA-soluble fraction of corneal endothelium on G-25 Sephadex that exhibits similar kinetics to the material studied radioautographically. It is not a pure fraction, as shown by the appearance of three peaks of radioactivity when Tris is used as eluent. Unfortunately, until now chemical analysis has been precluded by the paucity of the material.

The effect of ouabain in increasing the amount of the labeled material that can be extracted from the endothelium has led us to speculate that the fraction may contain a compound that is involved in ion transport. It can, in fact, be shown that ouabain appears to bind to a radioactive fraction, both through-out treatment on Sephadex and by electrophoresis, which would be consistent with mechanisms postulated for the inhibition of Na-K ATPase.

The behavior of the endothelial extract on electrophoresis shows the labeled macromolecule to be negatively charged, suggesting that it may have the properties of a cation exchanger. This characteristic is confirmed in the experiments with Na$^{22}$ on the Bio-Gel column.

We postulate that the molecule may possibly be synthesized in the Golgi apparatus of the corneal endothelium where it may bind sodium and, consequently, water. The marked lability of the complex is attributed to breakdown at the posterior cell membrane of the endothelial cells, resulting in release of ions and water. The unusual kinetics, the sodium binding and the swelling of Golgi vesicles in the presence of ouabain (S. A. Hodson, unpublished results) are the strongest indications we have in support of this postulate, but it does seem to warrant further investigation.

Supported in part by grants from the National Eye Institute 1-RO1-EY-00541-01 and the National Science Foundation GY-7480

## REFERENCES

1. ROGERS KT. Levels of (Na$^+$ and K$^+$)-activated and Mg$^+$-activated ATPase activity in bovine and feline corneal endothelium and epithelium. *Biochim Biophys Acta* **163**: 50, 1968.
2. HODSON SA. Macromolecular synthesis in corneal endothelium. *Exp Eye Res* **11**: 15, 1971.
3. RILEY MV. The role of the epithelium in control of corneal hydration. *Exp Eye Res* **12**: 128, 1971.
4. RILEY MV. Glucose oxygen utilization by the rabbit cornea. *Exp Eye Res* **8**: 193, 1969.

# THE ACTIVE CONTROL OF CORNEAL HYDRATION

S. DIKSTEIN* and D.M. MAURICE

Division of Ophthalmology, Stanford University Medical School, Stanford, California, USA

The transparency of the mammalian cornea depends upon the maintenance of its thickness. Under many conditions the tissue will swell by the uptake of fluid and become cloudy. There is considerable evidence that the hydration of the tissue is not a static condition but is the result of the balance of a physicochemical influx of water and a metabolically driven efflux.

The most direct evidence has been provided by experiments showing that the cornea of the enucleated rabbit eye swells if the eye is refrigerated; but, on incubation, the tissue returns to its original thickness (1, 2). In both studies, it was found that the reversal was dependent upon metabolic energy, and the fact that it operates against the swelling pressure of the corneal stroma indicates that it is an energy-requiring process.

The nature of the primarily transported material and the mechanism whereby its transfer is coupled to the metabolism of the corneal cells have not been elucidated. The only pump that has been identified in the rabbit cornea involves active transport of $Na^+$ and is located at the outer epithelial surface (3, 4). This pump tends to carry water with it into, rather than out of, the stroma.

Green (5, 6) has provided indirect evidence that this sodium pump controls tissue hydration via a mechanism which is accompanied by changes in the $Na^+$ concentration in the stroma. This in turn modifies the swelling properties of the polysaccharide of this connective tissue layer.

On the other hand, most workers believe that the active control is represented by a fluid pump located in the endothelial layer. The principal evidence for this has been provided by Mishima and Kudo (7), who have described techniques for excising the rabbit cornea, mounting it in a perfusion chamber and following changes in the thickness of the incubated tissue. The perfusion medium, most efficacious both in maintaining the normal thickness and in returning the swollen tissue to normal, was KEI solution, a tissue culture medium designed to replace the aqueous humor (8), which contains vitamins, cofactors and amino acids in addition to glucose and pyruvate.

The present paper outlines improved methods for mounting the cornea and determining its thickness. Experiments were designed to distinguish which components of the solution are essential for the temperature reversal, and which metabolic steps are directly involved in this process.

We have also shown that the isolated endothelium is capable of pumping fluid from

---

* Present address: Department of Applied Pharmacology, Hebrew University–Hadassah School of Pharmacy, Jerusalem, Israel.

the stroma into the aqueous humor, and therefore of controlling the corneal thickness.

This paper summarizes our conclusions (9, 10).

## METHODS AND RESULTS

*Metabolic studies.* The experimental techniques depend on a method of fixing the eye during the preparation of the cornea, in which it is anchored by means of its conjunctiva. This prevents the damage to the endothelium that can occur by wrinkling or folding of the cornea during its excision.

The cornea is mounted under a microscope so that its thickness can be measured with an accuracy of 1 or 2 μm by focusing in turn on its outer and inner surfaces. The endothelial surface can be perfused with any desired medium, and the temperature of the preparation can be controlled by means of a surrounding water jacket. The epithelial surface is covered with silicone oil to prevent any thinning of the cornea due to evaporation of water (Fig. 1 a).

With this system numerous substrates were tested for their ability to bring about a temperature reversal of the cornea to its original thickness. The presence of glutathione in the solution appeared to enhance the efficiency of the pumping system, and this was checked in later studies in which changes in thickness were compared in the two eyes of a single animal, one perfused with glutathione and one without.

Numerous energy-producing metabolites were directly compared at various concentrations. Adenosine was superior even to glucose in its ability to maintain the pump. Contrary to the experiences of other workers, the intermediates of the Krebs cycle did not appear to be active in this respect (Fig. 2). The presence of oxygen proved to be necessary, however, and the cornea swelled when it was absent. The presence of sodium and bicarbonate ions was also essential for the maintenance of corneal thickness and for the temperature reversal effect.

A number of inhibitors were dissolved in the perfusion fluid in order to try to identify the most important metabolic steps involved

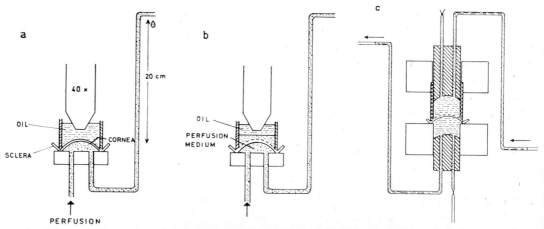

FIG. 1. Schematic illustration of techniques used to measure fluid flow across the endothelium. a) Cold-swollen cornea, with or without epithelium, covered with oil and mounted under microscope. Reduction of thickness on incubation observed by focusing on surfaces of tissue. b) De-epithelialized cornea covered with perfusion fluid under a layer of oil. Lowering of oil-water interface on incubation measured with microscope. c) De-epithelialized cornea mounted between two chambers. Measurement of fluid from one chamber to other noted by shift of capillary tube menisci.

504

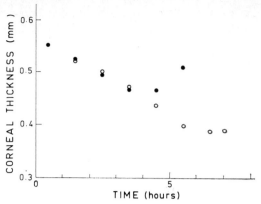

FIG. 2. Temperature reversal curves of two corneas of a rabbit; ○, perfused with 5 mM adenosine; ●, perfused with 2 mM succinate. Both were dissolved in the same media.

TABLE 1. *Approximate concentrations at which various inhibitors begin to affect the temperature reversal of corneal swelling*

| Inhibitor | Molar concentration |
| --- | --- |
| Actinomycin | $3 \times 10^{-7}$ |
| Puromycin | $> 10^{-4}$ |
| Ouabain | $10^{-7}$ |
| Potassium cyanide | $3 \times 10^{-5}$ |
| 2-desoxyglucose | $5 \times 10^{-3}$ |
| Sodium benzoate | $3 \times 10^{-4}$ |
| Antimycin | $10^{-10}$ |
| Oligomycin | $3 \times 10^{-8}$ |
| Iodoacetate | $2 \times 10^{-4}$ |

in driving the fluid pump. Whereas 0.2 mM dinitrophenol and 1 mM fluoroacetate had no effect on the temperature reversal, the cornea was sensitive to most of the other substances tested (Table 1). In some cases the cornea was sensitive to extremely low concentrations of inhibitor, as was shown most effectively by comparing the temperature reversal that oc-

curred in pairs of eyes with and without the addition of inhibitor. Our present working hypothesis on the biochemical control of the pump is summarized in Fig. 3.

*Location of pump.* Once a simplified perfusion system and nutrient medium had been developed it was possible to study the location of the pump. Three types of experiment showed that the endothelial layer was capable of pumping fluid from the stroma into the aqueous humor.

1) The epithelial layer was scraped off a

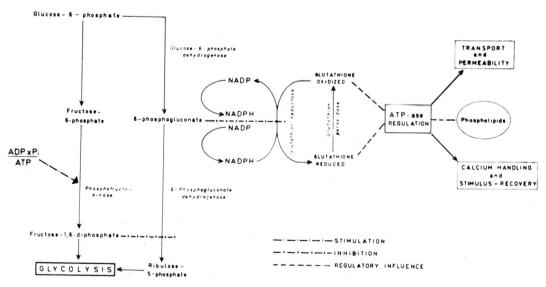

FIG. 3. Working hypothesis for the biochemical control of the pump. (Reproduced with permission from S. Dikstein, *Naturwissenschaften* **58**: 439, 1971.)

Green (5, 6, 15–17) has suggested that the normal thickness of the cornea is maintained by a mechanism entirely different from that proposed above. According to his view, the sodium pump in the epithelium raises the stromal concentration of this ion, the endothelium playing an entirely passive role as a barrier in maintaining this concentration. As a result, the amount of sodium bound by the stromal polysaccharide is increased and the attraction of the polyanion for water decreased, possibly as a result of a conformational change.

The main support for this hypothesis is indirect, and it has been criticized in detail elsewhere (10, 12). The principal objections are that the excised stroma will swell in salt solutions of any concentration, and tends to imbibe fluid *in vivo*. Above all, the existence of an endothelial pump releases one from the necessity of looking to the epithelium for the hydration control mechanism.

Supported by US Public Health Service Grant EY-00431.

## REFERENCES

1. DAVSON H. The hydration of the cornea. *Biochem J* **59**: 24, 1955.
2. HARRIS JE and NORDQUIST LT. The hydration of the cornea. I. Transport of water from the cornea. *Am J Ophthalmol* **40**: 100, 1955.
3. DONN A, MAURICE DM and MILLS NL. Studies on the living cornea *in vitro*. II. The active transport of sodium across the epithelium. *Arch Ophthalmol* **62**: 748, 1959.
4. GREEN K. Ion transport in isolated cornea of the rabbit. *Am J Physiol* **209**: 1311, 1965.
5. GREEN K. Relation of epithelial ion transport to corneal thickness and hydration. *Nature (Lond)* **217**: 1074, 1968.
6. GREEN K. Dependence of corneal thickness on epithelial ion transport and stromal sodium. *Am J Physiol* **217**: 1169, 1969.
7. MISHINA S and KUDO T. The *in vitro* incubation of rabbit cornea. *Invest Ophthalmol* **6**: 329, 1967.
8. WACHTL C and KINSEY VE. Studies on the crystalline lens. VIII. A synthetic medium for lens culture and the effects of various constituents on cell division in the epithelium. *Am J Ophthalmol* **46**: 288, 1958.
9. DIKSTEIN S and MAURICE DM. The metabolic basis of the fluid pump in the cornea. *J Physiol* **221**: 29, 1972.
10. MAURICE DM. The location of the fluid pump in the cornea. *J Physiol* **221**: 43, 1972.
11. DIKSTEIN S. Stimulability, adenosine triphosphatases and their control by cellular redox processes. *Naturwissenschaften* **58**: 439, 1971.
12. MAURICE DM. The cornea and sclera, in: Davson H (Ed), "The eye." New York, Academic Press, 1969.
13. MAURICE DM. The permeability to sodium ions of the living rabbit's cornea. *J Physiol* **122**: 367, 1951.
14. BERKLEY DA. Influence of intraocular pressure on corneal fluid pressure, tissue stress and thickness. *Exp Eye Res* **11**: 132, 1971.
15. GREEN K. Ion transport across the isolated rabbit cornea. *Exp Eye Res* **5**: 106, 1966.
16. GREEN K. Relationship of ion and water transport to corneal swelling, in: Langham M (Ed), "The cornea, macromolecular organization of a connective tissue." Baltimore, The Johns Hopkins Press, 1969.
17. GREEN K. Stromal cation binding after inhibition of epithelial transport in the cornea. *Am J Physiol* **218**: 1642, 1970.

# DISCUSSION

Dr. J. A. Zadunaisky (*USA*): I would like to ask Dr. Mishima if the transport of 3-O-methylglucose is, like glucose transport, temperature dependent.

Dr. S. Mishima (*Japan*): Yes, it is supposed to be, but we haven't measured it directly.

Dr. A. Spector (*USA*): Dr. Mishima, you showed a change in sodium concentration of approximately 7 to 9 mEq/liter. Do you think this is sufficient to account for the large influx of water during corneal swelling?

Dr. Mishima: This value is a change in concentration, not in total amount. If we assume a model of a pump-leak system in the endothelium and use all the values calculated for the hydraulic conductivity, reflection coefficient and sodium permeability of the endothelium, we arrive at a value of about 5 mEq/kg water, which is enough to counteract the swelling presence of 60 mm Hg.

Dr. M. V. Riley (*USA*): The ratio of counts as a function of ouabain concentration was illustrated as being less than 0.5 at zero ouabain concentration. What exactly does this ratio measure?

Dr. Mishima: This value is the ratio of counts per kg water in the medium and in the corneal water. The concentration you were referring to is that of glucose, not of ouabain, which is $10^{-5}$ M at all glucose concentrations. The illustration just shows that in the presence of ouabain, the uptake of D-glucose is not dependent on its concentration.

Dr. C. H. Dohlman (*USA*): Dr. Riley, where do you think the polysaccharide you described is synthesized and how is its synthesis related to water transfer from the cornea?

Dr. Riley: This molecule is synthesized in the Golgi apparatus where it binds a high concentra-tion of sodium. The molecule is packaged into vesicles which are then transported to the cell membrane and liberated into the aqueous humor. Here it is rapidly broken down either by contact with the aqueous or by enzymic degradation. When the molecule is in a degraded state, it can no longer bind sodium ions and they would therefore be removed from the cells. We haven't been able to identify the ion binding capacity precisely because at present we have no indication of the amount of substance that we are dealing with.

Dr. Spector: Dr. Riley, I wonder if you have thought about possible artefacts in this system regarding the specific handling of glucose. For example, the radioactive glucose you used could have been metabolized into any number of substances which were incorporated into your polysaccharide. Have you considered using $C_1$-labeled glucose instead of the uniformly labeled material? Also, did you try to remove the glucose with different kinds of detergent or with urea, to get some idea of whether you are really dealing with covalently-linked glucose? Finally, what evidence do you have that your polysaccharide binds only sodium?—why not potassium or other monovalent cations?

Dr. Riley: With regard to specific binding, we tried substituting potassium for sodium on the columns, but much to our disappointment, found no evidence for a preferential binding of sodium. However, it may not be necessary to argue for specific ion binding, since it is now known that cell membranes which are normally permeable to potassium, and not to sodium, may be altered structurally when subjected to very high osmotic pressures. A sudden break point occurs and they become sodium-permeable. Thus it seems possible that there may be a very high osmotic pressure created locally in the vesicles carrying the "sodium complex." If this could cause changes in the membrane characteristics, one could get pref-

509

erential sodium expulsion or sodium binding as a function of the osmotic pressure within the vesicle.

With regard to your first question, the use of $C_1$-labeled glucose is a good experiment and should be done.

In answer to your second question, we have tried to remove the glucose, not with detergents, but under various washing conditions. We got no clear answer because the molecule is very labile. It is synthesized very quickly in pulse experiments, and it breaks down very rapidly, too. This could be due mainly to an exchange of cold glucose for radioactive glucose, the latter perhaps being nonspecifically bound. But we still have no evidence that it can be shaken off.

DR. D. M. MAURICE (*USA*): I would like to address Dr. Zadunaisky in public after arguing with him so long in private discussions. I think there is something very strange about your epithelium experiments. We know the endothelium can pump, but you are saying that the epithelium is also pumping. The most extraordinary thing about your curves is that when the endothelial pump is working, your cornea is of normal thickness, but with your epithelial curves, the thickness falls to 0.2 mm and then ultimately to the dry value. This is all very strange.

DR. ZADUNAISKY: That isn't complete dryness. When we did these experiments, we were too impatient and didn't wait long enough. But we know that the thickness levels off. We have done other experiments starting at the normal level of thickness, and it remained that way until the cornea swelled. Then, afterward, it returned to normal, the same as you get with the endothelial pump. But the rate varies in different experiments; we don't get perfect results in every endothelial experiment, either.

DR. M. E. LANGHAM (*USA*): As you know, some of us have very different interpretations of what you've been hearing this morning. We have been trying to gain a better understanding of the forces that determine swelling and deturgescence in the stroma and now feel that the explanation lies in the interaction between the collagen fibers and the glycoprotein-mucopolysaccharide matrix. This system has several components that determine the expansive tendency. These are: a) the simple osmotic forces of small ions; b) the forces resulting from large macromolecules, which are expansive forces; and c) charges surrounding the macromolecules that can vary according to the configuration of the molecule. The endothelium, through its metabolic activity, is functioning to maintain the structural integrity of the system in terms of cohesiveness and permeability. We believe that the reason the epithelium is more sensitive to changes is because we are dealing with a stratified layer. Once this has been damaged and the interdigitations are destroyed, we have a funneling system in the extracellular space. But the endothelium, which is only a single cell layer, is held together by very complex interdigitation. We can get the same kind of experimental results shown by Dr. Zadunaisky: both the epithelium and the endothelium can deturgesce. Damage to the endothelium does not always cause corneal edema. Dr. Maumenee has some direct evidence of this from clinical studies.

DR. A. E. MAUMENEE (*USA*): I have had several patients with epithelial down-growths in whom I have measured the thickness of the cornea in the area over the downgrowth. Even in cases where at least half of the cornea has been covered, the stroma has maintained its normal thickness. I have other examples showing that the endothelium is not an absolute requirement for maintaining the normal thickness of the cornea. We all know that there is often some damage to the endothelium from the cryoprobe during cataract extraction, but still we see no edema. I don't think that the cornea will swell unless Descemet's membrane is damaged.

# GROWTH STIMULATING EFFECTS OF PROTEOLYTIC ENZYMES ON CORNEAL TISSUES

VIRGINIA L. WEIMAR and KENNETH H. HARAGUCHI

John E. Weeks Memorial Laboratory of Ophthalmology, Department of Ophthalmology, University of Oregon Medical School, Portland, Oregon, USA

## INTRODUCTION

Several pieces of evidence have suggested that a proteolytic enzyme (or enzymes) may play a role in the initiation of wound repair. Several years ago we showed that within 1 hr after injury there was an activation or release of a proteolytic enzyme (or enzymes) which appeared to trigger the following events: a) invasion of the cornea by polymorphonuclear leukocytes within 4 to 6 hr after injury (1); b) activation of corneal stromal cells to take up large quantities of the vital dye neutral red, beginning 4 hr after injury (2); c) the development of fibroblasts at the wound edge in the corneal stroma (3). Inhibition of this initial proteolytic activity prevented the appearance of all three of these events. They could all be restored in the wounded, protease-inhibited cornea by the topical application of one or two drops of 2% trypsin. All of these events were studied *in vivo*.

Ultimately we were able to show, in short-term studies *in vitro*, that the activation of neutral red uptake by the corneal stromal cells was initiated by an unknown factor (or factors) released from the epithelium by a protease (or proteases) (2).

Recently we developed and described an organ culture system, in totally defined chemical media, for the culture and maintenance of rabbit corneas for several days (4). This system has made possible the study of certain initial events which occur following injury under wholly controlled and defined conditions. In the organ culture system, as originally described, all corneas, normal and wounded alike, gradually became swollen and cloudy, although the corneal stromal cells remained normal in appearance. A modification of this organ culture system now maintains normal corneas in a thin, completely transparent, apparently normal state, for several days. Wounded corneas remain transparent except for a narrow zone around the lip of the wound. If such wounded corneas are maintained in this organ culture system, the opaque zone around the wound gradually clears.

In 1970, Rubin (5) described a nonviral factor, released from Rous sarcoma cells, which stimulated rapid and sustained overgrowth of chick embryo cultures. This factor could be mimicked with as little as 3 µg of crystalline trypsin per ml or with pronase. Burger (6) also found that low concentrations of ficin, trypsin or pronase in mouse fibroblast cultures could initiate cell division and escape from contact inhibition of growth.

In view of a) our previous results indicating that proteolytic enzymes may play a significant role in the initiation of wound repair and b) the growth-stimulating effects in cell cultures observed by Rubin with both trypsin and pronase, we have begun an extensive investigation of the possible role of proteolytic enzymes in wound repair.

In the study reported in this paper we have sought to determine, in organ cultures of rabbit corneas, if various types of proteolytic enzymes possess any growth stimulating effects on any of the three different cellular layers of the cornea.

Trypsin, α-chymotrypsin and pronase were selected for these studies. Trypsin and α-chymotrypsin have many similar physical characteristics but differ markedly in their specificities. Pronase, on the other hand, is a mixture of neutral and alkaline proteinases, carboxypeptidases and aminopeptidases.

### MATERIALS AND METHODS

New Zealand white rabbits, of either sex, and weighing approximately 2 kg, were used for all experiments.

All experiments were carried out in organ culture. The methods used will be described in detail elsewhere. The corneas were routinely cultured for 48 hr. In addition, some experiments were done in which the effects of pronase (at 5 µg/ml) were followed at 12, 24, 36, 48 and 60 hr.

Frozen sections, fixed with absolute methanol and stained with Giemsa were prepared as previously described (4).

A minimum of four eyes were tested for each concentration of each enzyme.

### RESULTS

*Epithelial cells.* All of the proteolytic enzymes tested, even at low concentrations (5 µg/ml), tended to cause loosening and detachment of the epithelial cells near the wound. (Compare Fig. 1, control media, with Fig. 2, pronase-treated). In areas away from the wound the epithelium tended to remain normal in appearance until enzyme concentrations of 20 µg/ml were reached. In every case, at 20 µg/ml, the outer layers of the epithelium were

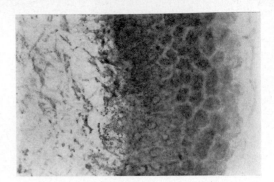

FIG. 1. Rabbit corneal epithelium near wound, control media, 48 hr. Giemsa. × 60.

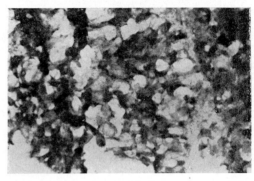

FIG. 2. Rabbit corneal epithelium near wound. Pronase, 5 µg/ml, 48 hr. Note loosening and detachment of epithelial cells. Giemsa. × 60.

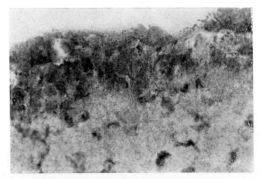

FIG. 3. Rabbit corneal epithelium away from wound area. Trypsin, 20 µg/ml, 48 hr. Note loss of epithelial cells and general disorganization of cells. Giemsa. × 60.

detached (Fig. 3). In addition, trypsin caused necrosis of the epithelial cells and sometimes complete loss of epithelium. The effect of

TABLE 1. *Epithelial cells*

| Concentration of enzyme (µg/ml) | Enzyme | | |
|---|---|---|---|
| | *α-chymotrypsin* | *Pronase* | *Trypsin* |
| 5 | Vigorous growth in wound. Loosening and detachment of cells near wound. Elsewhere no apparent effect. | Perhaps increased growth in wound. Loosening and detachment of cells near wound. Elsewhere no apparent effect. | Detachment and necrosis of cells in wound. Loosening and detachment of cells near wound. Elsewhere no apparent effect. |
| 10 | As above. | As above. | Quite variable. Often extensive loss and necrosis of epithelial cells distant from wound. |
| 20 | Overall loss of outer layers of epithelial cells. | Overall loss of outer layers of epithelial cells. Necrosis of cells common. | Extensive and sometimes total loss of epithelium. Necrosis of cells common. |

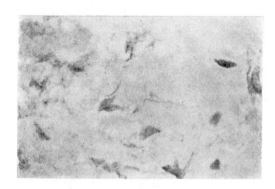

FIG. 4.   Corneal stromal cells along wound edge at level of anterior chamber, rabbit cornea, control media, 48 hr. Giemsa. × 60.

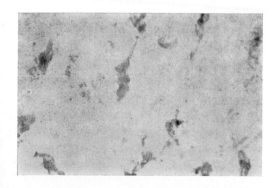

FIG. 5.   Corneal stromal cells along wound edge at level of anterior chamber, rabbit cornea, α-chymotrypsin (5 µg/ml), 48 hr. Giemsa. × 60.

trypsin was quite variable, in contrast to α-chymotrypsin and pronase. Even at 10 µg/ml trypsin sometimes produced a considerable loss of the outer layers of the epithelium.

In eyes with corneal wounds grown only in control media the epithelium grew partway down the wound and was solidly attached; its appearance was typical of that found in healing corneal wounds *in vivo*. α-chymotrypsin appeared to cause a vigorous growth of epithelial cells in the wound. Large numbers of completely disorganized epithelial cells were found in the wounds of pronase-treated corneas. Trypsin, on the other hand, caused loosening, detachment and necrosis of epithelial cells in the wound.

Table 1 summarizes the effects of the various proteolytic enzymes, at each concentration tested, on the epithelial cells.

*Corneal stromal cells.* In control media, fibroblasts developed along the wound edge, paralleling the downward growth of the epithelium (Fig. 4). Fibroblasts did not develop in areas in which the epithelium had not grown. α-chymotrypsin had no effect on the corneal stromal cells, either stimulating or toxic, at any concentration tested (Fig. 5).

Pronase profoundly enhanced the growth

**513**

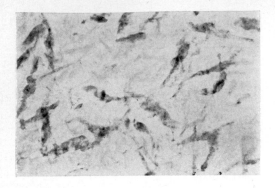

FIG. 6. Corneal stromal cells along wound edge at level of anterior chamber, rabbit cornea, pronase (5 µg/ml), 48 hr. Note profuse development of fibroblasts. Compare with Fig. 4, 5. Giemsa. × 60.

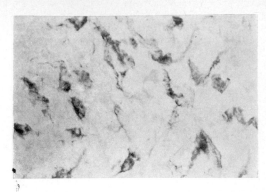

FIG. 8. Corneal stromal cells along wound edge at level of anterior chamber, rabbit cornea, trypsin (5 µg/ml), 48 hr. Note profuse development of fibroblasts. Compare with Fig. 4, 5, 6. Giemsa. × 60.

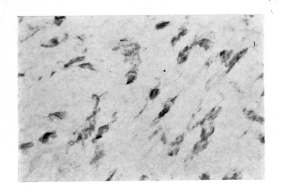

FIG. 7. Corneal stromal cells along wound edge at level of anterior chamber, rabbit cornea, pronase (20 µg/ml), 48 hr. Note continued profuse development of fibroblasts compared with control (Fig. 4). Giemsa. × 60.

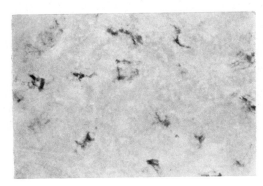

FIG. 9. Corneal stromal cells along wound edge at level of anterior chamber, rabbit cornea, trypsin (20 µg/ml), 48 hr. Most cells show necrosis or digestion. Compare with Fig. 7, 8. Giemsa. × 60.

TABLE 2. *Corneal stromal cells*

| Concentration of enzyme (µg/ml) | Enzyme | | |
|---|---|---|---|
| | a-chymotrypsin | Pronase | Trypsin |
| 5 | No effect | Vigorous growth | Vigorous growth |
| 10 | No effect | More vigorous growth than with 5 µg/ml | More growth than controls but also some necrosis |
| 20 | No effect | Vigorous growth (perhaps slightly less than with 10 µg/ml) | Necrosis and digestion occurring |

of fibroblasts along the wound edge, and at some distance from the wound edge, at all concentrations tested, although it was slightly less effective at 20 µg/ml than at either 5 µg/ml or 10 µg/ml (Fig. 6, 7). Pronase was growth stimulating to the corneal stromal cells even

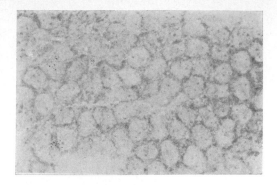

FIG. 10. Endothelial cells, rabbit cornea, control media, 48 hr. Giemsa. × 60.

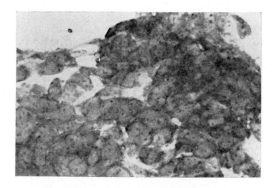

FIG. 11. Endothelial cells, rabbit cornea, trypsin (5 μg/ml), 48 hr. Note that endothelial cells contain larger, more numerous nucleoli than control cells, and are also stained much more intensely. Compare with Fig. 10. Giemsa. × 60.

in areas into which the epithelium had not yet grown.

Trypsin also markedly enhanced the growth of fibroblasts along the wound edge and away from it, and, as with pronase, even in areas into which the epithelium had not yet grown. Trypsin, in contrast to pronase, had a very limited effective concentration range. Trypsin caused corneal stromal cell necrosis and digestion at 20 μg/ml. At 10 μg/ml, trypsin caused some cell growth, but also some necrosis (Fig. 8, 9).

Table 2 summarizes the effects of each of the enzymes tested, at each concentration, on the corneal stromal cells.

*Endothelial cells.* α-chymotrypsin had neither a growth-stimulating nor a toxic effect on the endothelial cells. At 20 μg/ml α-chymotrypsin did cause a loosening and detachment of the endothelial cells from one another, but these cells appeared to be healthy and otherwise normal.

Pronase (at 5 and 10 μg/ml) had a possibly stimulating effect on the endothelial cells but in most cases they could not be distinguished from cells cultured in control media. At 20 μg/ml pronase was, however, highly toxic, causing almost total detachment of the endothelial cells or necrosis of those remaining.

Trypsin, in contrast to both α-chymotrypsin and pronase, had a progressively growth-stimulating effect on the endothelial cells (compare Fig. 10, normal, with Fig. 11, trypsin-treated). Even at 20 μg/ml the endothelial cells were firmly attached and dense in numbers.

Table 3 summarizes the effects of each enzyme, at each concentration tested, on the endothelial cells.

*Opacification.* The corneas remained thin

TABLE 3. *Endothelial cells*

| Concentration of enzyme (μg/ml) | Enzyme | | |
|---|---|---|---|
| | *α-chymotrypsin* | *Pronase* | *Trypsin* |
| 5 | No effect | Possibly slight stimulation | Growth stimulating |
| 10 | No effect | Possibly slight stimulation | Growth stimulating |
| 20 | Cells loosened and detaching but normal in appearance | Almost completely detached and necrotic | Growth stimulating |

TABLE 4. *Opacification of cornea*

| | |
|---|---|
| a-chymotrypsin | Cornea clear and thin at all concentrations (5, 10 and 20 μg/ml) although both epithelium and endothelium detaching at 20 μg/ml. |
| Pronase | Cornea clear although often swollen at 5 and 10 μg/ml. Totally opaque at 20 μg/ml (detachment and necrosis of both epithelium and endothelium occurring). |
| Trypsin | Cornea clear although often swollen at 5 and 10 μg/ml. Totally opaque at 20 μg/ml (endothelium attached and growing vigorously; epithelium almost totally detached or necrotic). |

and completely transparent in α-chymotrypsin at all concentrations tested, even though both the epithelial and endothelial cells were beginning to detach at 20 μg/ml.

Corneas cultured in 20 μg/ml of either trypsin or pronase were totally opaque. At 10 μg/ml of either enzyme the corneas were completely clear except for an opaque zone around the margins of the wound. At 5 μg/ml corneas cultured in either trypsin or pronase could not be distinguished macroscopically from corneas cultured in control media. The enzyme-treated corneas (even at 5 μg/ml) were, however, usually more swollen than the control corneas.

Table 4 summarizes the effect of each enzyme on the transparency of the cornea and the condition of epithelium and endothelium.

### DISCUSSION

The results clearly show that certain proteolytic enzymes, in low concentrations, may profoundly stimulate the growth of either the corneal stromal cells, or the endothelial cells, or both. The results further show that higher concentrations of these proteolytic enzymes may cause cell death and corneal opacification. None of the enzymes tested is a collagenase. However, it should be noted that pronase at high concentrations (2.5%) can cause complete liquefaction and dissolution of the cornea within 30 min at 37 C (Weimar, V. and Haraguchi, K. H., unpublished observations).

Since this study is preliminary, certain obvious questions remain to be answered:

1) Would the same effects be obtained with brief exposures of the cornea to these enzymes?

2) Is the presence of the epithelium necessary in order for pronase and trypsin to produce the enhanced corneal stromal cell growth?

3) Do these proteolytic enzymes act at the cell surface or within the cell? "Insoluble" trypsin, in particulate form, could be used to test this point.

4) What is the nature of the proteolytic enzymes of the corneal epithelium and the corneal stromal cells? What is their state of activation before and after injury?

Supported by Grant EY00238 National Eye Institute, US Public Health Service.

### REFERENCES

1. WEIMAR V. Polymorphonuclear invasion of wounded corneas. *J Exp Med* **105**: 141, 1957.
2. WEIMAR V. Activation of corneal stromal cells to take up the vital dye neutral red. *Exp Cell Res* **18**: 1, 1959.
3. WEIMAR V. Healing processes in the cornea, in: Duke-Elder S and Perkins ES (Eds) "The transparency of the cornea." Oxford, Blackwell Scientific Publications, 1960, p 111.
4. WEIMAR V and FELLMAN M. Connective tissue cell mobilization and migration following wounding. *Exp Eye Res* **9**: 12, 1970.
5. RUBIN H. Overgrowth stimulating factor released from Rous sarcoma cells. *Science* **167**: 1271, 1970.
6. BURGER MM. Proteolytic enzymes initiating cell division and escape from contact inhibition of growth. *Nature (Lond)* **227**: 170, 1970.

# COLLAGENOLYTIC ENZYMES
# IN CORNEAL PATHOLOGY*

STUART I. BROWN

Department of Ophthalmology, New York Hospital–Cornell University Medical Center, New York, New York, USA

Collagen is the major organic component of the cornea, comprising more than 60% of the dry weight of the tissue (1). The collagen molecule has a molecular weight of 300,000 and is composed of three helical polypeptide chains which are wound around a common axis forming a coiled chain (2). The helical structure of undenatured collagen in solution or fibrils is remarkably resistant to attack by proteolytic enzymes. Trypsin, chymotrypsin and pepsin may in time solubilize collagen fibrils by attacking the polar portions of the molecules or bonds between adjacent molecules but they do not change the helical structure of the molecules (3). A collagenase derived from *Clostridium histolyticum* was the first known enzyme that could attack the helical backbone of the collagen. It attacks and attaches to the molecule from either end and does not release its hold until the polypeptide chains are reduced almost to amino acids (4).

It has long been suspected that an enzyme is produced in animal tissues which could act on native collagen. Until relatively recently all efforts at isolating such an enzyme were futile. However, in the last 10 years intensive studies on the acid hydrolases and the isolation and characterization of a neutral collagenase have clarified the mechanisms of collagen degradation in animal tissues.

*Lysosomal enzymes.* Acid hydrolases which are usually of lysosomal origin can degrade collagen but only at a pH below 6.0. Consequently it is doubtful whether these enzymes could operate extracellularly in degrading collagen fibrils under physiologic conditions. The main function of the proteolytic acid hydrolases in connective tissues is generally considered to be associated with intracellular activity where the pH is acidic and the hydrolases can digest collagen debris as part of the process of phagocytosis (5).

*Collagenase.* In 1962, Gross and Lapiere (6) reported the first of a series of studies which demonstrated a collagenolytic enzyme in tissues that could operate under physiologic conditions. Collagenolytic activity was demonstrated and assayed by culturing tissue explants on opaque collagen gels. Lysis or clearing of the gel indicated collagen breakdown. The collagen which was heat-gelled was essentially fibrillar and provided a sensitive assay system when labeled with $C^{14}$. The first studies, which were carried out on the metamorphosing tadpole tail, showed that collagenase was produced mainly in the epithelial cells as well as in the underlying mesen-

* Address for reprints: Stuart I. Brown, M.D., 525 East 68th Street, New York, New York 10021, USA.

517

fibroblasts in the stroma may counterbalance collagenase breakdown. At the advancing cell border, collagenase is produced by the epithelium in addition to by the stromal cells.

Ulcerations of the stroma central to this advancing border may be explained by the production of collagenase in an area beyond the limits of the new vessels and where there are few or even no fibroblasts. These ulcers are almost never seen before 10 days and theoretically, in order to prevent ulcers, treatment with collagenase inhibitors should be started by seven days after the injury. Treatment should be continued until the epithelium has covered the cornea and the epithelial collagenase production has ceased. The stromal production of collagenase continues for a long time after epithelial healing but does not cause stromal dissolution, perhaps because of inhibition of this enzyme by serum proteins.

The method of collagenase destruction in corneal ulcers of eyes not burned with alkali is probably slightly different and involves selective enzymatic breakdown. If an epithelial defect is associated with stromal inflammation, the epithelium is induced to produce collagenase. Inflammatory enzymes produced in the stroma may hydrolyze the proteoglycan protection of the stromal collagen and, following this, the epithelial collagenase breaks down the stroma. Ulcers seem to heal when new blood vessels reach the inflamed area. The author speculates that further ulceration is stopped by the leakage of serum proteins from the new vessel which inhibits collagenase and stops further collagen breakdown.

Regardless of the type of corneal ulcer, one must be cautions of coincident treatment with corticosteroids. Brown et al. (28) found that corticosteroids potentiate collagenase activity by 15-fold. This may be the reason that certain ulcers rapidly progress to perforation after treatment with corticosteroids.

At present, clinical studies on the treatment of collagenase-induced corneal ulcers have been limited to the treatment of the various problems associated with the alkali-burned cornea (17, 18). Brown and Weller (21) reported preliminary studies indicating that perforations of alkali-burned human corneas may be prevented by topical treatment with cysteine (0.2 M). They also suggested treatment with collagenase inhibitors as an adjunct to corneal transplantation to prevent wound breakdown in the postoperative course.

*Clinical findings.* More than 120 eyes with severe injuries or ulcers were treated with 0.2 M cysteine applied topically six times a day. These corneas were diffusely opaque and completely denuded of epithelium after injury. Thirty-three of these burned eyes were treated and all but three healed without incident. One patient developed a corneal ulcer after an emergency cataract extraction while the patient was not on cysteine. This ulcer progressed in spite of initiation of cysteine therapy and eventually perforated. Two other eyes developed ulcers that eventually healed. There was a small control group of corneas with severe alkali burns which were not treated with cysteine. Five of the seven eyes not treated with cysteine perforated.

Four eyes with peripheral furrow ulcers were treated and all healed in three weeks. Seven descemetocele ulcers were also treated; six of these were of herpes simplex origin. None progressed and all eventually healed.

Recently we began treating dendritic ulcers with cysteine alone in order to determine whether stromal ulcerations can be prevented. Seven corneas with either large single or multiple ulcers were treated. The dendritic ulcers spread throughout the corneas but eventually all healed, usually 3 to 14 weeks after initiation of treatment with cysteine, and none extended into the stroma. Although this preliminary series comprised only seven

# STRUCTURAL MACROMOLECULES OF THE CORNEAL STROMA

## EMBRYONIC DEVELOPMENT AND BIOSYNTHESIS

M. MOCZAR and E. MOCZAR

Laboratoire de Biochimie du Tissue Conjonctif, Equipe de CNRS n° 53 and
Centre de Recherche d'Ophtalmologie, Groupe de Recherches U 86 de l'INSERM,
Fondation Ophtalmologique A. de Rothschild, Paris, France

Considerable evidence suggests that alterations in the structural organization of the corneal stroma are among the principal factors leading to scarring and opacification (1–7). Nevertheless our knowledge of this organization at the macromolecular level, even in the normal eye, is meager. The three principal types of macromolecule present in the corneal stroma are: 1) Proteoglycans. These are linear high molecular weight water-soluble acidic polymers. The term proteoglycan is defined here to mean glycosaminoglycan covalently linked to peptide residues and it replaces the older term mucopolysaccharide-protein complex. The disaccharide repeating unit characterizing keratan sulfate is galactose-N-acetyl-glucosamine galactose-glucosamine while the disaccharide characterizing chondroitin sulfate is glucuronic acid-N-acetyl galactosamine. 2) Structural glycoproteins. These are insoluble proteins containing covalently linked neutral sugars, amino sugars and sialic acid. 3) Collagen. This high molecular weight asymmetric fibril contains about 12 % hydroxyproline and thus belongs in the collagen family of structural proteins. In addition to this characteristic amino acid, corneal collagen also contains significant amounts of hydroxylysine-linked glucose and galactose.

Studies on variations in the relative proportions of these substances provide a convenient tool for studying the extracellular matrix of the corneal stroma (8–11). The present report describes two aspects of the structural organization of the stroma: a) changes in the chemical composition of the structural macromolecules during the development of the extracellular matrix and b) biosynthesis of the carbohydrate components of these macromolecules from radioactive precursors.

### EMBRYONIC DEVELOPMENT

Corneal stromas were extracted in $CaCl_2$ at pH 7.5 as described by Robert and Dische (12). This procedure yielded two soluble fractions: soluble glycoprotein-proteoglycan complex (CTC) and soluble collagen-glycoprotein-proteoglycan complex (CSC) and one insoluble polymeric stroma (PS) (13). Previous studies have shown that these fractions represent diffusible and polymeric forms of collagen, glycoproteins and proteoglycans (14). During embryonic and postnatal development the soluble components CTC and CSC decrease while polymeric stroma PS increases. At the same time, the carbohydrate content of the CSC fractions increases while that of the polymeric stroma decreases (15–17).

525

monosaccharides was determined. With the exception of hydroxylysine-linked sugars the specific activities were similar to the distribution of the sugars in the native molecule (Fig. 4). The highest incorporation was in the glycoproteins and the high molecular weight glycopeptide fractions.

## REFERENCES

1. SCHWARTZ W. Elektronmikroskopische Untersuchungen über die Differenzierung der Cornea und Skleralfibrillen des Menschen. *Z Zellforsch Mikrosk Anat* **38**: 78, 1953.
2. DOHLMAN CH. On the metabolism of the corneal graft. *Acta Ophthalmol (Kbh)* **35**: 303, 1957.
3. AURELL G. Healing process in the cornea with special regard to structure and metachromasia. *Acta Ophthalmol (Kbh)* **32**: 307, 1954.
4. ANSETH A. Glycosaminoglycans in corneal regeneration. *Exp Eye Res* **1**: 122, 1961.
5. ANSETH A and LAURENT TC. Polysaccharides in normal and pathological corneas. *Invest Ophthalmol* **1**: 195, 1962.
6. ANSETH A and FRANSSON LA. Studies on corneal polysaccharides. VI. Isolation of dermatan sulfate from corneal scar tissue. *Exp Eye Res* **8**: 302, 1969.
7. ROBERT L, SCHILLINGER G, MOCZAR M, JUNQUA S and MOCZAR E. Étude morphologique et biochimique du keratocone. II. Étude biochimique. *Arch Ophthalmol (Paris)* **30**: 143, 1970.
8. ROBERT L and ROBERT B. Structural glycoproteins of membranes and connective tissues: Biochemical and immunochemical properties, in: Peeters H (Ed), "Protides of the biological fluids." Amsterdam, Elsevier, 1967, v 15, p 143.
9. MOCZAR M, MOCZAR E and ROBERT L. Composition of glycopeptides obtained by proteolytic digestion of the media of porcine aorta. *Atherosclerosis* **12**: 31, 1970.
10. MOCZAR E and MOCZAR M. The glycopeptide pattern of the porcine and rabbit corneal stroma. *Comp Biochem Physiol* **36**: 547, 1970.
11. MOCZAR E and MOCZAR M. Distribution of carbohydrates in the insoluble network of connective tissue, in: Balazs EA (Ed), "Chemistry and molecular biology of the intercellular matrix." New York, Academic Press, 1970, p 243.
12. ROBERT L and DISCHE Z. Analysis of a sulfated sialoglucoglucosamino-galactomannosidoglycane from corneal stroma. *Biochem Biophys Res Commun* **10**: 209, 1963.
13. MOCZAR M and ROBERT L. Extraction and fractionation of the media of thoracic aorta. Isolation and characterization of structural glycoproteins. *Atherosclerosis* **11**: 7, 1970.
14. ROBERT AM, ROBERT B and ROBERT L. Chemical and physical properties of structural glycoproteins, in: Balazs A (Ed), "Chemistry and molecular biology of the intercellular matrix." New York, Academic Press, 1970, p 237.
15. MOCZAR M and MOCZAR E. Glycosylation de'hydroxylysine dans le stroma cornéen de veau. Étude du développement embryonnaire et postnatal. *CR Acad Sci [D] (Paris)* **271**: 1886, 1970.
16. SMITS G. Quantitative interrelationships of the chief components of some connective tissues during foetal and postnatal development in cattle. *Biochim Biophys Acta* **25**: 542, 1957.
17. ANSETH A. Glycosaminoglycans in the developing corneal stroma. *Exp Eye Res* **1**: 116, 1961.
18. MOCZAR E and MOCZAR M. Glycannes liés à la fraction insoluble de la cornée de roussette (*Scyliorhinus canicula L*). *Eur J Biochem* **13**: 28, 1970.
19. ROBERT L, REISS-BRION M, JUNQUA S and SALAÜN J. Sur la culture organotypique de cornées d'embryons de poulet. *CR Acad Sci [D] (Paris)* **269**: 1529, 1969.
20. ROBERT L and PARLEBAS J. Biosynthèse *in vitro* des glycoproteines de la cornée. *Bull Soc Chim Biol (Paris)* **241**: 1853, 1965.
21. BUTLER WT and CUNNINGHAM LW. Evidence for the linkage of a disaccharide to hydroxylysine in tropocollagen. *J Biol Chem* **241**: 3882, 1966.
22. MOCZAR E, MOCZAR M and ROBERT L. Isolation and characterization of the glycopeptides of the structural glycoproteins of corneal stroma. *Life Sci [II]* **8**: 757, 1969.
23. MOCZAR E and MOCZAR M. Micromethod for the determination of hydroxylysine and its glycosylated derivatives. *J Chromatogr* **51**: 277, 1970.

# DISCUSSION

DR. D. MISHIMA (*Japan*): We have heard some exciting reports dealing with two aspects of corneal pathology: first, the experimental approaches and second, the application of this knowledge to clinical problems.

DR. S. DIKSTEIN (*Israel*): I would like to ask Dr. Brown whether cysteine is specific in the inhibition of epithelial collagenase, or are other sulfhydryl compounds also active?

DR. S. I. BROWN (*USA*): We have found that dithiothreitol, which does not chelate calcium, is a rather potent inhibitor of collagenase. But when the sulfhydryl groups of dithiothreitol are blocked by iodoacetate, it no longer inhibits collagenase. We therefore think that cysteine inhibits the enzyme partly by chelating calcium and partly by cleaving disulfide linkages in the collagen molecule and, afterwards, probably binding at the sulfhydryl sites liberated.

DR. M. MOCZAR (*France*): We have some preliminary evidence suggesting that certain breakdown products of collagen, as well as other components of the stroma, may inhibit some of the degradative enzymes released during ulceration.

DR. A. SPECTOR (*USA*): I would imagine that if cysteine could be kept in constant contact with the corneal wound by means of a covering lens, it would be much more effective than instillation of drops for inhibiting collagenase.

DR. BROWN: We have in fact used cysteine with soft lenses but we are still not certain whether this combined treatment is any more effective than the use of drops alone.

Regarding Dr. Moczar's comment on the use of breakdown products from the stroma for inhibiting collagenase, one of the important problems is diffusion to the site of inhibition. We are also working on this, but as yet we haven't any clear-cut answers.

DR. V. L. WEIMAR (*USA*): We have been studying the role of proteolytic enzymes in wound repair, and at one time we tried to isolate keratocytes. Our first attempts to digest the collagen with collagenase were unsuccessful, and we later tried pronase. Somewhat to our surprise, we found that even at rather low concentrations, this enzyme completely digested the whole stroma. We were left with a highly viscous material, and although the keratocytes were liberated, they were so tightly trapped within the viscous fluid that we were unable to separate them. I therefore wonder about the specificity of collagenase, since it seems to me that other enzymes might also be acting—perhaps sequentially—on the native molecule. I would also like to point out that most collagenase inhibitors are active on other proteolytic enzymes as well.

Apart from this, it has been my impression that certain mucopolysaccharides, among them heparin, inhibit trypsin and perhaps other proteases.

DR. MISHIMA: The question of whether it is collagenase alone that degrades the collagen is a very important one. Is it possible that when the fibrils are no longer protected by the stromal proteoglycans, they are more susceptible to degradation?

DR. BROWN: In answer to Dr. Weimar's comment, we have tested purified preparations of heparin, chondroitin sulfate and keratan sulfate as possible inhibitors of collagenase and found that none of them was active. However, crude preparations of corneal proteoglycans completely inhibit collagenase. This provides a partial answer to Dr. Mishima's question since these results suggest that corneal glycosaminoglycans in their native state, that is, as proteoglycans, may in some way protect the collagen fibrils from attack by collagenase. Highly purified glycosaminoglycans, which are much lower in protein content and of much smaller molecular size than the proteoglycans, are apparently unable to play a protective role.

529

TABLE 5. *Relative frequency of the first senile cataract removal in nondiabetics and known diabetics living in Oxford, England; 1957–66*

| Age (years) | | Cataract extraction/1,000 population per year | | Ratio of rate of removal of cataract of known diabetics/ nondiabetics |
|---|---|---|---|---|
| | | Nondiabetics | Known diabetics | |
| 50 to 69 | Males | 0.49 | 2.40 | $4.9 \pm 2.1$ |
| | Females | 0.53 | 4.95 | $9.3 \pm 2.3$ |
| 70 + | Males | 2.32 | 7.39 | $3.2 \pm 1.2$ |
| | Females | 3.48 | 14.7 | $4.1 \pm 0.9$ |

There is no doubt that the number of people who are blind from cataract could be greatly reduced if surgery were available to them. There is also no doubt that a means of delay or prevention of cataracts would be even more valuable. This justifies research. I would like to indicate where research has been successful, the major problems which are being tackled now and what new aspects should be investigated.

*Cataract and diabetes.* Cataract in man is, by and large, called senile cataract when it occurs after 45 years of age. I agree with Sorsby (8) that this is a useless and possibly misleading label. In order to investigate cataract we must subdivide it into types. I will begin by suggesting a separate classification of "cataracts in diabetics." Many people have a particular interest in this type of cataract for they have worked with it. It is a cataract for which we know the initiating biochemical cause. Van Heyningen (9, 10) found that lenses of diabetic rats contained sorbitol which is not present in normal lenses. Sorbitol was formed in the lens from glucose but only when there was a high blood sugar. Kinoshita and co-workers (11) postulated and then proved that sorbitol in the lens increased osmotic pressure within the fibers. The fibers then swell and sometimes ultimately disrupt. This disruption of fibers and alteration of lens metabolism led directly to lens opacity in experimental animals. Whether the same sequence of events took place in man was, I think, clearly shown when Pirie and van Heyningen (12) found that the lens of the human diabetic, whether cataractous or not, contains sorbitol which is not present normally in the nondiabetic lens. Epidemiological studies showed that cataract extraction was surprisingly high in diabetics and also that diabetics have their cataracts extracted at an earlier age (3).

Diabetics make up 13% of all patients in Oxford having a cataract extracted. This is much higher than the percentage of diabetics in the adult population. Diabetics between 50 and 69 years of age are five to nine times as likely to have a cataract extracted as nondiabetics (Table 5). The discrepancy is less in the older group showing that diabetics have their cataracts removed at an earlier age.

It is now realized that cataract in diabetics is a larger problem in ophthalmology than it was earlier thought to be. The British Diabetic Association (13) published the results of an enquiry into the incidence of blindness due to diabetes. Registration of blindness in Britain is not compulsory and the object of the Association's enquiry was to find how many unregistered blind diabetics there might be in order to determine the true prevalence. This enquiry showed that about 40% of diabetics with registrable visual disability were in fact unregistered. Thus the official figures of incidence of blindness due to diabetes may need to be increased by 100%. This is startling enough but it is even more startling to read

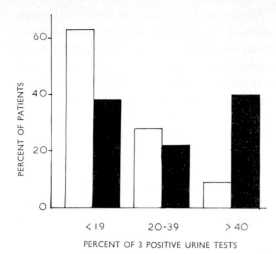

FIG. 2. Relation between control of diabetes and cataract extraction (each patient had had at least five urine tests). Sample size: 45 had cataract extraction (black columns) and 100 were randomly chosen patients (white columns).

that "There is thus approximately one diabetic blind from cataract for every three blind from retinopathy." (13). The proportion in Canada is one to four (14) and in Britain there may well be 2,000 diabetics blind from cataract alone. There are other societies in which the prevalence of diabetes is much greater such as that of the Pima Indians of the Arizona desert. Here, where half of the Indians over 30 years old are diabetic, the prevalence of cataract can also be expected to be higher.

There are two ways to delay or prevent the accumulation of sorbitol in the lens. One is to control the diabetes, since aldose reductase is active only when blood glucose is high. The other is to inhibit the enzyme. Efforts to correlate poor control of blood sugar with cataract have been only partly successful. A clear correlation was, however, found between frequency of high urinary glucose and cataract extraction (Fig. 2) (15).

Burditt and Caird (16) studied the relationship of diabetic control to lens opacities by analyzing 2,820 observations made by oph-thalmologists on the eyes of 1,827 diabetic patients. They found that the frequency of lens opacities in male diabetics and the chance of their development in older patients of both sexes were greater in those less well controlled, but there was no such difference in the progression of established opacities. Their study also provided evidence that bilateral lens opacities may disappear completely in as many as 10% of younger diabetics. No woman over 60 years of age whose diabetes was poorly controlled showed any sign of regression (0/27) but 14% of those whose diabetes was better controlled did regress (10/74). Here we have a metabolically initiated cataract which may constitute 13% of all those extracted in Oxford. This cataract would probably not deteriorate to the point where it had to be removed if the patient were able to maintain good control of his diabetes (17). Current research offers hope of finding an inhibitor to stop the formation of sorbitol which triggers the opacification of the lens.

*Protein, lens color and cataract.* Apart from cataract in diabetics, no other major group of cataracts has been classified biochemically. Yet, there are great biochemical differences between human cataracts which have been extracted. In Oxford, cataracts are classified

TABLE 6. *Incidence of different types of cataract extracted in Oxford or in Pakistan graded 1 to 4 by color*

| Grade | Color of lenses | Percent cataracts extracted[a] | |
|---|---|---|---|
| | | Oxford | Pakistan |
| 1 | Uniform pale yellow, nucleus not visible | 45 | 6 |
| 2 | Pale cortex with visible nucleus | 42 | 50 |
| 3 | Pale cortex with hazel-brown nucleus | 11 | 38 |
| 4 | Pale cortex with deep brown nucleus | 2 | 6 |

[a] Total sample no. of cataracts graded in Oxford was 328 and in Pakistan, 332.

**533**

3. CAIRD FI, HUTCHINSON M and PIRIE A. Cataract extraction in an English population. *Br J Prev Soc Med* **19**: 80, 1965.
4. *WHO Epidemiol Vital Statist Rep* **19**: 433, 1966.
5. FRANKEN S and MEHTA KR. Report from Christian Medical College, Ludhiana, India, 1969.
6. Vision and its disorders. Washington, US Department of Health, Education, and Welfare NINDB Monograph No 4, 1967, p 23.
7. DUANE TD. "Report on ophthalmic research, USA." Research to Prevent Blindness, Inc, 1965.
8. SORSBY A. The incidence and causes of blindness in England and Wales 1948–62. *Rep Public Health Med* No 114, London, HMSO, 1966.
9. VAN HEYNINGEN R. Formation of polyols by the lens of the rat with 'sugar' cataract. *Nature (Lond)* **184**: 194, 1959.
10. VAN HEYNINGEN R. The sorbitol pathway in the lens. *Exp Eye Res* **1**: 396, 1962.
11. KINOSHITA JH, MEROLA LO and DIKMAK E. Osmotic changes in experimental galactose cataracts. *Exp Eye Res* **1**: 405, 1962.
12. PIRIE A and VAN HEYNINGEN R. The effect of diabetes on the content of sorbitol, glucose, fructose and inositol in the human lens. *Exp Eye Res* **3**: 124, 1964.
13. Report on diabetic blindness in the UK. London, British Diabetic Association, 1970.
14. MACDONALD AE. Causes of blindness in Canada. *Can Med Assoc J* **92**: 264, 1965.
15. CAIRD FI, HUTCHINSON M and PIRIE A. Cataract and diabetes. *Br Med J* **2**: 665, 1964.
16. BURDITT AF and CAIRD FI. Natural history of lens opacities in diabetics. *Br J Ophthalmol* **52**: 433, 1968.
17. CAIRD FI, PIRIE A and RAMSELL TG. "Diabetes and the eye." Oxford, Blackwell Scientific Publications, 1969.
18. PIRIE A. Color and solubility of the proteins of human cataracts. *Invest Ophthalmol* **7**: 634, 1968.
19. HARDING JJ. Nature and origin of the insoluble protein of rat lens. *Exp Eye Res* **8**: 147, 1969.
20. DISCHE Z. Alterations of lens proteins as etiology in cataracts, in: Dardenne U (Ed), "Biochemistry of eye." Basel, Karger, 1968, p 413.
21. SPECTOR A and ZORN M. Studies upon the sulfhydryl groups of calf lens α-crystallins. *J Biol Chem* **242**: 3594, 1967.
22. TESTA M, FIORE C, BOCCI N and CALABRO S. Effect of the oxidation of sulfhydryl groups on lens proteins. *Exp Eye Res* **7**: 276, 1968.
23. BUCKINGHAM RH. Cross-links in protein from cataractous lenses. *Biochem J* **124**: 54, 1971.
24. FISHER RF. Elastic constants of the human lens capsule. *J Physiol (Lond)* **201**: 1, 1969.
25. KUCK JFR JR. The decrease in lens permeability with age in the rat, in: Dardenne U (Ed), "Biochemistry of the eye." Basel, Karger, 1968, p 388.
26. BELLOWS JG and CHINN H. Biochemistry of the lens. XV. Studies on the swelling of the isolated lens. *Am J Ophthalmol* **24**: 979, 1941.
27. PIRIE A. Difference in swelling and opacity formation between young and old lenses. *Nature (Lond)* **216**: 503, 1967.
28. PATTERSON JW and BUNTING KW. Sugar cataracts, polyol levels and lens swelling. *Doc Ophthalmol* **20**: 64, 1966.
29. GOLDMANN H. Senile changes of the lens and the vitreous. *Am J Ophthalmol* **57**: 1, 1964.
30. MACH H. Untersuchungen von Linseneiweiss und Mikroelektrophorese von wasserlöslichem Eiweiss im Altersstar. *Klin Monatsbl Augenheilkd* **143**: 689, 1963.
31. MARIANI G, SANTORI M and CARTA F. Modifications of adenosine triphosphate and of some enzymatic activities during the development of human senile cataract. *Exp Eye Res* **6**: 126, 1967.
32. CHARLTON JM and VAN HEYNINGEN R. An investigation into the loss of proteins of low molecular size from the lens in senile cataract. *Exp Eye Res* **7**: 47, 1968
33. BARBER GW. Free amino acids in senile cataractous lenses: possible osmotic etiology. *Invest Ophthalmol* **7**: 564, 1968.
34. THOFT RA and KINOSHITA JH. The effect of calcium on rat lens permeability. *Invest Ophthalmol* **4**: 122, 1965.
35. SRIVASTAVA SK and BEUTLER E. Increased susceptibility of riboflavin-deficient rats to galactose cataract. *Experientia* **26**: 250, 1970.
36. BAMJI MS. Glutathione reductase activity in red blood cells and riboflavin nutritional status in humans. *Clin Chim Acta* **26**: 263, 1969.
37. PIRIE A. Photooxidation of proteins and comparison of photo-oxidized proteins with those of the cataractous human lens. *Isr J Med Sci* **8**: 1567, 1972.
38. VAN HEYNINGEN R. The lens: metabolism and cataract, in: Davson H (Ed), "The eye," 2nd edn. London, Academic Press Inc, 1969, v 1, p 381.
39. WALEY SG. The lens: function and macromolecular composition, in: Davson H (Ed), "The Eye," 2nd edn. London, Academic Press Inc, 1969, v 1, p 299.
40. KUCK JFR JR. The lens, in: Graymore CN (Ed), "Biochemistry of the eye." London, Pergamon Press, 1970.

# MECHANISM OF DEVELOPMENT
# AND POSSIBLE PREVENTION OF SUGAR CATARACTS

## KENNETH H. GABBAY and JIN H. KINOSHITA

Cell Biology Laboratory, Endocrine Division, Department of Medicine, The Children's Hospital Medical Center, Department of Pediatrics, Harvard Medical School and The Howe Laboratory of Ophthalmology Massachusetts Eye and Ear Infirmary and Harvard Medical School, Boston, Massachusetts, USA

Sugar cataracts are observed clinically in diabetic and galactosemic patients. These sugar cataracts have been extensively studied in the laboratory because they can easily be reproduced in experimental animals. Diabetic cataract is reproduced in a number of animals by the induction of diabetes with alloxan or streptozotocin and the galactosemic cataract is induced in rats by feeding a diet rich in galactose. Other sugars besides glucose and galactose are cataractogenic in rats if their concentrations in the bloodstream can be kept sufficiently high for long periods. Thus far, xylose is the only other cataractogenic sugar which has been studied to any extent.

A number of theories have been proposed to explain the development of sugar cataracts. A lack of insulin has been thought to depress the rate of glucose metabolism in the diabetic lens. However, no major change in the rate of glucose metabolism has been observed in these lenses. In human galactosemic cataract the accumulation of galactose-1-phosphate has been suspected of altering some phase of carbohydrate metabolism, but no definite site of action has been established to account for the development of opacities. Galactose-1-phosphate inhibits the phosphoglucomutase reaction but this inhibition is not sufficient to prevent synthesis of essential polysaccharides

A hypothesis under consideration is that a common mechanism is responsible for the cataractous process in the various sugar cataracts. A common factor in hyperglycemia, galactosemia or xylosemia is the availability of an abnormally high concentration of these sugars in the aqueous humor. The ability of these sugars to penetrate into the lens appears to set off a sequence of events that initiates the cataractous process. Close similarities in the morphology and histopathology of these experimental sugar cataracts lend support to the hypothesis implicating a common mechanism. In these experimental sugar cataracts, opacities are first observed in the periphery or equatorial region of the lens. The first histopathological sign which occurs very early in these disorders, is the appearance of hydropic lens fibers caused by an accumulation of fluid. In the more advanced stages the swelling continues until the fibers liquify and rupture with the formation of interfibrillar clefts. This histological picture, observed in each of these forms of sugar cataracts suggests that differences in tonicity between the intralenticular and intraocular fluids cause a movement of water into the lens fibers. Thus, osmotic changes appear responsible for lens swelling

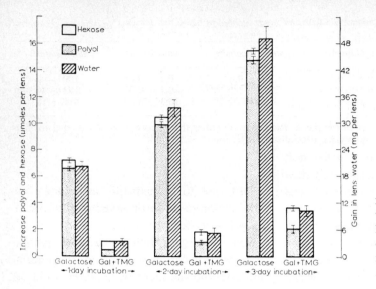

FIG. 2. Effect of $10^{-2}$ M tetramethylene glutaric acid (TMG) on a lens exposed to galactose for three days. (Reproduced with permission from KINOSHITA JH et al. *Biochim Biophys Acta* **158**: 472, 1968, Fig. 2.)

methylene glutaric acid (TMG), was especially effective in preventing the development of galactose cataracts *in vitro* (5). Lenses incubated in media containing TMG remain as clear as the normal controls, while their counterparts without TMG show high levels of dulcitol, swelling, loss of amino acids, electrolyte disequilibrium and opacification. These *in vitro* experiments indicate that the early changes observed in sugar-induced cataracts can be prevented by appropriate inhibitors of the enzyme aldose reductase (Fig. 2).

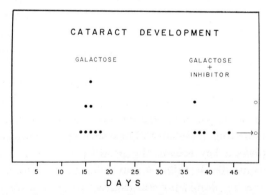

FIG. 3. The delaying effect of an orally fed aldose reductase inhibitor (AY-284) on the appearance of cataract in rats pair-fed a 40% galactose diet. The black circles denote the day of cataract appearance. Open circles indicate clear lenses.

While TMG has served a very useful function in *in vitro* experiments, it was ineffective in *in vivo* animal investigations. Recently, a more potent inhibitor of aldose reductase, Ayerst-284, has been developed. In lens cultures AY-284 was effective at a much lower concentration than TMG in preventing dulcitol accumulation and swelling of the lens in experiments similar to those illustrated in Fig. 2. In addition, AY-284 was effective in delaying the appearance of cataracts *in vivo*. In rats fed a 40% galactose diet containing AY-284, at least a 50% lowering of dulcitol accumulation in the lens was observed. Furthermore, in carefully controlled pair-fed experiments, the appearance of cataracts was strikingly delayed in the inhibitor-treated group. The dense nuclear cataracts in galactose-fed rats appeared at a median time of 16 days of galactose feeding (Fig. 3), while in the inhibitor-treated group the appearance of cataracts was delayed to a mean of 40 days. These results strongly suggest that prevention of sugar cataracts, both diabetic and galactosemic, may eventually be realized by oral or possibly topical administration of appropriate aldose reductase inhibitors. Furthermore, clarification of the mechanisms of diabetic and galactosemic cataract formation and the potential ability for preventive intervention may be of more general significance. Such an approach acquires additional importance, especially with the recent demonstration of the involvement of the sorbitol pathway in the formation of other diabetic and galactosemic tissue manifestations, namely, neuropathy and tubular nephropathy.

The authors would like to express their thanks to Drs. D. M. Dvornik and Robert A. Lehman of Ayerst Research Laboratories for their interest and cooperation.

Supported by Grants EY 17082, EY 00170 and EY 00304 from The National Eye Institute of The National Institutes of Health, by contract AT(30–1) 1368 from the United States Atomic Energy Commission and by a grant from Ayerst Research Laboratories. Dr. Gabbay is a recipient of a Medical Foundation Research Fellowship.

## REFERENCES

1. DUKE-ELDER WS.   Changes in refraction in diabetes mellitus. *Br J Ophthalmol* **9**: 167, 1925.
2. VAN HEYNINGEN R.   Metabolism of xylose by the lens. *Biochem J* **73**: 197, 1959.
3. WICK AN and DRURY DR.   Action of insulin on the permeability of cells to sorbitol. *Am J Physiol* **166**: 421, 1951.
4. KINOSHITA JH.   Cataracts in galactosemia. The Jonas S. Friedenwald Memorial Lecture. *Invest Ophthalmol* **4**: 786, 1965.
5. KINOSHITA JH, DVORNIK D, KRAML M and GABBAY KH.   The effect of an aldose reductase inhibitor on the galactose-exposed rabbit lens. *Biochim Biophys Acta* **158**: 472, 1968.

aspects should be pointed out. A statistically significant aggravation of galactose cataracts results from the administration of corticosteroids (12). Yet the lenses do not show the characteristic corticosteroid opacities. Instead they have the appearance of typical galactose cataracts. The same is seen in rabbits subjected to X-rays and naphthalene (7) and in rats subjected to X-rays and galactose (26). In both cases irradiation promotes typical naphthalene and galactose cataracts, respectively. It thus seems that subliminal lens hazards can aggravate the course of other cataracts without producing a different morphological type.

These findings may help us to elucidate some of the factors responsible for presenile cataracts, i.e., cataracts of a morphologically senile type at a presenile age. According to Otto Becker's early theory (27), senile opacities are a normal feature of aging, a kind of "physiological lens death" that cannot be avoided if the individual lives long enough. But why do signs of senile cataracts appear in some people before senescence? We think that an accumulation of subliminal lens hazards may accelerate the onset of senile opacities. This view is supported by many clinical observations. It was H. K. Müller who first led us to investigate this problem on a larger scale. He had noted presenile cataracts in several of his patients. Further inquiry revealed that they had been exposed for some time to cataractogenic agents, although the morphology of the opacities at first seemed to exclude these agents as the cause of the cataract. Among these patients were several who had for many years been on a diet highly deficient in proteins and vitamins. Another was a radiologist who had been exposed to more than the usual X-ray dosage for a long time. Although in the case of the radiologist no typical posterior subcapsular opacities were seen, the results of the above experiments pointed to subliminal cataractogenics as the causative factor in the development of presenile cata-

racts. Furthermore, not only do diabetics develop typical diabetic cataracts when young, but later in life these true diabetic opacities are no longer found. Instead, they now develop cataracts of the senile type, but earlier and more frequently than nondiabetics.

Also in the category of subliminal cataractogenics are many eye diseases which, by alteration of the aqueous and impairment of lens nutrition, can exert such an effect. For example, uveitis alone can cause complicated cataracts. If corticosteroid therapy is used, we must bear in mind that this may also act as a subliminal lens hazard. This then brings us to another important consequence of the above findings. In testing new drugs for their possible cataractogenic side effects, it is by no means sufficient to search for opacities after long-term administration of the substance to normal animals. We must also eliminate possible additive effects on the lens. This is especially important for drugs used in the treatment of eye diseases or systemic diseases that can by themselves affect the lens.

We have tested certain drugs in view of such potential subliminal effects (28). One was oxyphenbutazone which, apart from its many uses in ophthalmology, is frequently used against intraocular inflammations. White Wistar rats were subjected to a 40% galactose diet with oxyphenbutazone applied to the eye as an ointment. The lenses of the rats were photographed at intervals of two to three days (Fig. 1). These pictures were enlarged with a profile projector and the size of the opaque area was measured by planimetry. Expression of the opaque area as a percentage of the whole lens area provided absolute data on the progress of the opacity, which could be subjected to statistical analysis (Fig. 2). In the case of oxyphenbutazone, we did not find any additive effect of the drug on the formation of galactose-induced opacities. On the contrary, the animals treated with this drug seemed to show a slower progression of cata-

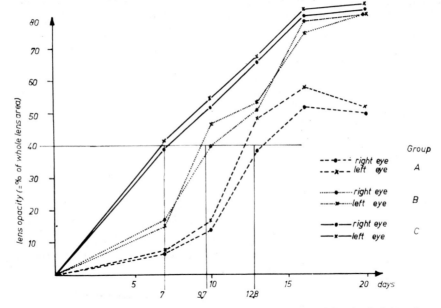

FIG. 1. Development of galactose cataracts in rabbits. Opacities of 40% (a), 60% (b) and 80% (c) of the lens area.

CC
WITH

A long hel
disproved
cause or c
some parts
changes in
tigated but
photosensit
gical condit
photo-oxida
The most pl
tidine, trypt
tyrosine. Ea
the brown
separated fr
less histidine

FIG. 2. Formation of lens opacities after galactose feeding and local administration of oxyphenbutazone (OPB) eye ointment. Group A: 5% OPB and 40% galactose diet; group B: 10% OPB and 40% galactose diet; group C: controls, 40% galactose diet.

Tota
Tota
Total
age
Total
dia

*a* Val

racts. Nevertheless, we thought this was a good example for demonstrating this testing procedure.

An investigation of the pattern of additive cataractogenic effects in suspected or established cataractogenics will help us to understand more about pathophysiological backgrounds of cataractogenesis. It will also enable us to work out test methods to detect undesirable drug side effects in new substances that are not known to be cataractogenic when acting alone on normal lenses.

REFERENCES

1. BLACK RL, OGLESBY RB, VON SALLMANN L and BUNIM JJ. Posterior subcapsular cataracts induced by corticosteroids in patients with rheumatoid arthritis. *JAMA* **174**: 166, 1960.
2. AXELSSON U. Glaucoma, miotic therapy and cataract. *Acta Ophthalmol* **46**: 83, 99, 831, 1968.

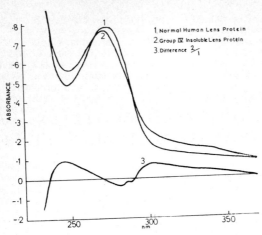

FIG. 1. Absorption spectra of 1) normal human lens protein, 2) Group IV (brown cataract) insoluble protein and 3) difference spectrum 2/1.

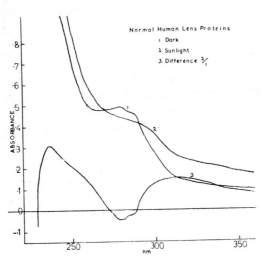

FIG. 2. Absorption spectra of normal human lens protein kept in 1) darkness, 2) the same after exposure to sun and 3) difference spectrum 2/1.

cataractous lenses resemble those of photo-oxidized proteins (5). I therefore investigated whether photo-oxidation of normal lens proteins exposed to sunlight would yield similar products. It is recognized that exposure to ultraviolet light of wavelength below 300 nm, which is the lower limit of sunlight, may cause different photo-oxidative changes. Because of initial insolubility or a developing insolubility on exposure to sunlight the proteins were dissolved in 6 M guanidinium hydrochloride at neutral pH. Controls were kept in darkness but otherwise under the same conditions. I examined not only proteins of the lens but also lysozyme, a protein rich in tryptophan, ribonuclease, a protein containing no tryptophan and serum albumin, a protein of low tryptophan content, and tryptophan itself.

All proteins turned golden brown after exposure to sunlight. Tryptophan first turned golden and then a deeper brown and deposited a black precipitate. The percent loss of amino acids in lens proteins compared with changes in serum albumin is shown in Table 2, and Table 3 shows changes in the tryptophan content of several different proteins after exposure to sunlight. The results vary probably because the intensity of sunlight is variable.

The most noticeable change in the absorption spectrum of bovine plasma albumin exposed to sunlight was a rise between 300 and 330 nm together with a loss of tryptophan

TABLE 2. *Percent loss of amino acids in proteins exposed to sunlight*

| | | Percent loss | | |
| Protein | Solvent | Histidine | Tryptophan | Tyrosine |
|---|---|---|---|---|
| Serum albumin | H$_2$O | 41, 8, 32, 6 | 46 | 3, 40, 35 |
| Serum albumin | 6 M guanidinium chloride | 48, 35, 50, 53 | 56 | 44, 71, 68 |
| Normal human lens | 6 M guanidinium chloride | 40, 31, 22 | 85, 36, 38 | nil |
| Human cortical cataract (Group I) | 6 M guanidinium chloride | 53, 51, 62, 60 | 62 | 30 |

Protein solutions were exposed to sunlight or kept in darkness for times varying from one to three weeks. Hours of sunlight were not measured. Each figure given for the percentage loss of an amino acid refers to a separate experiment.

TABLE 3. *Loss of tryptophan after exposure to sunlight*

| Preparation | Tryptophan (g/kg) | |
|---|---|---|
| | Darkness | Sunlight |
| Total normal human lens protein | 47 | 7 |
| Total normal human lens protein | 42 | 26 |
| Egg-white lysozyme | 36 | 18.5 |
| Bovine γ-crystallin | 37 | nil |
| Serum albumin | 6 | 3 |
| Serum albumin | 5 | 1 |
| Serum albumin in aqueous solution | 5.8 | 2.6 |

A solution of 10 mg of protein/ml in 6 M guanidium chloride at neutral pH (unless otherwise stated) was exposed to sunlight until the proteins showed a decrease in absorption at 280 nm and a rise at 320 nm.

absorption at 280 nm (Fig. 3). This suggested a formation of N′-formylkynurenine from tryptophan residues in this protein (6, 7). This substance is the first metabolic product of tryptophan breakdown. Fig. 4 shows all of the major products. N′-formylkynurenine is a transient metabolite, the formyl group being split off enzymatically to yield kynurenine. The absorption maximum of N′-formylkynurenine is 321 nm and that of kynurenine is 360 nm; this difference enables the two com-

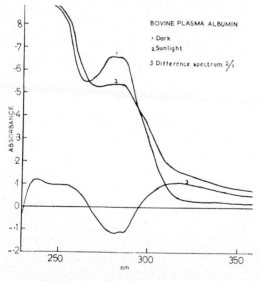

Some Pathways Involved in Tryptophan Oxidation.

FIG. 4. Some pathways involved in tryptophan oxidation.

pounds to be identified separately. For the purpose of comparison with proteins, N′-formylkynurenine was prepared by ozonization of tryptophan according to the method of Previero and Coletti-Previero (8).

Characteristic changes in the spectrum of N′-formylkynurenine take place after removal of the formyl group or reduction with boro-

FIG. 3. Absorption spectra of 1) bovine plasma albumin kept in darkness, 2) the same after exposure to sun and 3) difference spectrum 2/1.

| Substance | X | Y |
|---|---|---|
| N′-formylkynurenine | CHO | O |
| Kynurenine | H | O |
| γ (2-aminophenyl) homoserine | H | HOH |
| γ (2-formylaminophenyl) homoserine | CHO | HOH |

FIG. 5. N′-formylkynurenine and derivatives.

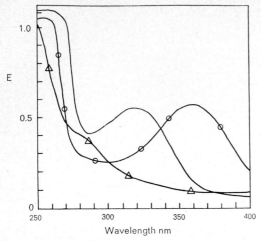

FIG. 6.   Absorption spectrum of N′-formylkynurenine and effect of hydrolysis with N HCl and of reduction with sodium borohydride. ——— N′-formylkynurenine H₂O, at pH 7, 0.03 mg/ml; O—O N′-formylkynurenine-treated N HCl at room temperature for 20 min and then neutralized, final concentration 0.03 mg/ml, phosphate bufferat pH 7; △—△ N′-formylkynurenine 0.03 mg/ml H₂O treated with sodium borohydride at room temperature for 20 min.

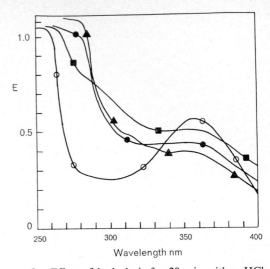

FIG. 8.   Effect of hydrolysis for 20 min with N HCl at room temperature on O N′-formylkynurenine 0.03 mg/ml, phosphate buffer at pH 7; ▲ photo-oxidized tryptophan 0.1 mg/ml, phosphate buffer at pH 7; ■ photo-oxidized lysozyme 0.4 mg/ml, 6 M guanidinium chloride containing phosphate buffer to pH 7; ● photo-oxidized normal human lens proteins 1.0 mg/ml, 6 M guanidinium chloride containing phosphate buffer at pH 7.

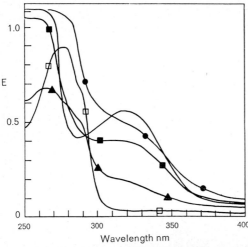

FIG. 7.   Absorption spectrum of photo-oxidized substrates compared with that of N′-formylkynurenine and of lysozyme. N′-formylkynurenine 0.03 mg/ml H₂O neutral; ▲ tryptophan photo-oxidized in sunlight 0.03 mg/ml H₂O neutral; ■ lysozyme photo-oxidized in sunlight 0.3 mg/ml 6 M guanidinium chloride; ● normal human lens proteins photo-oxidized in sunlight 0.4 mg/ml 6 M guanidinium chloride; □ lysozyme, kept in darkness 0.3 mg/ml, 6 M guanidinium chloride.

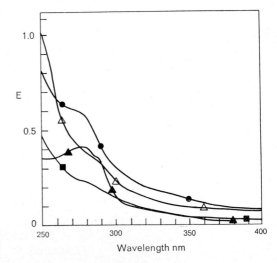

FIG. 9.   Effect of reduction with sodium borohydride on △ N′-formylkynurenine 0.03 mg/ml H₂O; ▲ photo-oxidized tryptophan 0.03 mg/ml, 0.03 M KHPO₄ at pH 7; ■ photo-oxidized lysozyme 0.4 mg/ml, 6 M guanidinium chloride; ● photo-oxidized normal human lens proteins 0.4 mg/ml, 6 M guanidinium chloride.

hydride (9, 10). Removal of the formyl group yields kynurenine with replacement of absorption at 320 nm by absorption at 360 nm. Reduction yields γ (2-formylaminophenyl) homoserine which has no absorption above 300 nm (Fig. 5).

The formyl group can be removed by treatment with N HCl for 20 min at room temperature. The carbonyl group can be reduced by addition of a trace of solid sodium borohydride at neutral pH allowing the reaction to proceed at room temperature for about 40 min (Fig. 5). Fig. 6 shows the spectral changes resulting from these reactions.

The absorption spectra of sun-exposed proteins were compared with that of N′-formylkynurenine (Fig. 7). When sun-exposed proteins were treated with N HCl for 20 min at room temperature their absorption changed to give a shoulder at 360 nm rather than at 320 nm (Fig. 8) and when reduced with borohydride both shoulders disappeared (Fig. 9).

Chromatography and electrophoresis of acid hydrolysates yielded further evidence that sunlight disrupts the indole ring of the tryptophan residues of proteins to yield N′-formylkynurenine. Tryptophan itself is unstable to acid hydrolysis and gives several fluorescent substances which have been identified as β-carbolines (11). Therefore acid hydrolysates of proteins cannot be used to identify fluorescent substances unless stringent controls are possible. β-carbolines, however, do not have the same chromatographic or electrophoretic behavior or the same color reactions as kynurenine or its derivatives. From amino acid analysis it is clear that kynurenine is not present in acid hydrolysates of normal proteins. Its detection in an acid hydrolysate is therefore an indication of the presence of kynurenine or N′-formylkynurenine in the intact protein.

N′-formylkynurenine prepared by ozonization of tryptophan (8) was used as a marker. Table 4 shows the electrophoretic behavior of the marker and other substances and their color reaction with the Ehrlich and Ekman reagents. Chromatographic examination in three solvents of acid hydrolysates of photo-oxidized lens proteins before and after reduction with borohydride showed that these hydrolysates contained kynurenine before reduction and γ (2-aminophenyl) homoserine after reduction (Table 5) (5).

The fluorescence spectrum of N′-formylkynurenine has not, as far as I am aware, been published. Our preparation showed an emission at 440 nm with excitation at 330 nm and 270 nm but it was not pure as shown by the molar extinction coefficient at 321 nm.

The fluorescence spectrum of proteins exposed to sunlight was similar to that of N′-formylkynurenine and showed a residual peak from tryptophan. Therefore fluorescence may be an added confirmation of the presence of N′-formylkynurenine in these proteins but a

TABLE 4.   *Electrophoresis of N′-formylkynurenine and derivatives[a]*

| | Distance travelled (cm) | Reaction with Ehrlich reagent | Reaction with Ekman reagent |
|---|---|---|---|
| N′-formylkynurenine | 10 | Orange | Negative[b] |
| Photo-oxidized tryptophan | 10 | Orange | Negative |
| Kynurenine | 11.8 | Orange | Purple |
| Reduced N′-formylkynurenine | 10.2 | Yellow | Negative |
| Reduced photo-oxidized tryptophan | 9.8 | Yellow | Negative |
| Reduced kynurenine | 14, 14.8 | Yellow | Purple |
| Tryptophan | 10.5 | Purple | Negative |

[a] Performed at 2.5 hr at 10/cm, 50 in A, Whatman 3 mm paper, pH 2.
[b] A false positive may develop since the formyl group is hydrolyzed by the reagent on the paper.

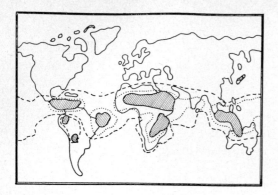

FIG. 10. World distribution of "sunburn" ultraviolet radiation corrected for latitude, cloud cover and altitude. Annual values for a 10 nm wide band of radiation centered on 307.5 nm (14). Shaded area 400 nm, .... 375 nm, – – – 350 nm.

pure preparation of this substance is essential.

The next point to consider is whether N′-formylkynurenine can be detected in the proteins of the cataractous lens. As we have seen there is considerable similarity in the absorption and fluorescence spectra of cataractous and sun-exposed lens proteins in that both seem to have lost the same amino acids. Work on this aspect is in progress. Kynurenine has been revealed chromatographically in acid hydrolysates of the brown proteins but the amount present is so small that it cannot account for the typtophan loss. None is present in hydrolysates of normal lens proteins.

It is reasonable to consider that if N′-formylkynurenine is formed in a protein it will react further. It may be hydroxylated; the formyl group may be removed or it may be part of a cross-linking system. These possibilities all make analysis difficult. However, in finding N′-formylkynurenine, I think we have for the first time identified a photo-oxidation product of proteins exposed to sunlight in the absence of photosensitizer.

To return to the original theory that sunlight may play a part in cataractogenesis, Teale and Weber (12) considered that light of 295 to 310 nm is almost specific for excita-

tion of tryptophan while Kinsey (13) found that 50% of the light of 310 nm reaches the lens. I found that filtering out light below 320 nm prevents browning of lens proteins. Experiments with dummy human heads which were performed by Urbach (14) in order to determine the conditions under which most sunlight reached the different head areas showed that the orbit was protected from overhead sun but when sun was reflected from sand, water or snow, the orbit received a much larger dose.

This brings us back to geographic ophthalmology. Fig. 10 shows a map of the world illustrating those areas where sunlight of the 10 nm band centered around 307.5 nm is the strongest. The values are corrected for latitude, cloud cover and altitude. Taking the black areas as 100%, the dotted lines enclose 94% and the dashed lines, 87%; but I cannot interpret the 100% in terms of light energy. We now need a map to show intensity of reflected sunlight but unless genetics and other factors play a large part it almost seems that the geographic ophthalmologists ought to be able to tell us biochemists whether sunlight is a factor in cataractogenesis.

## REFERENCES

1. DUKE-ELDER WS. The pathological action of light upon the eye. *Lancet* i: 1188, 1926.
2. SPIKES JD and LIVINGSTONE R. The molecular biology of photodynamic action. Sensitized photo-oxidations in biological systems. *Adv Rad Biol* 3: 29, 1969.
3. PIRIE A. Color and solubility of the proteins of human cataracts. *Invest Ophthalmol* 7: 634, 1968.
4. PIRIE A. Insoluble proteins of the lens. *Exp Eye Res* 8: 233, 1969.
5. PIRIE A. The effect of sunlight on proteins of the lens, in: Bellows JG (Ed), "Contemporary ophthalmology." Baltimore, Williams and Wilkins (in press).
6. MEHLER AH and KNOX WE. The conversion of tryptophan to kynurenine in liver. *J Biol Chem* 187: 431, 1950.
7. PIRIE A. Formation of N′-formyl kynurenine in proteins from lens and other sources exposed to sunlight. *Biochem J* 125: 203, 1971.
8. PREVIERO A and COLETTI-PREVIERO MA. Ozonolyse du tryptophane: Synthèse des peptides

DR. 
but I
in or
done
find
used
300 n
that 
with
starte
wron;
due—

DR. N
peopl
to mc
narro
I wou
incide
to vill

DR. N
becaus
We co
wouldr
the cit
hospita
first tir

DR. Pi
followii
physiol
people
cataract
in the
than 90
develop

DR. SPE
of aging
variety
simple c
cated by
diabetes
betic ca
the cata

DR. PIRI
was goin
your pap
triggered
though I
portant f
betic len:

de la N′-formylkynurenine. *CR Acad Sci [C] (Paris)* **264**: 633, 1967.

9. PREVIERO A and BORDIGNON E. Modifica controllata di triptofano, methionina, cistina et tirosina in peptidi naturale e proteine. *Gazz Chim Ital* **94**: 630, 1964.

10. PREVIERO A, COLETTI-PREVIERO MA and JOLLES P. Non enzymatic cleavage of tryptophyll peptide bonds in peptides and proteins. *Biochim Biophys Acta* **124**: 400, 1966.

11. TSCHESCHE R, JENNSEN H and RANGACHARI PN. Über Umsetzungsprodukte des L-Tryptophans bei der sauren Eiweisshydrolyse. *Ber Dtsch Chem Ges* **91**: 1732, 1958.

12. TEALE FWJ and WEBER G. Ultraviolet fluorescence of proteins. *Biochem J* **72**: 15, 1959.

13. KINSEY VE. Spectral transmission of the eye to ultraviolet radiations. *Arch Ophthalmol* **39**: 508, 1948.

14. URBACH F. "The biologic effects of ultraviolet irradiation." Oxford, Pergamon Press, 1969, p 635.

as yet found any difference in prevalence between diabetics and nondiabetics.

But in continuation of what I started to say before about the differences between juvenile and senile diabetic cataracts, we have not really proved that sorbitol itself is involved in senile cataracts. We have recently become interested in the interaction between sorbitol and proteins. Dr. Spector has already shown that sorbitol can cause irreversible changes in α-crystallin. I would like to postulate that in juvenile cataracts, only small amounts of sorbitol are required to produce cataract whereas in older individuals, whose lens proteins have undergone changes due to aging, much more sorbitol is required to interact with the α-crystallin. In fact, some of our work on diabetic retinopathy suggests that the damaging effect of sorbitol is not an osmotic one at all, but is due to specific interaction with protein.

DR. SPECTOR: I should add that it is not only sorbitol but also glucose that may be involved in the transformation of soluble lens proteins into insoluble macromoleculss. I really think we are dealing with several different mechanisms here. One is the so-called diabetic cataract, where it is an osmotic effect that initiates the process. In other cases, we have brown, light-induced cataracts and, finally, we have the senile cataract, which is a slow and continuous process involving perhaps either a sugar component or a protein or, more probably, both of these.

DR. H. R. KOCH (Germany): I think it is generally agreed that senile cataracts and typical diabetic cataracts are morphologically different. We have found that of the two enzymes responsible for the production of sorbitol, only the second one, polyol dehydrogenase, increases with age. This may explain why young people, who have a rather low level of polyol dehydrogenase, could get typical diabetic cataracts from an accumulation of sorbitol. In older patients with a higher level of the enzyme, more of the sorbitol is oxidized and hence they do not develop a typical "sorbitol cataract."

# AGGREGATION OF α-CRYSTALLIN AND ITS POSSIBLE RELATIONSHIP TO CATARACT FORMATION

ABRAHAM SPECTOR

Department of Ophthalmology, College of Physicians and Surgeons,
Columbia University, New York, New York, USA

Cataract, the insoluble lens proteins and the structural protein α-crystallin appear to be closely associated. The relationship of these two proteins to cataract has intrigued investigators since 1894 when Mörner (1) isolated, from beef lens, α-crystallin and the albuminoid which is an insoluble protein fraction. Early studies by Jess (2, 3) and Krause (4) indicated that the albuminoid fraction increased with aging and in cataractous lens. In both situations there was a concomitant decrease in the soluble protein. Moreover, this process appeared to occur to a much greater extent in the nucleus than in the cortical region of the lens.

Recent investigations have confirmed such observations and have shown that the albuminoid is not synthesized directly but arises from the insolubilization of the lens protein. In 1966, Fulhorst and Young (5) demonstrated that labeled amino acid is incorporated only into soluble protein in rat lens with the radioactivity appearing in the albuminoid fraction at a later time. Wannemacher and Spector (6) showed that the nuclear region of calf lenses is incapable of protein synthesis, and further investigation demonstrated that in older animals more than 50% of the lens can no longer support significant protein synthesis.

A significant decrease in the α-crystallin content of old lenses and cataractous lenses was noted by Jess (7) in 1922. A few years later, Woods and Burky (8), by using immunological techniques, were able to show that α-crystallin is related to the albuminoid fraction. A similar conclusion based on immunological investigations has been reported by others (9–12).

Chemical evidence also suggests a relationship between albuminoid and α-crystallin. Ruttenberg (11) obtained amino acid analyses of albuminoid which are comparable to α-crystallin. Peptide mapping by Thomann (13) and Waley (14) also suggest a close relationship between the albuminoid and α-crystallin.

There have also been reports which suggest that other lens proteins are present in the albuminoid fraction (12, 15). Dische (16) suggested that interaction between the albuminoid precursor protein and glycoproteins and glycolipoproteins of the lens fiber membrane may be involved in the insolubilization process. Most of these reports imply that the non-α-crystallin components represent a minor fraction of the total material. However, Lerman and co-workers (17) have presented evidence indicating the γ-crystallin and not α-crystallin is the major component of the

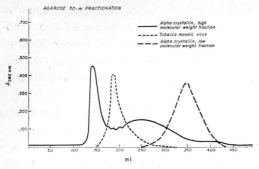

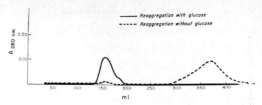

FIG. 4. The effect of glucose upon the reaggregation of the high molecular weight component (approximately $5 \times 10^7$ and greater) isolated from Agarose-50m.

FIG. 3. Fractionation of different sized α-crystallin populations on an Agarose-50m column (3.2 × 50 cm). The eluting buffer contained 0.1 M KCl, 0.01 M Tris, pH 7.6, and 0.001 M EDTA. The high molecular weight fraction from Agarose-15m and the low molecular weight fraction from Agarose-5m were utilized for this study.

this fraction with an unusually high molecular weight suggest that while only small amounts are present in calf nucleus, about 15% of the total soluble α-crystallin in nucleus from two-year-old cattle consists of this component and 30% or more in the nucleus of eight-year-old cattle. Amino acid composition and subunit profiles on sodium dodecylsulfate (SDS) gel electrophoresis again show no difference between these huge macromolecular aggregates and populations of α-crystallin more than 50 times smaller, but the presence of sugar was again detected.

After deaggregation in 7 M urea followed by reaggregation in the presence of 0.001 M sugar,* a profile similar to that of the original

material was obtained. Reaggregation in the absence of sugar yielded a low molecular weight profile (Fig. 4). Thus, the behavior of this fraction appears similar to the components isolated from Agarose-15m.

As the nuclear region of the lens ages there is thus a continuous increase in the concentration of high molecular weight α-crystallin aggregates. In the old bovine lens a significant proportion of this protein is represented by species with molecular weight in the order of 50 million or greater. Recently Benedek (28) suggested that scattering of light may be produced by microscopic variations in the index of refraction. The theory suggests that if large aggregates exist which have an index of refraction different from that of the average index of refraction of the lens and are distributed randomly, they will scatter light proportionately to their concentration. The scattering of light is known to be directly proportional to the size of the macromolecular aggregate. It follows that if the α-crystallin aggregates of high molecular weight are distributed randomly in sufficient concentration with a sufficiently different index of refraction from the average of the nuclear region of the lens, an opacity will develop. Recently Benedek (personal communication) measured

---

* The deaggregation and reaggregation were performed in the following manner. The α-crystallin was dissolved in a solution containing 7 M urea, 0.002 M phosphate buffer pH 7.0, 0.001 M mercaptoethanol. The urea was passed through a mixed bed ion exchanger MB-3 before use. The concentration of protein was usually between 2.5 to 4 mg/ml. The protein solution was dialyzed against 100- to 200-fold excess of the above buffer preparation for 9 hr, with two changes of solution after periods of 2 hr. The first dialysis was carried out at room temperature and all following dialyses at 4 C. The preparation was then dialyzed overnight (approximately 13 to 14 hr) against

water or water and 0.001 M glucose. This was followed by dialysis for 5 hr with two changes of solution against 0.1 M KCl, 0.01 M Tris, pH 7.6, 0.001 M EDTA with or without glucose.

the refractive index of the low molecular weight population of α-crystallin and obtained a value of 1.56, which differs significantly from values of 1.40 reported for the nuclear region by Huggert (29). As the lens ages its transparency is known to decreases (30, 31); and with sufficient aging an opacity will probably develop. Thus, it is possible that the gradual increase in the aggregate size of the α-crystallin is the cause of the nuclear opacity associated with aging.

Studies on different sized populations of the α-crystallin aggregates clearly show that there is a marked decrease in solubility with increase in size, suggesting that insolubilization will finally result from the production of very large aggregates. Thus, it is conceivable that the formation of the insoluble fraction may be caused by the gradual insolubilization of the very large α-crystallin aggregates which would, of course, contribute significantly to the overall scattering of light and to the development of opacity.

The relationship of glucose to the process of aggregation remains puzzling. While it is clear that glucose is capable of directing the aggregation of large macromolecules, the results obtained with subunits isolated from low molecular weight species of α-crystallin are variable. Such material obtained from young lenses does not yield high molecular weight species even in the presence of glucose and the deaggregated low molecular weight material from old lenses sometimes fails to produce the high molecular species on reaggregation in the presence of sugar. Other factors must therefore be involved. Li and Spector (32) recently observed a minor nondialyzable component of α-crystallin, which may be of importance in controlling the aggregation process. If it is assumed that the aggregation process leads to insolubilization, and that this is the major route for this process, then there should be appreciable amounts of glucose in the insoluble fraction.

However, our results suggest that there is little sugar in the albuminoid. If the bulk of the albuminoid is α-crystallin derived from the high molecular weight aggregates the sugar content should be higher. Thus, either the sugar is eliminated in the final stages of insolubilization or it is secondary to the total process.

Supported by grants from the National Institutes of Health of the U.S. Public Health Service and the John A. Hartford Foundation, Inc.

REFERENCES

1. MÖRNER CT. Untersuchungen der Protein Substanzen in den lichtbrechenden Medien des Auges. *Hoppe-Seyler Z Physiol Chem* **18**: 61, 1894.
2. JESS A. Beiträge zur Kenntnis der Chemie der normalen und der pathologisch veränderten Linse des Auges. *Z Biol* **61**: 93, 1913.
3. JESS A. Die Monoaminosäuren der Linsenproteine. *Hoppe-Seyler Z Physiol Chem* **110**: 266, 1920.
4. KRAUSE AC. "The biochemistry of the eye." Baltimore, Johns Hopkins Press, 1934.
5. FULHORST HW and YOUNG RW. Conversion of soluble lens protein to albuminoid. *Invest Ophthalmol* **5**: 298, 1966.
6. WANNENMACHER CF and SPECTOR A. Protein synthesis in the core of calf lens. *Exp Eye Res* **7**: 623, 1968.
7. JESS A. Die moderne Eiweisschemie im Dienste der Starforschung. *Arch F Ophthalmol (Paris)* **109**: 463, 1922.
8. WOODS AS and BURKY EL. Lens protein and its fractions. *JAMA* **89**: 102, 1927.
9. SIRCHIS J, FROMAGEOT P and BERNARD H. Similarity between alpha crystallin and the principal fraction $F_1$ of the insoluble crystalline lens of beef. *CR Soc Biol (Paris)* **243**: 2164, 1956.
10. RAO SS, MEHTA PD and COOPER SN. Antigenic relationship between insoluble and soluble lens proteins. *Exp Eye Res* **4**: 36, 1965.
11. RUTTENBERG G. The insoluble proteins of bovine crystalline lens. *Exp Eye Res* **4**: 18, 1965.
12. MANSKI W, BEHRENS M and MARTINEZ C. Immunochemical studies on albuminoid. **7**: 164, 1968.
13. THOMANN H. Structural chemistry studies on the assimilation of water-insoluble proteins in clear bovine lenses. *Albrecht von Graefes Arch Klin Ophthalmol* **165**: 219, 1962.
14. WALEY SG. The problem of albuminoid. *Eye Res* **4**: 293, 1965.
15. KRAUSE AC. Chemistry of the lens. 1. Composition of albuminoid and alpha crystallin. *Arch Ophthalmol* **8**: 166, 1932.
16. DISCHE Z. The glycoproteins and glycolipoproteins of the bovine lens and their relation to albuminoid. *Invest Ophthalmol* **4**: 759, 1965.

TABLE 2. *Soluble/insoluble protein fractions in human lenses, by age*

| Normal lenses | | | |
|---|---|---|---|
| Age (years) | Soluble protein (%) | Insoluble protein (%) | Average weight of lens (g) |
| 0 to 9 | 96.7 | 3.3 | 0.1167 |
| 10 to 19 | 97.1 | 2.9 | 0.1484 |
| 40 to 49 | 96.7 | 3.3 | 0.2130 |
| 50 to 59 | 90.9 | 9.1 | 0.2096 |
| 60 to 69 | 84.3 | 15.7 | 0.1840 |
| 70 to 79 | 82.6 | 17.4 | 0.2246 |
| 80 to 89 | 60.1 | 39.9 | 0.2328 |
| Brunescent and nigricant cataract | | | |
| 75 to 90 | 29.0 | 71.0 | 0.2255 |

TABLE 3. *Age-related changes in the concentration of α-, β- and γ-crystallins[a]*

| Species and age | α-crystallin (%) | β-crystallin (%) | γ-crystallin (%) |
|---|---|---|---|
| Human | | | |
| 10 to 19 years | 37 | 38 | 25 |
| 60 to 69 years | 55 | 33.6 | 11.4 |
| 80 to 89 years | 57.6 | 33.7 | 8.7 |
| Rat | | | |
| 5 to 6 weeks | 20 | 20 | 60 |
| 6 months | 38 | 42 | 20 |
| 11 months | 41 | 46 | 13 |

[a] Concentration expressed as percentage of total soluble proteins.

TABLE 4. *Amino acid composition of dogfish crystallins[a]*

| Amino acid | α-crystallin | β-crystallin | γ-crystallin | Albuminoid |
|---|---|---|---|---|
| Lysine | 7 | 7 | 3.4 | 4 |
| Histidine | 4 | 5 | 3.4 | 3.5 |
| Arginine | 11 | 12 | 20 | 14 |
| Aspartic acid | 15 | 14 | 17 | 17 |
| Threonine | 5 | 5 | 3 | 3.5 |
| Serine | 10 | 10 | 9 | 9 |
| Glutamic acid | 18 | 22 | 15 | 18 |
| Proline | 15 | 7 | 10 | 8 |
| Glycine | 8 | 13.5 | 12 | 14 |
| Alanine | 5 | 5 | 1.3 | 3.5 |
| Valine | 8 | 4 | 5 | 6 |
| Methionine | 4 | 4.3 | 7 | 7.4 |
| Isoleucine | 7 | 4.4 | 5 | 5.3 |
| Leucine | 9 | 5 | 2 | 4.5 |
| Tyrosine | 5 | 10 | 17 | 12 |
| Phenylalanine | 9 | 8 | 9.5 | 9 |
| Tryptophan | 2 | 3.5 | 2 | 3 |

[a] Expressed as residues per 20,000 g protein.

in the advanced human nuclear brunescent and nigricant cataract, the level of insoluble protein reaches 70% of the total protein concentration in the lens (Table 2). Furthermore, there is a considerable decrease in the relative concentration of the smaller protein molecules in the lens (γ-crystallin) with a corresponding increase in the concentration of the large soluble protein molecules (Table 3). Since scattering of light increases with the second power of the volume of the molecule (17), these large protein molecules (α-crystallin and albuminoid) have a greater ability to scatter light than the small molecules. Changes in the spatial order of the protein molecules may also occur resulting in independent scattering of light from each molecule. Hence, the transparency of the lens appears to be in part related to the structural lens proteins, particularly with respect to their relative concentrations. Loss of transparency in the lens with increasing age can be explained on the basis of 1) changes in the relative proportion of albuminoid to α-crystallin, resulting in an increased scattering of light; and 2) absorption of light in the blue region of the spectrum because of the presence of one or more fluorescent compounds. The advanced nuclear brunescent and nigricant cataract represents a condition in which these two processes have progressed to an extreme degree.

Previous communications from this laboratory have indicated that certain of the structural proteins in the ocular lens show an apparently high anomalous absorptivity at 280 nm (8, 18, 19). The structural proteins of the ocular lens in almost all species except birds consist of the soluble fractions known as the α, β and γ-crystallins and an insoluble portion frequently referred to as the albuminoid fraction. γ-crystallin derived from four species (rat, dogfish, cattle and human being) all demonstrate anomalously high molar absorptivities at 280 nm. A similar situation has also been noted in the insoluble (albuminoid) protein fractions derived from the rat and dogfish lens.

Absorption in the 280 nm region for proteins is mainly due to the tryptophan, tyrosine and phenylalanine residues. The $E_{280}^{1\%}$ values of most proteins are usually of the order of 10 to 15, particularly in those proteins containing relatively small amounts of tryptophan, as is the case with the lens proteins (Table 4).

Studies in this laboratory have demonstrated that the anomalously high absorptivity (at 280 nm) observed in γ-crystallin and in the albuminoid fraction of the ocular lens was due to the presence of a fluorescent compound (or compounds).

## MATERIALS AND METHODS

Fresh dogfish lenses were obtained at the Marine Biological Laboratory, Woods Hole, Massachusetts, and grouped according to age (i.e. size). Bovine lenses were obtained at the slaughterhouse within 1 hr after death and placed in refrigerated containers for transportation to the laboratory. Normal human lenses were obtained from the local eye bank within 12 hr of death. Advanced nuclear cataracts were obtained from the operating rooms of the Royal Victoria and Montreal General Hospitals. All of the lenses were either used as soon as they were obtained or were immediately frozen for use at a later time.

The lens capsules were carefully removed and the lenses were homogenized in de-ionized distilled water and centrifuged for 30 min at 600 × g at room temperature in order to remove the insoluble protein fractions from the dogfish and rat lenses. The insoluble protein fractions from the human and bovine lenses were removed by centrifugation at 12,000 × g, and were washed at least six times in 0.002 M phosphate buffer in order to remove any remaining soluble proteins. The soluble proteins present in the original supernatant fluid were centrifuged at 105,000 × g for 1 hr at room temperature and the resultant supernatant fluid was dialyzed overnight against de-ionized distilled water (pH 7.5) and separated into its constituent α, β and γ fractions by DEAE cellulose column chromatography (20).

The $E_{280}^{1\%}$ values of the soluble protein fractions and the sulfonated solubilized albuminoid

fraction (16) were determined in duplicate in quartz cuvettes in a Cary 14 recording spectrophotometer, and the protein concentrations were measured by the method of Lowry et al. (21).

Ionization of the phenolic groups in the tyrosine residues of γ-crystallin were studied in the Cary 14 spectrophotometer in order to measure the degree of the resulting hyperchromicity and bathochromic shift that occurs at alkaline pH. Identical concentrations of γ-crystallin were made up in six solutions of different pH varying from 6.5 to 13.0, and the ultraviolet (UV) absorption spectrum of each of these solutions was determined.

The fluorescent material was extracted from γ-crystallin and the insoluble protein fractions following 24-hr acid hydrolysis in 6 N HCl. After removing the hydrochloric acid by means of rotary evaporation in vacuum and repeated washings in 0.2 M acetic acid, the hydrolysate was passed through a phosphocellulose column, equilibrated and eluted with 0.2 M acetic acid. Desalting and final purification was accomplished on a P-2 Bio-Gel column by eluting with water. The tubes containing the fluorescent material were pooled and concentrated. UV spectra of the fluorogen were studied in the Cary 14 recording spectrophotometer and the fluorescence spectra were determined in the Aminco-Bowman spectrofluorimeter.

In order to rule out the possibility that the fluorescent material obtained following acid hydrolysis was a degradation product (e.g. of tryptophan), a second series of experiments were performed with albuminoid derived from human nuclear cataracts and from old dogfish lenses. One portion of the albuminoid was dissolved in 3% NaOH and fluorescence spectra were determined. A second portion of the albuminoid was subjected to pronase digestion for 24 hr at 45 C. The material was then passed through a Bio-Gel P-2 column and the fluorescent fractions were collected and pooled. Fluorescence spectra were determined on these fractions in the Aminco-Bowman spectrofluorimeter. UV absorption spectra on these fractions were determined in the Cary 14 spectrophotometer.

## RESULTS

$E_{280}^{1\%}$ values for rat, dogfish, bovine and human sulfonated albuminoid and the soluble crystallin fractions are shown in Table 5. In the rat and dogfish lens both γ-crystallin and derive from one or more of the tyrosine or tryptophan residues within the γ-crystallin molecule; that is, the fluorogen could be formed by means of a photo-oxidation reaction in which the process is initiated by prolonged exposure of the lens to UV light between 340 and 380 nm. While the cornea filters out almost all of the UV light up to 310 nm, the lens is exposed to the longer UV radiation. It is therefore conceivable that the initiating process in the formation of the fluorogen in the mammalian species could be prolonged exposure to long UV radiation which normally occurs throughout life. It is also known that tyrosinase is present in the lens and the enzyme could react with and oxidize one or more of the tyrosine residues in γ-crystallin. It is also possible that the fluorogen may play a role in the formation of the insoluble protein from one or more of the soluble lens protein precursors by means of C-S linkages.

The insoluble protein fraction of the lens has recently been defined as the water-insoluble derivative of the crystallins. It is generally accepted that both the relative and absolute concentration of albuminoid increases with age in most species. The albuminoid has also been characterized as consisting of one urea-soluble and one urea insoluble portion. The urea-insoluble fraction is obviously held together by covalent bonds such as S-S linkages and perhaps C-S linkages. The relative amount of urea-soluble and urea-insoluble albuminoid varies with the species under consideration. For example, in the bovine and human lenses most of the albuminoid is urea-soluble; while in the dogfish lenses there is a significant amount of the urea-insoluble albuminoid as well as urea-soluble albuminoid. In the bovine and human lenses in which the albuminoid is mainly of the urea-soluble form, most of the albuminoid appears to derive from α-crystallin although small but significant amounts of β- and γ-

crystallin are also present. In the rat and dogfish lenses, a considerable portion of the albuminoid is urea-insoluble, and that protein appears to derive mainly from γ-crystallin although small amounts of other crystallins have also been detected (15, 19, 22–33).

It is well known that the aging lens, contains a progressively increasing amount of fluorescent material. At least one fluorogen appears to be localized mainly in the γ-crystallin and albuminoid fraction. In the rat and dogfish lenses there is considerable evidence that the change from soluble to insoluble protein is associated with loss of SH groups. This and other data would indicate that one of the processes involved in the formation of the insoluble protein is the formation of disulfide bridges (15, 16, 19, 34–37). It is also possible that a portion of the urea-insoluble albuminoid fraction of the lens could arise from the reaction of a fluorogen with a thiol group, resulting in the formation of a C-S linkage. Reductive sulfonation dissolves most of the urea-insoluble albuminoid fraction, but the remainder could represent the fluorogen-linked portion of the protein. The process involved in the formation of the albuminoid fraction from its precursor soluble crystallins thus seems to involve S-S and perhaps C-S bond formation. In the latter case it is postulated that the fluorogen, which is closely associated with γ-crystallin, is involved in the process of polymerization and decreased solubility leading to the formation of a portion of the urea-insoluble albuminoid fraction. The remaining portion could result from the formation of disulfide bridges.

Supported by MRC Grant MA 3208.

## REFERENCES

1. Trokel S. The physical basis for transparency of the crystalline lens. *Invest Ophthalmol* 1: 493, 1962.
2. Krause AC. Chemical pathogenesis of cataract. *Am J Ophthalmol* 21: 1343, 1938.
3. Steinworth E and Munich W. Papierelektro-phoretische Untersuchungen über das Verhal-

ten verschiedener wasserlöslicher Organolipo-proteine des Kalbsauges. *Albrecht von Graefes Archklin Ophthalmol* **160**: 216, 1958.

4. LUDVIGH E and McCARTHY EF. Absorption of visible light by the refractive media of the human eye. *Arch Ophthalmol* **20**: 37, 1938.

5. WEALE RA. Light absorption by the lens of the human eye. *Opt Acta (Lond)* **1**: 107, 1954.

6. WALLS GL and JUDD HD. The intra-ocular colour-filters of vertebrates. *Br J Ophthalmol* **17**: 705, 1933.

7. LERMAN S. The role of albuminoid in aging and cataract formation. *Ann Inst Barraquer* **9**: 686, 1969.

8. LERMAN S. Characterization of the insoluble protein fraction in the ocular lens. *Can J Biochem* **47**: 1115, 1969.

9. FRANÇOIS J, RABAEY M and RECOULES N. A fluorescent substance of low molecular weight in the lens of primates. *Arch Ophthalmol* **4**: 142, 1961.

10. PIRIE A. Color and solubility of the proteins of human cataracts. *Invest Ophthalmol* **7**: 634, 1968.

11. COOPER GF and ROBSON JG. The yellow colour of the lens of man and other primates. *J Physiol (Lond)* **203**: 411, 1969.

12. LERMAN S, LOUIS D and HOLLANDER M. Characterization of a fluorogen in the ocular lens. *Can J Ophthalmol* **6**: 148, 1971.

13. LERMAN S, TAN AT, LOUIS D and HOLLANDER M. Anomalous absorptivity of lens proteins due to a fluorogen. *Ophthalmol Res* **1**: 338, 1970.

14. LERMAN S and FONTAINE J. The effect of aging on protein and RNA metabolism in the dog-fish lens. *Growth* **26**: 111, 1962.

15. LERMAN S. The structural proteins of the ocular lens. *Surv Ophthalmol* **12**: 112, 1967.

16. CLARK R, ZIGMAN S and LERMAN S. Studies on the structural proteins of the human lens. *Exp Eye Res* **8**: 172, 1969.

17. PHILIPSON B. Galactose cataract: Changes in protein distribution during development. *Invest Ophthalmol* **8**: 281, 1969.

18. LERMAN S, TUTTLE J and KOSER R. Composition and formation of insoluble protein in the dog-fish lens. *Biol Bull* **135**: 428, 1968.

19. LERMAN S, ZIGMAN S and FORBES WF. The insoluble protein fraction of the ocular lens. *Exp Eye Res* **7**: 444, 1968.

20. SPECTOR A. Methods of isolation of alpha, beta and gamma crystallins and their subgroups. *Invest Ophthalmol* **3**: 182, 1964.

21. LOWRY OH, ROSEBROUGH NJ, FARR AL and

RANDALL RJ. Protein measurement with the Folin phenol reagent. *J Biol Chem* **193**: 265, 1951.

22. ZIGMAN S and LERMAN S. The relationship between soluble and insoluble protein in the lens. *Biochim Biophys Acta* **154**: 423, 1968.

23. MEHTA P and LERMAN S. Immunochemical relationship between soluble and insoluble lens proteins. *Ophthalmol Res* **1**: 10, 1970.

24. LERMAN S. Species variations in the insoluble protein fraction of the lens. *Ann Ophthalmol* **1**: 73, 1969.

25. MEHTA PD and LERMAN S. Comparative studies of lens alpha crystallin from eight species. *Comp Biochem Physiol* **38A**: 637, 1971.

26. RUTTENBERG G. The insoluble protein of bovine crystalline lens. *Exp Eye Res* **4**: 18, 1965.

27. SRINWASA RAO S, MEHTA PD and COOPER SN. Antigenic relationship between insoluble and soluble lens protein. *Exp Eye Res* **4**: 36, 1965.

28. WALEY SG. The problem of albuminoid. *Exp Eye Res* **4**: 293, 1965.

29. MEHTA PD, COOPER SN and RAO SS. Identification of species specific and organ specific antigens in lens proteins. *Exp Eye Res* **3**: 192, 1964.

30. MEHTA PD and MAISEL H. Albuminoid of human and cynomolgus monkey lens. *Am J Ophthalmol* **63**: 967, 1967.

31. MANSKI W, BEHRENS M and MARTINEZ C. Immunochemical studies on albuminoid. *Exp Eye Res* **7**: 164, 1968.

32. CLAYTON RM, CAMPBELL JC and TRUMAN DES. A re-examination of the organ specificity of lens antigens. *Exp Eye Res* **7**: 11, 1968.

33. HARDING JJ. Nature and origin of the insoluble protein of rat lens. *Exp Eye Res* **8**: 147, 1969.

34. BJORK I. Studies on gamma-crystallin from calf lens. I. Isolation by gel filtration. *Exp Eye Res* **1**: 145, 1961.

35. KINOSHITA JH and MEROLA LO. The distribution of glutathione and protein sulfhydryl groups in calf and cattle lenses. *Am J Ophthalmol* **46**: 36, 1958.

36. LERMAN S, FORBES WF, ZIGMAN S and KIRMAN J. A study on gamma crystallin derived from the rat and dogfish lens. *Second Int Cong Ophthalmol Munich 1966*, New York, S. Karger, 1968, p 292.

37. DISCHE Z, BORENFREUND E and ZELMENIS G. Changes in lens proteins of rats during aging. *Arch Ophthalmol* **55**: 471, 1956.

TABLE 2.   *Reaction between pure calf $\gamma_1$-crystallin and UV tryptophan*

| Characteristics | Untreated | Treated |
|---|---|---|
| Color | White | Brown |
| Isoelectric point | 7.95 | $< 6.0$ |
| Mol wt | 21,500 | 21,500 |
| (SDS- acrylamide gel electrophoresis) | | $(+ 1,000$ to $2,000)$ |
| Binding sites for UV- tryptophan | $NH_2$ and SH groups of lysine, arginine, cysteine | |
| Moles of UV-tryptophan bound per mole protein | — | 6.0 |
| Electrophoretic mobility on acrylamide gels | More positive; moves only 1.03 cm toward + pole | More negative; moves 2.8 cm toward + pole |
| | Sharp peak at 278 nm | No distinct peak—absorption rises from 320 nm on down shoulder at 278 nm |
| Absorption of ultraviolet light | $E^{1cm}_{1\%} = 15$ | $E^{1cm}_{1\%} = 22$ |
| Absorption of visible light | 0 | Rapid rise from 500 nm down to 400 nm—no definite peak. |
| Fluorescence | | 1        2 |
| excitation | 278 nm | 278 nm    360 nm |
| emission | 330 nm | 330 nm    440 nm |
| Solubility | Less soluble in aqueous ethanol | More soluble in aqueous ethanol |

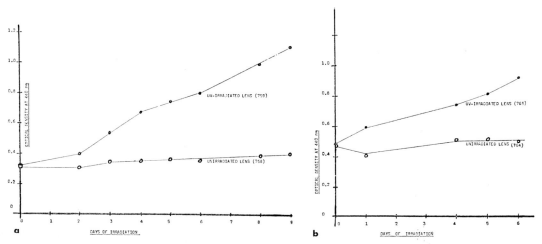

FIG. 1.   Pigmentation of human lenses as a result of near UV irradiation in Hank's balanced salt solution with penicillin and streptomycin with no additive. Absorption was read using a Cary 14 spectrophotometer. a) The lenses of a 54-year-old individual. b) The lenses of a 52-year-old individual.

added tryptophan became more intensely pigmented than those without (Fig. 2). Rabbit lenses irradiated in unaltered calf aqueous humor for 48 hr or longer were also stained yellow (Plate 1, B).

After pressure dialysis of the UV-irradiated

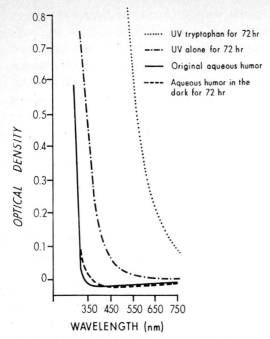

FIG. 2. Changes in the pigmentation of calf aqueous humor after near UV irradiation for 72 hr. A Cary 14 spectrophotometer was used to obtain the data.

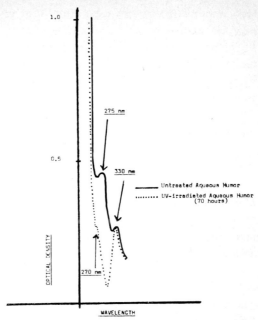

FIG. 4. Influence of near UV-irradiation on absorption of UV light by calf aqueous humor (diluted 1:10). The Cary 14 spectrophotometer was used to obtain the data.

TABLE 3. *Fluorescence at 440 nm of calf aqueous humor after excitation at 360 nm*

| Sample | Relative fluorescence (nm) |
|---|---|
| Unaltered aqueous humor | 390 |
| Aqueous humor UV-irradiated | 875 |
| Retentate (proteins) of unaltered aqueous humor | 30 |
| Retentate (proteins) of aqueous humor UV-irradiated | 100 |

Treatment consisted of exposure to near UV illumination (3,000 μw/cm²) for 48 hr.

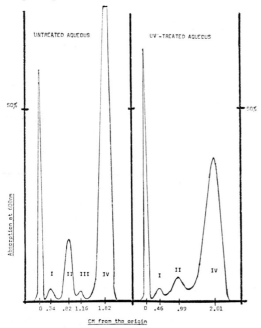

FIG. 3. Differences in electrophoretic mobility of UV-irradiated and unirradiated calf aqueous proteins on polyacrylamide gels. The curves were obtained using a Gilford densitometric attachment to a Gilford spectrophotometer.

aqueous humors containing added tryptophan, both the material passing through the dialysis membrane and the retentate were pigmented. However, when chemically unaltered UV-irradiated aqueous humors were pressure dialyzed, only the retentates (i.e. the proteins) were pigmented. Separated aqueous humor proteins irradiated after pressure dia-

**573**

# INDUCTION OF CATARACTS IN MICE BY EXPOSURE TO OXYGEN

STANLEY S. SCHOCKET, JOSEPH ESTERSON, BRADLEY BRADFORD, MORITZ MICHAELIS and RICHARD D. RICHARDS

Ophthalmology Research, University of Maryland School of Medicine, Baltimore, Maryland, USA

Oxygen at atmospheric and above-atmospheric pressures has been beneficially utilized in the treatment of various medical disorders in man (1). Unfortunately, oxygen usage is limited by its toxicity to human tissues (2). Manifestations of oxygen toxicity on the eye vary according to both the age and the species of animals studied. In man, these include retrolental fibroplasia in prematurity (3) and constriction of the retinal vessels and narrowing of the visual field in adults (4). In rabbits, degeneration of rods in the central retinal area is observed (5, 6). In dogs, retinal detachment and formation of cytoid bodies in the retina have been described (7). In albino guinea pigs, flattening of the corneal endothelium, loss of nuclei from the epithelium of the lens and edema of the inner plexiform layers occur on exposure to an oxygen-rich environment (8). Our own investigations have demonstrated mitotic abnormalities of lens epithelium cells in the mouse following hyperbaric oxygen exposure (9). The following report constitutes a detailed review of our previous work and documents, for the first time, cataract formation in the mouse eye induced by repeated exposure to hyperbaric oxygen.

## MATERIALS AND METHODS

In the first experiment, 78 female, 28-day Swiss albino mice were divided into 63 experimental and 15 control animals. The 63 mice were exposed for 3 hr to 100% oxygen at 3 atm in an eight cubic foot hyperbaric chamber (Dixie Manufacturing) previously described (10). Compression and decompression were carried out at the rate of 1 lb/min. A four-inch window allowed observation of the interior of the chamber. $CO_2$ was absorbed with soda lime and the rate of oxygen flow was maintained at 10 liters/min. A telethermometer was used to monitor the temperature of the interior of the tank, which was found to vary between 78 and 81 F. Control mice were similarly placed in the chamber and allowed to breathe room air for 4 hr. Control and experimental mice were sacrificed with an overdose of ether at the following times after decompression: 0 hr (Group A), 2 hr (Group B), 24 hr (Group C), 1 week (Group D), 2 weeks (Group E). The eyes were removed and flat mounts of the lenses prepared according to the methods of Howard (11) and Richards (12). After staining with hematoxylin and eosin, mitotic counts were performed under oil immersion magnification ($\times$ 900).

In the second experiment, 200 female, 30-day Swiss albino mice were utilized. Group 1 (100 animals) was divided into two equal groups which were exposed to oxygen at 3 atm for 2 hr and at varying pressures for an additional 1 hr during which compression and decompression of the chamber was carried out. Group 2 (50 animals) was exposed to 100% oxygen at 1 atm for 3 hr. Group 3 (50 animals) was allowed to breathe room air in the open hyperbaric chamber for 3 hr. Each group was exposed twice a week over a six-week period at different times of the day.

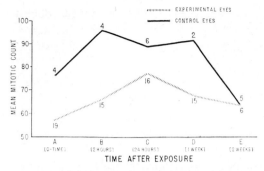

FIG. 1. Mean mitotic counts of mouse lens epithelial mount prepared at various times following a three-hour exposure to 100% oxygen at 3 atm pressure. Figures on graph indicate number of eyes examined.

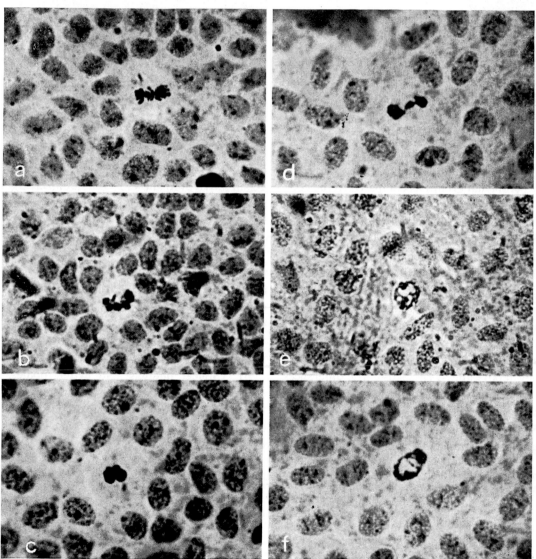

FIG. 2. a) Unusual arrangemement of chromosomes in metaphase of control animal. b, c) Amitotic division with multiple pyknotic nuclei. d) Trilobate condensation of nuclear chromatin metaphase in Group C. e, f) Vacuolation of nuclei from Group D.

# MEASUREMENT OF RETINAL ADHESION

HANAN ZAUBERMAN*

Retina Foundation, Boston, Massachusetts, USA

Research on retinal detachment has been focused mainly on the production of experimental detachments, the resulting physiopathological changes and techniques of re-attachment. However, the mechanism of retinal detachment cannot be completely understood without knowledge of the mechanism of normal retinal attachment. This aspect has not received much attention, probably because it has been assumed from gross observation that only a tenuous attachment exists between the retina and the pigment epithelium. Recent clinical observations and the results of histochemical and biochemical studies have led us to a study of the adhesion between retina and pigment epithelium in normal eyes.

*Clinical observations.* Evidence has accumulated from many sources suggesting that retinal detachment is less frequent in Negroes than in Caucasians (1–4). Yet the incidence of the retinopathy of detachment is similar for Caucasians and Africans (5), indicating that a factor preventing retinal detachment in the Negro, such as a stronger retinal adhesion, may be present. Furthermore, retinal holes are a common finding in "normal" fundi, the prevalence being between 5 and 10% (6, 7) of all eyes. Since most patients with holes do not develop retinal detachment, a "protective" factor must be involved, especially in Negro patients.

*Histochemical and biochemical studies.* A matrix substance interposed between the pigment epithelium and the outer segments has been shown histochemically to consist of acid mucopolysaccharides (8, 9). The matrix components have been identified as half-sulfated chondroitin sulfate and sialoglycans (10). It has been thought that this matrix serves as a glue between the sensory retina and the pigment epithelium.

On the basis of clinical, histochemical and biochemical data, it seemed reasonable to assume that the adhesiveness of the retina may play a role in the prevention of retinal detachment, and, conversely, that factors altering the adhesion may facilitate the detachment of the retina.

ADHESION OF THE RETINA *in vitro*

*Peeling experiments.* The force needed to peel the retina from the pigment epithelium in freshly enucleated cat eyes, at the rate of 5 mm/min, is small but measurable (11). Using rectangular 5-mm-wide strips of tissue extending from the optic nerve to the ora serrata, the force varied from 60 to 90 mg over the tapetum lucidum. Over the pigmented area, the adhesion was stronger, ranging between

* On leave of absence from the Department of Ophthalmology, Hadassah University Hospital, Jerusalem, Israel.

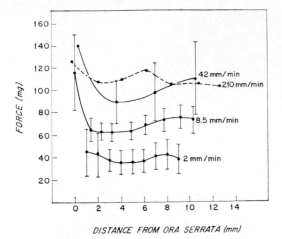

FIG. 1. Peeling force across the retinal strip vs. peeling rate.

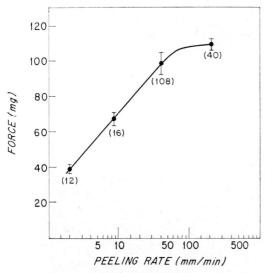

FIG. 2. Relation between peeling force and peeling rate. The number of experiments for each peeling rate is shown in brackets.

120 and 250 mg. This effect of pigmentation on the adhesive strength has also been noted in the rabbit eye (12).

The retina was peeled off albino rabbit eyes at low, medium and high rates as has been done to test adhesion in physical models. Rectangular strips of tissue, 6.5 mm wide, consisting of retina, pigment epithelium, choroid and sclera, and extending from the optic disk to the ora serrata at 12 or at 6

o'clock were cut from freshly enucleated eyes of albino rabbits after the vitreous had been carefully removed. The edge of the retina near the optic disk was glued to the rod of an instrument designed to peel off the retina at rates of 2, 8.5, 42.5 and 215 mm/min (Fig. 1). The force necessary to separate the retinal tissue was measured with a force transducer and a recorder. It increase with higher peeling rates according to a semilogarithmic relation (Fig. 2) (H. de Guillebon and H. Zauberman, in preparation).

*Traction experiments.* Another method was used to test the failure of the retinal adhesive joint in the undisturbed posterior segment of freshly enucleated owl monkey and rabbit eyes from which the vitreous had not been removed (H. Zauberman, H. de Guillebon and F. Holly, in preparation). Using localized traction exerted by means of a polyethylene tube (PE 10) glued to the retina in the equatorial area, the failure of the retinal adhesive joint was studied by exerting low (0.2 and 0.86 mm/min), medium (8.5 to 21.2 mm/min) and high traction (42.5, 85 and 425 mm/min) (Fig. 3).

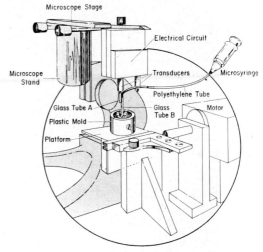

FIG. 3. Instrument to exert localized traction on the retina. The traction tube is connected to a transducer and recorder. The enucleated eye is on the platform and can be displaced at selected speed.

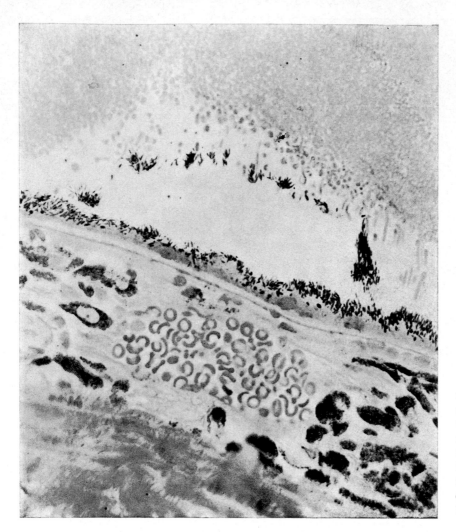

FIG. 7. At a traction rate of 8.5 mm/min, torn clumps of pigment remain attached to the outer segments, indicating cohesive failure in the pigment epithelium. Toluidine blue. × 460.

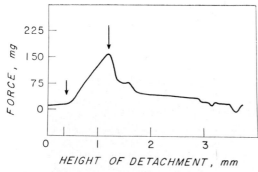

FIG. 8. Record of experiment at 8.5 mm/min. Baseline between the arrows corresponds to height of detachment; the peak of the record, to total traction force.

layer occured mainly between the outer segments of the photoreceptors and the villous processes of the pigment epithelium (Fig. 6). At a medium traction speed (8.5 mm/min), stretching and tearing of the pigment epithelium layer occurred in the cleavage area (Fig. 7).

*Force recordings.* The traction force was proportional to the height of detachment in all experiments at medium (Fig. 8) and high traction rates, but at low traction rates it was linear only when the height of detachment did not exceed 1.5 mm. Within the limits of

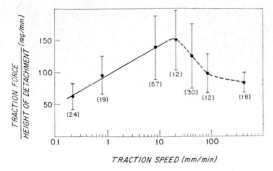

FIG. 9. Relationship between ratio of traction force to height of detachment and rate of traction. The numbers under each standard deviation indicate number of experiments for each traction.

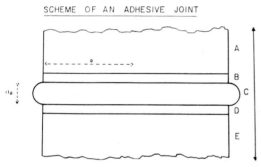

FIG. 10. Scheme of adhesive joint. A and E: solids; B and D: adherend surfaces; C: adhesive layer; O: radius of adhesive joint. (Adapted from Bikerman ref. 17.)

linearity, a ratio of traction force to height of detachment was obtained for each rate. This ratio was progressively higher with increasing traction speed, except for the high traction rate experiments, which resulted in chorioretinal separations. Fig. 9 shows a semilogarithmic relationship between the ratio and the rate of traction.

In five experiments in owl-monkey eyes, the retina was detached by traction at 8.5 mm/min, and then reapposed to the pigment epithelium. During renewed traction, no measurable force could be recorded.

*Interpretation of experimental data.* From the histologic (8, 9) and chemical (10) findings, it appears that the adhesive joint of the retina can be compared to an adhesive joint of two solids mediated by a thin layer of viscous substance (Fig. 10). For such a simple model the time needed to separate the two solids depends on the mechanical properties of the adhesive, such as viscosity and viscoelasticity' and on the geometry of the system. When traction is applied to the system, stresses are produced at various cross sections of the specimen. The behavior of the components of the system will determine the result. For the initial stage of pulling, the most significant in the process, the following equation to describe tackiness has been derived (13):

$$Ft = \frac{\eta 3\pi a^4}{4}\left(\frac{1}{h_1^{\,2}} - \frac{1}{h_2^{\,2}}\right)$$

where $F$ is the applied force, $t$ is the duration of the traction, $\eta$ is the viscosity of the adhesive liquid, $a$ is the radius of the specimen, and $h_1$ and $h_2$ are the initial and final thicknesses of the adhesive. This equation shows that there is no definite force opposing the breaking of the adhesive joint, the resistance to separation depending on the rate of separation. As $h$ is increased by a force attempting to separate the surfaces, a viscous flow of the adhesive toward the center will take place. The separation will occur within the adhesive material if the force applied is small and allows for such viscous flow (Fig. 6). This type of failure is cohesive rather than adhesive because the separation does not occur at the interface between the adherend and the adhesive. The phenomenon is rheological in nature. If the force applied to separate the surface is great and is exerted over a short time, a cohesive failure may take place in the adherend, because such an application of force does not allow viscous flow to occur (Fig. 7).

Vitreous traction is known to disrupt retinal adhesion and thus to play a major role in the development of retinal tears and detachments. It is conceivable that low traction rates cause large detachments without tears in the last

**589**

TABLE 2. *Effect of traction on the extent of detachment*

| | Experiment number | | | | | | | | | |
|---|---|---|---|---|---|---|---|---|---|---|
| | *1* | *2* | *3* | *4* | *5* | *6* | *7* | *8* | *9* | *10* |
| *In vivo* | | | | | | | | | | |
| Diameter of detachment (mm) | 0.6 | 0.9 | 0.6 | 0.6 | 0.75 | 0.6 | 0.75 | 0.75 | 0.6 | 0.75 |
| Height of detachment (mm) | 0.75 | 1.15 | 0.75 | 0.75 | 0.75 | 1.05 | 0.75 | 0.90 | 0.75 | 1.05 |
| *After death* | | | | | | | | | | |
| Time lapse after death (min) | 3 | 5 | 8 | 9 | 14 | 15 | 30 | 45 | 60 | 70 |
| Diameter of detachment (mm) | 3.0 | 4.2 | 3.6 | 4.8 | 5.0 | 5.0 | 3.0 | 3.0 | 4.2 | 4.8 |
| Height of detachment (mm) | 1.80 | 1.95 | 1.80 | 2.25 | 2.85 | 2.85 | 1.80 | 1.95 | 2.80 | 2.40 |
| *In vivo, multiple holes* | | | | | | | | | | |
| Diameter of detachment (mm) | | | | | | | | | | |
| 1st hole | 0.6 | 0.75 | 0.6 | 0.6 | | | | | | |
| 2nd hole | 0.7 | 0.6 | 0.75 | 0.75 | | | | | | |
| 3rd hole | 0.6 | 0.6 | 0.6 | 0.75 | | | | | | |
| 4th hole | 0.75 | 0.6 | 0.75 | 0.6 | | | | | | |

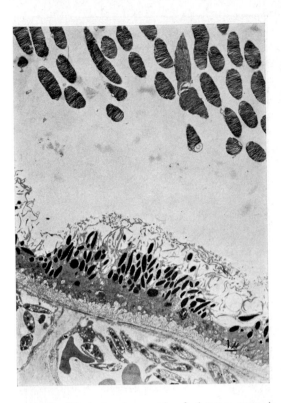

FIG. 15. Electron micrograph of cleavage area *in vivo*. Traction rate was 0.15 mm/min. Note stretching and tearing of pigment epithelium villous processes of albino rabbit. × 2,600.

Electron microscopic examination of the cleavage area affected by traction indicated stretching of the pigment epithelium *in vivo* (Fig. 15). After death, no such alteration of the pigment epithelium was observed (Fig. 16), indicating that a smaller force was needed to separate the layers.

It is evident from these results that retinal adhesion is stronger *in vivo* than shortly after death. Yet, no conclusion can be drawn as to the source of the stronger adhesion in life. Two hypotheses are worth considering. One is the possibility of a deterioration of the adhesive matrix produced by enzymes released after death. The second is that the adhesion deteriorates because a pump that removes fluid through the pigment epithelium ceases to function after death.

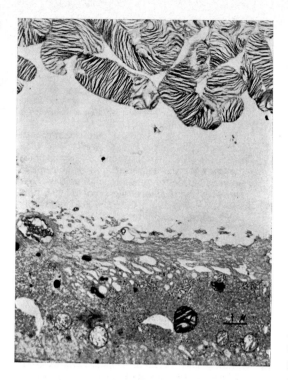

FIG. 16. Electron micrograph of cleavage area in albino rabbit after death. Traction rate: 0.15 mm/min. No obvious stretching of pigment epithelial processes.

*Degradation of retinal adhesion* in vivo. The detachments obtained in normal rabbits *in vivo* were consistently small. Similar traction experiments performed on eyes in which deterioration of adhesion was induced would be expected to result in larger detachments. Attempts to reduce the retinal adhesion were made by: a) curtailing the nutritional supply of the pigment epithelium by producing vascular occlusions, b) by trying to disturb transport enzymatically across the pigment epithelium and c) by attempting to alter the mucopolysaccharide matrix between the layers.

a) Occlusion of the choriocapillaris was obtained with a suspension of polystyrene-divinylbenzene beads (Dow Chemical Company) of 12 to 35 µm diameter, injected into a common carotid artery. After the injection, whitish conglomerates of particles were ob-

served in the arteries running through the myelinated fibers of the fundus, and an edematous area was seen around the disk. Traction experiments over an ophthalmoscopically normal-looking area of the posterior pole of the homolateral eye were performed at a rate of 0.15 mm/min within 1 to 2 hr after carotid injection in six eyes. In all instances, a large area of retina could be detached, indicating a deterioration of retinal adhesion. Ligature of the carotid artery also resulted in a similar deterioration of retinal adhesion in four homolateral eyes.

b) Ouabain (0.1 ml) injected into the vitreous cavity of four eyes at a concentration of $10^{-4}$ M caused a serious deterioration of adhesion when retinal traction was applied 12 hr after injection. However, it also gave rise to an inflammatory reaction in the anterior segment and vitreous, and a generalized edematous appearance of the fundus. Control experiments in which 0.1 ml of saline was injected into the fellow eyes did not alter retinal adhesion.

c) One-tenth milliliter of hyaluronidase (70 units) injected into the vitreous of six eyes resulted in vitreous liquefaction and a moderate deterioration of the adhesion when retinal traction was performed within 24 hr after injection (four eyes). Thereafter, the adhesion presented normal characteristics (two eyes).

Any pathological process resulting in a thickening of the matrix between the retina and the pigment epithelium would result in a weakening of the adhesion (H. Zauberman, H. de Guillebon and F. Holly, in preparation), and it is possible that occlusion of the choriocapillaris or enzymatic deterioration of the matrix could lead to alterations in retinal adhesion.

STRENGTHENING OF RETINAL ADHESION

Retinal adhesion is obviously amenable to reinforcement, and the application of different

**593**

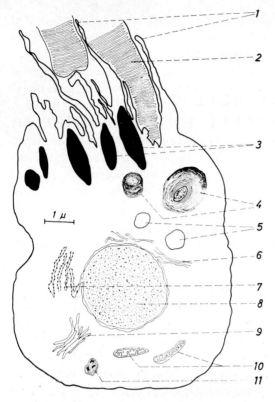

FIG. 1. Diagram of a generalized pigment epithelial cell showing: 1) microvillous extensions or apical processes of the cells, 2) rod outer segments, 3) pigment granules, 4) phagosomes or lamellar inclusion bodies, 5) oil droplets or lipofuscin bodies, 6) smooth endoplasmic reticulum, 7) rough endoplasmic reticulum, 8) nucleus, 9) Golgi complex, 10) mitochondria and 11) lysosomes.

enzymes exist in pigment epithelial cells? We recently demonstrated that sucrose homogenates from cattle eyes contain high activities of both β-galactosidase and N-acetyl-β-glucosaminidase (16), both with optimum activity at approximately pH 5. The second question, that of subcellular distribution of these enzymes, is far more complex. To date, the following organelles have been identified in pigment epithelial cells (Fig. 1): nuclei, mitochondria, endoplasmic reticulum (both smooth- and rough-surfaced), Golgi complex, lysosomes and lipid inclusion bodies. Organelles unique to pigment epithelial cells are the pigment granules and phagosomes.

Fractionation of sucrose-EDTA homogenates by differential centrifugation resulted in the isolation of nuclear, mitochondrial, lysosomal, microsomal and supernatant fractions, each defined according to the centrifugal force required for their sedimentation. As a check on the procedure used, cytochrome oxidase and acid phosphatase were used as reference enzymes for mitochondria and lysosomes, respectively. These enzymes were distributed as expected and the separation, although not perfect, is as efficient as possible, employing differential centrifugation alone. Three other enzymes were also

ment material? Second, if they are present, with what type of subcellular particle are they principally associated? In nearly all tissues the enzymes responsible for the degradation of both macromolecular substances and of intracellular organelles are found principally in the lysosomes (15). Approximately 40 of such enzymes have now been characterized, and with the exception of only two or three of them their most characteristic property is optimum activity between pH 4 to 6; hence the general term acid hydrolase.

*Distribution of acid hydrolases.* Do these

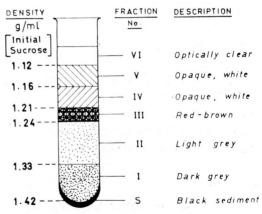

FIG. 2. Sucrose density-gradient centrifugation of the nuclear fraction of pigment epithelial cells.

examined, namely β-galactosidase, N-acetyl-β-glucosaminidase and esterase. The latter may play an important role in cleaving the retinol esters stored in pigment epithelial cells during the bleaching process. In these experiments, *p*-nitrophenyl stearate was used as the substrate since it is easily measured. However, preliminary experiments suggest that retinyl palmitate-cleaving activity is similarly distributed in pigment epithelial cells.

The "nuclear" fraction contained a higher proportion of so-called lysosomal enzymes than is commonly found in other tissues. However, in the case of pigment epithelial cells, this fraction, which sediments at 3,000 *g*-min, contains, in addition to nuclei, most of the pigment granules of the cell, as can be seen by visual inspection. It did not seem probable that pigment granules could be responsible for the excess acid hydrolase activity although the idea cannot be completely excluded. The only other organelles which might

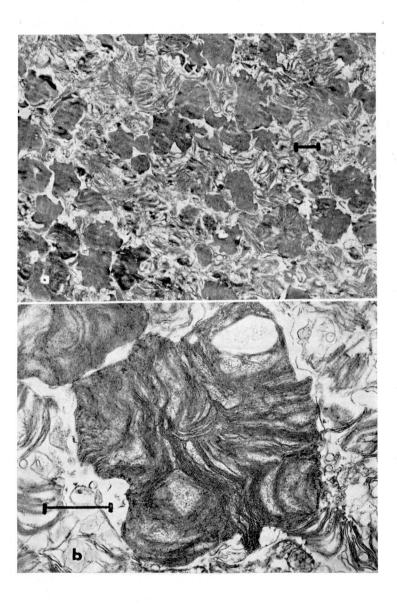

FIG. 3. Electron micrographs of fraction V isolated by sucrose density-gradient centrifugation. a) × 3,000. The bar represents 2 μm. b) × 16,000. The bar represents 1 μm.

3. YOUNG RW and BOK D. Participation of the retinal pigment epithelium in the rod outer segment renewal process. *J Cell Biol* **42**: 392, 1969.

4. YOUNG RW and BOK D. Autoradiographic studies on the metabolism of the retinal pigment epithelium. *Invest Ophthalmol* **9**: 524, 1970.

5. YOUNG RW. Shedding of discs from the rod outer segments in the rhesus monkey. *J Ultrastruct Res* **34**: 190, 1971.

6. MATSUBARA T, MIYATA M and MIZUNO K. Radioisotopic studies on renewal of opsin. *Vision Res* **8**: 1139, 1968.

7. HERRON WL, RIEGEL BW, MYERS OE and RUBIN ML. Retinal dystrophy in the rat—a pigment epithelial disease. *Invest Ophthalmol* **8**: 595, 1969.

8. ISHIKAWA T and YAMADA E. The degradation of the photoreceptor outer segment within the pigment epithelial cell of rat retina. *J Electron Microsc (Tokyo)* **19**: 85, 1970.

9. MACHEMER R and KROLL AJ. Experimental retinal detachment in the owl monkey. VII. Photoreceptor protein renewal in normal and detached retina. *Am J Ophthalmol* **71**: 690, 1971.

10. YOUNG RW. The renewal of rod and cone outer segments in the rhesus monkey. *J Cell Biol* **49**: 303, 1971.

11. KROLL AJ and MACHEMER R. Experimental retinal detachment in the owl monkey. III. Electron microscopy of retina and pigment epithelium. *Am J Ophthalmol* **66**: 410, 1968.

12. DOWLING JE and GIBBONS IR. The fine structure of the pigment epithelium in the albino rat. *J Cell Biol* **14**: 459, 1962.

13. BAIRATI A JR and ORZALESI N. The ultrastructure of the pigment epithelium and of the photoreceptor-pigment epithelium junction in the retina. *J Ultrastruct Res* **9**: 484, 1963.

14. SPITZNAS M and HOGAN MJ. Outer segments of photoreceptors and the retinal pigment epithelium. *Arch Ophthalmol* **84**: 810, 1970.

15. DE DUVE C and WATTIAUX R. Functions of lysosomes. *Annu Rev Physiol* **28**: 435, 1966.

16. BERMAN ER. Acid hydrolases of the retinal pigment epithelium. *Invest Ophthalmol* **10**: 64, 1971.

17. COLLINS FD, LOVE RM and MORTON RA. Studies on rhodopsin. 4. Preparation of rhodopsin. *Biochem J* **51**: 292, 1952.

18. McCONNELL DG. The isolation of retinal outer segment fragments. *J Cell Biol* **27**: 459, 1965.

19. FUTTERMAN S and SASLAW LD. The estimation of vitamin A aldehyde with thiobarbituric acid. *J Biol Chem* **236**: 1652, 1961.

20. ZORN M and FUTTERMAN S. Properties of rhodopsin dependent on associated phospholipid. *J Biol Chem* **246**: 881, 1971.

21. DOWLING JE and GIBBONS IR, in: Smelser GK (Ed), "The structure of the eye." New York, Academic Press, 1961, p 85.

22. KUWABARA T and GORN RA. Retinal damage by visible light: an electron microscopic study. *Arch Ophthalmol* **79**: 69, 1968.

23. SMITH RS and BERSON EL. Acute toxic effects of chloroquine on the cat retina: ultrastructural changes. *Invest Ophthalmol* **10**: 237, 1971.

# SYNTHESIS OF FATTY ACIDS BY NORMAL AND DIABETIC RETINAL TISSUE

SIDNEY FUTTERMAN and MARTHA H. ROLLINS

Department of Ophthalmology, University of Washington Medical School, Seattle, Washington, USA

## INTRODUCTION

Tissues of the central nervous system are not generally thought of as requiring insulin (1). The utilization of glucose by the brain is unresponsive to insulin. The glucose dependent electrical response of the retina to stimulation by light is essentially unaltered when glucose in the medium bathing the retina is reduced considerably below the physiological concentration (2). However, the possibility that some other aspect of retinal metabolism dependent upon insulin may be altered in diabetes is suggested by the gradual progression of retinopathic changes in animals made diabetic by various means (3, 4).

A few years ago, liver, lung and adipose tissues of alloxan-diabetic rats were found to have reduced capacities to desaturate stearate to oleate and to introduce double bonds in the pathways by which the essential fatty acids are metabolized through successive chain elongation and desaturation reactions (5–7). If similar defects in the biosynthesis of fatty acids were to occur in the retina, they might be expected in time to change sufficiently the fatty acid composition of structural lipids in lipoprotein membranes so as to alter membrane permeability and thereby to contribute to the development of diabetic retinopathy.

## MATERIALS AND METHODS

Particulate fractions of retinal tissue were prepared as previously described (8). Supernatant fluid fractions were prepared by homogenizing tissue in the proportion of 15 bovine retinas or 1 g of rabbit liver per 3 ml of isotonic KCl and centrifuging the homogenate for 1 hr at 105,000 $\times$ $g$ to remove particulate matter.

The methods used to analyze fatty acid composition, to fractionate methyl esters of fatty acids by thin layer chromatography on silica gel containing $AgNO_3$, to isolate individual methyl esters by gas chromatography, and to determine $C^{14}$ activity recovered in methyl ester fractions by liquid scintillation counting were those previously employed (9, 10). 1-$C^{14}$-acetate, 1,5-$C^{14}$-citrate, 1-$C^{14}$-acetyl-CoA and 1,3-$C^{14}$-malonyl-CoA were purchased from New England Nuclear Corporation.

Estimation of 1,5-$C^{14}$-acetate incorporation into long chain fatty acids was carried out in reaction mixtures (1 ml) containing 4 µmoles of ATP, 0.2 µmole of NADP, 0.8 µmole of $MnCl_2$, 0.1 µmole of CoA, 8 µmoles of cysteine, 20 µmoles of $KHCO_2$, 10 µmoles of isocitrate, 0.3 ml of isotonic phosphate buffer, pH 6.5, either 5 µmoles of 1,5-$C^{14}$-citrate (spec act 1.1 $\times$ 10⁵ count/min per µmole), or 2 µmoles of 1-$C^{14}$-acetate (spec act 1.1 $\times$ 10⁶ count/min per µmole), retinal supernatant fluid (4.7 mg dry wt) or liver supernatant fluid (6.1 mg dry wt) and, where indicated, 5 µmoles of unlabeled citrate or 2 µmoles of unlabeled acetate. After incubation under 5% $CO_2$ in $O_2$ at 37 C for 100 min, the fatty acids were extracted

TABLE 5. *Fatty acid composition (mole/100 ml) of normal and alloxan-diabetic rat retina*

| Fatty acid | | Normal | Diabetic |
|---|---|---|---|
| 16:0 | Palmitate | 19.6 | 25.6 |
| 18:0 | Stearate | 25.0 | 27.5 |
| 18:1 | Oleate | 9.8 | 12.7 |
| 18:2 | Linoleate | 0.7 | 1.6 |
| 20:4 | Arachidonate | 9.0 | 7.6 |
| 22:6 | Docosahexaenoate | 36.0 | 25.0 |

After induction of diabetes in male Sprague-Dawley rats and maintenance for 116 days without insulin, retinal tissue from six experimental and six control animals was analyzed for fatty acids. Minor components, with the exception of linoleate, were omitted. No selective loss of pericytes from the retinal capillaries was found. Data are from ref. 10.

the relative proportion of $C_{16}$ and $C_{18}$ fatty acids was increased. Impairment in polyenoic fatty acid synthesis by retinal tissue of diabetic animals was sufficient eventually to effect a modest alteration in the fatty acid composition of the retina.

## DISCUSSION

In general, the properties of the fatty acid synthesizing mechanism of retinal supernatant fluid with respect to the supplements required, optimal pH and product composition were quite similar to those properties that have previously been described for the fatty acid synthesizing system of liver (11). The stimulation by citrate of incorporation of acetyl groups from 1-C$^{14}$-acetyl-CoA into long chain fatty acids by retinal supernatant fluid suggests (14) that the acetyl-CoA carboxylase of retinal tissue is activated by citrate. In the retina, as in other tissues, citrate appears to serve a dual function: a) supplying acetyl groups, and b) accelerating the rate-limiting carboxylation step in fatty acid synthesis. The principal differences found between retina and liver could be adequately accounted for by the very much lower activities of acetate thiokinase and aconitase in retinal tissue than in liver.

*De novo* synthesis of saturated fatty acids and the chain elongation pathways of linoleate and linolenate metabolism were found to occur in the retina. The tissue fraction capable of the most rapid synthesis of fatty acids in retina, the microsomes, when prepared from alloxan-diabetic rat liver, has shown depressed desaturation of linoleic and α-linolenic acids (6, 15). The observed impairment in polyunsaturated fatty acid synthesis in retinal tissue of diabetic animals was sufficient eventually to effect a modest alteration in the fatty acid composition of the retina. These findings support the concept that the retina is a target for insulin. The possibility that impaired biosynthesis of fatty acids in the retina may contribute to the development of the retinopathic changes associated with diabetes remains to be explored.

Supported by United States Public Health Service Grant EY 00343 and a grant from the National Society for the Prevention of Blindness.

## REFERENCES

1. RENOLD AE and CAHILL GF JR. Diabetes mellitus, in: Stanbury JB and Fredrickson DS (Eds), "The metabolic basis of inherited disease." New York, McGraw-Hill, 1966, p 98.
2. AMES A III and GURIAN BS. Effects of glucose and oxygen deprivation on function of isolated mammalian retina. *J Neurophysiol* **26**: 617, 1963.
3. ENGERMAN RL and BLOODWORTH JMB JR. Experimental diabetic retinopathy in dogs. *Arch Ophthalmol* **73**: 205, 1965.
4. VAIL D. Account of "The Jules Gonin centennial celebration." *Am J Ophthalmol* **71**: 143, 1971.
5. BENJAMIN W and GELLHORN A. The effect of diabetes and insulin on the biosynthesis of individual fatty acids in adipose tissue. *J Biol Chem* **239**: 64, 1964.
6. MERCURI O, PELUFFO RO and BRENNER RR. Depression of microsomal desaturation of linoleic to γ-linolenic acid in the alloxan-diabetic rat. *Biochim Biophys Acta* **116**: 409, 1966.
7. FRIEDMANN N, GELLHORN A and BENJAMIN W. Synthesis of arachidonic acid from linoleic acid *in vivo* in diabetic rats. *Isr J Med Sci* **2**: 677, 1966.
8. ANDREWS JS and FUTTERMAN S. Metabolism of the retina. V. The role of microsomes in vitamin A esterification in the visual cycle. *J Biol Chem* **239**: 4073, 1964.

**604**

make adequate ophthalmoscopic examinations in our canine diabetic colony due to this complication. Attempts at cataract surgery in some of the animals have been unsuccessful in producing an adequate optical window for good visualization of the fundus.

Further research is indicated in an attempt to discover or develop a more satisfactory counterpart of human proliferative diabetic retinopathy. On the other hand, useful information will hopefully be obtained from background retinopathy cases, as the disease, at least in dogs, is virtually indistinguishable from that seen in mild background human disease (7).

## REFERENCES

1. PATZ A and MAUMENEE AE. Studies on diabetic retinopathy. I. Retinopathy in a dog with spontaneous diabetes mellitus. *Am J Ophthalmol* **54**: 532, 1962.
2. HAUSLER HR, SIBAY TM and CAMPBELL J. Retinopathy in a dog following diabetes induced by growth hormone. *Diabetes* **13**: 122, 1964.
3. ENGERMAN RL and BLOODWORTH JMB JR. Experimental diabetic retinopathy in dogs. *Arch Ophthalmol* **73**: 205, 1965.
4. VON SALLMANN L and GRIMES P. Eye changes in streptozotocin diabetes in rats. *Am J Ophthalmol* **71**: 312, 1971.
5. HAUSLER HR. Diabetic retinopathy. Newer concepts of its pathology and treatment. *Int Ophthalmol Clin* **7**: 39, 1967.
6. PATZ A, BERKOW JW, MAUMENEE AE and COX J. Studies in diabetic retinopathy. II. Retinopathy and nephropathy in spontaneous canine diabetes. *Diabetes* **14**: 700, 1965.
7. KUWABARA T and COGAN DG. Studies of retinal vascular patterns. *Arch Ophthalmol* **64**: 904, 1960.

fective way of controlling the disease. Now may I ask you the same question I asked about onchocerciasis? Since we will be interested in carrying out epidemiological studies, are we going to have any difficulty in diagnosing trachoma?

DR. COLLIER: I don't think that clinical diagnosis of trachoma is really that difficult now although there may be a few difficult cases. However, techniques for laboratory diagnosis are improving all the time. By culturing the trachoma agent in monolayers of cells, we are getting more and more positives. In the Gambia, where we are now working, I think we can isolate about 70% of the active cases by growing the monolayers in chick embryos. We hope to improve on this in the future.

DR. I. C. MICHAELSON (Israel): Did anything emerge on the nature of the local defense mechanism?

DR. COLLIER: We know that antibodies consisting of various types of immunoglobulins are locally produced. Both IgG and IgA have been reported in the conjunctival sac and again I think we should remember that it was the late Dr. Bernkopf, here in Jerusalem, who first found these antibodies in the eye. So this is probably part of the defense mechanism, but I think that cellular immunity, cell associated factors, also play a very significant role in immunity.

DR. MAUMENEE: I hate to belabor this, but I've been interested in immunology as far as corneal transplantation is concerned. Local immunity is usually not considered an important factor, although this point has been argued in many other conditions.

DR. COLLIER: All one can say is that people have put antigens into the eye and have been able to show that they exert protective effects. Therefore, some defense mechanism must have been stimulated. But the problem in the chalmydial group is very complicated because one would imagine that macrophages are an important part of local defense. We have recently shown that when the trachoma agent enters the macrophage, that is when the macrophage digests the elementary body, there is a mutually lethal effect. They literally kill each other. The destruction of macrophages by the trachomal elementary bodies may explain certain features of the pathology and perhaps the chronicity of the disease.

DR. MAUMENEE: Are there any other questions from the audience?

DR. R. STEIN (Israel): I believe that the chemotherapeutic approach will not help as long as there are reinfections and the hygienic state of the community is not improved.

DR. I. MANN (Australia): My experience is almost entirely clinical with the Aborigines in Australia. I have instituted various treatment campaigns. This is very difficult to do among primitive people because they don't believe in treatment. I have seen both in Australia and in other parts of the world the complete disappearance of active trachoma within a space of 10 or 15 years simply because of the institution of a water supply and the use of soap. I sometimes feel that trachoma is diminishing in severity, although diseases do fluctuate in intensity. It may be that by the time we have, on the one hand, raised the standard of hygiene and, on the other, produced the perfect antibiotic or the perfect immunological answer, the disease will have disappeared and we shall never know which factor was mainly responsible.

DR. MAUMENEE: I should like to ask Dr. Dohlman to report on his session on corneal

DR. MAUMENEE: Would anyone challenge me if I claim it is closer to one-tenth of a percent?

DR. MICHAELSON: To what extent do the newer methods of diagnosing disk changes help in differentiating between the real glaucomatous cases and those with straightforward hypertension?

DR. LINNÉR: I think some of the papers dealing with the disk and disk changes and the possibility of classifying what is a normal and what is an abnormal disk were very interesting. In this field we need more research before we can be sure of these classifications. I think this is a promising and important field for the future.

DR. STEIN: My question is what is the difference between glaucoma and hypertension, and not between a susceptible or nonsusceptible disk.

DR. LINNÉR: This is a very important point. A certain pressure level might, in one eye, lead to glaucomatous changes in the disk and to field changes, and in another eye might never lead to glaucoma. That is one of the reasons why it is so difficult to decide on a pressure value above which you have glaucoma and below which you don't.

DR. MAUMENEE: I think we had better move on to the problem of diabetic retinopathy.

DR. M. GOLDBERG (USA): Several important contributions were made in the session devoted to the treatment of diabetic retinopathy by photocoagulation. Of paramount importance was the observation that diabetic retinopathy has become a leading cause of blindness in many parts of the world and that the number of newly blind from this disease will surely increase in the future.

The erratic nature of diabetic retinopathy

surgery, with special reference to developing countries.

DR. C. H. DOHLMAN (USA): The corneal surgery session was a very exciting one with a number of excellent talks. There was one thing that became clear, not only from that session but also from the meeting as a whole, and that is a fantastic global need for penetrating keratoplasty. Mr. Wilson cited a figure of 15 million blind people. It is likely that half of them are due to corneal diseases and a good portion of these should be amenable to keratoplasty. We have to consider that keratoplasty is more demanding and more complicated than, say, cataract extraction. It is not so much the surgery itself as the follow-up which requires special knowledge. The steroid game has to be played correctly and the management is difficult to relegate to paramedical personnel.

Regarding preservation for lamellar keratoplasty, this is now well developed and cryopreserved tissue is now available for worldwide distribution. Dr. King at the International Eye Bank is doing that now but there may also be other organizations able to supply this material. There is, however, another means of increasing the supply of donor material and that is to change the existing laws. In several countries in Europe, for instance, surgeons are allowed to remove donor material from the dead body without specifically asking the next of kin. Such a law, if instituted, would immediately eliminate all donor problems. In the United States, for example, there are about 10 times more people dying than those receiving corneal transplants. So I think that ophthalmologists everywhere should lobby for changes toward more rational laws. And finally, there is the question of prosthesis, a very intriguing one. We can put a little plastic window in the cornea and the patient sees perfectly well; the only question is for how long. There is no doubt that great

strides have been made in this field during the last decade. Unfortunately, it isn't really so successful in those cases that really need it. In edema cases, and in others where results with keratoprosthesis are reasonably good, the same results could have been obtained with penetrating keratoplasty. On the other hand, in cases such as dry eyes or chemical burns, where we really need a good prosthesis, the results are still disappointing. So I think even though we are still far away from any mass application of prostheses, we should continue trying to improve them.

DR. MAUMENEE: It seems to me that the problem of penetrating keratoplasty in the developed and developing countries differs about as much as the incidence and prevalence of the diseases themselves. Whereas the cases we treat in the developed countries are usually due to edema following cataract, endothelial dystrophy, keratoconus and other favorable cases, patients with trachoma or anterior staphyloma following keratomalacia are unfavorable ones. Dr. Dahanda has reported improvement in vision up to 20/40 or better in only about 30% of 750 cases. In discussing keratoplasty in developing countries, I wonder if we aren't a bit more enthusiastic than we should be because we haven't had experience operating on patients with severe trachoma, keratomalacia and anterior staphyloma.

DR. DOHLMAN: This is perfectly true since in Europe and the United States, we are working on corneas which are essentially nonvascularized and thus less subject to immune reactions and other problems. I have recently read Dahanda's report myself, and although I agree that problems of corneal grafting in a developed country differ in many ways from those in developing countries, even if one-third of the eyes treated are saved, this may result in the restoration of useful sight to a million people.

DR. E. LINNÉR (*Sweden*): The diagnostic value of mass examination of a large part of the population was stressed, especially in high-risk groups such as family members in whom fully developed cases of glaucoma may be detected. It may also be possible to detect very early cases of chronic simple glaucoma by mass screening. However, at the present time pressure readings do not enable us to distinguish with sufficient accuracy between early chronic simple glaucoma and ocular hypertension. In the latter cases, true glaucoma will never develop. Further research is needed in this field. At the present time, our feeling is that there is no single parameter that can predict which eye with ocular hypertension will develop glaucoma. It is possible in developed countries to detect early field defects with small test targets.

It should be borne in mind that the therapy itself entails some risks. Therefore, with close supervision, one can withhold therapy in the face of moderate ocular hypertension. It must be remembered that every ophthalmologist must keep his patients under his own careful observation. In the future, new studies, such as the appearance of the disk, may have predictable value and I think that's all we can say as a conclusion.

DR. W. LEYDHECKER (*West Germany*): I think we agree about the facts but disagree on the practical conclusions to be drawn from them. We agree that there are eyes with a tension higher than normal which do not develop glaucoma within, say, 10 years. Now, what should a practitioner do when he finds such cases? He is told to keep the patient under close observation. The practical question is how can he be certain that the patient will not go to the next ophthalmologist or will not lose interest and avoid going to an ophthalmologist at all? The other big problem is to decide which are the minimum findings indicating the need to begin treatment.

detachment. If this is true, it may be that there is much overtreatment for prevention by photocoagulation.

Dr. Kurtz emphasized that holes can occur in one or both layers of the retina in retinoschisis. Dr. Treister indicated the degree to which highly myopic eyes, both phakic and aphakic, were at risk from retinal detachment. Dr. Lincoff rightly spoke on the indications and importance of emergency treatment in several categories of retinal detachment and how important this swift treatment was to the successful end result. Dr. Protonotarios set the standard for good functional results after retinal surgery and referred to eight cases of macular puckering as an unexplained complication. Dr. Friedman contrasted the favorable results of surgery without drainage of subretinal fluid with the less favorable results when the fluid was drained. Dr. Goldberg described several conditions leading to retinitis proliferans including retrolental fibroplasia, diabetes and sickle cell hemoglobin C disease. He showed how the proliferans fronds go toward the ischemic retina. Dr. Freilich described the use of hyperbaric oxygen chambers for retinal detachment surgery in patients with sickle cell C disease. He did not indicate, however, the impracticality and potential dangers of this treatment in inexperienced hands.

### ORGANIZATION FOR PREVENTION

DR. MAUMENEE: We will now proceed to the subject of Organization for Prevention: Between the Nations (J. François and I. C. Mann, chairmen) and Within the Nations (G. von Bahr and A. Nakajima, chairmen). May I ask these four chairmen to take their places on the platform and to present their reports. I would like to ask Dr. François to begin with the summary of his session.

DR. J. FRANÇOIS (*Belgium*): Dr. Tarizzo of the World Health Organization described how

this organization is attempting to define the overall problem of preventable blindness. Member states have been asked to provide available information on number, cause and age of onset of blindness. Infectious diseases and nutritional deficiencies are still the principal causes of preventable blindness in the world today.

Dr. Nizetic of the European office of the World Health Organization told us that the role of his office is to help the member states to achieve optimal eye health in the population. Epidemiological surveys and mass screenings represent powerful public health tools for assessing the state of eye health, thus providing a basis for achieving improved eye health. Positive findings on screening could lead to early detection, prevention, curative treatment and rehabilitation. My own report was a general outline of the technical assistance that some countries provide to developing countries in the field of ophthalmology. This assistance is of two types: first, integrated foreign aid—a beautiful example of which is Israel's foreign aid; and secondly, varied foreign aid such as that of Belgium, Britain, France, West Germany and Holland.

Mr. Wilson gave an impressive survey of what the International Society for the Blind, The Royal Commonwealth Society for the Blind and the American Foundation for Overseas Blind, are doing for the prevention of blindness.

Dr. Christy described the present role of missionary societies in the treatment of ophthalmic diseases. Their hospitals could be used effectively for preventive work if advice, inspiration, instruction and assistance could be given to their dedicated staffs.

Dr. King and Mr. Lawlor reported on the International Eye Foundation, which receives its main support from public donations. Its aim is the promotion of peace through the prevention and cure of blindness. It is dedicated to upgrading eye surgical care everywhere by sponsoring short term exchange fellowships and surgical teams. It also sends donor material for corneal grafting.

Dr. Scholtz told us that since 1958 MEDICO has provided opthalmic care in 11 countries; it attempts to teach the local doctors so that in time they can take over. It enters a country only by government invitation.

From the papers under discussion it may be concluded that: 1) Although much has already been done for the prevention of blindness, much more still remains to be done. 2) Regional or national plans of action should be formulated. 3) Before planning a program it is necessary to centralize all the information concerning the current activities. I think that WHO is already doing this. 4) Integrated aid is the most efficient method. The developed countries must not only assist the developing country with services, but should also train ophthalmologists, and if possible, promote research. Only this method can achieve the goal set up by Dr. Michaelson of: "serve, teach and leave."

DR. MAUMENEE: Thank you very much. Dr. Mann do you wish to add anything?

DR. MANN: I wish to thank Dr. François for having summarized this meeting so very well. Afterwards the reports from individual nations very clearly brought out the different levels of eye care available in various countries. I don't think I need summarize them because we have all been listening to papers on this subject. What we really need is more basic research, we need more collaboration in discovering the incidence of the diseases in the various countries and we need to initiate programs of treatment. But I say again what I always say in the trachoma sessions: that what we really need is more soap and water!

DR. MAUMENEE: Dr. Tarrizo, you had some very interesting comments to make about the 65 different definitions of blindness. Can you bring this down to something like the number of political organizations in the Israel parliament? Say to 14 or so?

DR. M. TARRIZO (*WHO, Switzerland*): The 65 definitions of blindness are those which are listed in the appendix to the 1966 Report on Blindness published by WHO. These definitions are actually different wordings of a much smaller number. The principles vary somewhat for different countries: some of them are objective measurements of vision and others are subjective interpretations of the individual's capacity to cope with normal life. WHO is now carrying out a study to get more meaningful definitions which we hope will be acceptable on an international scale. There will be separate definitions for visual impairment and for loss of vision.

DR. MAUMENEE: I thought that the gaussian curve that Dr. Nizetic presented was a very interesting way of defining visual loss. Could someone elaborate on this.

DR. TARRIZO: I would rather not go too deeply into the contents of the report because this might reflect the opinions of the consultants. The report will be circulated, as a matter of fact, to other interested parties for comments before it is submitted to the Assembly.

DR. MAUMENEE: Could you say something about the May and August 1972 meetings?

DR. TARRIZO: At the World Health Assembly held in Boston in 1969, a resolution was passed and adopted asking the World Health Organization a) to undertake a study on preventable and curable blindness in the world, b) to collect information, c) to assist in defining priorities and d) to make recommendations concerning future activities to be

**633**

carried out by WHO in collaboration with other government or nongovernment organizations in this field. In implementation of that resolution, details of the activities carried out so far and of the information collected have been collated.

The report will be prepared and will be submitted to the next World Health Assembly in May 1972. Then in August 1972, a study group on the prevention of blindness will be convened to assist the Organization in defining and developing this program. There is at present no program on the prevention of blindness, as such, within WHO. The approach of WHO to health problems in the world has always been public health oriented and the emphasis has been on acting on causes of diseases rather than on their manifestations or consequences. Thus, because blindness is something which can develop as a consequence of different causes requiring different methodological approaches, the prevention of blindness has so far been dealt with under different programs. One of these is the program for virus diseases which includes trachoma. Under nutrition, we deal with xerophthalmia and keratomalacia; and under parasitic diseases we are concerned with onchocerciasis. There are also other programs for other causes of blindness. But we do maintain and develop coordination both within the organization and among different programs.

DR. A. NAKAJIMA (*Japan*): May I just add that Japan has an enormous potential for international cooperation, but so far we have no great experience in this field. The only international cooperation program we have at the moment is with Thailand and we are prepared to expand this in the future. I have learned a great deal from this Congress that will help us in this respect.

DR. MAUMENEE: We welcome you into the fold, Dr. Nakajima.

DR. S. FRANKEN (*Netherlands*): This session is concerned with the organization for prevention and I feel that we haven't utilized this conference to the full extent for that purpose. I would like to give you two examples of what I mean. In the field of onchocerciasis there is a problem as to the best method of prevention, especially with respect to vector control or filaricides. The organizational efforts described so far today are not likely to provide the means of solving this problem, and attempts should be made to contact or to create other organizational fields capable of producing an answer. Similarly in keratomalacia, organizational help in addition to that described so far is required. Here at an organization of scientists, the problem is not the lack of knowledge regarding administration of vitamin A. It is the economic underdevelopment and social and cultural misconceptions regarding the right diet. The organization that can cope with these problems might be UNICEF or some other agency. This conference should take the necessary steps to broaden the scope of organizational help in these fields.

DR. MAUMENEE: Steps are being taken in this direction which you will hear more about later this morning. Meanwhile, we should like to hear the report of Dr. von Bahr, who was chairman of the session on Organization for Prevention: Within the Nations.

DR. G. VON BAHR (*Sweden*): Prevention of blindness has many aspects and most of them were illustrated at our session. The expression, prevention of blindness, has been used in various ways and may have different meanings in developed and in developing countries. The first meaning relates to preventing the disease from appearing or, if it has appeared, preventing the onset of functional loss. The second meaning implies limiting functional loss by active treatment. This has to be considered when we speak of organization for prevention of blindness because these two meanings lead to two different types of preventive activity.

The first group of preventive activities includes genetic counseling; prenatal care; adequate nutrition, especially for children; eradication of vectors of infectious diseases; systematic health examinations and health care from birth onwards; preventive vaccination programs; legislation requiring eye protection in industrial work; prohibition of fireworks and other explosives; and general education in hygiene and the risk of accidents to the eye in childhood and in sport. In some developed countries these measures have already been partially or even completely undertaken by the state authorities, government or public health institutions, as well as by schools. For many of these preventive measures, the role of the ophthalmologist is mainly to serve as initiator and advisor. He should stimulate the undertaking of the necessary epidemiological surveys. But most of the measures have to be carried out by others. It therefore follows that national associations for the prevention of blindness should include not only ophthalmologists but also other specialists concerned with conditions affecting vision.

The second group of activities includes mainly curative measures, and applies principally to developing countries. This means the expansion or the setting up (if they do not already exist) of eye services of all kinds and the increasing of staff, both medical and auxiliary.

We must realize that for many measures named under the first group of preventive activities, the role of the ophthalmologist is mainly to serve as an initiator and an advisor. We have to make the diagnosis and therefore aid in providing reliable statistics on frequency and causes of blindness in the various countries, and also to give advice on what to do in order to eliminate them. However, most of the practical measures have to be undertaken by others. International as well as national organizations should assist wherever possible. The WHO is a center for close collaboration with other international organizations such as the International Association for the Prevention of Blindness and the World Council for the Welfare of the Blind and UNICEF. It is also recommended that most countries should have local national associations for the prevention of blindness and should include not only ophthalmologists but also other specialists concerned with conditions affecting vision. They in turn should cooperate with other organizations and institutions for public health.

Mr. Chairman, may I make a plea for our Association for the Prevention of Blindness and ask that all of you sign the application for membership. Thank you.

### OPHTHALMIC TEACHING

DR. MAUMENEE: I propose that we now discuss the reports on ophthalmic teaching.

DR. THOMAS: I would like to know from the experts whether we should train multi-disciplinary para-medical staff who, in addition to detecting eye diseases, can also investigate cases of, for example, a parasitic infection?

DR. MICHAELSON: I think the first stage is to develop our para-ophthalmological possibilities and find our way during the next year or two. As you know, some steps have already been taken in that direction. I think that it is probably not wise to attempt to combine paramedical disciplines at this stage.

DR. W.J. HOLMES (*Hawaii*): In Indonesia there are about 100 well trained eye nurses who have had regular nursing training plus an additional year or more of training in eye care. They are well able to detect and take

**635**

care of close to 70 or 80% of the common eye conditions. They can remove foreign bodies, treat chalazions and sties and detect serious eye conditions and refer them to the eye specialist. These eye nurses are strategically located throughout the islands of Indonesia as well as in central Java. Here then is positive proof that paramedical personnel who are not multidisciplinary, but specifically trained for ophthalmology, indeed have their place, and I have been told that these paramedical personnel have helped considerably in reducing the incidence of severe eye disease.

I would also like to comment on health education of the public. Some years ago in Indonesia, there was a public health campaign using posters and folders to inform the public of the dangers of xerophthalmia and how it could be prevented. If this could be done on a larger scale, I feel it would be even more effective.

DR. MAUMENEE: I'm sure that it is not necessary to become a physician to do most of the things that the physicians waste their time doing today. I believe very strongly that anything that a physician does routinely should be done by allied or paramedical personnel. The physician's training leads him to judgment and he should spend his time in diagnosis and decision-making rather than in routine duties. So, I'm sure that what you just said can be done in the future, but at the beginning, we should not train paramedical personnel for the complicated tasks. There is a large gap between a beginning and an ideal. So far we are rather far down the ladder, so the more simply we begin, the better off we will be.

CONTRIBUTIONS OF BASIC RESEARCH

DR. MAUMENEE: I would now like to call on the chairmen of the sessions on basic research in corneal opacification, cataract and retinal diseases (D.M. Maurice, S.I. Brown, S. Mishima, M.E. Langham, A. Spector, A. Pirie, M.V. Riley and T. Kuwabara). The first subject is corneal opacification and I see that Dr. Maurice is ready with his report.

DR. D.M. MAURICE (*USA*): The basic physiologist or biochemist generally expects only long-term results from his researches and considers himself very fortunate if he can do anything immediately useful for the prevention of blindness. I think this has been exemplified in our session on corneal opacification which concerned itself almost entirely with the biological and physiological mechanisms whereby the cornea maintains its normal thickness and transparency. I think this basic research has borne fruit. For example, I think we are already improving methods of assessing donor corneas and improving the methods of storing corneas. Also we are now able to excise the cornea and keep it alive under perfused conditions for up to 12 hr; this has proved a great help in assessing the effect of fungicides and other drugs on the cornea.

Apart from this, the Congress has stimulated me in another way. I have always assumed that trachoma and keratomalacia were not medical problems but entirely social problems. We basic scientists always have glaucoma and cataract forced on our attention by the ophthalmologists. We are never told about keratomalacia or xerophthalmia. I have the impression that this problem is far from being solved and I would like to reverse the usual question and instead ask the clinicians present if there is anything that we, the basic physiologists and biochemists, can do to help in the problem of xerophthalmia?

DR. VENKATASWAMY: This is a good point, Dr. Maurice. In the discussion on keratomalacia, at least some workers questioned, whether vitamin A alone is responsible for keratomalacia. We don't know and we are very badly in need of biochemists to solve this problem for us.

MR. RODGER: It is such a pleasure to get a scientist offering help that I can't resist this opportunity. I have been very interested in Dohlman's recent work on the precorneal tear film and the effect of mucus on the surface of the cornea. I think there may be some relationship here to xerophthalmia. I would like to ask whether you are in a position to associate changes in mucus with xerophthalmia? If you do get an alteration in the consistency of the mucus which covers the eye, might not that be a starting point in keratomalacia?

DR. MAUMENEE: May I ask two questions on this? One, has there ever been a case of keratomalacia or xerophthalmia in a patient who did not have vitamin A deficiency? No! (from the audience).

Secondly, do all patients with the same degree of vitamin A deficiency develop the same degree of xerophthalmia? No! (from the audience).

DR. MAURICE: In answer to Dr. Rodger, I am sure I could do something about this, and I'm sure Dr. Dohlman could do it better! The question is, would this really be helpful in curing the disease?

DR. A. CHATTERJEE (India): I would like to say that India can be divided into two zones: one, the wheat-eating zone, and the other, rice-eating. It is a well known fact that in the rice-eating areas, there is considerable keratomalacia. I have been working for the last 10 years in Punjab, a wheat-eating zone, and I haven't yet seen a single case of keratomalacia.

DR. MAUMENEE: I shall now ask Dr. Mishima to report on the session on Corneal Opacification.

DR. S. MISHIMA (Japan): This session brought out many examples of how basic research can be applied to clinical medicine. Drs. Dohlman and Brown, working independently on the problem of corneal ulceration, have shown that collagenase released from damaged epithelial cells is able to attack stromal collagen fibrils after the protective envelope of glycoprotein or proteoglycan has been removed. This invariably leads to corneal ulcerations. However, the whole process can be prevented in one of three ways: a) administration of collagenase inhibitors such as sodium EDTA or cysteine; b) prevention of epithelial contact with the corneal ulcer by use of gluedon contact lenses and c) formation of a conjunctival flap. Another important point was the potentiating effect of steroids on collagenase; these hormones should be used with caution, especially in cases of corneal ulceration.

DR. MAUMENEE: I should like to ask two questions. Firstly, could you summarize the degree of effectiveness of the collagenase inhibitors in the treatment or prevention of corneal ulcers? Secondly, it is my impression that glued-on lenses are used very little now that we have soft contact lenses available.

DR. DOHLMAN: Regarding the efficacy of collagenase inhibitors, the results of a double-blind study carried out by our group using calcium EDTA suggest that it is highly effective. However, considerably more work needs to be done in order to find out which collagenase inhibitor is really the best one for clinical use. At the present time, we cannot say that these drugs will eradicate all corneal ulcerations.

I agree with you about glued-on lenses. They have, in the long run, been disappointing because they tend to loosen after a year or two, and sometimes sooner. Epithelium then grows in and the lens has to be removed or

DR. T. KUWABARA (*USA*): The papers in this session reflected the progress that has recently been made in our understanding of the structure and function of the retina. Dr. Lincoff showed the structural details of retinal adhesion after cryosurgery and Dr. Zauberman reported on the physical force of retinal adhesion in both normal and pathological conditions. It appears that in life processes, pumping mechanisms in the pigment epithelial cells, for example, play a very important role in promoting this adhesion. Drs. Berman and Bach reported on the distribution of hydrolytic enzymes in isolated fractions from pigment epithelial cells and identified the particles in each fraction by electron microscopy.

Several papers were presented on diabetic retinopathy. Dr. Futterman showed that the synthetic activity of long chain fatty acids by the microsomal fraction of the retina was depressed in experimentally induced diabetes. Dr. Gabbay demonstrated the intracellular accumulation of sorbitol in diabetic retinas and in peripheral nerves. He also discussed the role of aldose reductase in this process. Dr. Patz described the vascular changes in the retina in diabetic animals, and Drs. Yanko, Michaelson and Cohen showed some remarkable retinal changes in sucrose-fed rats. These experiments were based on the observation that whereas diabetes was rare among Yemenites in their native country, many of them developed the diabetic syndrome after immigrating to Israel. The principal cause seems to be related to changes in their dietary habits.

We do not yet know whether the basic studies reported in this session can be applied directly to clinical problems. However, the information gained is extremely important for our understanding of the pathogenesis of retinal diseases. I feel that the information presented at this symposium will be utilized by scientists all over the world to pursue their basic researches in all fields of ophthalmology.

DR. MAUMENEE: One of the most extensively investigated aspects of diabetic retinopathy is the thickening of the capillary basement membrane. These pathological changes have been observed by many electron microscopists. Now, I would like to ask whether this thickening may be related to sorbitol accumulation in the retina, or do you perhaps think that the basement membrane changes may be an artifact in electron microscopy?

DR. KUWABARA: This is a very important question and a difficult one to answer. For one thing, basement membrane thickening is not confined to the retina; it is observed in the whole microcapillary system. Moreover, the thickening itself is not specific for diabetes; it is observed in many other pathological states. It is my feeling at the present time that basement membrane thickening per se is not directly related to the pathogenesis of the diabetic condition itself.

CHAIRMAN'S SUMMARY

DR. MAUMENEE: We have heard some wonderful statements at this conference. Dr. Thomas really went to the heart of the problem when he said that if we could only get to the citizens in many parts of the world to teach them hygiene and give them medical advice, then we would be doing a great deal in preventive medicine.

Dr. Bisley pointed out that in the area where he worked, there was a community where trachoma was extremely scarce. When he went to look at the children and find out why, he discovered that there was a stream of water running close to the school. The teacher made the children wash their faces before they came to school in the morning and wash their faces again when they went home. So, in such a simple way as this, trachoma was reduced tremendously.

I have somehow always had the impression that Ph.D. scientists lived in ivory towers and weren't inclined to interest themselves in practical research. But now, I realize that they are really human beings, sincerely interested in diseases, and would like to join the common folk (the physicians) in a combined effort to find the causes and the means to eradicate many diseases. This is very exciting and wonderful news.

Dr. Rambo pointed out that this was the first meeting he has ever attended where he saw an ophthalmologist with a heart for prevention. He thought that their main interests were in cataract extractions and glaucoma operations. When he talked about prevention, they shied away from him. So he is very excited to know that perhaps now they would like to do something for prevention after all.

So, I think from this point of view the meeting has been most exciting. And to sum it up, I found that meeting old friends and making new ones with people around the world has been extremely valuable. It has been wonderful for me to study at closer hand the genius of Dr. Michaelson in organizing such a conference and bringing us all together. It has also been exciting to see this new country, its development and all that is going on, and to feel the warm hospitality of our Israel hosts. I really thank them for all they have done for us.

Progress in the prevention of blindness means a multidisciplinary approach—the collaboration of scientists, public health workers and administrators. I think this kind of team approach will be one theme which will come out of this meeting.

All of us feel that there is a very pressing need for a central registry where we can coordinate some of our activities. We feel that there are many ophthalmologists who would volunteer for this work. There are, in addition, scientists, nurses and others who would like to join this effort. Certainly there are many agencies already working in this area, but probably overlapping in their services. If there were a central agency to coordinate all these activities, we would surely advance much more rapidly.

All of us feel that there is a need for action now and that all the factors coming together are building up. There is closer communication, I think, between nations. There is more interest at the national level, wealthy nations help those nations that are not so wealthy and I think the physicians participating in these efforts have found them extremely rewarding.

I know you will all agree with me when I say that this conference has been so successful that we should begin planning for another in the very near future. I, for one, think it is almost impossible to repeat a conference as good as this one has been, but I think we should try. The only way we can be certain of this is to have Dr. Michaelson organize it all over again!

Please let us also know of any changes in original data, such as a change of address, a new publication or an alteration in your status or facilities. These will be circulated, so should be typed.

If any communication is indecipherable it will have to be retyped before taking photostats. If this is done the communication will be headed RETYPE, for if indecipherable it may have to be edited and those on the Agency files will want to know if they are reading the original document or not. The kind of improved communication at which the Central Agency aims should not only make for improved efficiency, but should prevent duplication of effort, act as a spur and stimulate our thinking.

If you are ever in doubt as to whom you should contact for special knowledge, where to find a certain reference or paper, how to get a combined research project of any kind going, or anything else of this nature, the Central Agency will do all it can to help. With each communication you send us, please include an addressed envelope (stamped if in U.K.) which will be of great help, for we have no funds. Finally, many people must have been inadvertently omitted, so please send the name and address of anyone whom you know would like to join us, even if he is in another field, such as nutrition, statistics or economics.

Name
Year of birth
Postal address
Nationality
Present post held
Past posts (that might be helpful)
Medical school(s) and degree(s)—in brief
Aspect of onchocerciasis in which most experienced
Other (non-oncho) medical or scientific skills or experiences
Availability for field work *in any one year*
  1. Duration
  2. Preferred month(s)
Facilities for teaching (if relevant)
  1. Junior salaried posts and duration
  2. Attachments (nonsalaried) and duration
  3. Accommodation details for 1 or 2 above
  4. Anything else.
Any suggestions or opinions e.g., concerning the idea of a Central Agency, whether the agency should organize seminars or conferences or not, to be run by its own members or not, etc.

*To be returned to F. C. Rodger, Princess Margaret Hospital, Swindon, Wilts., U.K.*

Please attach separately a list of your publications with titles and full references, preferably in chronological order so additions can be readily made as new papers appear.

## XEROPHTHALMIA CLUB

The manifesto and present membership follow

February 1972

Dear Colleague,

This Club was formed at the Seminar on the Prevention of Blindness held in Jerusalem, August 1971, because it was felt that those concerned with preventing blindness in children, due to malnutrition, would be more effective if they kept in touch, than if they were each working in isolation.

The Club will promote measures which could help to prevent and cure malnutritional blindness, particularly xerophthalmia and keratomalacia in young children. For nearly 50 years this has been known to be due, basically, to lack of vitamin A and of the provitamin carotene in food, often aggravated by other factors such as infection or lack of protein.

At present there is no organization that unites ophthalmologists, pediatricians, pathologists, biochemists, nutritionists, health educators, agriculturalists, horticulturalists and Societies for the Prevention of Blindness. All these should be concerned with the blindness in children due to xerophthalmia.

The immediate arrangements are these:

1) The Xerophthalmia Club consists of individuals, not organizations, and can embrace anyone, anywhere in the world, who subscribes to the purpose outlined.

2) Professor H.A.P.C. Oomen has agreed to be Chairman.

3) The Royal Commonwealth Society for the Blind, Director Mr. John Wilson, has agreed to provide administrative help, and, within its overall program, to stimulate world interest in this problem, to help in coordinating information and to promote demonstration projects such as the Nutrition Centre already established at the Government Erskine Hospital, Madurai, South India.

4) Dr. A. Pirie has agreed to be Secretary, acting as post box, receiving information and sending it out, together with requests for action.

These arrangements are temporary; direction should finally be in the hands of those who encounter xerophthalmia in their daily work.

Different countries and even different areas within one country have different problems, but it seems probable that xerophthalmia is still neglected and unrecognized, confused and submerged in the diagnoses of measles blindness, gonorrhea blindness, protein calorie malnutrition or tuberculosis, or hidden behind the nutritional misery which is a consequence of mass displacement due to war and other disasters.

Many cases may go undetected. Alertness to the possibility of blindness in infants and young children is essential. The important thing is to give vitamin A at once without waiting for a further diagnosis by experts. It is true that more care is now given to child malnutrition and thus more children survive. Sadly, this means in practice that more blind children survive because xerophthalmia was not diagnosed in time.

The World Health Organization considers xerophthalmia blindness to be one of three main causes of preventable blindness (the others are trachoma and onchocerciasis) to be tackled in future programs.

Because of these things we are forming this "Xerophthalmia Club" to ask for information from those who have to deal with problems of blinding diseases in children and may have some successes or failures to report, and to send out information by way of a bulletin of case histories, information on programs of prevention, meetings concerned with xerophthalmia and so on.

We ask for your cooperation and support.

But if you think this is not an important hazard in your area, what are your real hazards? If you consider that measles is the cause of blindness in small children, can you explain why measles never causes blindness in the West? Do you ever meet acquired corneal blindness in children? Was this blindness caused by xerophthalmia or was it gonorrhea? Is the use of unfortified skim milk powder as an infant food a hazard in your area?

Would you be prepared to give advice on how to attack the problem, for example by

– collecting epidemiological data,
– reporting representative case histories,
– discussing modes of prevention and treatment,
– indicating approaches to nutrition education,

**647**

Dr. I. Ben Sira, Eye Department, Hadassah University Hospital, Jerusalem

## AUSTRALIA
Prof. Ida Mann, 56 Hobbs Avenue, Nedlands, 6009 W.A.

## EUROPE
**Denmark**

Dr. Nizetic, WHO Regional Ofice for Europe, 8 Scherfigsvej, D.K. 2100 Copenhagen

**Switzerland**

Dr. J. M. Bengoa, Chief, Nutrition Unit, WHO, 1211 Geneva 27

Dr. E. M. DeMaeyer, Medical Officer, Nutrition Research, WHO, 1211 Geneva 27

Dr. M. Tarizzo, WHO, 1211 Geneva 27

**United Kingdom**

Dr. W. R. Aykroyd, St. Anne's House, Charlbury, Oxfordshire

Dr. D. P. Choyce, 9 Drake Road, Westcliff-on-Sea, Essex

Dr. G. J. Ebrahim, Institute of Child Health, 30 Guildford Street, London WC1

Dr. A. Pirie, Nuffield Laboratory of Ophthalmology, 20 Walton Street, Oxford, OX2 6AW

Mr. N. W. Pirie, Rothampsted Experimental Station, Herpenden, Herts

Dr. F. C. Rodgers, Princess Margaret Hospital, Okus Road, Swindon, Wilts

Mr. J. F. Wilson, CBE, Director, Royal Commonwealth Society for the Blind, Heath Road, Haywards Heath, Sussex

**Netherlands**

Dr. Johanna ten Doesschate, V. Ketwich Verschuurlaan 153a, Groningen

Dr. S. Franken, University Eye Clinic, Hofstede de Grootkade 36, Groningen

Dr. H. A. P. C. Oomen, Royal Tropical Institute, Mauritskade 63, Amsterdam-Oost

Dr. R. L. H. Sampimon, Secretary to Prof. Weve Stichting, Oudwijk 37, Utrecht

**Italy**

Prof. G. B. Bietti, Clinica Oculistica, Universita di Roma, Via Cesare Beccaria 18, Rome

## AMERICA
**Mexico**

Dr. Adolfo Chavez, Chief Nutrition Division, National Nutrition Institute, Tlalpan, Mexico 22

**Guatemala**

Dr. G. Arroyave, Division of Physiological Chemistry, Institute of Nutrition for Central America and Panama, P.O. Box 1188, Guatemala City

Dr. Ivan D. Beghin, INCAP, P.O. Box 1188, Guatemala City

**El Salvador**

Dr. Humberto Escapini, Clínical Medicas, 25, A.N. 640, San Salvador

**United States**

Dr. J. W. Ferree, American Foundation for Overseas Blind, 22 West 17th Street, New York, N.Y. 10011

Dr. W. J. Holmes, 280 Alexander Young Building, Honolulu, Hawaii

Dr. C. Kupfer, National Eye Institute, Department of Health, Bethesda, Md. 20014

Prof. A. E. Maumenee, Wilmer Institute, Johns Hopkins Hospital, Baltimore, Md. 21205

Dr. D. Maurice, 12125 Joandra, Los Altos, Cal. 94022

Dr. V. Rambo, 6026 Germantown Avenue, Philadelphia, Pa. 19144

Prof. M. L. Sears, Department of Ophthalmology, Yale University, School of Medicine, New Haven, Conn.

Dr. L. J. Teply, Food Conservation Division, UNICEF, United Nations, New York

Dr. D. Weeks, Executive Director, Research to Prevent Blindness, 598 Madison Avenue, New York

**Canada**

Dr. J. N. Thompson, Department of National Health and Welfare, Ottawa 3, Ontario

# AUTHOR INDEX

Aiello, L. M., 316
Anderson, D. R., 362
Anseth, A., 526
Auerbach, E., 482
Aviel, E., 146, 240

Bach, G., 595
Barkai, S., 404
Becker, Y., 90, 114, 196, 205
Ben-Sira, I., 63, 136, 149, 172,
    189, 240, 261, 452
Berman, E. R., 582, 595, 617
Bietti, G. B., 49, 81, 104, 118,
    255, 350
Bisley, G. G., 35, 53, 62, 225
Blumenthal, M., 386, 388
Bradford, B., 576
Brown, S. I., 517, 529
Byer, N. E., 397, 443

Capella, J. A., 278
Cass, E. E., 626
Charamis, J., 419
Chatterjee, N., 35, 219, 555, 637
Choyce, D. P., 123, 149, 265,
    621, 623
Christy, N. E., 28, 230, 555
Cohen, A. M., 612, 617, 618
Collier, L. H., 94, 118, 623, 624
Crawford, J. S., 468

David, R., 146, 240
Delthil, S., 453
Dikstein, S., 503, 529
Dobree, J. H., 149, 308, 328, 324
Dohlman, C. H., 159, 191, 286,
    287, 509, 625, 626, 637

Esterson, J., 576

Feiler, V., 404, 409
Feitelberg, I., 35, 64
Fison, L., 395, 442, 443, 444, 631
François, J., 11, 21, 34, 353, 388,
    632, 638

Franken, S., 223, 634
Freilich, D. B., 438
Friedman, M. W., 423
Futterman, S., 601, 617

Gabbay, K. H., 537, 555, 583,
    606
Ghione, M., 104
Goldberg, M. F., 291, 327, 427,
    629, 630, 631
Gorin, G., 327, 380, 387, 388
Grover, D., 570
Gunders, A. E., 119, 138, 149

Halberg, G. P., 59
Haraguchi, K. H., 511
Hart, R. W., 365
Hayakawa, M., 487
Hockwin, O., 542
Hodson, S. A., 499
Holmes, W. J., 44, 635
Hudson, J. R., 390, 442, 443
Hyams, S., 404

Intini, C., 104
Isetta, A. M., 104
Ivry, M., 404

Jedwab, E., 404

Kalevar, V., 159
Kaufman, H. E., 192, 211, 218,
    278, 286
King, J. H. Jr., 256, 273, 286
Kinoshita, J. H., 537
Kirsch, R. E., 362, 388
Klein, M., 328
Koch, H.-R., 542, 556
Kolker, A. E., 330, 337, 386, 387
Kornzweig, A. L., 296, 327, 328
Krakowski, D., 404
Kupfer, C., 72, 324, 554, 555
Kurz, O., 411
Kuwabara, T., 617, 618, 640

Lagraulet, J., 133
Langham, M. E., 35, 191, 365,
    510
Lawlor, J. J., 30
Lemmingson, W., 303
Lerman, S., 382, 563
Levitt-Hadar, J., 205
Levy, R., 110
Leydhecker, W., 346, 387, 388,
    628
Lincoff, H., 329, 442, 443, 617
Linnér, E., 374, 628, 629
Lowe, R. F., 342
Luntz, M. H., 55

Mann, I., 40, 624, 633
Maumenee, A. E., 8, 386, 510,
    621, 622, 623, 624, 625, 626,
    627, 628, 629, 630, 631, 632,
    633, 634, 635, 636, 637, 638,
    639, 640, 642, 644
Maurice, D. M., 503, 510, 554,
    636, 637
Maythar, B., 110, 404
Merin, S., 255, 268
Michaelis, M., 576
Michaelson, I. C., 7, 34, 57, 78,
    401, 442, 444, 612, 624, 626,
    629, 630, 631, 635, 644
Mishima, S., 487, 509, 529, 637
Moczar, E., 525
Moczar, M., 525, 529

Nakajima, A., 50, 634
Nawratzki, I., 68, 449, 455, 480,
    481, 482
Neuman, S., 205
Neumann, E., 119, 138, 404, 442,
    443, 444, 449, 481

Oliver, M., 449
Olson, J. A., 150, 179, 191, 621
Olurin, O., 377
Oomen, H. A. P. C., 175
Orr, H. T., 499

Patz, A., 319, 328, 610, 618
Pirie, A., 35, 530, 547, 554, 555, 582, 583, 617, 618, 639
Polack, F. M., 278
Potts, A. M., 454
Protonotarios, P., 250, 255

Quana'a, P., 78, 118

Rambo, V., 34, 191, 219, 554
Reif, J., 411
Réthy, I., 460, 481, 482
Richards, R. D., 576
Riley, M. V., 499, 509, 554, 582
Rizzuti, A. B., 77, 269, 286
Rodger, F. C., 130, 143, 149, 621, 622, 637
Rollins, M. H., 601
Romano, A., 215, 409

Sachs, U., 452
Samuels, L., 386
Schappert-Kimijser, J., 54
Scharf, J., 404
Schlossman, A., 59, 66, 78
Schocket, S. S., 576
Scholz, R. O., 32

Schultz, J. B., 570
Sears, M. L., 187, 246, 255, 325, 327, 328, 387
Seelenfreund, M. H., 438
Shenken, E., 43
Shusterman, M., 328, 443
Slatt, B., 68, 78
Sloane, A. E., 480, 481, 627
Soldari, M., 104
Sourdille, J., 453
Spalter, H. F., 321, 328
Spector, A., 509, 529, 554, 555, 557, 582, 583, 638, 639
Stein, H. A., 68
Stein, R., 215, 218, 255, 327, 328, 401, 409, 442, 624, 629
Steiner-Freud, J., 69
Stohlman, Y., 78

Tarizzo, M. L., 17, 87, 633
Ten Doesschate, J., 78, 164
Theodossiadis, G., 328, 419
Thomas, H. M., 34, 149, 622, 635
Ticho, U., 189, 240, 261
Treister, G., 414
Trevor-Roper, P. D., 259, 286
Tsibidas, P., 250

Vassiliades, J., 250
Venkataswamy, G., 46, 61, 170, 234, 255, 626, 636
von Bahr, G., 10, 37, 634
von Noorden, G. K., 445, 476, 480, 481, 482, 483

Waubke, Th. N., 311
Weigelin, E., 542
Weimar, V. L., 511, 529
Wilson, J., 12, 25, 642
Wolff, J. E., 388
Wyatt, H., 78
Wybar, K., 462, 472, 482, 483

Yanko, L., 612
Yassur, S., 172, 452
Yassur, Y., 63, 136, 172, 189, 452
Yulo, T., 570

Zachs, U., 172
Zadunaisky, J. A., 509, 510, 617
Zaifrani, S., 172, 452
Zauberman, H., 443, 582, 617
Zigman, S., 570
Zinger, L., 404

# SUBJECT INDEX*

Aldose reductase
  Diabetic retinopathy 606, 640
  Inhibitor 537, 638, 639
  Purification and immunological identification
    in retina 606
Amblyopia
  Classification, diagnosis, natural history 445,
    460, 480, 627
  Congenital cataract 468
  Experimental 476
  Prevalence, in Australia among Aborigines 40
    in Hawaii 44
    in Italy 49
  Prevention when caused by incomplete cataract
    468
  Register 629
  Screening 449, 452, 453, 627
  Stimulus deprivation 462
  Treatment 454, 455, 460, 480, 627
American Foundation for Overseas Blind 25
Aqueous humor proteins
  Effect of near-UV radiation 570
Australia
  Aborigines, prevalence of amblyopia, cataract,
    trachoma 40
  Prevention of blindness 40
Auxiliary ophthalmic personnel, training of 59,
    61, 66, 68, 69

Basic research, contributions of 636
Blindness
  Cataract in India 219
  Causes including onchocerciasis, malnutrition
    and trachoma 17
  Cost in USA 638
  Definition 17
  Life expectation in India if due to cataract 626
  Prevalence 12, 17

Cataract
  Aggregation of α-crystallin 557
  Cataractogenesis, new aspects 542

Classification 638
Combined glaucoma operation 250
Congenital cataract and amblyopia 468
Congenital rubella and cataract 450
Diabetic cataract, aldose reductase and sorbitol
  in 638
Diet and cataract 626
Induction by exposure to oxygen 576
Photo-oxidized proteins in 547
Possible prevention in sugar cataract 537
Subliminal factors in 542, 638
Cataract in India
  Cause of blindness 46, 626
  Cost of cataract operation 46
  Number receiving surgery 626
  Surgery in eye camps 46, 234
Collagenase
  In corneal ulceration 637
  Inhibitors 637, 638
Cornea
  Endothelium in relation to dehydration and
    nutrition 487
  Growth stimulating effects of proteolytic en-
    zymes 511
  Hydration, active control of 503
  Synthetic activity of the endothelium 499
Corneal grafting, in developing countries
  Combined graft and cataract surgery 259
  Cryopreserved donor tissue 278
  Donor material, availability of 30, 46, 273,
    625, 626
  Number requiring corneal grafting 625
  Prognosis in phakic and aphakic patients 278,
    625
  Total keratoplasty, role of 261
Corneal opacification
  Polysaccharide chemistry 523
Corneal stroma
  Structural macromolecules 525
α-crystallin
  Aggregation of, and its possible relationship to
    cataract formation 557, 639

Diabetic retinopathy
  Capillary aneurysms 296

---

\* Numbers refer to first page of the article in which
the subject is discussed.

653

Cause of blindness   291, 629
Classification   291
Control study   629
Experimental: sucrose fed rats   610, 612, 640
Factors related to development
    Age   291
    Duration   291
    Fundal appearance   630
    Metabolic control   291, 630
Maculopathy in maturity onset diabetes   321
Natural history   291
Pathogenesis   291
Regression   291
Rest in therapy   308, 630
Retinal microcirculation following photoco-agulation   303
Shunt vessels   296
Synthesis of fatty acids   601
Treatment
    by argon laser   319, 324, 327
    by light coagulation   308, 311, 324, 325, 327
    by ruby laser   316, 327
Visual loss, mechanism of   291

Endothelium, corneal, in relation to dehydration and nutrition   487
Epithelial tissue, role of vitamin A   150
Eye banks   30, 46, 273
Eye camps   46, 234
Eye injuries   44

Fatty acids
    Synthesis by normal and diabetic retinal tissue   601, 640
Fluorescence
    Lens proteins   563
Foreign aid
    American Foundation for Overseas Blind   25
    Governmental technical assistance   21
    International Eye Foundation   30
    Missionary societies   28
    Ophthalmological services of MEDICO   32
    Royal Commonwealth Society for the Blind   25
    World Health Organization   17

Glaucoma
    Primary angle-closure glaucoma
        Latent irido-cyclitis   380
        Prevention and early treatment   342
        Screening for   346, 350
    Primary open-angle glaucoma   28
        Diagnosis   374, 386
        Family study   337, 386

Natural history   14
Ocular hypertension, relation to   330, 386, 628
Optic disk in   353, 362, 386, 629
Prevalence   628
Screening for   346, 350, 386, 628
Therapy   365, 374
    Aspects in developing countries   377
    Prolonged-release medication   382

Herpes cornea
    Effects of distamycin A and congocidine on replication of virus   205
    Medical therapy   211
    Molecular biology of herpes simplex virus   196
    Natural history and diagnosis   192
    Surgical treatment   215

International Association for Prevention of Blindness   17, 25, 37
International Conference for Prevention of Blindness in 1974,   642
International Eye Foundation   30
International Organization against Trachoma   17
India
    Auxiliary ophthalmic personnel 61
    Cost of cataract operation   46
    Eye camps   46, 234
    Malnutrition and blindness   46
    Ophthalmic personnel   34
    Ophthalmic services   46
    Prevalence of cataract   46, 626
    Village hospitals   230

Keratomalacia   159
Keratoprosthesis, present status   265, 269, 625

Lens proteins
    Effects of near-UV radiation   570
    Fluorescence   563
Liberia
    Ophthalmology in   34

Malawi
    Regional organization of eye clinics   240
MEDICO, Medical International Cooperation Organization   32
Missionary societies and prevention of blindness   25
Mobile eye units   21, 25, 34, 43, 55, 219, 223, 225

National Eye Institute, Bethesda   72
Netherlands, prevention of blindness in   54
Newfoundland, prevention of blindness in   43

Nursing training in blindness prevention   21

Nystagmus, significance in suspected blindness in infancy   472

Ocular hypertension and treatment   330, 386, 628

Onchocerciasis
  Blindness from   123, 133
  Cataract   622
  Cause of blindness   17
  Central agency for   645
  Control and treatment   17, 21, 25, 123, 143, 146, 622, 623, 634
  Diagnosis   119, 130, 622
  Epidemiology   17, 123, 130, 133, 622
  Glaucoma   622
  International study group   643
  Natural history   123, 130
  Parasitology, Onchocercus volvulvus   119, 622

Ophthalmologists in developing countries   34, 46, 57

Paramedical personnel   17, 30, 32, 34, 62, 63, 64, 68, 240, 635
  International study group   643

Photocoagulation in diabetic retinopathy   308, 311, 316, 319, 324, 325, 327

Photo-oxidation of proteins and comparison with those of cataractous human lens   547, 638

Pigment epithelium
  Role of enzymes in retinal detachment   595, 640

Prevention of blindness
  Definition   34, 37, 634
  Main causes
    Amblyopia   445
    Cataract   219
    Diabetic retinopathy   291
    Glaucoma   330
    Herpes cornea   190
    Onchocerciasis   119
    Opacification of cornea   487
    Trachoma   81
    Xerophthalmia   150
  Multidisciplinary attack   34
  Representative endeavors
    Australia   40
    Hawaii   44
    India   46
    Italy   49
    Japan   50
    Kenya   53
    Netherlands   54
    Newfoundland   43
    South Africa   55

Research   34, 72
  World prevention of blindness conference   643

Regional organization of eye clinics in Malawi   240

Resolution of conference   642

Retina, aldose reductase in   606

Retinal adhesion, measurement   584, 640

Retinal detachment
  National study in prevention   401, 442
  Natural history of detachment retinopathy   397, 404, 442
    Retinoschisis   411
    Time factor in the hole-detachment phase   242
  Possible role of pigment epithelial enzymes   595
  Prevalence
    Australia, among Aborigines and whites   40
    Israel   401
  Prevention of detachment retinopathy
    Hole stage   310, 397, 401
    Myopic aphakic eyes   415
    Pre-hole stage   395, 397
    Results of preventive treatment   404
  Proliferative retinopathy with retinal detachment   427

Retrolental fibroplasia   44

Royal Commonwealth Society for the Blind   21, 25, 46

Sorbitol
  Diabetic cataract   638, 639

South Africa
  Prevention of blindness   55

Sucrose feeding
  Diabetic retinopathy   612

Sugar cataracts
  Mechanism of development and possible prevention   537

Swaziland
  Prevention of blindness   56

Teaching of ophthalmology
  Auxiliary personnel   66, 68
  Nursing personnel   57, 61, 68
  Ophthalmologists   57
  Orthoptists   61, 68
  Para-ophthalmic personnel   57, 61, 62, 63, 64

Trachoma
  Agent
    Local antibodies   110, 624
    Molecular biology   114
    Transmission   94

Cause of blindness   17, 81
Chemotherapy   87, 94, 104, 623, 644
  Rifampicin   90, 623
Classification   81
Clinical aspects   81
Control   21, 25, 34, 94
Diagnosis   81, 624
Geographical distribution   81
Immunity   104, 110
International study group   643
Mass therapy   94
Pathology   81
Prevalence   17, 40, 81, 94
  India   46
  Italy   49
  South Africa   19, 55
Research   17, 21
Vaccine-therapy   94, 104

UV radiation
  Effects on lens and aqueous humor proteins
  570

Vitamin A
  Deficiency and xerophthalmia   17, 150, 159
  Role in maintaining epithelial tissues   150

World Council for the Welfare of the Blind   25
World Health Organization and prevention of
  blindness   17, 632, 633, 634
  Regional office in Europe   17
World Prevention of Blindness Committee   25

Xerophthalmia
  Cause of blindness   17
  Clinical aspects   159, 164, 175, 179, 187, 621
  Epidemiological aspects   17, 170, 172, 187
  International study group   642
  Keratomalacia   159, 164, 170, 172, 189
  Mucus, changes in   637
  Prevention   25, 159, 164, 175, 179, 187, 621
  Protein deficiency   159
  Surgical treatment in severe forms of kerato-
    malacia   189
  Vitamin A   636
Xerophthalmia Club   647